Integrative Pediatrics

Integrative Pediatrics
Art, Science, and Clinical Application

Hilary McClafferty, MD, FAAP
Associate Professor, Department of Medicine
Director, Pediatric Integrative Medicine in Residency
Co-Director, Fellowship in Integrative Medicine
University of Arizona Center for Integrative Medicine
University of Arizona College of Medicine
Tucson, Arizona

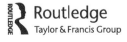
Routledge
Taylor & Francis Group

First published 2017
by Routledge
2 Park Square, Milton Park, Abingdon, Oxon OX14 4RN

and by Routledge
711 Third Avenue, New York, NY 10017

Routledge is an imprint of the Taylor & Francis Group, an informa business

British Library Cataloguing-in-Publication Data
A catalogue record for this book is available from the British Library

ISBN: 978-1-4987-1671-0 (Hardback)
ISBN: 978-1-138-19607-0 (Paperback)
ISBN: 978-1-4987-1672-7 (Ebook)

To Kylie and Liam

Contents

Foreword by Andrew Weil

With its focus on preventive health, engagement of the individual's innate healing capacity, and goals of minimizing invasive procedures and use of prescription medications, integrative medicine is a natural fit for pediatrics. Coming from the world of pediatric emergency medicine, Hilary McClafferty would seem an unlikely champion for the field, but, in fact, she has been a most effective one. I first met Hilary when she was a Fellow in the University of Arizona Center for Integrative Medicine, Class of 2005. She raised her hand during one of my lectures to ask about the use of integrative medicine in children. I replied, "Pediatric integrative medicine is the way of the future," knowing very well that at the time the field was in its infancy and needed the efforts of committed pediatrician advocates to advance it.

She took this encouragement to heart and since completing the Fellowship has become involved in local, national, and international initiatives to introduce research and clinical and educational programs on integrative pediatrics into mainstream medicine. One of the most innovative she leads is the Pediatric Integrative Medicine in Residency (PIMR) program at the University of Arizona Center for Integrative Medicine, which has just completed a three-year pilot run involving more than 500 pediatric residents at leading academic institutions. These residents received foundational training in integrative pediatrics embedded in their conventional medical training. The first initiative of its kind in pediatrics, PIMR has grown to include other first-rate pediatric residencies around the country and was recently launched at three children's hospitals in Germany.

Hilary has also been a highly effective leader within the American Academy of Pediatrics, where she is immediate past chair of the Section on Integrative Medicine, a group with the ambitious mission of raising awareness about the field throughout the 66,000-member Academy. In this role, she also created an integrative medicine model for physician self-care and wellbeing and led development of the first policy statement on physician wellness for the Academy. She expects this work to catalyze an array of educational initiatives that will continue to grow in scale and impact. Hilary is currently leading the update of the Academy's Clinical Report on Pediatric Integrative Medicine, an in-depth review of the literature in the field that serves as a guidepost for the Academy and its diverse membership.

As a leader of the Fellowship in Integrative Medicine at the University of Arizona and as a founding member of the American Board of Integrative Medicine, Hilary is known and admired for her creativity and collaborative spirit and her commitment to mentoring upcoming faculty and students. What most people may not know about her is that her passion for integrative pediatrics stems in part from deeply personal experiences in the healthcare system, where as a mother who is also a physician she has lived firsthand the challenges of advocating for a child and a family dealing with chronic disease. From her years of navigating the healthcare system with a foot in both worlds and from her early work in acute care, she has drawn rich lessons that inform her teaching every day.

Hilary tells me that her primary goals in writing this book are to document the progress that has occurred in this emerging field and to highlight areas where research gaps remain. Her hope is that it will serve to guide integrative pediatrics to its rightful place in the forefront of the day-to-day care of children of all ages.

Andrew Weil, MD
Lovell-Jones Endowed Chair in Integrative Rheumatology
Clinical Professor of Medicine
University of Arizona College of Medicine

Foreword by James E. Dalen

This is one of the rare textbooks with a single author, Dr. Hilary McClafferty, a very experienced pediatrician and leader in the emergence of integrative medicine. She serves as chair of the American Academy of Pediatrics Section on Integrative Medicine, and at the University of Arizona Center for Integrative Medicine designed and directs an internationally distributed online integrative medicine curriculum for pediatric residents.

Integrative Pediatrics: Art, Science, and Clinical Application demonstrates how the various aspects of integrative medicine can enhance pediatric care. It stresses prevention by emphasis on nutrition, physical activity, mind–body medicine, sleep, and environmental health.

A very important section of the text is her evidence-based evaluation of complementary therapies, including dietary supplements, which may be helpful in pediatric care. She carefully points out which of these therapies have been validated by appropriate research, and which have not.

This text, by introducing the principles of integrative medicine, can enhance the clinical skills of practicing pediatricians and expand therapeutic options for children and adolescents.

James E. Dalen, MD, MPH, ScD (hon)
Executive Director, Weil Foundation
Dean Emeritus, University of Arizona College of Medicine

About the Author

Hilary McClafferty is Board certified in pediatrics, pediatric emergency medicine, and integrative medicine. She is Associate Professor in the Department of Medicine at the University of Arizona College of Medicine in Tucson, Arizona, a founding Board member of the American Board of Integrative Medicine, a leader of the Fellowship in Integrative Medicine and Director of the international Pediatric Integrative Medicine in Residency Program at the University of Arizona Center for Integrative Medicine. She is certified in clinical hypnosis, trained in medical acupuncture, and speaks and teaches internationally on integrative medicine topics including pediatrics, mind–body medicine, environmental health, and physician wellness and resilience.

Acknowledgments

My sincere thanks and gratitude go out to all the children and families who have been my great teachers through the years, and to my inspired colleagues in pediatric integrative medicine who are working together to improve the health and wellbeing of children around the world. My thanks extend to Dr. Weil and my colleagues and students at the University of Arizona Center for Integrative Medicine, Tucson, for their creative energy and dedication to creating a paradigm shift in healthcare.

Part 1

Integrative Medicine: A New Frontier in Pediatrics

1 Introduction to Pediatric Integrative Medicine

Children are born with a natural capacity to thrive, ideally supported by parents who provide food, shelter, companionship, education, and unconditional love. The clinician's role has historically been that of trusted guide and dedicated child advocate in the medical arena. Rapid changes in the business of medicine and an emphasis on productivity over patient-centered care have stripped pediatric practice of some of its richness, resulting in a lost sense of collaboration for many clinicians. Parents have been similarly affected by the "commercialization" of medicine and seek a deeper connection with providers who can deliver more personalized care, expanded treatment options, and accurate information about emerging therapies that may improve their child's health. Pediatric integrative medicine can serve to reconnect clinician, child, and parent and can be defined as a modern approach to children's health in that it respects the strengths of conventional medicine while embracing emerging research in preventive health and management of chronic illness. The field includes topics such as nutrition, physical activity, sleep, stress management, mental health, environmental influences, and social relationships across every stage of development. One of the newest concepts in the field is inter-professionalism, which emphasizes the value of an interdisciplinary team approach. The practice of pediatric integrative medicine has potential to bring the heart back to pediatric practice by creating a child-centered model of care, infusing the medical encounter with forward looking, evidence-based therapies, and prioritizing health across the lifespan.

Some of the principles of integrative medicine practice include:

- Emphasis on preventative health and lifestyle
- Support of the individual's innate healing response
- Focus on the therapeutic relationship between patient, family, and clinician
- Consideration of health in all dimensions (body, mind, and spirit)
- Family-centered care
- Cultural competency
- Use of all appropriate evidence-based therapies

(Maizes, Rakel, and Niemiec 2009)

These principles are well aligned with the medical home model and will hopefully pave the way for creation of an "integrative medical home," a model that places whole childcare squarely in the mainstream of healthcare.

Historically, expansion of the field of integrative medicine has been hampered by those preying on the fears of parents willing to accept any therapy, no matter how unscientific, in the effort to help their child. A guiding principle of this book will be to convey a balanced approach to the field and to stress the importance of evidence-based therapies. The goal is to raise awareness about the field of integrative pediatrics and its enormous potential to improve healthcare for children. The title of the book reflects three important elements that together can help clinicians maximize whole child health. These include: the art of medicine practiced with compassion and awareness, a firm foundation of scientific evidence, and the skillful clinical application of all appropriate therapies. When combined, these elements exceed the sum of their parts and describe a modern approach to pediatrics that blends appropriate conventional and complementary therapies in a child-centered model with the potential to optimize children's health from preconception through adulthood.

What's in a Name?

As the field of integrative medicine has evolved, the language used to define it has adapted accordingly. Here the term integrative will be used to reflect an evidence-based *blending* of conventional and complementary approaches. Popularity of the term *complementary and alternative therapy* (CAM) is waning as concerns have mounted about the lack of evidence underpinning alternative therapies, defined as *treatments used in place of conventional medicine*. This change is reflected in the name change of the former National Center for Complementary and Alternative Medicine (NCCAM) to the National Center for Complementary and Integrative Health (NCCIH) in 2014 (National Institutes of Health 2014; NCCIH 2014).

The following example compares conventional, complementary, integrative, and alternative approaches in a child with migraine headache.

Examples of Treatment Approaches for an Adolescent with Migraine Headache

- **Conventional:** Traditional history and physical by an MD or DO, prescription medication as needed, comprehensive physical once per year, 'sick' visits as needed, hospital admission if necessary.
- **Complementary:** "Complements" conventional treatment. May include nutrition counseling, judicious use of dietary supplements such as butterbur, vitamin D, and omega-3 fatty acids, mind–body therapies such as guided imagery, yoga, clinical hypnosis, or biofeedback, probiotics, and bioenergetics treatments such as acupuncture.
- **Integrative:** Emphasis on preventive health, conventional treatment as needed, evidence-based complementary therapies as appropriate. In the integrative model, complementary therapies might be appropriately used alone, but openness to blending both conventional and evidence-based complementary therapies for the highest benefit of the patient is the overarching theme. This approach might include dietary review, possible symptom-driven elimination diet, stress management skills, and counseling on sleep and environmental triggers. All evidence-based therapies would be considered.
- **Alternative:** Alternative medicine refers to use of non-evidence-based therapies *in place of* conventional medicine. This approach will not be covered in this text.

Functional medicine is an emerging field primarily based on molecular biology and metabolic pathways with an emphasis on laboratory testing and use of replacement

Table 1.1 National Center for Complementary and Integrative Health Classifications

Practice	Examples
Whole medical systems	Homeopathy, naturopathy, Ayurveda, traditional Chinese medicine
Mind–body medicine	Meditation, prayer, mental healing, creative therapy (art, music, dance)
Biologically based practices	Dietary supplements, botanical medicine
Manipulative and body-based practices	Chiropractic, osteopathy, massage
Energy therapies	Biofield therapies (Qi gong, reiki, therapeutic touch), Bioelectromagnetics (electromagnetic fields)

supplements. There is currently a relative paucity of evidence supporting this approach in pediatrics, and for this reason functional medicine will not be covered in detail in this work. Research is active in this field and will be important for pediatricians and others caring for children to follow.

Many integrative therapies that have been gradually accepted into the Western biomedical model originated in long-established cultural healing traditions. A lack of standardized definitions associated with this rich history can create challenges to clear communication among conventionally trained health professionals. One approach historically used is the NIH NCCIH classification developed by the former NCCAM Advisory Board, noted in Table 1.1. This approach has recently been updated and streamlined to include three main categories: mind and body practices, natural products, and other complementary health approaches (https://nccih.nih.gov/health/integrative-health#types).

Organization and Overview

The main categories of integrative medicine discussed in the text include those with the current strongest evidence in children. Part 1 includes an overview of the field, and introduces the topic of clinician self-care and its important influence on patient outcome. Part 2 covers the foundations of healthy lifestyle habits in pediatrics including:

- Nutrition
- Selected dietary supplements
- Physical activity
- Mind–body therapies, spirituality in medicine
- Sleep
- Environmental health

Part 3 covers evidence-based complementary therapies including:

- Botanicals
- Manual medicine (therapeutic massage, osteopathy, craniosacral therapy)
- Aromatherapy
- Homeopathy

- Whole medical systems (traditional Chinese medicine, naturopathy)
- Bioenergetic therapies (acupuncture, therapeutic touch, healing touch)

Part 4 covers integrative approaches to a variety of common pediatric conditions in the areas of:

- Preventive care
- Allergy and asthma
- Dermatology
- Gastroenterology
- Infectious disease (URI and otitis media)
- Mental health
- Neurodevelopmental disorders
- Obesity and metabolic disorders
- Integrative intake

Why Do Parents Use Integrative Medicine for their Children?

Reasons for the use of integrative medicine vary and can include a desire to support the child's natural healing process, a wish to explore all treatment options, preference for less invasive treatments, and reduction of pain, stress, and suffering. An increased range of cost-effective treatment options, cultural preference, and lack of access to conventional care may be other important reasons. Integrative medicine holds special potential to improve care in children by expanding treatment options, introducing new approaches to chronic conditions and prioritizing health and wellness from preconception through adulthood.

Why is Pediatric Integrative Medicine Relevant to Modern Pediatric Practice?

The use of integrative therapies is high in children and in adolescents, requiring awareness on the part of all practitioners caring for these patients. Data from the 2012 National Health Interview Survey (NHIS) found that nearly 12% of children used complementary therapies in the prior year (about one in nine), similar to the overall prevalence recorded in the 2007 NHIS survey. Prevalence increases to approximately 50% in children living with a chronic illness (Black et al. 2015).

Dietary supplements (other than vitamins and minerals) were again the most commonly used approaches. The 2012 survey showed an increase from 3.9% in 2007 to 4.9% of children using dietary supplements, and a significant increase in pediatric use of yoga, fish oil, and melatonin. Therapies used most frequently were reported as natural products (3.9%), chiropractic and osteopathic (2.8%), deep breathing (2.2%), yoga (2.1%), homeopathy (1.3%), traditional healers (1.1%), massage (1.0%), diet-based therapies (0.8%), and progressive relaxation (0.5%). Use remained higher in children whose parents had also used complementary or alternative therapies, in children with more than one health condition, and in children who did not use, or whose families could not afford, conventional care. Fish oil was the most commonly used supplement in 2012, as compared to echinacea in 2007. Melatonin was the second most commonly used supplement in 2012. The conditions where complementary therapies were most commonly used remained constant from 2007 and included back or neck pain (6.7%), head or chest cold (6.6%), anxiety/stress (4.8%), other types of musculoskeletal conditions (4.2%), ADHD (2.5%), and insomnia (1.8%) (Barnes, Bloom, and Nahin 2008; NCCIH 2012).

What do the Statistics Imply?

High prevalence of use of integrative and complementary therapies reinforces the need for pediatricians and other practitioners caring for children to be current on research in integrative medicine and familiar with reliable sources of information to best serve the needs of their patients. The statistics also suggest that children and their families, especially children living with chronic illness, may not be fully served in the conventional health model. Many turn to integrative therapies to fill the gap, citing concerns about medication side effects and lack of access to care that is consistent with their values (Birdee et al. 2010).

The relatively high use of integrative medicine in the pediatric population often goes unrecognized, in part because of low disclosure rates (less than 50% in several studies) by parents who may fear a negative reaction from their child's clinician (Kemper et al. 2008).

Parents should be encouraged to discuss integrative therapies with their clinician, especially to avoid unwanted drug–supplement interactions. Conversely clinicians should feel comfortable discussing the subject and be able to offer accurate information and identify reliable resources to help guide parents.

As noted by Culbert and Olness (2009) in *Integrative Pediatrics*, other factors driving interest in pediatric integrative medicine reflect the sharp increase in the prevalence of chronic illnesses reaching into progressively younger age groups, prescription drug use, and the upturn in stress-related disorders in children.

Asthma

Asthma is the most prevalent chronic inflammatory pediatric illness in the U.S. and has increased from a prevalence of 3.6 to 13.6 over the past 30 years, 1980–2010. Lifetime prevalence of 13.6 in ages 18 and under in 2010 has increased from a prevalence of 3.6% in 1980 (Winer et al. 2012; NHIS National Health Interview Survey [NHIS] Data 2010; Centers for Disease Control and Prevention 2010).

Obesity

Childhood obesity has more than tripled in the past 30 years. In 2008 more than one-third of children and adolescents were overweight or obese, and one in six children aged 6–19 years were overweight or obese, a 45% increase in the past 10 years (Centers for Disease Control and Prevention 2015).

Diabetes

The prevalence of type-2 diabetes has increased significantly in U.S. children, keeping pace with increasing prevalence of obesity and showing an estimated tenfold increase in the last decade, with higher rates in children of American Indian, African American, Mexican American, and Pacific Islander descent (Mayer-Davis 2008).

Attention-Deficit/Hyperactivity Disorder

Attention-deficit/hyperactivity disorder in children aged 5–17 years has increased in prevalence from 6.9% to 9.0% in the periods from 1998–2000 through 2007–2009, indicating that approximately 1 in 12 children have been diagnosed with ADHD, with highest prevalence in lower socioeconomic groups and in the Midwest and Southern United States (Akinbami et al. 2011).

Autism Spectrum Disorders

Autism spectrum disorders now affect 1 in approximately every 68 American children (1 in 42 boys, 1 in 189 girls), a more than twenty-fold increase since the 1980s.

Despite numbers almost beyond comprehension, a clear etiology remains elusive (Lee, Thomas, and Lee 2015; Section On Complementary and Integrative Medicine et al. 2012).

Premature Birth

Premature birth (less than 37 weeks' gestation) affects one in eight babies born in the U.S. each year, contributing to one-third of all infant deaths. Premature births are estimated to cost greater than $26 billion annually. The causes of premature birth are multi-factorial and closely linked to prenatal care and poor maternal nutritional status (Centers for Disease Control and Prevention 2012).

Cancer

The prevalence of leukemia and cancers of the brain and central nervous system make cancer the leading cause of death by disease among U.S. children of 1–14 years of age. The causes of childhood cancer remain unclear (National Cancer Institute 2014).

Mental Health Disorders

Mental health disorders in children are increasing and were estimated to impact 13%–20% of U.S. children in a given year between 1994 and 2011 as reported by the U.S. CDC.

Suicide was the second leading cause of death for ages 12–17 in 2010. On any given day approximately 2% of school-aged children and about 8% of adolescents are estimated to meet criteria for major depression (Centers for Disease Control and Prevention 2005–2011).

Review of these statistics reflects startling shifts in a broad range of conditions, often accompanied by a sharp uptick in prescription medicine use. For example, an estimated 2.8 million children under 19 years received stimulant medication in the U.S. in 2008, a number that has increased steadily since 1996, primarily in the adolescent age group (Zuvekas and Vitiello 2012).

Strengths and Challenges of Integrative Medicine

Strengths

One of the main strengths of integrative medicine is its focus on preventive health. A policy of incremental intervention while maximizing healthy lifestyle approaches has the potential to reduce the need for prescription medications and to help lay a solid foundation of health. Another strength of integrative medicine is its inherent flexibility with the ability to tailor treatments to children of nearly any age, including those living with chronic health conditions. The field promotes the child's inherent capacity for self-regulation and healing (if not always cure), regardless of diagnosis. Other important strengths emphasized in integrative medicine are cultivation of self-control, resiliency, and self-efficacy, traits that have been shown to have significant impact on quality of life and health outcomes. Caretaker health, including parents, family members, and the medical team members has an important impact on health outcomes, and for this reason is also considered a foundation of the integrative medicine approach.

Another strength of pediatric integrative medicine is that it can be practiced in nearly any setting, from outpatient to the intensive and neonatal intensive care settings, including:

- Pre-natal consults
- Well child visits
- Home setting
- Acute care
- Complex chronic illness
- Behavioral and mental health issues
- Inpatient medicine
- Palliative care
- Hospice care

Obstacles

In addition to the stigma related to a history of unethical promotion of alternative therapies to parents of ill children, other challenges include a lack of outcomes research, inadequate insurance reimbursement, and disparate funding for child and maternal preventive health. A lack of training opportunities for clinicians is another obstacle, although this is gradually changing. Strongly skeptical colleagues and those complementary practitioners who take extreme positions (for example anti-vaccination) have each polarized the field in different ways, slowing meaningful progress on research, educational, and clinical fronts to benefit children's healthcare.

Ethical and legal considerations are a critical concern in integrative medicine. The guiding principles of **beneficence** (promote the wellbeing of the patient), **nonmalfeasance** (do no harm), and **patient autonomy** (does the patient have enough information to make an informed decision) must be applied in every encounter (Gilmour et al. 2011a).

Variability in training, licensure, and credentialing is another challenge. It is paramount that clinicians (and parents) have a full understanding of the state of the evidence surrounding individual therapies, an understanding of the qualifications of all practitioners, a clear understanding of the proposed treatment plan, and awareness of all potential risks and benefits (Gilmour et al. 2011b).

Table 1.2 Approach to CAM Therapies in Children Based on Efficacy and Safety

		Efficacy	
		Yes	No
Safety	Yes	Recommend	Tolerate
	No	Monitor closely or discourage	Discourage

In general, according to the National Center for Complementary and Integrative Health, physicians may provide complementary therapies such as nutritional counseling, herbal medicine, biofeedback, and hypnotherapy because they are authorized by state law to diagnose and treat disease. Psychologists are licensed in all states and commonly provide mind–body therapies and teach therapies such as biofeedback, guided imagery, hypnosis, and stress management, including cognitive behavioral therapy, mindfulness based stress reduction and others. However, states may or may not allow other licensed clinicians, conventional or complementary, to provide such therapies, or may not have laws addressing the question at all. Currently, four complementary practices are widely licensed in the United States: acupuncture, naturopathy, massage, chiropractic. A fifth, homeopathy, is licensed in only three states.

Difficulty in evaluating therapies for safety and efficacy is another important obstacle, especially with the lack of pediatric outcome studies available. One approach is to use a hierarchy of evidence, which means the greater the potential harm, the better the strength of evidence required before endorsement of the therapy can be made. Cohen and Kemper have developed a useful model to assess efficacy and safety of individual treatment approaches, shown in Table 1.2 (Kemper and Cohen 2004).

Policy

A paradigm change in priorities for national pediatric healthcare is needed to interrupt the ineffective cycle that places millions of children at a staggering financial, physical, mental, and emotional disadvantage often before they are even born. Research exists to help us intelligently address critical time windows in early life that determine the foundations of lifelong health. Clinicians caring for children must be the advocates that translate this science into positive action. In addition, the prevalence of neurodevelopmental disorders, attention-deficit/hyperactivity disorder, obesity, type-2 diabetes, metabolic syndrome, inflammatory bowel disease, asthma, and arthritis, premature birth and other conditions has literally changed the landscape of pediatrics, impacting millions of children, families, and clinicians. The old models of medical education and insurance reimbursement are outdated and unable to keep pace with the realities of pediatric practice. New approaches are urgently needed.

Given the complex realities of health policy, a thoughtful, informed, and well-coordinated approach will be needed to move the field of pediatric integrative medicine forward.

Medicine, and by association integrative medicine, is influenced by scientific advances, healthcare economics, and strategically positioned policy makers. To be effective, clinicians who advocate for children must be present at the highest levels of the healthcare debate. It is a fact that children bear a disproportionate burden of poverty, and have long been shortchanged in healthcare funding. According to 2010 statistics from the U.S. Bureau of the Census, children comprise 24% of the total population, yet they represent 36% of the country's poor. In 2010, an estimated 16.4 million children were living in poverty, with highest rates in Black and Hispanic children (Census 2010).

It is shortsighted to treat child healthcare policy as separate from the adult healthcare system. In fact, preventive child health is a fiscal issue with huge impact on the adult healthcare system. Imagine the healthcare savings in a generation of children where food quality is maximized and healthy weight is the norm, mastery of self-regulation skills is taught from preschool onward, policies are in place to limit and prevent exposures to harmful or potentially harmful environmental toxins, prescription drug use is minimized, and emerging research can be harnessed in areas such as nutrition, neuroscience, and environmental health, and social connections can be translated into positive change for children.

Disparities in delivery of healthcare must be eliminated in order to meet the needs of families at every income level, to include those with children with special healthcare needs, and evenhandedly distributed to every racial and ethnic background. (Selected Findings from the 2010 National Healthcare Quality and Disparities Reports [Agency for Healthcare Research and Quality 2010].)

Given the complexity of the issues involved, it would be understandable for clinicians to feel overwhelmed, or to doubt that change is possible. However, pediatricians have a track record of successful advocacy and examples of successful policy change exist. Federal and state advocacy efforts through the 66,000-member American Academy of Pediatrics and other organizations are ongoing to protect funding for children's healthcare by fighting cuts in Medicaid, Children's Health Insurance Program (CHIP) and the Special Supplemental Nutrition Program for Women, Infants, and Children and for maintaining federal healthcare subsidies under the Affordable Care Act for those who reside in U.S. states that have not created their own health insurance exchanges. Bright Futures, a collaboration between the American Academy of Pediatrics, Maternal and Child Health Bureau, and the Health Resources and Services Administration is an existing national program that promotes preventive health for all children and has important overlaps with the principles of integrative medicine (American Academy of Pediatrics [a]).

The Center on the Developing Child at Harvard University also offers an important example of this advocacy work with focus areas that have significant intersection with pediatric integrative medicine priorities. Their stated mission is "to drive science-based innovation that achieves breakthrough outcomes for children facing adversity." Their goal is "to create meaningful change in policy and practice that produces sustainably larger impacts on the learning capacity, health, and economic and social mobility of vulnerable young children" (Harvard University).

In addition to groundbreaking work on the negative effects of toxic stress on the developing brain, the Center identifies three foundations of health:

Sound appropriate nutrition: beginning with preconception nutritional status. This is well aligned with one of the fundamental priorities in integrative medicine that uses healthy nutrition as a main tool of preventive health.

Stable responsible relationships: prioritizing nurturing interactions with caring adults that enhance learning and help children develop resilience and a well-regulated stress response system that lay the groundwork for robust mental health through adult life.

Priorities in integrative medicine include cultivation of resilience, effective stress management, self-efficacy, and non-pharmacologic approaches to robust mental health.

Safe physical surroundings: free of physical, chemical, and structural hazards that encourage families to exercise and make social connections in a healthy and safe environment.

The **Harvard's Center on the Developing Child's** work in these three core areas aligns well with the guiding principles of integrative medicine and with recommendations the 2012 Institute of Medicine (IOM) report "Best Care at Lower Cost: The Path to Continuously Learning Health Care in America" which identifies three significant imperatives for change in the healthcare system: rising complexity of the healthcare system, unsustainable cost increase, and outcomes that are below the system's potential (Institute of Medicine 2012).

To deliver care that matches the needs of the modern healthcare system, the IOM calls for practitioners with a broader set of:

- Knowledge (nutrition, physical activity, mind–body, spirituality, environmental health)
- Attitudes (awareness of how personal, cultural, spiritual beliefs impact treatment and recommendations, appreciation of importance of self-care)
- Skills (communicate, listen, skilled at modeling and teaching behavior change)
- Relationships (openness to an inter-professional team-based approach and ability to partner with the patient and family's own human experience to benefit the patient)

Ultimately all healthcare is personal and must be approached in that spirit. Parents want the best for their children, and when they have better information, delivered by clinicians with higher awareness, they are able to provide care for their children that ideally will translate into lifelong health. Some of the most important partners in advocacy are parents, especially those with children affected by serious health conditions.

Education

Education about integrative medicine is an investment in children's health that involves both academic and community-based clinicians, insurance carriers, policy makers, and philanthropists.

What is the Current State of Education in the Field?

Education in the field of integrative medicine accelerated after publication of the 2005 Institute of Medicine report recommending that health professional schools include education on complementary medicine at all training levels. (Institute of Medicine. Complementary and Alternative Medicine in the United States. Available online: http://www.iom.edu/reports/2005/complementary-and-alternative-medicine-in-the-united-states.aspx)

Currently more than 60 major academic centers have educational and clinical programs connected through the Academic Consortium for Integrative Medicine & Health (formerly The Consortium of Academic Health Centers for Integrative Medicine).

Pediatric integrative medicine is supported by the American Academy of Pediatrics, which established a Provisional Section on Complementary, Holistic and Integrative

Medicine in 2006. This Section is now formally recognized, and was renamed the Section on Integrative Medicine in 2011. Pediatricians as a group have shown high interest in learning about integrative medicine and are frequently questioned about integrative medicine options for children. Of 1607 (856 completed) members, 87% had been asked about complementary therapies in the 3 months prior to the survey. Most common inquiries were about dietary supplements, followed by questions about chiropractic and nutrition. And 39% of surveyed pediatricians indicated that they, or their family members, used some type of complementary therapy in the year preceding the survey. Seventy-three percent of these surveyed agreed they should provide patients information about all possible treatment options. And nearly 50% had concerns about medical liability with regards to CAM (Kemper et al. 2008; American Academy of Pediatrics [b]; Kemper and O'Connor 2004).

The Special Interest Group on Physician Health and Wellness is housed in the AAP Section on Integrative Medicine deliberately due to the important correlations between physician wellness and patient outcomes, and as a result of the group's focus on preventive health and use of tools such as mindfulness in burnout prevention and cultivation of resilience, discussed in more detail in the following chapter. Many pediatricians themselves are interested in learning new approaches to treat children, and they are aware of the toll burnout takes on their personal and professional wellbeing (McClafferty et al. 2014).

Other medical education developments include launch of the University of Arizona Center for Integrative Medicine Pediatric Integrative Medicine in Residency (PIMR) program in 2012. The program is a 100-hour online curriculum designed to introduce integrative pediatrics into conventional pediatric training and is modeled after the IMR in Family Medicine (Lebensohn et al. 2012, McClafferty et al. 2015).

The PIMR curriculum provides an overview of fundamental topics in integrative pediatrics, including: nutrition, evidence-based dietary supplements, mind–body medicine, spirituality in medicine, physical activity, culturally based medical practices such as traditional Chinese medicine and Ayurveda, manual medicine, resident self-care and environment and health, along with case-based approaches to common pediatric conditions. Development of the first U.S. physician Board in Integrative Medicine in 2014 is another important step forward for the field overall.

Conclusion

In summary, overarching goals in pediatric integrative medicine include enhancement of the child's natural capacity to thrive and a desire to restore the richness of collaboration to the healthcare relationship. This requires a strong connection with parents and children, education, and focus on the foundations of preventive health, thoughtful blending of conventional and complementary therapies, and deliberate harnessing of emerging research in preventive health, nutrition, toxic stress, neuroplasticity, epigenetics, and environmental health in the service of improving children's lifelong health. When motivated clinicians, patients, and parents organize and work together, real change in the health of this and future generations of children will be inevitable.

References

"Academic Consortium for Integrative Medicine & Health." https://www.imconsortium.org

Agency for Healthcare Research and Quality. 2010. "Child and Adolescent Healthcare." http://www.ahrq.gov/research/findings/nhqrdr/nhqrdr10/children.html.

Akinbami, L. J., X. Liu, P. N. Pastor, and C. A. Reuben. 2011. "Attention deficit hyperactivity disorder among children aged 5–17 years in the United States, 1998–2009." *NCHS Data Brief* (70): 1–8.

American Academy of Pediatrics. [a] "Bright Futures." https://brightfutures.aap.org/Pages/default.aspx.

American Academy of Pediatrics. [b] "Periodic Survey #49 Complementary and Alternative Medicine (CAM) Therapies in Pediatric Practices." http://www.aap.org/en-us/professional-resources/Research/Pages/PS49_Executive_Summary_Complementaryand AlterowsComplementaryandAlternativeMedicineCAMTherapiesinPediatric.aspx.

Barnes, P. M., B. Bloom, and R. L. Nahin. 2008. "Complementary and alternative medicine use among adults and children: United States, 2007." *Natl Health Stat Report* (12): 1–23.

Birdee, G. S., R. S. Phillips, R. B. Davis, and P. Gardiner. 2010. "Factors associated with pediatric use of complementary and alternative medicine." *Pediatrics* 125(2): 249–56. doi: 10.1542/peds.2009-1406.

Black, L. I., T. C. Clarke, P. M. Barnes, B. J. Stussman, and R. L. Nahin. 2015. "Use of complementary health approaches among children aged 4–17 years in the United States: National Health Interview Survey, 2007–2012." *Natl Health Stat Report* (78): 1–19.

Centers for Disease Control and Prevention. 2005–2011. "Mental Health Surveillance Among Children." Last Modified May 17, 2013. http://www.cdc.gov/mmwr/preview/mmwrhtml/su6202a1.htm?s_cid=su6202a1_w.

Centers for Disease Control and Prevention. 2010. "2010 National Health Interview Survey (NHIS) Data." http://www.cdc.gov/asthma/nhis/2010/data.htm.

Centers for Disease Control and Prevention. 2012. "National Prematurity Awareness Month." http://www.cdc.gov/features/prematurebirth/

Centers for Disease Control and Prevention. 2015. "Childhood Obesity Facts."

Gilmour, J., C. Harrison, L. Asadi, M. H. Cohen, and S. Vohra. 2011a. "Complementary and alternative medicine practitioners' standard of care: responsibilities to patients and parents." *Pediatrics* 128(Suppl 4): S200–5. doi: 10.1542/peds.2010-2720J.

Gilmour, J., C. Harrison, L. Asadi, M. H. Cohen, and S. Vohra. 2011b. "Referrals and shared or collaborative care: managing relationships with complementary and alternative medicine practitioners." *Pediatrics* 128(Suppl 4): S181–6. doi: 10.1542/peds.2010-2720G.

Harvard University Center on the Development Child. http://developingchild.harvard.edu/about/.

Institute of Medicine. 2005. "Complementary and Alternative Medicine in the United States." http://www.iom.edu/reports/2005/complementary-and-alternative-medicine-in-the-united-states.aspx

Institute of Medicine. 2012. "Best Care at Lower Cost: The Path to Continuously Learning Health Care in America." http://iom.nationalacademies.org/Reports/2012/Best-Care-at-Lower-Cost-The-Path-to-Continuously-Learning-Health-Care-in-America.aspx?utm_source=feedburner&utm_medium=feed&utm_campaign=Feed%3A+IomTopicHealthServices CoverageAndAccess+(IOM+Topic%3A+Health+Services+Coverage+and+Access).

Kemper, K. J., and M. Cohen. 2004. "Ethics meet complementary and alternative medicine: new light on old principles." *Contemp Pediatr* 21(3): 61.

Kemper, K. J., and K. G. O'Connor. 2004. "Pediatricians' recommendations for complementary and alternative medical (CAM) therapies." *Ambul Pediatr* 4(6): 482–7. doi: 10.1367/A04-050R.1.

Kemper, K. J., S. Vohra, R. Walls, Complementary Task Force on, Medicine Alternative, Holistic Provisional Section on Complementary, and Medicine Integrative. 2008. "American Academy of Pediatrics. The use of complementary and alternative medicine in pediatrics." *Pediatrics* 122(6): 1374–86. doi: 10.1542/peds.2008-2173.

Lebensohn, P., B. Kligler, S. Dodds, C. Schneider, S. Sroka, R. Benn, P. Cook, M. Guerrera, T. Low Dog, V. Sierpina, R. Teets, D. Waxman, J. Woytowicz, A. Weil, and V. Maizes. 2012. "Integrative medicine in residency education: developing competency through online curriculum training." *J Grad Med Educ* 4(1): 76–82. doi: 10.4300/JGME-04-01-30.

Lee, P. F., R. E. Thomas, and P. A. Lee. 2015. "Approach to autism spectrum disorder: Using the new DSM-V diagnostic criteria and the CanMEDS-FM framework." *Can Fam Physician* 61(5): 421–4.

Maizes, V., D. Rakel, and C. Niemiec. 2009. "Integrative medicine and patient-centered care." *Explore (NY)* 5(5): 277–89. doi: 10.1016/j.explore.2009.06.008.

Mayer-Davis, E. J. 2008. "Type 2 diabetes in youth: epidemiology and current research toward prevention and treatment." *J Am Diet Assoc* 108(4 Suppl 1): S45–51. doi: 10.1016/j.jada.2008.01.018.

McClafferty, H., O. W. Brown, Medicine Section on Integrative, Practice Committee on, Medicine Ambulatory, and Medicine Section on Integrative. 2014. "Physician health and wellness." *Pediatrics* 134(4): 830–5. doi: 10.1542/peds.2014-2278.

McClafferty, H., S. Dodds, A. J. Brooks, M. G. Brenner, M. L. Brown, P. Frazer, J. D. Mark, J. A. Weydert, G. M. G. Wilcox, P. Lebensohn, and V. Maizes. 2015. "Pediatric Integrative Medicine in Residency (PIMR): Description of a new online educational curriculum." *Children* 2(1): 98–107. doi: 10.3390/children2010098.

National Cancer Institute. 2014. "Cancer in Children and Adolescents." http://www.cancer.gov/cancertopics/factsheet/Sites-Types/childhood

National Center for Complementary and Integrative Health. "Children's Use of Complementary Health Approaches, 2012 Survey Results." https://nccih.nih.gov/health/providers/digest/child-use?nav=cd

National Center for Complementary and Integrative Health. 2012. "Complementary, Alternative, or Integrative Health: What's In a Name?" https://nccih.nih.gov/health/integrative-health#types

National Center for Complementary and Integrative Health. 2014. "Complementary, Alternative, or Integrative Health: What's In a Name?"

National Institutes of Health [NIH]. 2014. "The NIH Almanac." http://www.nih.gov/about/almanac/organization/NCCIH.htm.

Section on Complementary and Integrative Medicine, Council on Children with Disabilities, American Academy of Pediatrics, M. Zimmer, and L. Desch. 2012. "Sensory integration therapies for children with developmental and behavioral disorders." *Pediatrics* 129(6): 1186–9. doi: 10.1542/peds.2012-0876.

U.S. Bureau of the Census. 2010. "Income, Poverty, and Health Insurance Coverage in the United States: 2010." http://www.npc.umich.edu/poverty/.

Winer, R. A., X. Qin, T. Harrington, J. Moorman, and H. Zahran. 2012. "Asthma incidence among children and adults: Findings from the Behavioral Risk Factor Surveillance system asthma call-back survey—United States, 2006–2008." *J Asthma* 49(1): 16–22. doi: 10.3109/02770903.2011.637594.

Zuvekas, S. H., and B. Vitiello. 2012. "Stimulant medication use in children: A 12-year perspective." *Am J Psychiatry* 169(2): 160–6.

2 Self-Care: Cultivating Healthy Resilience

Introduction

Burnout is highly prevalent in the healthcare system and takes a steep toll on physicians and other members of the healthcare team. Mounting research on the serious physical, mental, and social effects of long-term stress, shift work, and sleep disruption (Siedsma and Emlet 2015) points to the need for a shift from the outdated model of endurance and stoicism to a modern approach to physician health that capitalizes on research advances in nutrition, key dietary supplements, physical activity, sleep, environmental health, and mind–body approaches. Integrative medicine offers a useful blueprint for progress. (McClafferty et al. 2014) Some of the most compelling research in physician health and wellness has accumulated in the mind–body medicine arena, particularly in mindfulness and compassion training, discussed in more detail below.

Understanding Burnout

Most commonly measured by the Maslach Burnout Inventory, burnout is assessed by measurement of emotional exhaustion, depersonalization, and sense of personal accomplishment (Maslach and Leiter 2008). Symptoms of burnout are seen at every stage of medical training, peaking during training and in mid-career (Dyrbye et al. 2013; Pantaleoni et al. 2014), offering the opportunity to anticipate predictable stressors and act accordingly.

The prevalence of burnout in pediatricians has been shown to mirror rates in other specialties, with highest rates in specialties such as oncology, intensive care, neonatal intensive care, and pediatric surgery (Kushnir and Cohen 2008; Leigh, Tancredi, and Kravitz 2009).

The prevalence of substance abuse disorders, especially abuse of alcohol, in American physicians is high and significantly associated with burnout, depression, suicidal ideation, decreased quality of life, lower career satisfaction, and recent medical errors. A 2015 survey of 7288 physicians showed that 12.9% of male physicians and 21.4% of female physicians met the criteria for alcohol abuse or dependence, which highlights the importance of early and effective intervention (Oreskovich et al. 2015).

Many factors contribute to burnout; some of the most common include:

- **Individual stressors** such as fatigue, excessive work hours, difficult patients, coping with death or bad outcomes, threat of malpractice suits, bullying, financial worries, isolation, lack of effective stress management skills, and competing family expectations.

- **Hospital or practice-based stressors** such as competition, job insecurity or uncertainty, management conflicts, loss of personal control, time pressures, electronic medical records, productivity and performance demands, and unsupportive work environments. Organizational leadership has been shown to have a significant impact on physician burnout, especially the elements of good communication, efficiency of the organization, level of flexibility and autonomy, and workload expectations. A study by Shanafelt et al. summarized leadership qualities of physician leaders correlated with lower burnout as the ability to "inform, engage, inspire, develop, and recognize" (Shanafelt et al. 2015).

- **Stressors embedded in the "culture of medicine"** such as the expectation of unrealistic endurance, a code of silence regarding errors, vicarious traumatization (second victim phenomenon), pressure to publish or obtain ongoing grant funding, fear of vulnerability being perceived as weakness, and, paradoxically, reduction of resident duty hours with resulting increase in faculty work hours and stress (Blum et al. 2011; Wong and Imrie 2013).

Burnout has been described as occurring gradually in many cases, although symptoms may manifest abruptly and may be accompanied by anxiety or depression. One of the most concerning statistics in the burnout literature is the rate of physician suicidal ideation and completed suicide. It is an unacceptable fact that an estimated 300–400 U.S. physicians complete suicide annually. Women physicians are at special risk, with suicide rate 130% higher than women in the general population (relative risk ratio 2.7). Male physicians have been shown to have a rate 40% higher than men in general (relative risk ratio 1.41) (Schernhammer 2005; Schernhammer and Colditz 2004). Suicide linked to drug abuse has the highest rates in specialties such as anesthesia where access to drugs of potential abuse is higher (Rose and Brown 2010).

Disaster response medicine is another area identified with high stress and burnout in clinicians. Those who care for children in extreme situations such as poverty, war, genocide, terrorism, school shootings, or catastrophic natural disasters such as hurricanes, tornadoes, floods, and earthquakes often witness terrible suffering and loss with inadequate access to supplies and medical support.

Although The Federation for State Physician Health Programs was developed in response to demand for programs tailored to physicians struggling with drug addiction or alcohol abuse (JAMA 1973), and The Federation of State Physician Health Programs (FSPHP 2016) recognition of burnout in oneself or in a colleague can be complicated due to fear of stigma, pressure to continue to work, and the lack of effective support programs.

PTSD, Second Victim, and Lessons Learned from the Military

Research in soldiers suffering from PTSD has some overlap with clinician burnout, especially in physicians suffering vicarious traumatization, or "second victim trauma." Second victims are healthcare providers who are traumatized by work events in a way that is not always immediately evident. They may be involved in an unanticipated adverse patient event, in a medical error or injury, or other unanticipated occurrence including loss of a patient, and may feel personally responsible for the outcome. This can lead to erosive feelings of guilt, failure, and doubt of their medical skills (Scott et al. 2009).

There are some overlapping themes in the experience of PTSD treatment in the military that offer food for thought for diagnosing and approaching treatment for physicians diagnosed with high levels of burnout. Murphy et al. determined a pattern of step-wise progression in cohorts of soldiers being evaluated for PTSD treatment that offers some ideas for understanding and approaching burnout symptoms in clinicians. These themes include a progression from experiencing symptoms without understanding, to a sense of control and autonomy (Murphy et al. 2014).

Theme 1: Recognizing that Something is Wrong

Often the first symptoms noticed are physical rather than psychological; for example, pain that may reach a crisis point until symptoms cannot be ignored. In part the delay to seek treatment originates in an ingrained culture of stoicism, carrying on despite significant difficulties.

Theme 2: Overcoming Internal Stigma

A common finding with perception of shame was concern about peer judgment, but more often the shame was associated with internal rather than external stigma, related to the difficulty of admitting vulnerability. Input from a trusted witness increased acceptance that the situation was serious and they needed to seek help.

Theme 3: Finding an Explanation

"Why me?" Getting a psychological explanation for the symptoms and a diagnosis was a crucial step for the soldiers in the process of seeking and accepting help. In Murphy's study this was often noted as the pivotal step on the road to healing.

Theme 4: Not Being Alone

Learning that they were not alone led to normalization. This acceptance created the opportunity of a safe, non-judgmental space for progress to occur. Connection also led to a sense of hope, relief, and acceptance.

Theme 5: Control

An external locus of control was often associated with anxiety and depression. Help-seeking behavior shifted the focus from external to an internal locus of control about treatment options. This cultivated a feeling of autonomy over treatment approaches. The flexibility of an individualized approach was important, tailored to the individual's needs. This facilitated communication and in-depth discussion about an individual's access and barriers to care and a desire to help others overcome similar situations.

In summary, key factors to engaging in health-seeking behaviors for PTSD included:

- Recognition that something was wrong
- Overcoming internal stigma

- Finding an explanation
- Finding connection
- Shifting from external to internal locus of control
- Participation in development of programs to reduce stigma for peers

Mirroring progress in the military, increasing awareness about the prevalence of burnout in the medical culture is an important first step to prevention. Concrete steps to change outdated patterns in the culture of medicine are needed for both clinicians in practice and those coming after. Systems-based changes are slowly taking shape in the form of the 2009 Joint Commission guidelines mandating an approach to physician health that is separate from disciplinary actions (Commission 2009).

Progress in the field of pediatrics has been catalyzed in part by new Accreditation Council for Graduate Medical Education (ACGME) core competencies in the area of professionalism that call for the trainee to embody characteristics of compassion, empathy, emotional intelligence, and self-awareness, with the underlying goal of earlier identification of burnout symptoms and more structured acquisition of self-regulation skills (Hicks et al. 2010).

Development of the Special Interest Group on Physician Health and Wellness in the American Academy of Pediatrics is another step designed to promote broad education and policy change.

Shifting to Burnout Prevention and Cultivating Clinician Wellness

It seems intuitive that meaningful healthcare reform should begin from inside the system, led by healthy and resilient clinicians and inter-professional team members rather than be shaped by outside forces. Multiple studies have documented the high rates of burnout in medicine, yet relatively few have reported effective approaches to preventive wellness. Factors that have been identified include:

- Greater sense of control
- Absence of role conflict
- A sense of fair treatment
- Positive social support
- Appropriate rewards (financial, institutional, and social)
- Alignment of values between individual and workplace

(Maslach and Leiter 2008; Hinami et al. 2012)

Using an integrative medicine approach as a blueprint encourages a focus on multiple dimensions of health and specifically targets systemic inflammation associated with chronic stress. Elements of this approach are tailored to the individual's needs, interests, and readiness to make changes and include the topics of: nutrition, selected dietary supplements, enjoyable physical activity, sleep, environmental health, and mind–body approaches. An overview of supporting evidence for an integrative approach to physician wellness is reviewed below. Individual topics are covered in more detail in Part 2 Foundations of Health.

Healthy Lifestyle

Studies show that preventive wellness behaviors in physicians are additive (Shanafelt et al. 2012), associated with longer telomeres (Sun et al. 2012), and can even impact quality of patient counseling and patient outcome (Howe et al. 2010).

Nutrition: The Mediterranean diet pattern overlaps in many ways with the "prudent diet" widely discussed in the literature, which includes fruits, vegetables, whole grains, legumes, nuts, fish, and low-fat dairy, has been shown in multiple large population-based studies to reduce cardiovascular risk and rates of chronic inflammatory-illness-related mortality. The Mediterranean diet pattern emphasizes a plant-centered diet that is rich in vegetables and fruits, whole grains, nuts, seeds, legumes, fish, and olive oil, and water, with moderate dairy, coffee, tea, optional alcohol, and chocolate. This approach is low in processed foods, red meat, and sugary beverages. (Moderate alcohol intake is generally included for adults who already choose to drink alcohol, unless individual contraindications exist.) (Jacobs and Tapsell 2015)

In addition to reduction in cardiovascular risk, another important benefit identified in association of the Mediterranean diet pattern is increased telomere length in peripheral blood leukocytes, a recognized biomarker of aging. For example, results from the Nurses' Health Study involving 4676 healthy nurses showed significant correlation between adherence to a Mediterranean diet pattern and longer telomere length (Crous-Bou et al. 2014).

Selected dietary supplements including: adequate omega-3 fatty acids, associated with reduction of triglyceride levels and promotion of cardiovascular health (Leslie et al. 2015); vitamin D widely associated with bone health, modulation of oxidative stress and systemic inflammation, and under active study as a protective agent in atherogenesis (Holick 2005; Carvalho and Sposito 2015).

Healthy restorative sleep is associated with a range of significant health benefits, whereas shift work, often a necessity in medical training and practice, has been associated with increased risk of obesity, metabolic syndrome (Roth 2012; Wang et al. 2014), and breast cancer in women (Wang et al. 2013).

Elevated cholesterol and hypertriglyceridemia have also been reported in several studies on shift work, as has a correlation with reduction in physical activity and increase in sedentary behavior (Loprinzi 2015b, a).

Physical Activity

The myriad benefits of physical activity have been widely reported, yet many physicians in practice and in training do not exercise regularly. Large survey studies in U.S. surgeons tracking health behaviors showed that preventive wellness behaviors including the addition of regular exercise were additive in predicting quality of life and job satisfaction (Shanafelt et al. 2012).

Telomere length is also impacted by sedentary habits, and even modest increases in physical activity were associated with increased telomere length in a large survey (n = 7813) in the Nurses' Health Study (Du et al. 2012).

Environmental Health

Environmental exposures such as to phthalates, known endocrine-disrupting chemicals, are another consideration in the healthcare setting. This is an active area of research covered in more detail in Chapter 8 (Environmental Health) (Grady and Sathyanarayana 2012).

Mind–Body Therapies

Ideally a clinician would maintain a positive, calm emotional state, carry a healing intention, and maintain focus in the present moment in every patient encounter. In reality, medical practice is often chaotic, time pressured, and highly complex, straining the capacity of even the most caring individual over the course of a busy day, let alone a training rotation or throughout years of practice. It is imperative that clinicians learn and maintain effective self-regulation skills to help buffer them from the wear and tear of high levels of chronic stress. Emerging research shows stress to be a highly detrimental element in burnout associated with significant physiological and mental health effects such as alteration of immune function, upregulation of inflammatory markers, metabolic syndrome, diabetes, cardiovascular disease, and depression (Shonkoff 2012; Silverman and Sternberg 2012; Downs and Faulkner 2015).

Mind–body medicine is a cornerstone of integrative medicine with great potential for reducing stress and improving health. Although there is a wide variety of mind–body therapies, one of the best-studied mind–body therapies to date is mindfulness. The concept of mindfulness meditation is not new, but was not formally introduced into the medical arena until the early 1980s by Jon Kabat-Zinn, PhD (Kabat-Zinn 1982).

Mindfulness has been described as "the intentional self-regulation of attention from moment to moment" and has been shown to be effective in improving quality of life, reductions in pain perception, anxiety, and depression in a variety of patient populations (Merkes 2010).

The use of mindfulness and mindfulness-based stress reduction in addressing physician burnout has been shown to improve measures of empathy and sense of personal accomplishment, as well as reducing depersonalization and emotional exhaustion (Ludwig and Kabat-Zinn 2008; Fortney and Taylor 2010).

Mindfulness has also been shown to increase telomerase activity in peripheral blood mononuclear cells, associated with increased telomere length (Schutte and Malouff 2014). Unknowns in the use of mindfulness include the specific neural mechanism involved (Tang, Holzel, and Posner 2015), and the "dose" of mindfulness adequate to address burnout symptoms. Studies investigating the use of abbreviated mindfulness interventions have shown benefit in reduction of burnout symptoms (Fortney et al. 2013), as have interventions designed using a hybrid in-person and group telephone approach (Bazarko et al. 2013).

Other studies have used mindfulness or mindfulness-based stress reduction as part of a group-oriented intervention with encouraging success (West et al. 2014).

Empathy Versus Compassion

One of the important nuances in clinician self-care is the distinction between empathy and compassion. Empathy (the ability to *share, experience, participate in the feelings of another while knowing that the feeling isn't yours*) can be valuable in the medical interaction, but an excess of empathy has been associated with burnout and has also been associated with reduced emotional connectedness (Klimecki et al. 2014).

In fact, imaging studies show that the brain of the person *experiencing* the *feeling of empathy* activates the same brain regions of the person who is *experiencing the suffering*, therefore empathic suffering is considered a true experience of suffering—which can become overwhelming with repeated exposure (Engen and Singer 2015).

Compassion in this context should be differentiated from empathy, and has been defined as the emotional feeling that arises when witnessing another's suffering coupled with the motivation to alleviate the suffering. Compassion training is garnering active research interest in clinician self-care, in part due to the prevalence of compassion fatigue in clinical caregivers (Goetz, Keltner, and Simon-Thomas 2010).

Compassion fatigue is thought to result from a combination of secondary post-traumatic stress and symptoms of burnout, and has been inversely associated with emotional intelligence and adaptive coping skills (Fernando and Consedine 2014a; Zeidner et al. 2013).

Studies have shown that those with higher trait emotional intelligence can be buffered against negative emotion. Therefore it may be that those healthcare workers who are more vulnerable to compassion fatigue can be identified and taught self-regulation skills that encourage cultivation of higher levels of emotional intelligence. This is in part the basis for research interest in the field of compassion training and compassion-based cognitive therapy (Zeidner et al. 2013; Raab 2014).

A simplified explanation of compassion training is that of learning to first generate the emotional state of loving-kindness for oneself (self-compassion) through a series of imagery and positive memories, then learning to extend this feeling of care and loving-kindness to others. A range of studies show that even short-term training in compassion has been associated with positive benefits such as pro-social behavior and resilience. Imaging studies have shown a correlation between positive affects associated with compassion and increased activity in brain regions associated with reward and affiliation, providing a buffer of positive affect to negative stimuli (Weng et al. 2013).

The idea that compassion can be learned as a self-regulation skill for clinicians holds tremendous potential for helping preserve their emotional resilience over the arc of training and practice (Fernando and Consedine 2014b). Understanding the neural processes involved in this approach is an area of active study (Mascaro et al. 2015; Klimecki et al. 2013; Engen and Singer 2015; Weng et al. 2013).

Finding the Right Fit

Interest in the application of the mind–body therapies in the clinical setting is high, despite the complexity of medical practice, challenging patients, and ubiquitous time pressures (Siedsma and Emlet 2015). Some of the familiar challenges involved in applying consistent self-care are the familiar juggle of work and family expectations, sedentary habits ingrained after years of school, sleep disruption, reluctance to expose vulnerability, and the presence of chronic stress. Approaches to self-care are needed that are individualized, effective, and sustainable to help reluctant clinicians begin to make meaningful change—and can help the clinician understand, adopt, and model healthy lifestyle behaviors that may make them more effect in the clinical setting (Frank, Breyan, and Elon 2000; Howe et al. 2010).

Preventive Wellness Steps

Concrete steps a clinician can take toward preventive wellness include the following.

Step 1. Recognition of Symptoms: "Taking Stock"

It is important for the clinician to reinforce the positive, and provide a "shame-free" place for considering their health and wellbeing, including: weight management, cardio-vascular health, reproductive health, endocrine, and especially mental health including PTSD, anxiety, depression, and other serious (and treatable) mental health concerns.

- General health assessment
- Physical assessment, "get the numbers"
- BMI
- Blood pressure, labs
- Caloric intake
- Sleep quality
- Physical activity
- Evaluate number and type of medications

Step 2. Useful Tools for Evaluating Burnout

- Maslach inventory
- Wheel of Life exercise

Step 3. Values Clarification: Assess Strengths and Accomplishments

- Who am I? Why am I here?
- What do I deeply value?
- What really matters to me?
- How do you define your life?
- What is the meaning of your story?
- Recognition of burnout can lead to rich insights: what have you learned?

Step 4. Process: Skills Needed for an Integrative Medicine Approach to Be Successful

- Time
- Generous listening
- Motivational interviewing
- Incremental intervention, focus on lifestyle changes first
- Mastery of self-regulation skill(s)
- Recognizing positive progress, enhancement of sense of self-efficacy

Step 5. Content: Knowledge Needed for Success

What is entailed and why is it relevant to clinician health? This approach is designed to shift the focus from burnout to preventive health by harnessing emerging research in neuroscience, nutrition, physical activity, environmental health, mind–body medicine, spirituality, and social support to directly benefit the clinician.

- Nutrition
- Selected dietary supplements (omega-3 fatty acids, vitamin D for example)
- Physical activity
- Mind–body therapies
- Sleep
- Environmental awareness

Step 6. Cultivating Resilience (Commonly Requires Adversity as a Catalyst)

Resilience:

- The power or ability to return to the original form, position, etc., after being bent, compressed, or stretched; elasticity
- Ability to recover readily from illness, depression, adversity, or the like; buoyancy
- Amount of potential energy stored in an elastic material when deformed
- Ability of an ecosystem to return to its original state after being disturbed

(Merriam Webster)

Resilience is a trait under active study in physician health and wellness, and can be applied to an individual, an organization, or the culture of medicine itself. It is important to note that while cultivation of resilience is important, it should not imply an unending reserve of endurance as is often unrealistically expected in medical training. Therefore, an individual's cultivation of resilience would ideally parallel meaningful steps in the organization and overarching culture of medicine to help clinicians develop a healthy hardiness and reserve that would serve them throughout a satisfying and meaningful medical career. One of the key components in resilience research is the idea of preserving mental and physical capacity in the face of high stressors, and of growing stronger for the experiences, combining the idea of "bouncing back" with a positive spiral of growth. Some of the common characteristics identified in resilient physicians include: the capacity for mindfulness, self-awareness and monitoring, consistent limit setting, and skills for constructive engagement as opposed to withdrawal at work. Building a positive community at work is a critical component of physician resilience and has been shown to improve quality patient care and patient satisfaction (Zwack and Schweitzer 2013; Epstein and Krasner 2013; Lister, Ledbetter, and Warren 2015). Less quantifiable, yet gaining increasing research interest in physician health and wellness, are the qualities of optimism (Jeste et al. 2015) and grit (perseverance and passion for long-term goals) (Duckworth et al. 2007; Eskreis-Winkler et al. 2014; Robertson-Kraft and Duckworth 2014).

Physician Coaching

One emerging trend is that of a physician coach to help develop and implement a sustainable plan for long-term health (Gazelle, Liebschutz, and Riess 2015; Schneider, Kingsolver, and Rosdahl 2014).

Some of the Goals of a Coaching Relationship

- Grow beyond perceived limits
- Expand your options
- Provoke discussion and deeper understanding of career trajectory
- Open to new approaches to health and healing
- Increase adaptability
- Tap into creativity and innovation
- Create opportunities that enhance a sense of control and career gratification

Summary

Clinician health and wellness is a critical component of medical practice that will ideally be prioritized from the earliest stages of pre-medical training. Every clinician, administrator, and member of the inter-professional healthcare team can benefit from a conscious and well-organized approach to health and wellbeing with the goals of creating engaged and caring clinicians and care teams, and improving patient outcomes. Mind–body approaches that enhance self-regulation show significant potential as life-skills that can help reduce burnout and compassion fatigue, and promote career satisfaction in conjunction with modern preventive lifestyle measures.

References

Bazarko, D., R. A. Cate, F. Azocar, and M. J. Kreitzer. 2013. "The impact of an innovative mindfulness-based stress reduction program on the health and well-being of nurses employed in a corporate setting." *J Workplace Behav Health* 28(2): 107–33. doi: 10.1080/15555240.2013.779518.

Blum, A. B., S. Shea, C. A. Czeisler, C. P. Landrigan, and L. Leape. 2011. "Implementing the 2009 Institute of Medicine recommendations on resident physician work hours, supervision, and safety." *Nat Sci Sleep* 3: 47–85. doi: 10.2147/NSS.S19649.

Carvalho, L. S., and A. C. Sposito. 2015. "Vitamin D for the prevention of cardiovascular disease: are we ready for that?" *Atherosclerosis* 241(2): 729–40. doi: 10.1016/j.atherosclerosis.2015.06.034.

Commission, The Joint. 2009. *Comprehensive Accreditation Manual for Hospitals: The Official Handbook, 2009*. Oakbrook Terrace, IL.

Crous-Bou, M., T. T. Fung, J. Prescott, B. Julin, M. Du, Q. Sun, K. M. Rexrode, F. B. Hu, and I. De Vivo. 2014. "Mediterranean diet and telomere length in Nurses' Health Study: population based cohort study." *BMJ* 349: g6674. doi: 10.1136/bmj.g6674.

Downs, C. A., and M. S. Faulkner. 2015. "Toxic stress, inflammation and symptomatology of chronic complications in diabetes." *World J Diabetes* 6(4): 554–65. doi: 10.4239/wjd.v6.i4.554.

Du, M., J. Prescott, P. Kraft, J. Han, E. Giovannucci, S. E. Hankinson, and I. De Vivo. 2012. "Physical activity, sedentary behavior, and leukocyte telomere length in women." *Am J Epidemiol* 175(5): 414–22. doi: 10.1093/aje/kwr330.

Duckworth, A. L., C. Peterson, M. D. Matthews, and D. R. Kelly. 2007. "Grit: perseverance and passion for long-term goals." *J Pers Soc Psychol* 92(6): 1087–101. doi: 10.1037/0022-3514.92.6.1087.

Dyrbye L. N., P. Varkey, S. L. Boone, D. V. Satele, J. A. Sloan, and T. D. Shanafelt. 2013. "Physician satisfaction and burnout at different career stages." *Mayo Clin Proc* 88(12): 1358–67.

Engen, H. G., and T. Singer. 2015. "Compassion-based emotion regulation up-regulates experienced positive affect and associated neural networks." *Soc Cogn Affect Neurosci* doi: 10.1093/scan/nsv008.

Epstein, R. M., and M. S. Krasner. 2013. "Physician resilience: what it means, why it matters, and how to promote it." *Acad Med* 88(3): 301–3. doi: 10.1097/ACM.0b013e318280cff0.

Eskreis-Winkler, L., E. P. Shulman, S. A. Beal, and A. L. Duckworth. 2014. "The grit effect: predicting retention in the military, the workplace, school and marriage." *Front Psychol* 5: 36. doi: 10.3389/fpsyg.2014.00036.

Fernando, A. T., 3rd, and N. S. Consedine. 2014a. "Beyond compassion fatigue: the transactional model of physician compassion." *J Pain Symptom Manage* 48(2): 289–98. doi: 10.1016/j.jpainsymman.2013.09.014.

Fernando, A. T., 3rd, and N. S. Consedine. 2014b. "Development and initial psychometric properties of the Barriers to Physician Compassion questionnaire." *Postgrad Med J* 90(1065): 388–95. doi: 10.1136/postgradmedj-2013-132127.

Fortney, L., C. Luchterhand, L. Zakletskaia, A. Zgierska, and D. Rakel. 2013. "Abbreviated mindfulness intervention for job satisfaction, quality of life, and compassion in primary care clinicians: a pilot study." *Ann Fam Med* 11(5): 412–20. doi: 10.1370/afm.1511.

Fortney, L., and M. Taylor. 2010. "Meditation in medical practice: a review of the evidence and practice." *Prim Care* 37(1): 81–90. doi: 10.1016/j.pop.2009.09.004.

Frank, E., J. Breyan, and L. Elon. 2000. "Physician disclosure of healthy personal behaviors improves credibility and ability to motivate." *Arch Fam Med* 9(3): 287–90.

FSPHP. 2016. "The Federation of State Physician Health Programs." Accessed September 12. http://www.fsphp.org/History.html.

Gazelle, G., J. M. Liebschutz, and H. Riess. 2015. "Physician burnout: coaching a way out." *J Gen Intern Med* 30(4): 508–13. doi: 10.1007/s11606-014-3144-y.

Goetz, J. L., D. Keltner, and E. Simon-Thomas. 2010. "Compassion: an evolutionary analysis and empirical review." *Psychol Bull* 136(3): 351–74. doi: 10.1037/a0018807.

Grady, R., and S. Sathyanarayana. 2012. "An update on phthalates and male reproductive development and function." *Curr Urol Rep* 13(4): 307–10. doi: 10.1007/s11934-012-0261-1.

Hicks, P. J., D. J. Schumacher, B. J. Benson, A. E. Burke, R. Englander, S. Guralnick, S. Ludwig, and C. Carraccio. 2010. "The pediatrics milestones: conceptual framework, guiding principles, and approach to development." *J Grad Med Educ* 2(3): 410–8. doi: 10.4300/JGME-D-10-00126.1.

Hinami, K., C. T. Whelan, R. J. Wolosin, J. A. Miller, and T. B. Wetterneck. 2012. "Worklife and satisfaction of hospitalists: toward flourishing careers." *J Gen Intern Med* 27(1): 28–36. doi: 10.1007/s11606-011-1780-z.

Holick, M. F. 2005. "The vitamin D epidemic and its health consequences." *J Nutr* 135(11): 2739S–48S.

Howe, M., A. Leidel, S. M. Krishnan, A. Weber, M. Rubenfire, and E. A. Jackson. 2010. "Patient-related diet and exercise counseling: do providers' own lifestyle habits matter?" *Prev Cardiol* 13(4): 180–5. doi: 10.1111/j.1751-7141.2010.00079.x.

Jacobs, D. R., Jr., and L. C. Tapsell. 2015. "What an anticardiovascular diet should be in 2015." *Curr Opin Lipidol* 26 (4): 270–5. doi: 10.1097/MOL.0000000000000184.

JAMA. 1973. "The sick physician. Impairment by psychiatric disorders, including alcoholism and drug dependence." *JAMA* 223(6): 684–7.

Jeste, D. V., B. W. Palmer, D. C. Rettew, and S. Boardman. 2015. "Positive psychiatry: its time has come." *J Clin Psychiatry* 76(6): 675–83. doi: 10.4088/JCP.14nr09599.

Kabat-Zinn, J. 1982. "An outpatient program in behavioral medicine for chronic pain patients based on the practice of mindfulness meditation: theoretical considerations and preliminary results." *Gen Hosp Psychiatry* 4(1): 33–47.

Klimecki, O. M., S. Leiberg, C. Lamm, and T. Singer. 2013. "Functional neural plasticity and associated changes in positive affect after compassion training." *Cereb Cortex* 23(7): 1552–61. doi: 10.1093/cercor/bhs142.

Klimecki, O. M., S. Leiberg, M. Ricard, and T. Singer. 2014. "Differential pattern of functional brain plasticity after compassion and empathy training." *Soc Cogn Affect Neurosci* 9(6): 873–9. doi: 10.1093/scan/nst060.

Kushnir, T., and A. H. Cohen. 2008. "Positive and negative work characteristics associated with burnout among primary care pediatricians." *Pediatr Int* 50(4): 546–51. doi: 10.1111/j.1442-200X.2008.02619.x.

Leigh, J. P., D. J. Tancredi, and R. L. Kravitz. 2009. "Physician career satisfaction within specialties." *BMC Health Serv Res* 9: 166. doi: 10.1186/1472-6963-9-166.

Leslie, M. A., D. J. Cohen, D. M. Liddle, L. E. Robinson, and D. W. Ma. 2015. "A review of the effect of omega-3 polyunsaturated fatty acids on blood triacylglycerol levels in normolipidemic and borderline hyperlipidemic individuals." *Lipids Health Dis* 14: 53. doi: 10.1186/s12944-015-0049-7.

Lister, E. D., T. G. Ledbetter, and A. M. Warren. 2015. "The engaged physician." *Mayo Clin Proc* 90(4): 425–7. doi: 10.1016/j.mayocp.2015.02.005.

Loprinzi, P. D. 2015a. "The effect of shift work on red blood cell distribution width." *Physiol Behav* 142: 121–5. doi: 10.1016/j.physbeh.2015.01.020.

Loprinzi, P. D. 2015b. "The effects of shift work on free-living physical activity and sedentary behavior." *Prev Med* 76: 43–7. doi: 10.1016/j.ypmed.2015.03.025.

Ludwig, D. S., and J. Kabat-Zinn. 2008. "Mindfulness in medicine." *JAMA* 300(11): 1350–2. doi: 10.1001/jama.300.11.1350.

Mascaro, J. S., A. Darcher, L. T. Negi, and C. L. Raison. 2015. "The neural mediators of kindness-based meditation: a theoretical model." *Front Psychol* 6: 109. doi: 10.3389/fpsyg.2015.00109.

Maslach, C., and M. P. Leiter. 2008. "Early predictors of job burnout and engagement." *J Appl Psychol* 93(3): 498–512. doi: 10.1037/0021-9010.93.3.498.

Merkes, M. 2010. "Mindfulness-based stress reduction for people with chronic diseases." *Aust J Prim Health* 16(3): 200–10. doi: 10.1071/PY09063.

McClafferty, H., O. W. Brown, Medicine Section on Integrative, Practice Committee on, Medicine Ambulatory, and Medicine Section on Integrative. 2014. "Physician health and wellness." *Pediatrics* 134(4): 830–5. doi: 10.1542/peds.2014-2278.

Murphy, D., E. Hunt, O. Luzon, and N. Greenberg. 2014. "Exploring positive pathways to care for members of the UK Armed Forces receiving treatment for PTSD: a qualitative study." *Eur J Psychotraumatol* 5. doi: 10.3402/ejpt.v5.21759.

Oreskovich, M. R., T. Shanafelt, L. N. Dyrbye, L. Tan, W. Sotile, D. Satele, C. P. West, J. Sloan, and S. Boone. 2015. "The prevalence of substance use disorders in American physicians." *Am J Addict* 24(1): 30–8. doi: 10.1111/ajad.12173.

Pantaleoni J. L., E. M. Augustine, B. M. Sourkes, and L. K. Bachrach. 2014. "Burnout in pediatric residents over a 2-year period: a longitudinal study." *Acad Pediatr* 4(2): 167–72.

Raab, K. 2014. "Mindfulness, self-compassion, and empathy among health care professionals: a review of the literature." *J Health Care Chaplain* 20(3): 95–108. doi: 10.1080/08854726.2014.913876.

Robertson-Kraft, C., and A. L. Duckworth. 2014. "True Grit: trait-level perseverance and passion for long-term goals predicts effectiveness and retention among novice teachers." *Teach Coll Rec (1970)* 116(3).

Rose, G. L., and R. E. Brown, Jr. 2010. "The impaired anesthesiologist: not just about drugs and alcohol anymore." *J Clin Anesth* 22(5): 379–84. doi: 10.1016/j.jclinane.2009.09.009.

Roth, T. 2012. "Appropriate therapeutic selection for patients with shift work disorder." *Sleep Med* 13(4): 335–41. doi: 10.1016/j.sleep.2011.11.006.

Schernhammer, E. 2005. "Taking their own lives: the high rate of physician suicide." *N Engl J Med* 352(24): 2473–6. doi: 10.1056/NEJMp058014.

Schernhammer, E. S., and G. A. Colditz. 2004. "Suicide rates among physicians: a quantitative and gender assessment (meta-analysis)." *Am J Psychiatry* 161(12): 2295–302. doi: 10.1176/appi.ajp.161.12.2295.

Schneider, S., K. Kingsolver, and J. Rosdahl. 2014. "Physician coaching to enhance well-being: a qualitative analysis of a pilot intervention." *Explore (NY)* 10(6): 372–9. doi: 10.1016/j.explore.2014.08.007.

Schutte, N. S., and J. M. Malouff. 2014. "A meta-analytic review of the effects of mindfulness meditation on telomerase activity." *Psychoneuroendocrinology* 42: 45–8. doi: 10.1016/j.psyneuen.2013.12.017.

Scott, S. D., L. E. Hirschinger, K. R. Cox, M. McCoig, J. Brandt, and L. W. Hall. 2009. "The natural history of recovery for the healthcare provider 'second victim' after adverse patient events." *Qual Saf Health Care* 18(5): 325–30. doi: 10.1136/qshc.2009.032870.

Shanafelt, T. D., G. Gorringe, R. Menaker, K. A. Storz, D. Reeves, S. J. Buskirk, J. A. Sloan, and S. J. Swensen. 2015. "Impact of organizational leadership on physician burnout and satisfaction." *Mayo Clin Proc* 90(4): 432–40. doi: 10.1016/j.mayocp.2015.01.012.

Shanafelt, T. D., M. R. Oreskovich, L. N. Dyrbye, D. V. Satele, J. B. Hanks, J. A. Sloan, and C. M. Balch. 2012. "Avoiding burnout: the personal health habits and wellness practices of US surgeons." *Ann Surg* 255(4): 625–33. doi: 10.1097/SLA.0b013e31824b2fa0.

Shonkoff, J. P. 2012. "Leveraging the biology of adversity to address the roots of disparities in health and development." *Proc Natl Acad Sci U S A* 109(Suppl 2): 17302–7. doi: 10.1073/pnas.1121259109.

Siedsma, M., and L. Emlet. 2015. "Physician burnout: can we make a difference together?" *Crit Care* 19: 273. doi: 10.1186/s13054-015-0990-x.

Silverman, M. N., and E. M. Sternberg. 2012. "Glucocorticoid regulation of inflammation and its functional correlates: from HPA axis to glucocorticoid receptor dysfunction." *Ann N Y Acad Sci* 1261: 55–63. doi: 10.1111/j.1749-6632.2012.06633.x.

Sun, Q., L. Shi, J. Prescott, S. E. Chiuve, F. B. Hu, I. De Vivo, M. J. Stampfer, P. W. Franks, J. E. Manson, and K. M. Rexrode. 2012. "Healthy lifestyle and leukocyte telomere length in U.S. women." *PLoS One* 7(5): e38374. doi: 10.1371/journal.pone.0038374.

Tang, Y. Y., B. K. Holzel, and M. I. Posner. 2015. "The neuroscience of mindfulness meditation." *Nat Rev Neurosci* 16(4): 213–25. doi: 10.1038/nrn3916.

Wang, F., K. L. Yeung, W. C. Chan, C. C. Kwok, S. L. Leung, C. Wu, E. Y. Chan, I. T. Yu, X. R. Yang, and L. A. Tse. 2013. "A meta-analysis on dose-response relationship between night shift work and the risk of breast cancer." *Ann Oncol* 24(11): 2724–32. doi: 10.1093/annonc/mdt283.

Wang, F., L. Zhang, Y. Zhang, B. Zhang, Y. He, S. Xie, M. Li, X. Miao, E. Y. Chan, J. L. Tang, M. C. Wong, Z. Li, I. T. Yu, and L. A. Tse. 2014. "Meta-analysis on night shift work and risk of metabolic syndrome." *Obes Rev* 15(9): 709–20. doi: 10.1111/obr.12194.

Weng, H. Y., A. S. Fox, A. J. Shackman, D. E. Stodola, J. Z. Caldwell, M. C. Olson, G. M. Rogers, and R. J. Davidson. 2013. "Compassion training alters altruism and neural responses to suffering." *Psychol Sci* 24(7): 1171–80. doi: 10.1177/0956797612469537.

West, C. P., L. N. Dyrbye, J. T. Rabatin, T. G. Call, J. H. Davidson, A. Multari, S. A. Romanski, J. M. Hellyer, J. A. Sloan, and T. D. Shanafelt. 2014. "Intervention to promote physician well-being, job satisfaction, and professionalism: a randomized clinical trial." *JAMA Intern Med* 174(4): 527–33. doi: 10.1001/jamainternmed.2013.14387.

Wong, B. M., and K. Imrie. 2013. "Why resident duty hours regulations must address attending physicians' workload." *Acad Med* 88(9): 1209–11. doi: 10.1097/ACM.0b013e31829e5727.

Zeidner, M., D. Hadar, G. Matthews, and R. D. Roberts. 2013. "Personal factors related to compassion fatigue in health professionals." *Anxiety Stress Coping* 26(6): 595–609. doi: 10.1080/10615806.2013.777045.

Zwack, J., and J. Schweitzer. 2013. "If every fifth physician is affected by burnout, what about the other four? Resilience strategies of experienced physicians." *Acad Med* 88(3): 382–9. doi: 10.1097/ACM.0b013e318281696b.

Part 2

Foundations of Health

3 Nutrition

Introduction

In the ideal scenario, nutrition would be emphasized as a priority in every well child visit, beginning with the prenatal visit. In reality, many conventionally trained practitioners receive minimal education about everyday nutrition and feel unprepared to knowledgably counsel patients on the subject (Devries et al. 2014).

Other obstacles in introducing nutrition into the medical encounter are the lack of insurance reimbursement for time spent in nutrition counseling, and time pressures common in the typical medical visit (Lenders et al. 2014).

The potential positive impact of evidence-based nutrition interventions on long-term health, especially in children, suggests that every clinician should be equipped to be an effective counselor in this area and have time for meaningful counseling routinely covered by insurance. In the integrative medicine approach nutrition is considered fundamental to health and is emphasized accordingly.

The intent of this chapter is to focus on several core themes in children's nutrition rather than attempting an exhaustive review of specialized areas. These themes include: recognition and maintenance of healthy weight, the building blocks of nutrition, integrating nutrition into the well child visit, the Mediterranean diet, and 'healthy-prudent' diet patterns. Examples of selected food sensitivities are also covered. Pediatric obesity and its associated comorbidities are discussed in Chapter 21.

Nutrition Policy and Child Health

Healthy weight is a critical predictor of lifelong health, yet large population surveys show large gaps between recommended dietary guidelines and consumer eating patterns (Britten et al. 2012b).

The USDA Healthy Eating Index-2010 measure confirms that only half of U.S. children 2–17 years meet federal diet quality standards (designed to measure quality in terms of how well diets meet the recommendations of the 2010 Dietary Guidelines for Americans), missing the critical benefit of sound nutrition in early life (USDA Centre for Nutrition Policy and Promotion 2013). Not surprisingly, gaps were largest in the 'Greens, Beans, and Whole Grain' categories (Britten et al. 2012a).

Challenges and Obstacles

Challenges related to these nutritional gaps are serious and include: socioeconomic considerations leading to lack of access to fresh and wholesome food, cutbacks in federal and state funding for nutrition programs, ingrained nutritional habits and behaviors, cultural patterns, and significant competition from well-funded marketing and advertising campaigns directed to children. For example, a 2015 study by Kunkel et al. analyzed food advertisements appearing in children's television programs and showed no improvement in direct advertising to children despite an industry-wide pledge of self-regulation of direct marketing to children. Analysis of the commercial content in 2014 by researchers showed that 80% of the foods advertised to children were products with poor nutrition quality (Kunkel, Castonguay, and Filer 2015).

Web-based and smart phones are also important sources of direct-to-children advertising. For example, a study by Ustjanauskas showed that 3.4 *billion* food advertisements appeared on frequently visited children's websites in 2009–2010 with the vast majority advertising unhealthy foods (Ustjanauskas, Harris, and Schwartz 2014).

$4.6 billion was spent on fast food marketing and advertising directly to children in 2012, up from $4.2 billion in 2009, including advertising in television markets, and social media such as Facebook, Twitter, YouTube, mobile website banner ads, smartphone applications, and text message advertising (Harris, Schwartz, and Munsell 2013).

Critical Time Windows

It has been shown that healthy weight is programmed early and may be influenced by both maternal and paternal body-mass-index among other factors (Weng et al. 2013).

One of the first windows of opportunity to promote healthy weight occurs with the decision whether or not to breastfeed. The World Health Organization, the Institute of Medicine, and the American Academy of Pediatrics (AAP) strongly endorse breast milk as the optimal food for newborns and infants. In fact, in the 2012 AAP policy, breastfeeding is described as a medical priority for infants rather than a lifestyle choice by the parent. The AAP recommends exclusive breastfeeding for about 6 months and continued use of breast milk in conjunction with solid foods after they are introduced (American Academy of Pediatrics 2012).

Duration of breastfeeding has been inversely correlated with risk of overweight; for example, each month of breastfeeding has been associated with an estimated 4% risk reduction of overweight. In addition, a 15%–30% reduction in adolescent and adult obesity rates has been documented if any breastfeeding occurred in infancy compared to no breastfeeding in infancy. The AAP report reviews the important immune modulatory factors of breast milk and its protective effect against a diverse range of illnesses including: otitis media and upper respiratory infections, gastrointestinal infections, necrotizing enterocolitis, sudden infant death syndrome, allergic disease, celiac disease, inflammatory bowel disease, type-1 diabetes, childhood leukemia and lymphoma (American Academy of Pediatrics 2012).

One of the most important steps the clinician can take in the prenatal and newborn visits is to encourage and support the parents in successful breastfeeding (Handa and Schanler 2013).

A recent trend in the use of pasteurized donor human milk through the Human Milk Banking Association of North America (HMBANA) is promising for those mothers who are unable, or who choose not to, breast feed, and is being increasingly used in premature infants. Due caution must be exercised regarding sourcing due to possible contamination. Only carefully regulated and known sources should be used (Vickers et al. 2015).

Healthy Weight

Strategies for Prevention

Nutrition recommendations in the U.S. Dietary Guidelines 2010 for Americans do not currently include guidelines for children under the age of 2 years (USDA Centre for Nutrition Policy and Promotion 2010). However, recommendations of the IOM committee (Institute of Medicine 2011) do include guidelines to measure and record growth parameters at every well visit, which is important for the early detection of overweight. IOM guidelines recommend discussion and intervention in children with growth measurements at or above the 85th percentile for age, rapid rate of weight gain, and in parents who are overweight or obese. Since September 2010, consensus from the AAP and CDC recommends use of the WHO growth curves for all children younger than 24 months because they more accurately reflect growth of healthy breastfed infants and more accurately identify overweight and obese infants. Consistent education in well child visits about healthy infant weight is important, especially if parents' culture has differing opinions about what constitutes a healthy weight in babies and young children.

This matters because healthy weight in infancy and childhood is a critical determinant of healthy weight in both adolescence and adulthood. Duration of obesity (from childhood through adulthood) has also been correlated with progressively increased risk of comorbidities such as type-2 diabetes, the metabolic syndrome, and nonalcoholic fatty liver disease. Other comorbidities include serious cardiovascular risk factors such as hypertension, and carotid and abdominal aortal vascular wall thickening (Dhuper, Buddhe, and Patel 2013).

Childhood Obesity Statistics

Although the rate of increase of pediatric obesity has flattened, the combined prevalence of overweight and obesity in U.S. children is 30%, with 1 out of every 10 children under the age of 6 being obese (Ogden et al. 2014; Centers for Disease Control and Prevention [b]).

Of significant concern, a 2011 Institute of Medicine report on Early Childhood Obesity Prevention Policy released in June 2011 indicated that almost 10% of infants and toddlers and 20% of children between the ages of 2 and 5 years already meet criteria for overweight or obesity, highlighting the urgent need for early effective education and effective interventions.

In the search for the critical time windows for healthy weight interventions, three weight trajectories were identified by Li et al. in a survey of 1739 children younger than 2 years and followed through to 12 years of age. These included: early onset overweight (10.9%), late onset overweight (5.2%), and never overweight (83.9%) (Li et al. 2007).

A similar study by Pryor et al. in 1678 children 6–12 years identified two main overweight trajectories (early and late onset) and identified the several associated risk factors. Risk factors common to both groups included parental overweight, history of preschool overweight, and large for gestational age. Characteristics specific to the early onset group included short nighttime sleep duration, maternal overprotection, and immigrant status (Pryor et al. 2015).

Other predictors of overweight that have been widely reported include diet and activity patterns, television and technology time, poverty and food insecurity, harsh parenting styles, and peer victimization (bullying) (Foster et al. 2015).

Research is active in pediatric obesity-overweight prevention, reviewed in more detail in Chapter 21, Obesity and Metabolic Conditions:

Key Points in Maintenance of Healthy Weight in Children

- Obesity is programmed early, both prenatally and in infancy.
- Obesity tracks through childhood and adolescence into adult life.
- Overweight and obesity puts children and adolescents at risk for serious physical and psychological comorbidities.
- Breastfeeding is protective against overweight.
- Early and repeated intervention in well visits is important for prevention of overweight.
- Nutrition counseling should be accompanied by family education on healthy lifestyle measures starting before the age of 2 years.

Foundations of Nutrition

The following section will give an overview of carbohydrates, fats, and proteins with an eye to shaping a healthy diet pattern. The breakdown of categories is somewhat artificial, as relatively few foods contain only one nutritional component. In addition, understanding nutrition building blocks and regulating portion size, as well as balancing the proportions of nutrients, is important. The current guidelines from the USDA reflect a recommended ratio of 50%–60% carbohydrates, 25%–30% protein, and 25%–30% healthy fats at each meal (Table 3.1).

Combining whole foods in healthy proportions is the key to healthy nutrition.

Carbohydrates

Carbohydrates make up a relatively high percent of the pediatric diet and are needed to provide ready fuel to support growth and physical activity. The quality of carbohydrates is important and is determined in part by the fiber content of the food. The proportion of fiber determines the effects of the carbohydrate on blood glucose. This effect is often compared using the glycemic index, a measure of the rise in blood glucose caused by the food in a 2-hour time frame as compared to a control of 50 grams

Table 3.1 USDA Guidelines of Ratio and Proportions Per Meal

Building Block	Proportion
Carbohydrates	50%–60%
Protein	25%–30%
Healthy Fats	25%–35%
*Saturated Fats	10%

*Fat percentages may be higher for children 12 months and younger depending on growth velocity and weight (USDA Centre for Nutrition Policy and Promotion 2010).

of pure glucose. Glycemic load is another measurement used to categorize carbohydrate quality. Glycemic load is defined as the glycemic index multiplied by grams of available carbohydrate divided by 100 (GL = GI × g/100). Both glycemic index and glycemic load estimate the impact of carbohydrates on insulin levels, insulin sensitivity, and inflammatory markers. Large, longitudinal population surveys have shown that diets high in glycemic index/glycemic load (sugary, lower fiber) are associated with a significantly higher risk of type-2 diabetes in adults (Bhupathiraju et al. 2014), and increasingly children, especially as they enter puberty (Reinehr 2013).

A priority in pediatric nutrition after infancy and weaning is to focus on high quality, nutritious carbohydrates. This would include foods with a denser carbohydrate structure that would allow slower absorption and slower rise in postprandial glucose levels. Good examples of this type of carbohydrate include steel cut oatmeal, minimally processed or unprocessed whole grain breads, quinoa, rye, barley, vegetables, whole fruits (not fruit juice), and beans. The distinction between whole fruit and fruit juice is especially important for young children who are frequently given fruit juice. The difference is made by the fiber content found in the whole fruit, which slows the rise of blood glucose. For example, an orange has been estimated to have twice as much fiber and half as much sugar as a glass of fresh squeezed orange juice.

Conversely, foods such as baked potatoes, corn flakes, processed white bread, pastries, soda, and sugary snacks are less dense carbohydrates and therefore rapidly converted to glucose, causing a jump in postprandial glucose levels and triggering insulin release. These types of foods are high on the glycemic index and associated with increased inflammation and risk of cardiovascular disease, type-2 diabetes and other serious chronic illnesses (Chiu et al. 2011).

More on Fiber and Inflammation

An important emerging topic in nutrition research involves the influence of fiber on inflammatory diseases. Dietary fiber is metabolized by gut microbes into short-chain fatty acids, which attenuate the inflammatory pathways in macrophages, and in dendritic cells, and promote the development of regulatory T cells along with their actions related to maintaining the integrity of gut epithelium (Velasquez-Manoff 2015).

For example, recent animal studies have shown that high dietary fiber can regulate the lungs' immune system, resulting in reduction of airway inflammation (Huffnagle 2014).

These studies add to the growing body of research linking the gut microbiome to a variety of inflammatory-driven conditions, and reinforce the importance of fiber in the diet from an early age.

Fructose

Fructose is a carbohydrate that has been shown to have properties of special concern because of its selective hepatic metabolism. Fructose is frequently consumed by children in foods and beverages containing high fructose corn syrup; in fact, it has been estimated that children and adolescents are among those ingesting as much as 30% of their diet as fructose and other added non-nutritive sugars. Beverages containing high fructose corn syrup have been identified as an independent risk factor for metabolic syndrome due to the accumulation of fat in the liver associated with nonalcoholic fatty liver disease (Basaranoglu et al. 2013; Sellmann et al. 2015).

Examples of high fructose foods include:

- Sweetened soda
- Fruit juice and fruit juice blends
- Many types of breakfast cereals
- Yogurt with fruit flavor
- Salad dressings/condiments
- Breads, pastries, and baked goods
- Candy
- Nutrition and energy bars
- Meal supplement drinks
- Agave syrup

Sweet Beverages

Sugar-sweetened and artificially sweetened beverages have both been identified with health issues in pediatrics, including overweight and obesity (Hu 2013; Green and Murphy 2012).

Both sweetened and artificially sweetened sodas should be avoided in children. Research from large population surveys also identifies a link between high fructose corn syrup and asthma in children. This may be related to the development of advanced glycation end products (DeChristopher, Uribarri, and Tucker 2015), with receptor of advanced glycation end products (RAGE) acting as a mediator of asthma linked to oxidative stress and upregulation of inflammation (Uribarri et al. 2015; Schmidt 2015).

Dental caries have also been conclusively linked to sugar-sweetened beverage consumption (soda, fruit juice and fruit drinks, sports and energy drinks, sweetened teas and coffee drinks). Patterns of sugar-sweetened beverage intake in infancy have been closely correlated with its intake in later childhood, suggesting that parent and pediatricians should focus on developing behaviors that restrict consumption of these non-nutritive drinks in children from an early age (Park et al. 2014).

In general the American Academy of Pediatrics endorses clean fresh water and non-sweetened, fortified reduced fat milk as preferred beverages, unless milk intolerance is present (Patel and Ritchie 2013).

It is important that children are introduced to a wide variety of high quality carbohydrate foods that are rich in fiber and low in sugar, and to healthy low sugar beverages early in life, so that they may have the opportunity to become used to these flavors and textures as part of a healthy dietary pattern (Miller and Cassady 2015).

Fats

Review of the 2015 U.S. Dietary Guidelines: Lifting the Ban on Total Dietary Fat (Mozaffarian and Ludwig 2015) reviews the wide array of functions fats perform in the body. Most foods actually contain a combination of fats. As a group they provide efficient energy; are integral to cell membrane structure and function; critical to brain and nervous system health; needed for fat-soluble vitamins (A, D, E, and K); act as regulators and components of many hormones; help regulate body temperature; support internal organs; and act as immune system modulators.

When considering the different types of fats, one way to differentiate is through the concept that form dictates function.

Saturated fat is solid at room temperature. Common sources are red meat, dairy fat, and tropical oils. Saturated fat is primarily an energy source and has been shown to raise serum cholesterol. It is no longer considered "forbidden," but should be used in moderation. The term "saturated" refers to a lack of double bonds in a fatty acid chain, making the molecule stiffer and less susceptible to oxidation.

Monounsaturated fats are liquid at room temperature but thicken when refrigerated. They contain one double bond in their long fatty acid carbon chains, thus the term "monounsaturated." Oleic acid is the most common type of monounsaturated fat. Olive oil and canola oil are common sources of oleic acid. The American Heart Association identifies foods high in monounsaturated fats include: olive and canola oil, peanut oil, safflower oil, avocado and many types of seeds and nuts.

Polyunsaturated fats are liquid at room temperature. Common examples of polyunsaturated fatty acids are the omega-3 and omega-6 fatty acids. These are considered essential fatty acids (not produced by the body) and contain two or more double bonds in their long fatty acid carbon chains. The omega-3 and -6 fatty acids are commonly found in the cell membrane where both add structural flexibility. Broadly omega-3 fatty acids are considered anti-inflammatory and omega-6 pro-inflammatory, although both serve important physiologic functions. Fatty acids in the diet have a substantial impact on: cell signaling, gene expression, circulating inflammatory markers, and adipose tissue synthesis among other things. They are discussed in more detail in Chapter 4, Key Dietary Supplements.

According to the American Heart Association, foods high in polyunsaturated fats include those rich in omega-3 fatty acids such as oily fish (salmon, mackerel, sardines, and others), soybean oil, corn oil, sunflower oil, nuts and seeds—especially walnuts and sunflower seeds, tofu, and soybeans. Another type of polyunsaturated omega-3 fatty acid is alpha-linoleic acid, found in especially high concentration in flax seeds.

Trans fatty acid: Small amounts of trans fats do occur naturally in beef and some dairy foods (ruminant trans fats), but an estimated 80% of trans fats in the U.S. diet comes from artificially produced, partially hydrogenated vegetable oil modified for the purpose of increasing commercial food shelf life (Ganguly and Pierce 2015).

Trans fats are linked to coronary artery disease, increase in total cholesterol, and lowering of HDL cholesterol. Foods containing trans fats include margarine, icing, many commercial baked goods, and many brands of potato chips (Arcand et al. 2014).

Mandatory declaration of trans fat content was instituted in the U.S. and Canada in 2003, yet careful reading of food labels is important regarding trans fats because legally foods can be labeled as "no trans fats"—if only one serving is eaten. If more than one serving is eaten, the trans fats have the potential to deliver an unhealthy dose. This type of marketing is confusing to consumers and skirts the intent of healthy recommendations. Efforts for reform and increased awareness in this area are active internationally (Hendry et al. 2015).

Diets proportionately rich in monounsaturated (such as olive oil) and polyunsaturated fats (such as omega-3 fatty acids) have been associated with reduced overall mortality, improved cardiovascular health, and reduction in obesity and its associated comorbidities. Translated into pediatric practice, a child whose primary dietary fat sources reflect a balance of "healthy fats" and minimal intake of unhealthy fats (such as artificially produced trans fats) will reduce risk for future cardiovascular and other serious chronic health conditions.

Protein

The building blocks of proteins are amino acids, which catalyze biochemical reactions as enzymes and serve as transport and storage sources for molecules. Protein is needed for manufacture of all cell membranes, needed to build healthy muscle cells, cartilage, and collagen, nails, and bone. According to the 2010 USDA Dietary Guidelines for Americans 2010 report, the typical American diet generally contains adequate protein for healthy children (USDA Centre for Nutrition Policy and Promotion 2013). Common sources of protein are meats, poultry, seafood, beans and other legumes, nuts, dairy, eggs, soy beans, tofu and other soy foods, broccoli, and quinoa.

From Nutrition Building Blocks to a Healthy Diet

The next challenge for the clinician is helping the family organize the basic building blocks of nutrition into a healthy nutritional pattern over the various stages of the child's growth and development. Emerging research on the benefits of the Mediterranean diet pattern and prudent diets can help significantly simplify this challenge (if healthy food is available to the family). Trends in improving coverage of fresh and nutritious foods with state and federal food programs such as SNAP, WIC, and the NSLP are important steps in providing significant health benefits to millions of children in the U.S. through access to whole healthy foods.

- **SNAP** (Supplemental Nutrition Assistance Program) (http://www.fns.usda.gov/snap/supplemental-nutrition-assistance-program-snap)
- **WIC** (Women, Infants, and Children) (http://www.fns.usda.gov/wic/wic-benefits-and-services)
- **NSLP** (National School Lunch Program) (http://www.fns.usda.gov/nslp/national-school-lunch-program)

Both the Mediterranean and prudent diet patterns include a plant-based emphasis, rich in a variety of fruits and vegetables, legumes, whole grains, nuts, seeds, berries, and lean protein with an emphasis on fish. The Mediterranean diet emphasizes olive oil as main cooking oil, and suggests dairy in moderation. Soy can be included as a protein option for vegetarians. Low intake of red meat and low- to no intake of processed foods, especially processed meats, are a common denominator of both dietary patterns (Jacobs and Tapsell 2015).

Accruing research on the benefits of the Mediterranean diet (Tognon et al. 2014) and prudent diet pattern in children (Kaikkonen, Mikkila, and Raitakari 2014) show them to have an important inverse association with overweight and obesity and a protective effect against inflammatory-mediated chronic conditions such as cardiovascular disease and type-2 diabetes. Other studies have shown reduction in allergy and asthma symptoms in school children adhering to a Mediterranean diet pattern (Arvaniti et al. 2011; Garcia-Marcos et al. 2013).

This beauty of the healthy whole food approach is that it includes a wide range of protective phytonutrients in their natural forms. Whole food is amazingly complex and it has proven extremely difficult to study the isolated active elements of many foods, especially in children.

More on Phytonutrients

Flavonoids are part of the polyphenol family with powerful health effects. These are found in tea, berries, chocolate, cinnamon, red wine, and grapes among other foods. More than 4000 different flavonoids have been identified and associated with significant health benefits. Research is active around their potential to affect epigenetic cellular mechanisms; for example, to modulate DNA methylation and histone acetylation important in chronic illness and in cancer (Busch et al. 2015).

Flavanols are a subset of the flavonoid family associated with improvement in lipid profiles and reduction in platelet aggregation. Catechins found in green tea are a good example of this category, especially epigallocatechin-gallate or EGCG, a potent antioxidant that has been shown in multiple studies to have protective cardiovascular and anticancer actions (Wang, Tang, and Wang 2015).

Green tea is also under study for its antibacterial effect in oral health, and for antiviral properties, which have been shown to be protective against influenza (Narotzki et al. 2012; Kim, Quon, and Kim 2014).

Few studies on green tea exist in children, although children in many cultures drink it daily (ideally in decaffeinated form). Of note, as reviewed in Natural Standards Comprehensive Database, due to caffeine content green tea should be avoided in pregnant or nursing mothers and in children or adults taking anti-arrhythmics, benzodiazepines, on antidepressants such as monoamine oxidase inhibitors, or mood stabilizers such as lithium, cough or cold preparations containing caffeine, or any cardiac or other drug such as theophylline that may be potentiated by caffeine. Other cautions include patients on quinolone antibiotics, beta-lactam antibiotics, clozapine, birth control pills, warfarin, and chemotherapy—although reported side effects are rare.

Soy Isoflavones

A second subset of flavonoids with particular relevance to prepubescent girls are the soy isoflavones: genistein, daidzein, and glycitein found in soy beans and whole soy products. These have weak estrogenic properties thought to interact with estrogen receptors. Studies have shown that intake of whole soy foods in prepubertal girls has been correlated with reduction in breast cancer prevalence later in life (Warri et al. 2008; Messina and Hilakivi-Clarke 2009).

The isoflavones have also been associated with reduction in low density lipoprotein cholesterol, fasting glucose levels and proinflammatory cytokines with potential for important immunomodulatory effects (Ponzo et al. 2015; Tezuka and Imai 2015).

Other "superfoods" used as spices and seasonings that can be added to a healthy whole food diet and which have shown benefit in the pediatric population include curcumin (covered in Chapter 9, Botanicals), which is under active study for its powerful anti-inflammatory and antioxidant effects in inflammatory bowel disease (Vecchi Brumatti et al. 2014; Suskind et al. 2013) and in cancer treatment (Wolff et al. 2012; Feitelson et al. 2015).

Dietary gaps can be filled with selected supplements on an individualized basis. A

Table 3.2 BMI Categories in Children

Weight Status Category	Percentile Range
Underweight	Less than the 5th percentile
Healthy weight	5th percentile to less than the 85th percentile
Overweight	85th to less than the 95th percentile
Obese	Equal to or greater than the 95th percentile

selection of some of the more commonly used dietary supplements such as omega-3 fatty acids, probiotics, and vitamin D are reviewed in the following chapter.

Nutrition: Practical Integration

Even if a registered dietician or health coach is part of the team reinforcing nutrition education, it is important for clinicians to have a solid foundation in nutrition basics. An organized approach to discussion of the subject can be very useful in the clinical setting. One approach is outlined below.

1. Establish an early baseline for body-mass-index, follow regularly, and intervene early with concerns. The U.S. Centers for Disease Control and Prevention has a useful body-mass-index calculator for children aged 2–19 years (Table 3.2). Many electronic medical record programs now have built in graphing (Centers for Disease Control and Prevention [a]).
2. Obtain a thorough nutritional history. This also provides useful insight into the day-to-day functioning of the family. It can be very helpful to ask what the patient eats on a typical day, whether mealtimes are organized and enjoyable, or stressful. Other important information is who is generally responsible for shopping and cooking, and what positive behaviors are already in place that can be maximized.
3. Review the proper nutrient proportions (carbohydrates 50%–60%, protein 25%–30%, healthy fats 25%–35% with saturated fats ~10%).* These apply generally in healthy children with no special medical conditions such as malabsorption or other serious illnesses. This pattern should be generally followed at each meal and snack to maintain a healthy balance of nutrients and a steady energy supply throughout the day.
4. Relate an estimate of average calories needs per day based on age and gender (Tables 3.3 and 3.4).

Practical Integration of Nutrition into Pediatric Practice

- Understand the child's nutritional baseline and BMI for age.
- Review the child's average daily calorie needs.
- Blend the nutritional building blocks (carbohydrates, fiber, fats, proteins).
- Distribute the approximate calories proportionally throughout the day.
- Limit processed foods and sugary beverages. Discourage use of food as a reward.
- Emphasize the Mediterranean or prudent diet patterns to simplify meal planning.

Additional caveats include the following.

* Source: 2010 Dietary Guidelines for Americans: http://www.cnpp.usda.gov/dietaryguidelines.htm

Table 3.3 Daily Energy Needs (in Calories Per Day) for Boys

Boys	Not Active	Somewhat Active	Very Active
2–3 years	1000–1200	1000–1400	1000–1400
4–8 years	1200–1400	1400–1600	1600–2000
9–13 years	1600–2000	2400–2800	2800–3200
14–18 years	2000–2400	2400–2800	2800–3200

Sources: United States Department of Agriculture. 2010. "Dietary Guidelines for Americans." http://www.cnpp.usda.gov/ DietaryGuidelines.htm; National Institutes of Health. 2010. "Parent Tips: Calories Needed Each Day." http://www.nhlbi.nih.gov/health/public/heart/obesity/wecan/downloads/calreqtips.pdf

Table 3.4 Daily Energy Needs (in Calories Per Day) for Girls

Girls	Not Active	Somewhat Active	Very Active
2–3 years	1000	1000–1200	1000–1400
4–8 years	1200–1600	1600–2000	1400–1800
9–13 years	1400–1600	1600–2000	1800–2200
14–18 years	1800	2000	2400

Sources: United States Department of Agriculture. 2010. "Dietary Guidelines for Americans." http://www.cnpp.usda.gov/ DietaryGuidelines.htm; National Institutes of Health. 2010. "Parent Tips: Calories Needed Each Day." http://www.nhlbi.nih.gov/health/public/heart/obesity/wecan/downloads/calreqtips.pdf

Food Allergy and Sensitivity

Food allergy and food sensitivity can be expressed through a wide range of clinical manifestations. In the most serious form, anaphylaxis might be the first manifestation of allergy, while food sensitivity can present as variably as abdominal complaints or subtle behavior changes, for example in a child with IBS or ADHD respectively. Data from large population studies shows that the prevalence of food allergy has been steadily increasing in children in the U.S. and other developed countries (Platts-Mills 2015).

According to the U.S. CDC an estimated 3.9% of children under 18 years old have a reported food allergy, an increase of 18% over the 10-year period between 1997 and 2006 in children of all ages (Branum and Lukacs 2009). The 2011 Guidelines for the Diagnosis and Management of Food Allergy in the United States: Report of the National Institute of Allergy and Infectious Disease (NIAID) reinforce several important points in pediatrics and provide a comprehensive road map to immunoglobulin E (IgE)-mediated food reactions (Boyce et al. 2011).

One of the most important is that tests for food-specific IgE can assist in diagnosis, but should not be relied on as the only method of diagnosis due to risk of false positive or false negative result. Medically monitored food challenge is currently the most definitive test for food allergy. The report also notes that large panel IgE testing can also be misleading, and recommendation is for targeted testing based on clinical symptoms. Several diagnostic tests are specifically *not* recommended, including food IgG/IgG4, applied kinesiology, provocation neutralization, hair analysis, and electrodermal testing (Burks et al. 2011).

The report also notes that children with moderate to severe atopic dermatitis, and children younger than 5 years old, should be considered for food allergy evaluation for milk, egg, peanut, wheat, and soy, if at least one of the following caveats are present: atopic dermatitis persists after optimal medical management or reliable history of reaction to a specific food immediately after ingestion.

Milk, eggs, peanuts, tree nuts, fish, shellfish, soy, and wheat are the eight foods that have been reported to account for the vast majority (>90%), of allergic reactions. In children milk, soy, egg, wheat and peanut account for more than 80% of all reactions (Ramesh 2008).

It is estimated that approximately 85% of children with IgE-mediated allergies to milk, soy, egg, and wheat outgrow their sensitivity by 3 years of age. Outgrowing peanut allergy is far less common. Research is active in the mission of finding safe approaches to sensitize patients with peanut allergy (Ramesh 2008).

Food Allergy and Asthma

Children with true food allergy are more than twice as likely to have asthma and other allergies. This is important to remember because children with the dual symptoms of asthma and food allergy are at higher risk of anaphylactic shock and possible death. Auto-injectable epinephrine pens should be prescribed for children at risk for severe reaction and be available at home, school, and throughout all other activities (Bock, Munoz-Furlong, and Sampson 2007).

Diagnosis

Diagnosis of food allergy can be challenging. Accurate history and a symptom diary can be very helpful in less severe cases; for example, to record reports of oral swelling or tingling or redness, urticaria, respiratory symptoms such as hoarseness, tightness of the throat or wheezing after food ingestion. Lab tests typically include allergy skin prick tests or food-specific serum immunoglobulin E (IgE) testing, although it is important to realize that these tests alone do not diagnose an allergy, or represent the potential severity of an allergy as noted above. They also do not provide the food dose that might be a trigger. If a history of anaphylaxis is present, testing for food-specific IgE is the recommended approach. Oral food challenges are a third diagnostic approach. Any testing for food allergy in children must be done under closely supervised conditions in a setting where full pediatric specific emergency care can be delivered if needed (Pansare and Kamat 2010; Sicherer et al. 2010). Peanut allergy has increased in prevalence over the past 10–15 years in many developed countries and now affects an estimated 1%–3% of children (Dyer et al. 2015; Wood and Sampson 2014).

Important work is ongoing in the development of allergy prevention guidelines through collaboration between leading organizations (Fleischer et al. 2015) following encouraging results from the Learning Early About Peanut Allergy (LEAP) study, a randomized controlled trial in infants 4–11 months with severe eczema, egg allergy, or both. In the study, early introduction of peanuts compared to avoidance until 60 months of age showed significant reduction in the development of peanut allergy in the study population (Du Toit et al. 2015).

Although this approach has shown promise in a closely supervised, randomized controlled trial, several significant questions remain to be answered, including: varying doses of peanut protein, length of treatment necessary to achieve effect or the potential risks of intermittent consumption or early discontinuation of the oral sensitization regimen (Fleischer et al. 2015).

Complementary Approaches to Peanut Allergy

Interest in a Chinese herbal preparation containing a blend of nine herbs that has shown efficacy in treatment in animal models of peanut allergy is high. It is under study as herbal formula 2 (FAHF-2) that appears to suppress histamine and T-helper cell (TH2) release and upregulate T-helper cells (TH1) action. A small double-blind, dose-escalation phase 1 study showed good safety and efficacy. Further human studies are underway (Li and Brown 2009).

Eosinophilic Esophagitis

Eosinophilic esophagitis, a chronic T-helper cell 2–mediated disease of the esophagus distinguished by esophageal eosinophilic infiltration, is another atopic condition seen in both children and adults. Tissue remodeling leads to the physical hallmarks of dysphagia, food impaction, and gastroesophageal reflux in adults. Symptoms in children can be more variable depending on age and can include irritability, vomiting, feeding problems, and abdominal pain. Patients with eosinophilic esophagitis often have other allergic and atopic conditions including allergic rhinitis, asthma, eczema, and hypersensitivity to various foods. Etiology in children seems to be food-driven antigen in origin. Milk, egg, wheat, and soy have been identified as the four main triggers of childhood eosinophilic esophagitis, with milk being the leading trigger (Arias et al. 2014).

Studies of a targeted elimination diet in children have shown good efficacy (Straumann et al. 2012), and an empiric elimination diet omitting milk, egg, soy, wheat, peanuts, tree nuts, fish, and shellfish has been shown to eliminate symptoms and tissue infiltration in 74% of pediatric patients with the diagnosis (Kagalwalla et al. 2006). The etiology of the condition is an area of active study, thought to be a combination of genetic susceptibility and environmental triggers (Benitez et al. 2015).

Emerging research suggests that eosinophilic esophagitis is accompanied by a distinctive shift in the esophageal microbiome, consistent with microbiome shifts seen in other diseases such as IBD and obesity (Harris et al. 2015; Benitez et al. 2015).

Celiac Disease and Gluten Sensitivity

Immunologic Non-IgE-mediated Disease

Prevalence of celiac disease is increasing, and is now estimated to affect 1%–3% of the Western population. Although a food-related condition, celiac disease differs from food allergies in that it is related to human leukocyte antigen (HLA) genotype. Diagnosis can be made through well-validated testing such as endomysial antibodies, (EMA-IgA) or small bowel biopsy (Rubio-Tapia et al. 2012).

Adoption of a strict gluten-free diet is the treatment of celiac disease. Conversely nonceliac gluten sensitivity remains a controversial topic with a less clear treatment approach, which can be challenging for both patient and practitioner (Branchi et al. 2015).

Elimination Diet

In cases of food allergy or sensitivity, elimination diet can be a useful first-line approach to narrow the suspect list of food triggers and has potential as a helpful clinical tool when skin prick testing or IgE testing are inconclusive. In more complex cases, referral to an experienced allergist can be helpful in evaluating the potential benefit of an elimination diet trial. Elimination diet requires significant attention and commitment on the part of the family to be sure to avoid possible exposure by hidden ingredients or foods that may have been cross-contaminated in processing. Another important consideration in children is that if multiple food elimination is undertaken, a careful and organized reintroduction of foods is done to confirm findings and avoid unnecessary dietary restriction.

There are no hard and fast rules to the elimination diet, which can range from elimination of one substance to a whole food group. The timetable can also be variable (Boyce et al. 2011).

One approach is with the six food elimination diet (cow's milk, soy, wheat, egg, peanuts and tree nuts, and seafood), with close attention to nutrition labels for packaged foods. An elimination diary is used to track symptoms including gut-related, condition-specific, and lifestyle factors such as sleep, energy level, and behavior changes. Foods can be reintroduced after 2 weeks. One food at a time is given every 3 days, with continued use of the diary to record symptoms. If the food is tolerated, move on to introduction of the next food. Ideally if a food is tolerated, after its 3-day trial the child should still wait until the full trial is complete before they start eating it again. This will allow each food to be tested individually.

Environmental Toxins

Environmental toxicants are a real concern in the food and beverage supply for children. Significant classes of toxicants include the endocrine-disrupting chemicals, especially pesticides, and chemicals used in the production of plastics such as bisphenol A and the various phthalates. These topics are covered in detail in Chapter 8, Environmental Health.

References

American Academy of Pediatrics, Section on Breastfeeding. 2012. "Breastfeeding and the use of human milk." *Pediatrics* 129(3): e827–41. doi: 10.1542/peds.2011-3552.

Arcand, J., M. J. Scourboutakos, J. T. Au, and M. R. L'Abbe. 2014. "Trans Fatty acids in the Canadian food supply: an updated analysis." *Am J Clin Nutr* 100(4): 1116–23. doi: 10.3945/ajcn.114.088732.

Arias, A., J. Gonzalez-Cervera, J. M. Tenias, and A. J. Lucendo. 2014. "Efficacy of dietary interventions for inducing histologic remission in patients with eosinophilic esophagitis: a systematic review and meta-analysis." *Gastroenterology* 146(7): 1639–48. doi: 10.1053/j.gastro.2014.02.006.

Arvaniti, F., K. N. Priftis, A. Papadimitriou, M. Papadopoulos, E. Roma, M. Kapsokefalou, M. B. Anthracopoulos, and D. B. Panagiotakos. 2011. "Adherence to the Mediterranean type of diet is associated with lower prevalence of asthma symptoms, among 10–12 years old children: the PANACEA study." *Pediatr Allergy Immunol* 22(3): 283–9. doi: 10.1111/j.1399-3038.2010.01113.x.

Basaranoglu, M., G. Basaranoglu, T. Sabuncu, and H. Senturk. 2013. "Fructose as a key player in the development of fatty liver disease." *World J Gastroenterol* 19(8): 1166–72. doi: 10.3748/wjg.v19.i8.1166.

Benitez, A. J., C. Hoffmann, A. B. Muir, K. K. Dods, J. M. Spergel, F. D. Bushman, and M. L. Wang. 2015. "Inflammation-associated microbiota in pediatric eosinophilic esophagitis." *Microbiome* 3: 23. doi: 10.1186/s40168-015-0085-6.

Bhupathiraju, S. N., D. K. Tobias, V. S. Malik, A. Pan, A. Hruby, J. E. Manson, W. C. Willett, and F. B. Hu. 2014. "Glycemic index, glycemic load, and risk of type 2 diabetes: results from 3 large US cohorts and an updated meta-analysis." *Am J Clin Nutr* 100(1): 218–32. doi: 10.3945/ajcn.113.079533.

Bock, S. A., A. Munoz-Furlong, and H. A. Sampson. 2007. "Further fatalities caused by anaphylactic reactions to food, 2001–2006." *J Allergy Clin Immunol* 119(4): 1016–8. doi: 10.1016/j.jaci.2006.12.622.

Boyce, J. A., A. Assa'ad, A. W. Burks, S. M. Jones, H. A. Sampson, R. A. Wood, M. Plaut, S. F. Cooper, M. J. Fenton, S. H. Arshad, S. L. Bahna, L. A. Beck, C. Byrd-Bredbenner, C. A. Camargo, Jr., L. Eichenfield, G. T. Furuta, J. M. Hanifin, C. Jones, M. Kraft, B. D. Levy, P. Lieberman, S. Luccioli, K. M. McCall, L. C. Schneider, R. A. Simon, F. E. Simons, S. J. Teach, B. P. Yawn, and J. M. Schwaninger. 2011. "Guidelines for the diagnosis and management of food allergy in the United States: summary of the NIAID-sponsored expert panel report." *Nutr Res* 31(1): 61–75. doi: 10.1016/j.nutres.2011.01.001.

Branchi, F., I. Aziz, D. Conte, and D. S. Sanders. 2015. "Noncoeliac gluten sensitivity: a diagnostic dilemma." *Curr Opin Clin Nutr Metab Care* doi: 10.1097/MCO.0000000000000207.

Branum, A. M., and S. L. Lukacs. 2009. "Food allergy among children in the United States." *Pediatrics* 124(6): 1549–55. doi: 10.1542/peds.2009-1210.

Britten, P., L. E. Cleveland, K. L. Koegel, K. J. Kuczynski, and S. M. Nickols-Richardson. 2012a. "Impact of typical rather than nutrient-dense food choices in the US Department of Agriculture Food Patterns." *J Acad Nutr Diet* 112(10): 1560–9. doi: 10.1016/j.jand.2012.06.360.

Britten, P., L. E. Cleveland, K. L. Koegel, K. J. Kuczynski, and S. M. Nickols-Richardson. 2012b. "Updated US Department of Agriculture Food Patterns meet goals of the 2010 dietary guidelines." *J Acad Nutr Diet* 112(10): 1648–55. doi: 10.1016/j.jand.2012.05.021.

Burks, A. W., S. M. Jones, J. A. Boyce, S. H. Sicherer, R. A. Wood, A. Assa'ad, and H. A. Sampson. 2011. "NIAID-sponsored 2010 guidelines for managing food allergy: applications in the pediatric population." *Pediatrics* 128(5): 955–65. doi: 10.1542/peds.2011-0539.

Busch, C., M. Burkard, C. Leischner, U. M. Lauer, J. Frank, and S. Venturelli. 2015. "Epigenetic activities of flavonoids in the prevention and treatment of cancer." *Clin Epigenetics* 7(1): 64. doi: 10.1186/s13148-015-0095-z.

Centers for Disease Control and Prevention [a]. Adapted from "Healthy Weight: About BMI for Children and Teens." http://www.cdc.gov/healthyweight/assessing/bmi/childrens_bmi/about_childrens_bmi.html.

Centers for Disease Control and Prevention [b]. "BMI Percentile Calculator for Child and Teen."

Chiu, C. J., S. Liu, W. C. Willett, T. M. Wolever, J. C. Brand-Miller, A. W. Barclay, and A. Taylor. 2011. "Informing food choices and health outcomes by use of the dietary glycemic index." *Nutr Rev* 69(4): 231–42. doi: 10.1111/j.1753-4887.2011.00382.x.

DeChristopher, L. R., J. Uribarri, and K. L. Tucker. 2015. "Intakes of apple juice, fruit drinks and soda are associated with prevalent asthma in US children aged 2–9 years." *Public Health Nutr*: 1–8. doi: 10.1017/S1368980015000865.

Devries, S., J. E. Dalen, D. M. Eisenberg, V. Maizes, D. Ornish, A. Prasad, V. Sierpina, A. T. Weil, and W. Willett. 2014. "A deficiency of nutrition education in medical training." *Am J Med* 127(9): 804–6. doi: 10.1016/j.amjmed.2014.04.003.

Dhuper, S., S. Buddhe, and S. Patel. 2013. "Managing cardiovascular risk in overweight children and adolescents." *Paediatr Drugs* 15(3): 181–90. doi: 10.1007/s40272-013-0011-y.

Du Toit, G., G. Roberts, P. H. Sayre, H. T. Bahnson, S. Radulovic, A. F. Santos, H. A. Brough, D. Phippard, M. Basting, M. Feeney, V. Turcanu, M. L. Sever, M. Gomez Lorenzo, M. Plaut,

G. Lack, and Leap Study Team. 2015. "Randomized trial of peanut consumption in infants at risk for peanut allergy." *N Engl J Med* 372(9): 803–13. doi: 10.1056/NEJMoa1414850.

Dyer, A. A., V. Rivkina, D. Perumal, B. M. Smeltzer, B. M. Smith, and R. S. Gupta. 2015. "Epidemiology of childhood peanut allergy." *Allergy Asthma Proc* 36(1): 58–64. doi: 10.2500/aap.2015.36.3819.

Feitelson, M. A., A. Arzumanyan, R. J. Kulathinal, S. W. Blain, R. F. Holcombe, J. Mahajna, M. Marino, M. L. Martinez-Chantar, R. Nawroth, I. Sanchez-Garcia, D. Sharma, N. K. Saxena, N. Singh, P. J. Vlachostergios, S. Guo, K. Honoki, H. Fujii, A. G. Georgakilas, A. Bilsland, A. Amedei, E. Niccolai, A. Amin, S. S. Ashraf, C. S. Boosani, G. Guha, M. R. Ciriolo, K. Aquilano, S. Chen, S. I. Mohammed, A. S. Azmi, D. Bhakta, D. Halicka, W. N. Keith, and S. Nowsheen. 2015. "Sustained proliferation in cancer: Mechanisms and novel therapeutic targets." *Semin Cancer Biol* doi: 10.1016/j.semcancer.2015.02.006.

Fleischer, D. M., S. Sicherer, M. Greenhawt, D. Campbell, E. Chan, A. Muraro, S. Halken, Y. Katz, M. Ebisawa, L. Eichenfield, H. Sampson, G. Lack, G. Du Toit, G. Roberts, H. Bahnson, M. Feeney, J. Hourihane, J. Spergel, M. Young, A. As'aad, K. Allen, S. Prescott, S. Kapur, H. Saito, I. Agache, C. A. Akdis, H. Arshad, K. Beyer, A. Dubois, P. Eigenmann, M. Fernandez-Rivas, K. Grimshaw, K. Hoffman-Sommergruber, A. Host, S. Lau, L. O'Mahony, C. Mills, N. Papadopoulos, C. Venter, N. Agmon-Levin, A. Kessel, R. Antaya, B. Drolet, and L. Rosenwasser. 2015. "Consensus communication on early peanut introduction and the prevention of peanut allergy in high-risk infants." *J Allergy Clin Immunol* doi: 10.1016/j.jaci.2015.06.001.

Foster, B. A., J. Farragher, P. Parker, and E. T. Sosa. 2015. "Treatment Interventions for Early Childhood Obesity: A Systematic Review." *Acad Pediatr* 15(4): 353–61. doi: 10.1016/j.acap.2015.04.037.

Ganguly, R., and G. N. Pierce. 2015. "The toxicity of dietary trans fats." *Food Chem Toxicol* 78: 170–6. doi: 10.1016/j.fct.2015.02.004.

Garcia-Marcos, L., J. A. Castro-Rodriguez, G. Weinmayr, D. B. Panagiotakos, K. N. Priftis, and G. Nagel. 2013. "Influence of Mediterranean diet on asthma in children: a systematic review and meta-analysis." *Pediatr Allergy Immunol* 24(4): 330–8. doi: 10.1111/pai.12071.

Green, E., and C. Murphy. 2012. "Altered processing of sweet taste in the brain of diet soda drinkers." *Physiol Behav* 107(4): 560–7. doi: 10.1016/j.physbeh.2012.05.006.

Handa, D., and R. J. Schanler. 2013. "Role of the pediatrician in breastfeeding management." *Pediatr Clin North Am* 60(1): 1–10. doi: 10.1016/j.pcl.2012.10.004.

Harris J., M. Schwartz, C. Munsell, et al. 2013. Fast Food Facts 2013: Measuring Progress in Nutrition and Marketing to Children and Teens. In *Yale Rudd Center for Food Policy and Obesity*.

Harris, J. K., R. Fang, B. D. Wagner, H. N. Choe, C. J. Kelly, S. Schroeder, W. Moore, M. J. Stevens, A. Yeckes, K. Amsden, A. F. Kagalwalla, A. Zalewski, I. Hirano, N. Gonsalves, L. N. Henry, J. C. Masterson, C. E. Robertson, D. Y. Leung, N. R. Pace, S. J. Ackerman, G. T. Furuta, and S. A. Fillon. 2015. "Esophageal microbiome in eosinophilic esophagitis." *PLoS One* 10(5): e0128346. doi: 10.1371/journal.pone.0128346.

Hendry, V. L., E. Almiron-Roig, P. Monsivais, S. A. Jebb, S. E. Neelon, S. J. Griffin, and D. B. Ogilvie. 2015. "Impact of regulatory interventions to reduce intake of artificial trans-fatty acids: a systematic review." *Am J Public Health* 105(3): e32–42. doi: 10.2105/AJPH.2014.302372.

Hu, F. B. 2013. "Resolved: there is sufficient scientific evidence that decreasing sugar-sweetened beverage consumption will reduce the prevalence of obesity and obesity-related diseases." *Obes Rev* 14(8): 606–19. doi: 10.1111/obr.12040.

Huffnagle, G. B. 2014. "Increase in dietary fiber dampens allergic responses in the lung." *Nat Med* 20(2): 120–1. doi: 10.1038/nm.3472.

Institute of Medicine (IOM). Early Childhood Obesity Prevention Policies. Washington, D.C.: The National Academies Press; 2011.

Jacobs, D. R., Jr., and L. C. Tapsell. 2015. "What an anticardiovascular diet should be in 2015." *Curr Opin Lipidol* 26(4): 270–5. doi: 10.1097/MOL.0000000000000184.

Kagalwalla, A. F., T. A. Sentongo, S. Ritz, T. Hess, S. P. Nelson, K. M. Emerick, H. Melin-Aldana, and B. U. Li. 2006. "Effect of six-food elimination diet on clinical and histologic outcomes in eosinophilic esophagitis." *Clin Gastroenterol Hepatol* 4(9): 1097–102. doi: 10.1016/j.cgh.2006.05.026.

Kaikkonen, J. E., V. Mikkila, and O. T. Raitakari. 2014. "Role of childhood food patterns on adult cardiovascular disease risk." *Curr Atheroscler Rep* 16(10): 443. doi: 10.1007/s11883-014-0443-z.

Kim, H. S., M. J. Quon, and J. A. Kim. 2014. "New insights into the mechanisms of polyphenols beyond antioxidant properties; lessons from the green tea polyphenol, epigallocatechin 3-gallate." *Redox Biol* 2: 187–95. doi: 10.1016/j.redox.2013.12.022.

Kunkel, D. L., J. S. Castonguay, and C. R. Filer. 2015. "Evaluating industry self-regulation of food marketing to children." *Am J Prev Med* 49(2): 181–7. doi: 10.1016/j.amepre.2015.01.027.

Lenders, C. M., D. D. Deen, B. Bistrian, M. S. Edwards, D. L. Seidner, M. M. McMahon, M. Kohlmeier, and N. F. Krebs. 2014. "Residency and specialties training in nutrition: a call for action." *Am J Clin Nutr* 99(5 Suppl): 1174S–83S. doi: 10.3945/ajcn.113.073528.

Li, C., M. I. Goran, H. Kaur, N. Nollen, and J. S. Ahluwalia. 2007. "Developmental trajectories of overweight during childhood: role of early life factors." *Obesity (Silver Spring)* 15(3): 760–71. doi: 10.1038/oby.2007.585.

Li, X. M., and L. Brown. 2009. "Efficacy and mechanisms of action of traditional Chinese medicines for treating asthma and allergy." *J Allergy Clin Immunol* 123(2): 297–306; quiz 307–8. doi: 10.1016/j.jaci.2008.12.026.

Messina, M., and L. Hilakivi-Clarke. 2009. "Early intake appears to be the key to the proposed protective effects of soy intake against breast cancer." *Nutr Cancer* 61(6): 792–8. doi: 10.1080/01635580903285015.

Miller, L. M., and D. L. Cassady. 2015. "The effects of nutrition knowledge on food label use. A review of the literature." *Appetite* 92: 207–16. doi: 10.1016/j.appet.2015.05.029.

Mozaffarian, D., and D. S. Ludwig. 2015. "The 2015 US Dietary Guidelines: lifting the ban on total dietary fat." *JAMA* 313(24): 2421–2. doi: 10.1001/jama.2015.5941.

Narotzki, B., A. Z. Reznick, D. Aizenbud, and Y. Levy. 2012. "Green tea: a promising natural product in oral health." *Arch Oral Biol* 57(5): 429–35. doi: 10.1016/j.archoralbio.2011.11.017.

Ogden, C. L., M. D. Carroll, B. K. Kit, and K. M. Flegal. 2014. "Prevalence of childhood and adult obesity in the United States, 2011–2012." *JAMA* 311(8): 806–14. doi: 10.1001/jama.2014.732.

Pansare, M., and D. Kamat. 2010. "Peanut allergy." *Curr Opin Pediatr* 22(5): 642–6. doi: 10.1097/MOP.0b013e32833d95cb.

Park, S., L. Pan, B. Sherry, and R. Li. 2014. "The association of sugar-sweetened beverage intake during infancy with sugar-sweetened beverage intake at 6 years of age." *Pediatrics* 134(Suppl 1): S56–62. doi: 10.1542/peds.2014-0646J.

Patel, A. I., and L. Ritchie. 2013. "Striving for meaningful policies to reduce sugar-sweetened beverage intake among young children." *Pediatrics* 132(3): 566–8. doi: 10.1542/peds.2013-1799.

Platts-Mills, T. A. 2015. "The allergy epidemics: 1870–2010." *J Allergy Clin Immunol* 136(1): 3–13. doi: 10.1016/j.jaci.2015.03.048.

Ponzo, V., I. Goitre, M. Fadda, R. Gambino, A. De Francesco, L. Soldati, L. Gentile, P. Magistroni, M. Cassader, and S. Bo. 2015. "Dietary flavonoid intake and cardiovascular risk: a population-based cohort study." *J Transl Med* 13: 218. doi: 10.1186/s12967-015-0573-2.

Pryor, L. E., M. Brendgen, R. E. Tremblay, J. B. Pingault, X. Liu, L. Dubois, E. Touchette, B. Falissard, M. Boivin, and S. M. Cote. 2015. "Early risk factors of overweight developmental trajectories during middle childhood." *PLoS One* 10(6): e0131231. doi: 10.1371/journal.pone.0131231.

Ramesh, S. 2008. "Food allergy overview in children." *Clin Rev Allergy Immunol* 34(2): 217–30. doi: 10.1007/s12016-007-8034-1.

Reinehr, T. 2013. "Type 2 diabetes mellitus in children and adolescents." *World J Diabetes* 4(6): 270–81. doi: 10.4239/wjd.v4.i6.270.

Rubio-Tapia, A., J. F. Ludvigsson, T. L. Brantner, J. A. Murray, and J. E. Everhart. 2012. "The prevalence of celiac disease in the United States." *Am J Gastroenterol* 107(10): 1538–44; quiz 1537, 1545. doi: 10.1038/ajg.2012.219.

Schmidt, A. M. 2015. "Soluble RAGEs—Prospects for treating & tracking metabolic and inflammatory disease." *Vascul Pharmacol* doi: 10.1016/j.vph.2015.06.011.

Sellmann, C., J. Priebs, M. Landmann, C. Degen, A. J. Engstler, C. J. Jin, S. Garttner, A. Spruss, O. Huber, and I. Bergheim. 2015. "Diets rich in fructose, fat or fructose and fat alter intestinal barrier function and lead to the development of nonalcoholic fatty liver disease over time." *J Nutr Biochem* doi: 10.1016/j.jnutbio.2015.05.011.

Sicherer, S. H., T. Mahr, Allergy American Academy of Pediatrics Section on, and Immunology. 2010. "Management of food allergy in the school setting." *Pediatrics* 126(6): 1232–9. doi: 10.1542/peds.2010-2575.

Straumann, A., S. S. Aceves, C. Blanchard, M. H. Collins, G. T. Furuta, I. Hirano, A. M. Schoepfer, D. Simon, and H. U. Simon. 2012. "Pediatric and adult eosinophilic esophagitis: similarities and differences." *Allergy* 67(4): 477–90. doi: 10.1111/j.1398-9995.2012.02787.x.

Suskind, D. L., G. Wahbeh, T. Burpee, M. Cohen, D. Christie, and W. Weber. 2013. "Tolerability of curcumin in pediatric inflammatory bowel disease: a forced-dose titration study." *J Pediatr Gastroenterol Nutr* 56(3): 277–9. doi: 10.1097/MPG.0b013e318276977d.

Tezuka, H., and S. Imai. 2015. "Immunomodulatory effects of soybeans and processed soy food compounds." *Recent Pat Food Nutr Agric* 7(2): 92–9.

Tognon, G., A. Hebestreit, A. Lanfer, L. A. Moreno, V. Pala, A. Siani, M. Tornaritis, S. De Henauw, T. Veidebaum, D. Molnar, W. Ahrens, and L. Lissner. 2014. "Mediterranean diet, overweight and body composition in children from eight European countries: cross-sectional and prospective results from the IDEFICS study." *Nutr Metab Cardiovasc Dis* 24(2): 205–13. doi: 10.1016/j.numecd.2013.04.013.

United States Department of Agriculture [USDA] Center for Nutrition Policy and Promotion. "Dietary Guidelines for Americans." Last Modified 2010. http://www.cnpp.usda.gov/DietaryGuidelines.

United States Department of Agriculture [USDA] Center for Nutrition Policy and Promotion. 2013. "USDA Diet Quality of Children Age 2–17 Years as Measured by the Healthy Eating Index–2010." http://www.cnpp.usda.gov/sites/default/files/nutrition_insights_uploads/Insight52.pdf.

Uribarri, J., M. D. Del Castillo, M. P. de la Maza, R. Filip, A. Gugliucci, C. Luevano-Contreras, M. H. Macias-Cervantes, D. H. Markowicz Bastos, A. Medrano, T. Menini, M. Portero-Otin, A. Rojas, G. R. Sampaio, K. Wrobel, K. Wrobel, and M. E. Garay-Sevilla. 2015. "Dietary advanced glycation end products and their role in health and disease." *Adv Nutr* 6(4): 461–73. doi: 10.3945/an.115.008433.

Ustjanauskas, A. E., J. L. Harris, and M. B. Schwartz. 2014. "Food and beverage advertising on children's web sites." *Pediatr Obes* 9(5): 362–72. doi: 10.1111/j.2047-6310.2013.00185.x.

Vecchi Brumatti, L., A. Marcuzzi, P. M. Tricarico, V. Zanin, M. Girardelli, and A. M. Bianco. 2014. "Curcumin and inflammatory bowel disease: potential and limits of innovative treatments." *Molecules* 19(12): 21127–53. doi: 10.3390/molecules191221127.

Velasquez-Manoff, M. 2015. "Gut microbiome: the peacekeepers." *Nature* 518(7540): S3–11. doi: 10.1038/518S3a.

Vickers, A. M., S. Starks-Solis, D. R. Hill, and D. S. Newburg. 2015. "Pasteurized donor human milk maintains microbiological purity for 4 days at 4 degrees C." *J Hum Lact* 31(3): 401–5. doi: 10.1177/0890334415576512.

Wang, J., L. Tang, and J. S. Wang. 2015. "Biomarkers of dietary polyphenols in cancer studies: current evidence and beyond." *Oxid Med Cell Longev* 2015: 732302. doi: 10.1155/2015/732302.

Warri, A., N. M. Saarinen, S. Makela, and L. Hilakivi-Clarke. 2008. "The role of early life genistein exposures in modifying breast cancer risk." *Br J Cancer* 98(9): 1485–93. doi: 10.1038/sj.bjc.6604321.

Weng, S. F., S. A. Redsell, D. Nathan, J. A. Swift, M. Yang, and C. Glazebrook. 2013. "Estimating overweight risk in childhood from predictors during infancy." *Pediatrics* 132(2): e414–21. doi: 10.1542/peds.2012–3858.

Wolff, J. E., R. E. Brown, J. Buryanek, S. Pfister, T. S. Vats, and M. E. Rytting. 2012. "Preliminary experience with personalized and targeted therapy for pediatric brain tumors." *Pediatr Blood Cancer* 59(1): 27–33. doi: 10.1002/pbc.23402.

Wood, R. A., and H. A. Sampson. 2014. "Oral immunotherapy for the treatment of peanut allergy: is it ready for prime time?" *J Allergy Clin Immunol Pract* 2(1): 97–8. doi: 10.1016/j.jaip.2013.11.010.

4 Key Dietary Supplements: Omega-3 Fatty Acids, Vitamin D, and Probiotics

Introduction and Background

Dietary supplements are a multi-billion-dollar industry in the U.S. with more than 29,000 herbal dietary supplements products alone on the market (Tsourounis and Bent 2010).

The 2012 National Health Interview Survey (NHIS) study reported that 17.7% of adults and 4.9% of children in the U.S. use non-vitamin, non-mineral dietary supplements (Clarke et al. 2015), consistent with previous reports. The 2012 NHIS data reiterated higher prevalence seen in children aged 12–17 over those aged 4–11 years, and higher prevalence in children whose parents had more than a high school education (Barnes, Bloom, and Nahin 2008). An estimated 50% of children living with chronic health conditions use complementary therapies, with dietary supplements the most common category of use (Birdee et al. 2010). Use of dietary supplements is also surprisingly high in infancy. A 2011 study by Zhang et al. using data from the FDA and CDC Infant Practices Feeding Study II indicated that approximately 9% of infants were given dietary botanical supplements or teas in the first 12 months of life, including newborns. Mothers who used dietary supplements themselves were more likely to use them in their infants (Zhang, Fein, and Fein 2011). Parents turn to dietary supplements for their children for various reasons, for example a desire to avoid prescription medication, but may not have a full understanding of the product's risks or benefits. A high number of parents also fail to disclose use of natural products in their children to their pediatrician for fear of censure or ridicule (Birdee et al. 2010). An important first step for the clinician is to invite open and respectful conversation about all therapies the child may be receiving in order to focus on the child's safety and avoid unwanted drug–supplement interactions. To this end there are several resources for the clinician's use, noted below. One of the first steps is to have a clear understanding of how dietary supplements are defined and regulated.

The United States Food and Drug Administration (FDA) defines dietary supplements as follows:

"A dietary supplement is a product intended for ingestion that contains a 'dietary ingredient' intended to add further nutritional value to (supplement) the diet. A 'dietary ingredient' may be one, or any combination, of the following substances:

- A vitamin
- A mineral
- An herb or other botanical
- An amino acid

- A dietary substance for use by people to supplement the diet by increasing total dietary intake
- A concentrate, metabolite, constituent, or extract

Dietary supplements may be found in many forms such as tablets, capsules, softgels, gelcaps, liquids, or powders. Some dietary supplements can help ensure that you get an adequate dietary intake of essential nutrients; others may help you reduce your risk of disease." (FDA 2015)

The FDA is responsible for taking action against any adulterated or misbranded dietary supplement product after it reaches the market. (http://www.fda.gov/AboutFDA/Transparency/Basics/ucm195635.htm)

This equates dietary supplements with the standards used for food products, requiring less stringent regulation than for prescription or even over-the-counter medications. The 1994 Dietary Supplement Health and Education Act (DSHEA) added further guidelines, establishing responsibility on the part of the manufacturer to ensure the product information is clearly labeled as a dietary supplement, and has not been adulterated or misbranded (103rd Congress of the United States 1994).

Additionally, products sold as dietary supplements may not claim to treat, prevent, or cure any disease, although it should be noted that products on the market prior to the 1994 DSHEA are exempt even from these guidelines. (http://www.fda.gov/Food/DietarySupplements/)

Manufacturers of dietary supplements must register their facilities with the FDA and report all serious adverse events but are not required to get pre-market approval of their products. Strengthening of FDA safety regulations was introduced in 2007 in the form of Current Good Manufacturing Practices (CGMPs), which mandate that dietary supplements are processed, labeled and packaged in accordance with stricter guidelines (http://www.fda.gov/Food/GuidanceRegulation/CGMP/ucm079496.htm). This is a step forward and consumers should be counseled to look for the GMP seal, but still be aware that this does not imply efficacy or safety. The FDA voluntary reporting system MedWatch is available for reporting concerns and adverse events, a helpful but reactive system. (http://www.fda.gov/Safety/MedWatch/default.htm)

In contrast, products sold in Canada require pre-market approval by Health Canada and are subject to the Natural Health Products Regulations established in 2004. This requires pre-market product license, compliance with specific labeling and packaging requirements and good manufacturing practices, along with evidence supporting safety and efficacy. (http://www.hc-sc.gc.ca/dhp-mps/prodnatur/about-apropos/index-eng.php)

The European Commission has adopted similarly stringent pre-market regulations for natural product labeling and sale. (http://ec.europa.eu/food/safety/labelling_nutrition/claims/index_en.htm)

In reality, dietary supplements should meet the highest safety and efficacy criteria before even being considered for use in the pediatric population, yet reports of adverse events continue to accrue, reminding us of the importance of development of safety standards that specifically consider the pediatric population (Gardiner et al. 2013).

Ultimately it is a joint responsibility between parent and clinician to ensure the safety of the child. Given the high prevalence of dietary supplement use in children, clinicians must be able to counsel patients on potential beneficial or harmful effects, quality control issues, and potential supplement–drug interactions. Useful resources include:

- National Center for Complementary & Integrative Health (NCCIH) formerly NCCAM: https://nccih.nih.gov/health/supplements
- Consumer Lab: http://www.consumerlab.com
- Natural Standard: http://www.naturalstandard.com
- American Botanical Counsel: http://abc.herbalgram.org/site/PageServr

Omega-3 Fatty Acids, Probiotics, and Vitamin D

The 2012 NHIS survey showed that fish oil and probiotics were among the most common non-vitamin, non-mineral supplements used by children. Based on this prevalence, the following material will cover omega-3 fatty acids, selected probiotics, and vitamin D, which has strong supporting evidence for its use in children. Background information and doses provided are guidelines only. Individual patient recommendations will vary. Seven other botanical dietary supplements with growing evidence for pediatric use are reviewed in Chapter 9. These include butterbur, chamomile, curcumin, echinacea, melatonin, peppermint, and St. John's wort.

Omega-3 Fatty Acids

The two main groups of essential fatty acids include the omega-3 and omega-6 fatty acids, both polyunsaturated fats. Essential fatty acids by definition must come from the diet and are not produced in the body. In the broadest terms, omega-3 fatty acids are considered more anti-inflammatory, while omega-6 fatty acids are considered more pro-inflammatory. The balance of omega-3 versus omega-6 in the diet is important because they compete for the same desaturase enzyme, meaning the more pro-inflammatory omega-6 fatty acids consumed, the less ability the body has to make use of the beneficial omega-3 fatty acids present. The typical Western diet contains a high ratio of omega-6 fatty acids and has been associated with higher incidence of cardiovascular disease, cancer, inflammatory and autoimmune illness, whereas a lower ratio of omega-6 and a higher ratio of omega-3 fatty acids has been found to have a protective effect (Mozaffarian and Wu 2012).

The primary omega-3 polyunsaturated fatty acids are eicosapentaenoic acid (EPA) (20:5n-3, EPA) and docosahexaenoic acid (DHA) (22:6n-3, DHA). These play a key role in gene expression and metabolic regulation via PPARS, peroxisomal proliferator activated receptors made up of transcription proteins involved in complex metabolic pathways related to immune function, lipid metabolism, and conditions such as obesity and type-2 diabetes (Wahli and Michalik 2012) and have been shown to have a beneficial effect on body weight and insulin resistance (Khan et al. 2014), and lowering of triglycerides (Mozaffarian and Wu 2012). Lower levels of the omega-3 fatty acids have also been correlated with shortened telomeres in adults with cardiovascular disease, a marker of cellular aging (Farzaneh-Far et al. 2010).

Omega-3 Fatty Acids in Children

The omega-3 fatty acids, especially DHA, play an important role in children's health from the earliest stages of development through maternal transfer via the placenta. DHA has been clearly associated with prolongation of gestation beyond 34 weeks, and is integral to development of organs and tissues rich in fatty acids, including the brain, nervous system, retinal membrane synapses, rods, cones, renal cortex, and testes among others. Maternal stores of DHA can reduce 50% during pregnancy and not return to pre-pregnancy levels until 6 months postpartum (Mozurkewich and Klemens 2012).

Maternal Supplementation and Disease Prevention

Studies evaluating improved visual and cognitive outcomes in children who received DHA supplementation in utero are inconclusive, although study size, quality, and confounding variables such as nutrition, social stimulation, medications, and illness play important roles (Makrides et al. 2014).

Maternal DHA supplementation for the modulation of allergic disease is an area showing promise. Studies evaluating the benefit of DHA supplementation show evidence of reduction in the prevalence of eczema/atopic dermatitis, asthma and other allergic conditions through modulation of the T-helper cell type 1 and 2 pathways (De Giuseppe, Roggi, and Cena 2014).

Postpartum

Postpartum DHA is passed from mother to infant in the breast milk. DHA levels in breast milk have been shown to correlate with maternal DHA stores. The current minimum recommended DHA supplement dose for pregnant and lactating women according to the International Society for the Study of Fatty Acids and Lipids is 200 mg per day (Koletzko et al. 2007).

Since 2002, synthetic DHA and ARA (arachidonic acid), extracted with hexane, have become integral ingredients in infant formula. The USDA banned the use of synthetic DHA and ARA in organic baby formula in 2010. Despite significant research interest in this area, claims of improvement in visual, neural, or developmental outcomes in infants receiving DHA supplementation either through breast milk or through formula enhanced with DHA have not been consistently demonstrated. Research in this area remains active (Hoffman, Boettcher, and Diersen-Schade 2009).

Beyond infancy, the omega-3 fatty acids have not been extensively studied in children, although improvement in insulin sensitivity, reduction in triglycerides, and mixed reports of protective benefit in reduction of blood pressure in males have been reported. There are mixed results for their use in weight loss in obese children in small studies (Bonafini et al. 2015).

There is some evidence that physiologic effects of omega-3 fatty acids may be sex specific in children. DHA and EPA have also been shown to have different effects on metabolic markers in children; however, more research is needed to clarify recommendations (Damsgaard et al. 2014).

Low levels of omega-3 fatty acids have been identified in certain mental health conditions. For example, a study examining red blood cell fatty acid profiles in a case-controlled study of depressed adolescents (n = 150) and controls (n = 161) found a reduced omega-3 fatty acid content, especially DHA, in depressed adolescents' red blood cell fatty acid profiles (Pottala et al. 2012).

Large systematic reviews have shown mixed results in omega-3 fatty acid supplementation in children with ADHD, in part due to variability of diagnostic criteria, study design, type and dose of omega-3 fatty acid, and individual variation in baseline red blood cell fatty acid levels (Gillies et al. 2012).

However, several studies have shown benefit, and cumulative evidence support Center for Evidence-Based Medicine level-1 evidence for their use in ADHD (as opposed to children with ADHD and concomitant primary disorders such as learning disorders) at a dose range of 1–2 g daily (with a mix of DHA and EPA). Research continues to be active in this area (Bloch and Mulqueen 2014).

FOOD SOURCES AND SUPPLEMENTS

The highest concentrations of EPA/DHA are found in fish (especially fatty fish such as wild caught salmon, cod, mackerel, tuna, sardines, and herring). Plant sources of omega-3 fatty acids such as alpha-linoleic acid (ALA) are found in lower concentrations and are converted to EPA and DHA in the body, although it is not an efficient process. Some of the best plant-based sources include flax, walnuts, and chia seeds. In reality, some children may not find fish or these plant-based food sources palatable and subsequently fall short of daily nutritional requirements. A wide range of child-friendly omega-3 fatty acid supplements can be found commercially in liquid, softgel, chewable, and capsule forms. Vegetarian supplements are also widely available, harvested from microalgae, which is a plant-based source of marine omega-3 EPA and DHA.

SAFETY AND SIDE EFFECTS

Omega-3 fatty acid supplements are generally well tolerated other than occasional gastrointestinal side effects such as eructation. Adverse effects are rare. Omega-3 fatty acids in high doses may have anti-platelet function (Mozaffarian and Wu 2012).

DOSING

The Institute of Medicine has set an acceptable macronutrient distribution range (AMDR) for total omega-3 fatty acid intake at 0.6–1.2 g per day for ages 1 and up. However, these may be conservative figures. For cardiovascular health, most experts recommend 1–2 g of EPA + DHA per day for adults. For elevated triglycerides, the adult dose is 4 g EPA + DHA per day (Institute of Medicine 2002). Omega-3 supplements (both vegetarian and non-vegetarian) available in the U.S. are relatively free of detectable levels of mercury, polychlorinated biphenyls (PCBs) and organochlorine (OC) pesticides as most are molecularly distilled to remove toxins.

DOSAGE SUMMARY *

- Pregnant and lactating women: at least 200 mg/day of DHA to facilitate fetal brain and nervous system development.
- Infants: ideally DHA is passed to the infant via breast milk.
- Children: 1 year and older 0.6–1.2 g per day.
- Adults: 2–3 g per day; 4 g per day recommended for treatment of hypertriglyceridemia.

---

* Source: http://www.issfal.org/statements/pufa-recommendations/statement-4

Prebiotics and Probiotics and Synbiotics

Probiotics are live microorganisms with immunomodulating effects, while prebiotics are nondigestible carbohydrates that selectively stimulate growth and activity of probiotic bacteria. Oligosaccharides are a primary type of prebiotic compound and are remarkable in that they are resistant to the host's digestive enzymes, yet still susceptible to fermentation by the colonic microbiobes. Synbiotics refer to a combination of pre and probiotics used together (Wasilewski et al. 2015).

Research on the microbiome has increased exponentially over the past decade yet many questions have yet to be answered about the use and efficacy of probiotics, especially in children. Some of the challenges include matching probiotic strain with the condition, dose, and duration of treatment. Three main groups of probiotics typically come from the *Lactobacillus*, *Bifidobacterium*, and *Streptococcus* groups. Some of the most commonly studied strains in children include *Lactobacillus* GG, *Bifidobacterium lactis*, and *Streptococcus thermophiles*. Another frequently studied type is the yeast *Saccharomyces boulardii*. The infant gut appears to be populated with bacteria in utero rather than be sterile at birth as previously believed (Prince et al. 2015, Neu and Rushing 2011). In fact, microbes have been identified in amniotic fluid, placenta, in fetal membranes, umbilical cord blood, and in meconium (West, Jenmalm, and Prescott 2015). Further population of the gastrointestinal tract occurs rapidly and type of bacteria present is determined by type of birth (vaginal versus cesarean delivery), exposure to perinatal antibiotics, colonization of the birth canal, and other factors. By the end of the first month of life many breastfed infants have a predominance of Bifidobacteria present. Rapidly accruing research ties the gut microbiome to defense mechanisms and immune modulation, gut mucosal maintenance and nutrient absorption and defense against bacterial pathogens. Use of probiotics may provide benefit in cases when the ratio of beneficial bacteria is out of balance due to causes such as infection, antibiotic treatment or genetic predisposition to atopic conditions (Thomas et al. 2010).

Conditions in children where probiotics have shown best efficacy include the following.

Acute Infectious Diarrhea

Two Cochrane reviews have concluded safety and efficacy in shortening duration and frequency of diarrhea in children (Allen et al. 2010).

Shortened hospital stay was also noted in one large study group. A variety of probiotic strains demonstrated benefit, including 10–20 billion cells daily of *Lactobacillus* GG. Adverse events were very rare (Bernaola Aponte et al. 2013).

Conversely, data on the use of probiotics in antibiotic-associated diarrhea, including that due to *Clostridium difficile*-associated colitis, remains mixed in large randomized controlled trials, although probiotics are frequently added as adjunct treatment (Issa and Moucari 2014).

Atopic Dermatitis

Large randomized double-blind placebo-controlled studies of oral probiotic in pregnant and in nursing mothers or to infants under 3 months of age have been reliably shown to prevent atopic disease, especially eczema in high-risk infants. Interestingly, mixtures of probiotics were most effective. No positive effect was seen in single strains of either Lactobacilli or Bifidobacteria in these studies (Zuccotti et al. 2015).

No significant benefit has yet been shown for probiotic use in other allergic/atopic conditions such as asthma, wheezing, or allergic rhinitis. Research is ongoing.

Necrotizing Enterocolitis

Probiotic use is becoming increasingly prevalent in the neonatal intensive care unit setting to prevent necrotizing enterocolitis (NEC). A 2104 Cochrane Database Review found conclusive benefit in randomized controlled trials of enteral probiotic supplementation for reduction in incidence of severe NEC and all-cause mortality. Questions about most effective strains, dose, and duration remain to be answered (AlFaleh and Anabrees 2014).

Irritable Bowel Syndrome

Evidence exists in randomized controlled trials for benefit of VSL#3 (a combination of eight probiotic strains: *Bifidobacterium breve, B. longum, B. infantis, Lactobacillus acidophilus, L. plantarum, L. paracasei, L. bulgaricus,* and *Streptococcus thermophilus*), and for *Lactobacillus* GG, although again dose and duration are yet to be fully understood (Sandhu and Paul 2014; Tiequn, Guanqun, and Shuo 2015).

Inflammatory Bowel Disease

Randomized controlled trials to date support the use of probiotics including VSL#3 in induction and maintenance of remission in ulcerative colitis and in treatment of antibiotic-associated pouchitis. No consistent benefits have been seen in the treatment of Crohn's disease (Ghouri et al. 2014).

Psychobiotics: Emerging Science

Research is active in the exploration of the role of probiotics in microbiota-gut-brain axis largely mediated via the vagus nerve. Studies have shown that cortisol, secreted under stress conditions and regulated by the hypothalamic-pituitary-adrenal axis, modulates cytokine secretion and also impacts the type and function of microbes present in the gut. It has also been shown that intestinal bacteria can produce a wide variety of neurohormones such as serotonin and gamma-aminobutyric acid (GABA), which in turn impact the microbiota-gut-brain network. This work will be especially relevant to those suffering from conditions such as irritable bowel syndrome and depression that involve mental and physical symptoms. Research is scant in children in this evolving area (Wasilewski et al. 2015; Mayer, Tillisch, and Gupta 2015).

Safety and Side Effects

Probiotics are generally recognized as safe, although rare cases of sepsis have been reported in immunosuppressed patients, premature infants, patients with short gut syndrome, those with indwelling central catheters, and patients with disease of a cardiac valve (Doron and Snydman 2015).

Dosage

Research on optimal probiotic strains for specific illnesses in both children and adults is active. Guidelines from the World Gastroenterology Organization are a useful starting point, although likely to change as research accrues (Guarner et al. 2012).

Vitamin D

Contrary to its name, vitamin D is actually a fat-soluble steroid hormone with a wide range of physiologic effects. These include key roles in the regulation of blood calcium and phosphorus, bone metabolism, and a range of metabolic, neural, and immune functions. The primary natural source of vitamin D is from direct synthesis in the skin. This occurs when the precursor 7-dehydrocholesterolin in epidermal cells is synthesized to vitamin D3 after exposure to UVB in sunlight. Vitamin D2 (ergocalciferol) is the other natural source, found in plants, and the form most commonly used to fortify foods in the U.S. (Holick 2005).

Once synthesized in the skin or ingested as food or supplement, the vitamins D3 and D2 are transported to the liver, where they are hydroxylated to form calcitriol or 25-hydroxyvitamin D [25(OH)D]. This is the major circulating form of vitamin D. Increased sun exposure or increased intake of vitamin D increases serum concentrations of [25(OH)D], which is also the form tested in the blood test used to check vitamin D status. From the liver the calcitriol [25(OH)D] is sent to the kidney, where a second hydroxylation takes place creating 1 alpha, 25-dihydroxyvitamin D [1,25(OH)2D]—the most potent form of vitamin D. The primary effects of vitamin D are related to the activity of this compound, which has been shown to regulate more than 200 genes (either directly or indirectly) through vitamin D nuclear hormone receptors that exist in many tissues including small intestine, colon, osteoblasts, activated T and B lymphocytes, pancreas beta islet cells, and in organs such as the brain, heart, gonads, prostate, breast, and in muscle (Lee, So, and Thackray 2013; Holick 2008).

Interpretation of optimal blood levels varies. A main point of disagreement between the Institute of Medicine (IOM) and the Endocrine Society guidelines are the cutoff for sufficient levels. IOM guidelines indicate 20 ng/mL as sufficient for most individuals in the general population, while the Endocrine Society recommends 30 ng/mL. The AAP guidelines align most closely with the IOM (Holick et al. 2011; Rosen, Abrams and Committee on 2012; Institute of Medicine 2010) (Table 4.1).

Table 4.1 American Academy of Pediatrics Vitamin D Status Guidelines (in ng/mL)

Status	ng/mL
Severe deficiency	< 5
Mild to moderate deficiency	5–15
Insufficiency	16–20
Sufficiency	21–100
Excess	101–149
Intoxication	> 150

Source: Misra, M., D. Pacaud, A. Petryk, P. F. Collett-Solberg, M. Kappy, Drug, and Society Therapeutics Committee of the Lawson Wilkins Pediatric Endocrine. 2008. "Vitamin D deficiency in children and its management: review of current knowledge and recommendations." *Pediatrics* 122(2): 398–417.

Children in the U.S. have almost universally low vitamin D levels (Mansbach, Ginde, and Camargo 2009), therefore attention to serum levels in children is very important. Vitamin D is recommended for all newborns, with exclusively breastfed infants at highest risk of deficiency, especially if they have increased skin pigmentation or receive little sun exposure. Breast milk generally provides only 25 IU of vitamin D per liter, which is insufficient for an infant if this is the sole source of nutrition. Older infants and toddlers exclusively fed milk substitutes and weaning foods that are not vitamin D fortified are also at an increased risk of vitamin D deficiency. The American Academy of Pediatrics recommends that all infants that are not consuming at least 500 mL (16 ounces) of vitamin D-fortified formula or milk be given a vitamin D supplement of 400 IU/day (Perrine et al. 2010).

Preterm infants are also at high risk of vitamin D deficiency (Misra et al. 2008). Current AAP recommendations include 200–400 IU/day in very low birth weight infants < 1500 g (Abrams and Committee on 2013).

Other conditions with an association to vitamin D deficiency include (Lee, So, and Thackray 2013, Thacher and Clarke 2011, Bener et al. 2014):

- Fat malabsorption syndromes (cystic fibrosis, pancreatitis, celiac disease, short gut syndrome, Crohn's disease).
- Renal disease.
- Obesity.
- Asthma, allergy, atopy.
- Cardiovascular disease.
- Some cancers (breast, colorectal, prostate).
- Vegan or strict vegetarian diet, unless getting enough sun exposure.
- Some antiepileptic drugs (phenytoin, carbamazepine, phenobarbital and others) induce cytochrome P450 and can increase metabolism of vitamin D leading to decreased levels.
- Human immunodeficiency virus/acquired immunodeficiency syndrome.

There also is active research interest in the role of vitamin D in the inflammatory-mediated mechanism of depression (Jo et al. 2015). Severely insufficient vitamin D impairs calcium absorption and can lead to rickets in children and osteomalacia in adults due to poor mineralization of the collagen matrix (Holick 2005). Metabolically, low vitamin D has been correlated with diabetes, prediabetes, metabolic syndrome, and obesity in both children and adults, although causality has not been determined (Rosen, Adams et al. 2012).

Small preliminary studies show that correcting vitamin D improves insulin sensitivity in obese adolescents (Peterson, Tosh, and Belenchia 2014). Ultimately, the importance of maintaining vitamin D levels in the sufficient range seems evident in children of all ages and health conditions given the broad physiologic impact of vitamin D.

FOOD SOURCES OF VITAMIN D

Very few foods are naturally high in vitamin D: cod liver oil, fatty fish such as salmon, tuna, and mackerel are among the best natural sources. Portobello, maitake, and morel and other mushrooms have good amounts. Beef liver, cheese, and egg yolks provide small amounts. In the U.S., fortified foods provide most of the vitamin D in the diet.

For example, almost all of the U.S. milk supply is fortified with 400 IU of vitamin D per quart. All infant formula in the U.S. also contains at least 400 IU/L of vitamin D. Foods made from milk, like cheese and ice cream, are usually not fortified. Vitamin D is frequently added to breakfast cereals and to some brands of orange juice, yogurt, margarine, and soy beverages.

VITAMIN D SUPPLEMENTATION

Data from supplementation studies indicates that vitamin D intakes of at least 800–1000 IU/day are required by adults living in temperate latitudes to achieve serum 25 (OH)D levels of at least 32 ng/mL. Many adults and children require supplementation to reach and maintain optimal levels. Although general guidelines exist, correction and supplementation of vitamin D must be guided by testing of individual blood levels, especially in children to avoid overdose. Follow-up 12 weeks after dose adjustments are made is the recommended timeline. Difficulty reaching or maintaining adequate levels in a child or adolescent should prompt endocrine consult.

Institute of Medicine recommended vitamin D dietary allowance (IU/day) (Institute of Medicine 2010) is:

* 400 IU in infants through 12 months
* 600 IU for ages 1 year to 70 years
* 800 IU for aged 70 years and over

Both vitamin D2 (ergocalciferol) and vitamin D3 (cholecalciferol) are available in supplement form. There is compelling evidence to support vitamin D3 as the more effective form in raising human blood levels (Heaney et al. 2011).

Supplements come in a variety of child-friendly preparations including drops, solution, capsule, tablet, and rapid melt tablet. Many children's vitamins also have 400 or more IU per tablet.

SAFETY AND SIDE EFFECTS

Vitamin D is considered safe at recommended doses. Very high doses have been associated with hypercalcemia, which can cause loss of appetite, nausea and vomiting in some people. Treatment is discontinuation of supplement and follow-up of blood levels until normalized. Serious cases may require hospitalization. (National Institutes of Health, Office of Dietary Supplements: http://ods.od.nih.gov/factsheets/VitaminD-HealthProfessional)

References

103rd Congress of the United States. 1994. Dietary Supplement Health and Education Act.

Abrams, S. A., and Nutrition Committee on. 2013. "Calcium and vitamin D requirements of enterally fed preterm infants." *Pediatrics* 131(5): e1676–83. doi: 10.1542/peds.2013-0420.

AlFaleh, K., and J. Anabrees. 2014. "Probiotics for prevention of necrotizing enterocolitis in preterm infants." *Cochrane Database Syst Rev* 4: CD005496. doi: 10.1002/14651858. CD005496.pub4.

Allen, S. J., E. G. Martinez, G. V. Gregorio, and L. F. Dans. 2010. "Probiotics for treating acute infectious diarrhoea." *Cochrane Database Syst Rev* (11): CD003048. doi: 10.1002/14651858. CD003048.pub3.

Barnes, P. M., B. Bloom, and R. L. Nahin. 2008. "Complementary and alternative medicine use among adults and children: United States, 2007." *Natl Health Stat Report* (12): 1–23.

Bener, A., M. S. Ehlayel, H. Z. Bener, and Q. Hamid. 2014. "The impact of Vitamin D deficiency on asthma, allergic rhinitis and wheezing in children: an emerging public health problem." *J Family Community Med* 21(3): 154–61. doi: 10.4103/2230-8229.142967.

Bernaola Aponte, G., C. A. Bada Mancilla, N. Y. Carreazo, and R. A. Rojas Galarza. 2013. "Probiotics for treating persistent diarrhoea in children." *Cochrane Database Syst Rev* 8: CD007401. doi: 10.1002/14651858.CD007401.pub3.

Birdee, G. S., R. S. Phillips, R. B. Davis, and P. Gardiner. 2010. "Factors associated with pediatric use of complementary and alternative medicine." *Pediatrics* 125(2): 249–56. doi: 10.1542/peds.2009-1406.

Bloch, M. H., and J. Mulqueen. 2014. "Nutritional supplements for the treatment of ADHD." *Child Adolesc Psychiatr Clin N Am* 23(4): 883–97. doi: 10.1016/j.chc.2014.05.002.

Bonafini, S., F. Antoniazzi, C. Maffeis, P. Minuz, and C. Fava. 2015. "Beneficial effects of omega-3 PUFA in children on cardiovascular risk factors during childhood and adolescence." *Prostaglandins Other Lipid Mediat* doi: 10.1016/j.prostaglandins.2015.03.006.

Clarke, T. C., L. I. Black, B. J. Stussman, P. M. Barnes, and R. L. Nahin. 2015. "Trends in the use of complementary health approaches among adults: United States, 2002–2012." *Natl Health Stat Report* (79): 1–16.

Damsgaard, C. T., M. B. Eidner, K. D. Stark, M. F. Hjorth, A. Sjodin, M. R. Andersen, R. Andersen, I. Tetens, A. Astrup, K. F. Michaelsen, and L. Lauritzen. 2014. "Eicosapentaenoic acid and docosahexaenoic acid in whole blood are differentially and sex-specifically associated with cardiometabolic risk markers in 8–11-year-old danish children." *PLoS One* 9 (10): e109368. doi: 10.1371/journal.pone.0109368.

De Giuseppe, R., C. Roggi, and H. Cena. 2014. "n-3 LC-PUFA supplementation: effects on infant and maternal outcomes." *Eur J Nutr* 53 (5): 1147–54. doi: 10.1007/s00394-014-0660-9.

Doron, S., and D. R. Snydman. 2015. "Risk and safety of probiotics." *Clin Infect Dis* 60(Suppl 2): S129–34. doi: 10.1093/cid/civ085.

Farzaneh-Far, R., J. Lin, E. S. Epel, W. S. Harris, E. H. Blackburn, and M. A. Whooley. 2010. "Association of marine omega-3 fatty acid levels with telomeric aging in patients with coronary heart disease." *JAMA* 303 (3): 250–7. doi: 10.1001/jama.2009.2008.

Food and Drug Administration (FDA). 2015. "What is a dietary supplement?" http://www.fda.gov/AboutFDA/Transparency/Basics/ucm195635.htm

Gardiner, P., D. Adams, A. C. Filippelli, H. Nasser, R. Saper, L. White, and S. Vohra. 2013. "A systematic review of the reporting of adverse events associated with medical herb use among children." *Glob Adv Health Med* 2(2): 46–55. doi: 10.7453/gahmj.2012.071.

Ghouri, Y. A., D. M. Richards, E. F. Rahimi, J. T. Krill, K. A. Jelinek, and A. W. DuPont. 2014. "Systematic review of randomized controlled trials of probiotics, prebiotics, and synbiotics in inflammatory bowel disease." *Clin Exp Gastroenterol* 7: 473–87. doi: 10.2147/CEG.S27530.

Gillies, D., JKh Sinn, S. S. Lad, M. J. Leach, and M. J. Ross. 2012. "Polyunsaturated fatty acids (PUFA) for attention deficit hyperactivity disorder (ADHD) in children and adolescents." *Cochrane Database Syst Rev* 7: CD007986. doi: 10.1002/14651858.CD007986.pub2.

Guarner, F., A. G. Khan, J. Garisch, R. Eliakim, A. Gangl, A. Thomson, J. Krabshuis, T. Lemair, P. Kaufmann, J. A. de Paula, R. Fedorak, F. Shanahan, M. E. Sanders, H. Szajewska, B. S. Ramakrishna, T. Karakan, N. Kim, and Organization World Gastroenterology. 2012. "World Gastroenterology Organisation Global Guidelines: probiotics and prebiotics October 2011." *J Clin Gastroenterol* 46(6): 468–81. doi: 10.1097/MCG.0b013e3182549092.

Heaney, R. P., R. R. Recker, J. Grote, R. L. Horst, and L. A. Armas. 2011. "Vitamin D(3) is more potent than vitamin D(2) in humans." *J Clin Endocrinol Metab* 96(3): E447–52. doi: 10.1210/jc.2010-2230.

Hoffman, D. R., J. A. Boettcher, and D. A. Diersen-Schade. 2009. "Toward optimizing vision and cognition in term infants by dietary docosahexaenoic and arachidonic acid supplementation: a review of randomized controlled trials." *Prostaglandins Leukot Essent Fatty Acids* 81(2–3): 151–8. doi: 10.1016/j.plefa.2009.05.003.

Holick, M. F. 2005. "The vitamin D epidemic and its health consequences." *J Nutr* 135(11): 2739S–48S.

Holick, M. F. 2008. "The vitamin D deficiency pandemic and consequences for nonskeletal health: mechanisms of action." *Mol Aspects Med* 29(6): 361–8. doi: 10.1016/j.mam.2008.08.008.

Holick, M. F., N. C. Binkley, H. A. Bischoff-Ferrari, C. M. Gordon, D. A. Hanley, R. P. Heaney, M. H. Murad, C. M. Weaver, and Society Endocrine. 2011. "Evaluation, treatment, and prevention of vitamin D deficiency: an Endocrine Society clinical practice guideline." *J Clin Endocrinol Metab* 96(7): 1911–30. doi: 10.1210/jc.2011-0385.

Institute of Medicine (IOM). Dietary Reference Intakes for Energy, Carbohydrate, Fiber, Fat, Fatty Acids, Cholesterol, Protein, and Amino Acids (Macronutrients). Washington, D.C.: The National Academies Press; 2005.

Institute of Medicine, Food and Nutrition Board. 2010. Dietary Reference Intakes for Calcium and Vitamin D. Washington, D.C.: National Academy Press.

Issa, I., and R. Moucari. 2014. "Probiotics for antibiotic-associated diarrhea: do we have a verdict?" *World J Gastroenterol* 20(47): 17788–95. doi: 10.3748/wjg.v20.i47.17788.

Jo, W. K., Y. Zhang, H. M. Emrich, and D. E. Dietrich. 2015. "Glia in the cytokine-mediated onset of depression: fine tuning the immune response." *Front Cell Neurosci* 9: 268. doi: 10.3389/fncel.2015.00268.

Khan, S. A., A. Ali, S. A. Khan, S. A. Zahran, G. Damanhouri, E. Azhar, and I. Qadri. 2014. "Unraveling the complex relationship triad between lipids, obesity, and inflammation." *Mediators Inflamm* 2014: 502749. doi: 10.1155/2014/502749.

Koletzko, B., I. Cetin, J. T. Brenna. 2007. "Consensus Statement: Dietary fats for pregnant and lactating women." *Brit J Nutr* 98(5): 873–7. doi: 10.1017/S0007114507764747

Lee, J. Y., T. Y. So, and J. Thackray. 2013. "A review on vitamin d deficiency treatment in pediatric patients." *J Pediatr Pharmacol Ther* 18(4): 277–91. doi: 10.5863/1551-6776-18.4.277.

Makrides, M., J. F. Gould, N. R. Gawlik, L. N. Yelland, L. G. Smithers, P. J. Anderson, and R. A. Gibson. 2014. "Four-year follow-up of children born to women in a randomized trial of prenatal DHA supplementation." *JAMA* 311(17): 1802–4. doi: 10.1001/jama.2014.2194.

Mansbach, J. M., A. A. Ginde, and C. A. Camargo, Jr. 2009. "Serum 25-hydroxyvitamin D levels among US children aged 1 to 11 years: do children need more vitamin D?" *Pediatrics* 124(5): 1404–10. doi: 10.1542/peds.2008-2041.

Mayer, E. A., K. Tillisch, and A. Gupta. 2015. "Gut/brain axis and the microbiota." *J Clin Invest* 125(3): 926–38. doi: 10.1172/JCI76304.

Misra, M., D. Pacaud, A. Petryk, P. F. Collett-Solberg, M. Kappy, Drug, and Society Therapeutics Committee of the Lawson Wilkins Pediatric Endocrine. 2008. "Vitamin D deficiency in children and its management: review of current knowledge and recommendations." *Pediatrics* 122(2): 398–417. doi: 10.1542/peds.2007-1894.

Mozaffarian, D., and J. H. Wu. 2012. "(n-3) fatty acids and cardiovascular health: are effects of EPA and DHA shared or complementary?" *J Nutr* 142(3): 614S–625S. doi: 10.3945/jn.111.149633.

Mozurkewich, E. L., and C. Klemens. 2012. "Omega-3 fatty acids and pregnancy: current implications for practice." *Curr Opin Obstet Gynecol* 24(2): 72–7. doi: 10.1097/GCO.0b013e328350fd34.

Neu, J., and J. Rushing. 2011. "Cesarean versus vaginal delivery: long-term infant outcomes and the hygiene hypothesis." *Clin Perinatol* 38(2): 321–31. doi: 10.1016/j.clp.2011.03.008.

Perrine, C.G., A. J. Sharma, M. E. Jefferds, M. K. Serdula, K. S. Scanlon. 2010. "Adherence to vitamin D recommendations among US infants." *Pediatrics* 125(4): 627–32. doi: 10.1542/peds.2009-2571.

Peterson, C. A., A. K. Tosh, and A. M. Belenchia. 2014. "Vitamin D insufficiency and insulin resistance in obese adolescents." *Ther Adv Endocrinol Metab* 5(6): 166–89. doi: 10.1177/2042018814547205.

Pottala, J. V., J. A. Talley, S. W. Churchill, D. A. Lynch, C. von Schacky, and W. S. Harris. 2012. "Red blood cell fatty acids are associated with depression in a case-control study of adolescents." *Prostaglandins Leukot Essent Fatty Acids* 86(4–5): 161–5. doi: 10.1016/j.plefa.2012.03.002.

Prince, A. L., D. M. Chu, M. D. Seferovic, K. M. Antony, J. Ma, and K. M. Aagaard. 2015. "The perinatal microbiome and pregnancy: moving beyond the vaginal microbiome." *Cold Spring Harb Perspect Med* 5(6). doi: 10.1101/cshperspect.a023051.

Rosen, C. J., S. A. Abrams, J. F. Aloia, P. M. Brannon, S. K. Clinton, R. A. Durazo-Arvizu, J. C. Gallagher, R. L. Gallo, G. Jones, C. S. Kovacs, J. E. Manson, S. T. Mayne, A. C. Ross, S. A. Shapses, and C. L. Taylor. 2012. "IOM committee members respond to Endocrine Society vitamin D guideline." *J Clin Endocrinol Metab* 97(4): 1146–52. doi: 10.1210/jc.2011-2218.

Rosen, C. J., J. S. Adams, D. D. Bikle, D. M. Black, M. B. Demay, J. E. Manson, M. H. Murad, and C. S. Kovacs. 2012. "The nonskeletal effects of vitamin D: an Endocrine Society scientific statement." *Endocr Rev* 33(3): 456–92. doi: 10.1210/er.2012-1000.

Sandhu, B. K., and S. P. Paul. 2014. "Irritable bowel syndrome in children: pathogenesis, diagnosis and evidence-based treatment." *World J Gastroenterol* 20(20): 6013–23. doi: 10.3748/wjg.v20.i20.6013.

Thacher, T. D., and B. L. Clarke. 2011. "Vitamin D insufficiency." *Mayo Clin Proc* 86(1): 50–60. doi: 10.4065/mcp.2010.0567.

Thomas, D. W., F. R. Greer, Nutrition American Academy of Pediatrics Committee on, Hepatology American Academy of Pediatrics Section on Gastroenterology, and Nutrition. 2010. "Probiotics and prebiotics in pediatrics." *Pediatrics* 126(6): 1217–31. doi: 10.1542/peds.2010-2548.

Tiequn, B., C. Guanqun, and Z. Shuo. 2015. "Therapeutic effects of Lactobacillus in treating irritable bowel syndrome: a meta-analysis." *Intern Med* 54(3): 243–9. doi: 10.2169/internalmedicine.54.2710.

Tsourounis, C., and S. Bent. 2010. "Why change is needed in research examining dietary supplements." *Clin Pharmacol Ther* 87(2): 147–9. doi: 10.1038/clpt.2009.241.

Wahli, W., and L. Michalik. 2012. "PPARs at the crossroads of lipid signaling and inflammation." *Trends Endocrinol Metab* 23(7): 351–63. doi: 10.1016/j.tem.2012.05.001.

Wasilewski, A., M. Zielinska, M. Storr, and J. Fichna. 2015. "Beneficial effects of probiotics, prebiotics, synbiotics, and psychobiotics in inflammatory bowel disease." *Inflamm Bowel Dis* 21(7): 1674–82. doi: 10.1097/MIB.0000000000000364.

West, C. E., M. C. Jenmalm, and S. L. Prescott. 2015. "The gut microbiota and its role in the development of allergic disease: a wider perspective." *Clin Exp Allergy* 45(1): 43–53. doi: 10.1111/cea.12332.

Zhang, Y., E. B. Fein, and S. B. Fein. 2011. "Feeding of dietary botanical supplements and teas to infants in the United States." *Pediatrics* 127(6): 1060–6. doi: 10.1542/peds.2010-2294.

Zuccotti, G., F. Meneghin, A. Aceti, G. Barone, M. L. Callegari, A. Di Mauro, M. P. Fantini, D. Gori, F. Indrio, L. Maggio, L. Morelli, L. Corvaglia, and Neonatology Italian Society of. 2015. "Probiotics for prevention of atopic diseases in infants:systematic review and meta-analysis." *Allergy*. doi: 10.1111/all.12700.

5   Physical Activity

In addition to forming a basis for lifelong health, physical activity can provide flexible non-pharmacologic approaches to help in the treatment of many of the chronic medical conditions prevalent in pediatrics such as obesity, metabolic syndrome, and asthma. Despite these benefits, patterns of physical activity in children have declined dramatically over time as sedentary time has increased. This is due to a number of factors, including societal shifts to a more suburban society and intrusion of technology into day-to-day life (Jones et al. 2013; Downing, Hnatiuk, and Hesketh 2015).

Other obstacles to regular physical activity include: cultural norms (especially in girls after puberty), overweight and obesity, poverty, safety concerns, disabilities, loss of school recess time and PE, lack of adult supervision, and sedentary role models. Lack of willpower, low self-esteem, embarrassment, fear of injury, and negative peer pressure are other considerations.

Given the mounting evidence of the serious detrimental effects of sedentary life in childhood, the American Academy of Pediatrics has taken the steps of addressing these issues in formal policy statements highlighting the importance of designing communities that encourage and support natural physical activity (Committee on Environmental and Tester 2009), limiting television and technology time (2 hours or less over the age of 2 years and no daily screen time under the age of 2 years) (American Academy of Pediatrics, Committee on Public 2001), emphasizing the importance of free play (Ginsburg et al. 2007), and endorsing a guideline of 60 minutes of physical activity per day (Council on Sports, Fitness, and Council on School 2006).

But despite these widely publicized policies, and a range of high-profile public campaigns such as Let's Move, change has been slow in stemming the prevalence of overweight and obesity in children and in (re)introducing regular enjoyable physical activity into the day-to-day life of children and adolescents.

Physical Activity: Impressive Benefits

The benefits of physical activity in children are hard to overstate. In addition to improving cardiovascular fitness, regular aerobic physical activity has been shown to have important benefits in children such as (Langford et al. 2015; Field 2012):

- Decreased blood pressure and resting heart rate
- Increased high density lipoprotein (HDL) cholesterol
- Improved glucose tolerance and decreased insulin resistance
- Decreased triglycerides

- Decreased inflammation
- Weight reduction
- Stimulation of growth factors and improvement in bone mineral density
- Improved psychological wellbeing
- Improved academic performance
- Reduction in peer victimization (bullying)
- Increased physical endurance

The addition of age-appropriate resistance training adds the benefits of increased muscle strength and mass, improved tendon and ligament strength, increased lean body mass, and improved HDL and glucose tolerance. Flexibility training adds the potential to reduce risk of injury and to improve balance and coordination (American Academy of Pediatrics Council on Sports et al. 2008).

An area of emerging study in adults is the impact of physical fitness on telomere length, a marker of biological aging. A positive correlation has been shown in older adults (Soares-Miranda et al. 2015).

Studies are currently limited in children, although overweight adolescents in an intensive multidisciplinary treatment program that included supervised physical activity showed a statistically significant lengthening of telomeres in the treatment group. Longer baseline telomere length was a positive predictor for more substantial decrease in body weight (Garcia-Calzon et al. 2014).

The Importance of Good Role Models

The impact of active role models on children has been well documented. For example, physical activity and television viewing habits of parents have shown to be highly predictive of these behaviors, even in preschoolers, and preferentially modeled after the gender-matched parents (Abbott et al. 2015).

Multiple studies show that adult screen time is a predictor of child and adolescent screen time (Minges et al. 2015).

Yet a majority of American adults remain sedentary, with the CDC reporting that only approximately one in five adults meets the 2008 physical activity guidelines of 150 minutes per week of physical activity. Differences in day-to-day levels of physical activity based on geography, gender, race and ethnicity, and education level impact activity levels and are mirrored in the pediatric population (Centers for Disease Control and Prevention).

Clinicians are a second category of important role models for an active lifestyle. Studies support the finding that physicians who are themselves physically active feel more confident counseling patients about healthy lifestyle approaches (Howe et al. 2010), and are in turn more effective in counseling their patients in healthy lifestyle change (Lobelo and de Quevedo 2014).

Such modeling has been shown to increase a patient's willingness to follow through with activity recommendations, and also has been shown to lead to better outcome measures (Shai et al. 2012).

One promising approach in improving physician counseling behavior was demonstrated in a small yet innovative study in Canadian family physicians that used a 3-hour educational experiential workshop as a training tool. Components of the workshop included evaluation of the physicians' baseline physical activity, experiential motivational interviewing to encourage activity, and development of personal exercise prescriptions (Windt et al. 2015).

Participants in this study showed a significant increase in self-reported knowledge and confidence in counseling skills after the workshop and at 1 month follow-up (p < 0.01 for both measures). Increase in exercise counseling and exercise prescription writing for patients also significantly increased. An important part of the intervention was providing tools to the attendees to use in clinical practice which included a way to assess and record patient physical activity (Sallis 2011) and an "Exercise is Medicine" Canada prescription pad along with resources to refer patients for further exercise consult. The strength of this study was identified as the combination of education with tools for immediate implementation in clinical practice (Lobelo and de Quevedo 2014).

Physical Activity in the Well Visit

Clinicians approaching the topic of physical activity in the pediatric visit can consider some of the following questions to help understand the child's needs:

* What are the patient and family's past experience with exercise?
* Current medical conditions or risk for other conditions?
* Patient and family goals for exercise?
* Patient's expectations?

Social or environmental barriers to consider include:

* Access to safe and well-supervised after school and/or community recreation programs?
* Regular physical education class in school?
* Does the child get regular recess time?
* Ability to walk or bike to school?
* Excessive homework demands?
* Pressure from over-competitive parents, teachers, or coaches?

Accumulating studies show that a multipronged approach involving individuals, families, school, and communities are needed to create significant change, making it important for the clinician to get a full understanding of the child's situation to be the most effective counselor and advocate for the importance of regular enjoyable physical activity in the child's life (Martin et al. 2014).

Early Steps

Families new to the habit of physical activity may experience early success by simply being encouraged to incorporate enjoyable physical activity naturally into the day's activities. Some examples include walking or biking to and from school, use of stairs over elevators, gardening, family hikes, swimming, age-appropriate scavenger hunts, camping, or time at a local park or playground. Recommendations from the AAP Committee on Sports Medicine suggest the following as age-appropriate guidelines:

Infants and toddlers: Ample time for free play and age-appropriate exploration in a supervised environment. No screen time under 2 years of age.

Preschoolers (4–6 years): Ample time for free play, limited screen time to less than 2 hours per day. Reduction in sedentary transportation in strollers and cars, encouragement of age-appropriate family walks if possible (Carson et al. 2015).

Elementary school (6–9): Free play and early emphasis on fundamental skill acquisition. Encouragement of a good variety of activities to develop motor skills, visual tracking, and balance. Non-pressured age-appropriate team skills with an emphasis on fun rather than competition.

Middle school (10–12 years): Focus on enjoyable activities with friends and family. Skill development, tactics and strategy can be introduced successfully, team sports now better comprehended. Wide variation in developmental stage and size make it important to avoid injury in sports where contact is possible such as football, basketball, or hockey. High-repetition weight training with light weights can be initiated under supervised conditions using proper technique.

High school: Sports can play a significant role in socialization. Personal preference is important, and a range of activities can be enjoyed including free play, recreational activities, transportation as in walking or biking to and from school, chores, activities at age-appropriate work, as well as planned exercise, personal training, sports competitions, and family activities.

Ideally, children and adolescents should get 60 or more minutes of daily enjoyable physical activity that is age appropriate, enjoyable, and easily accessible. Most of the exercise should be aerobic, at either moderate or vigorous effort. Muscle-strengthening activities should be included at least three times per week; for example, during free play such as climbing, or in supervised high-resistance weight lifting with light weights in appropriate age groups.

Weight training raises special questions that are addressed in an AAP Policy on the topic. In summary (American Academy of Pediatrics Council on Sports et al. 2008), the report recommends a medical evaluation prior to starting strength training, use of low-resistance exercises, gradual addition of weight as tolerated to 8–15 repetitions, use of all muscle groups, proper technique through the range of motion of each joint, done two to three times per week—no more than four times per week in sessions of 20–30 minutes each. Weight training should generally be accompanied by enjoyable aerobic conditioning for overall fitness.

Physical Activity in Schools

Given the number of hours that children spend in and around school, this offers a critical platform for physical activity initiatives. The World Health Organization Health Promoting Schools (HPS) framework was established in the late 1980s in recognition of the interdependent relationship between good health and education. The program emphasized health curriculum, healthy activities embedded into the school culture, and engagement with families and the broader community to encourage and support healthy initiatives. Work is active in this area to bring successful physical activity programs into schools. One example is the SPARK Physical Education program (Sports, Play, and Active Recreation for Kids) developed in the 1990s for both elementary and middle/high school students which has been adapted in a variety of settings. The program consists of a structured physical education curriculum taught by teachers in three 30-minute classes per week that involve cardiovascular fitness and skill building. A second component of the program is a self-management curriculum to promote physical activity outside of school. Three core topics include self-monitoring (of physical activity), self-evaluation (weekly goal setting including progress and problems), and self-reinforcement (positive self-talk, making activities enjoyable, increasing social support). Simple reinforcement rewards such as water bottles and pencils may be offered to motivate progress. Monthly newsletters and parent reinforcement and sign-off of weekly goal sheets can be included. Self-management workshops encouraged group participation and help in problem solving classmates obstacles (Sallis et al. 1993).

Other studies of fitness-oriented PE classes have shown benefit in overweight middle school children where activities are focused on lifestyle and fitness rather than competitive or team sports. Improvements included loss of body fat, improvement in fasting insulin level, and improvement in cardiovascular fitness (Carrel et al. 2005). Some initiatives have been directed at increasing and encouraging physical activity during recess and lunchtime using specific programming (reduction of allowable sitting time during breaks and lunch and extension of each break time by 5 minutes) and equipment (balls, jump ropes, hoops, cricket sets, and other toys) to increase time spent in moderate to vigorous activity (Parrish et al. 2015) or through introduction of novel moveable structures to facilitate movement and creative play (Hyndman et al. 2014).

An emerging trend mirroring the peak in interest in standing office desks in adults are classrooms using sit-to-stand desks, which have shown a significant decrease in sitting time in early studies in primary schools in Australia (Clemes et al. 2015).

A group of schools in Winston-Salem, North Carolina have introduced Read and Ride programs where stationary bikes are provided for the full class during reading time.

Innovative interventions that involve a multidimensional approach to increasing physical activity that involve the individual, family, school, and community are likely to be most effective (Martin et al. 2014; Dobbins et al. 2013).

One important issue to be aware of in the school setting is the presence of "fat bias" on the part of teachers and physical activity teachers and peers toward overweight and obese children. A survey study of 62 school-based PE and 177 non-PE teachers in Australia found that both teacher groups endorsed a strong feeling of weight stigmatization towards overweight or obese children, with PE teachers endorsing more bias. Teachers of obese or overweight children in this study had lower expectations for obese children across physical, academic, and social skills. Reasons for overweight were viewed as the child's responsibility and attributed to insufficient physical activity, overeating, poor eating habits, and lack of willpower (Lynagh, Cliff, and Morgan 2015).

Studies in the U.S. are evaluating similar questions about how best to recognize and reduce bias towards overweight students in relation to physical activity in schools (Greenleaf, Martin, and Rhea 2008).

Tailoring Physical Activity to the Child's Needs

Tailoring physical activity to children's needs and interests can take some trial and error. Chronic medical conditions can make the problem more challenging, but also create a new range of new options to explore such as yoga and tai chi which are low impact, well tolerated and can be practiced at home once the basic skills are learned. Regardless of diagnosis or activity chosen, the goal in every child is to build strength and overall fitness gradually within the framework of their condition and to avoid injury or overexertion that may cause a setback, or derail their fitness goals (Field 2012).

Some conditions with the most promising supporting research for the benefit of physical activity include overweight-obesity, diabetes, childhood asthma, depression, anxiety, and ADHD.

Overweight/Obesity

Studies evaluating the effect of exercise in overweight/obese children often consist of a variety of interventions rather than isolated physical activity, making interpretation more difficult. Even though weight loss is not always involved, aerobic physical activity in overweight children has been clearly shown to reduce triglycerides, and improve cardiovascular fitness, blood pressure, LDL cholesterol, and increase lean body mass (Vasconcellos et al. 2014).

Increased bone strength is an additional benefit of physical activity for all children, especially in adolescents (Pitukcheewanont, Punyasavatsut, and Feuille 2010).

Studies are ongoing to determine optimal 'dose' and timing of age-appropriate physical activity. Intermittent weight training has also been shown to increase lean body mass (Kelley and Kelley 2008).

Diabetes

Physical activity has been shown to be effective in both type-1 and type-2 diabetes in children with proper supervision and attention to risk factors associated with hypo- and hyperglycemia. Physiologic benefits seen in an overview of studies include: improved insulin sensitivity, decreased central adiposity, reduced low-density lipoproteins and triglycerides, increased high-density lipoproteins, and decreased blood pressure (Giannini, Mohn, and Chiarelli 2006; Giannini et al. 2007; Field 2012).

Asthma

A small randomized 6-week trial of monitored aerobic training (30 minutes of treadmill three times per week) in 33 children aged 6–17 years showed statistically significant improvement in functional capacity, maximal respiratory pressure, and improvement in quality of life and asthma-related symptoms such as sensation of dyspnea in the treatment group. Although serum inflammatory cytokines were measured, no significant change was noted in this study group (Andrade et al. 2014).

Another randomized study involving 105 children 11–12 years old in a 12-week indoor intermittent training program involving high- and low-intensity exercises and a variety of aerobic activities (total 60 minutes three times per week) found significant improvement in forced expiratory volume, dyspnea index, and improvement in quality of life measures, body mass index, and decreased fat mass in the treatment group (Latorre-Roman, Navarro-Martinez, and Garcia-Pinillos 2014).

A 2013 Cochrane Database Systematic Review of the benefit of swimming in asthmatic children and adolescents found good correlation with improvement in lung function and cardiopulmonary fitness (Beggs et al. 2013).

Mental Health: Depression and Anxiety

Large meta-analyses have shown mixed reviews in the protective effect of physical activity and depression in adolescents, although activity offers a range of positive effects such as increased fitness and opportunity for social connection.

For example, a large prospective study in more than 496 adolescent girls found that regular physical activity offered some protective effect against the onset of minor and major depression over the course of a 6-year study. Physical activity was also correlated with more social connectedness, self-efficacy, and enjoyment. Conversely, presence of depressive symptoms significantly reduced evidence of future physical activity (Jerstad et al. 2010).

A 2010 meta-analysis of 2789 students aged 11–14 found an association between the level of physical activity and decreased depressive symptoms, with a decrease of approximately 8% noted for every additional hour of weekly exercise (Rothon et al. 2010).

A subsequent meta-analysis of nine studies involving 581 children and adolescents found a small but significant protective effect of physical activity on depression.

Although there was wide variation in the interventions, aerobic activity on at least 3 days per week was the most common intervention (Brown et al. 2013).

However, a longitudinal study of 736 adolescents followed for 3 years found no protective effect of physical activity against depression, concluding that physical activity may not serve as a strong protective factor against depression in adolescents aged 14–17 (Toseeb et al. 2014).

ADHD

Systematic review and meta-analysis of eight randomized controlled trials involving 249 children with ADHD found that aerobic exercise had a moderate to large effect in improving symptoms of inattention, hyperactivity, impulsivity, and associated anxiety, executive function, and social disorders (Cerrillo-Urbina et al. 2015).

Yoga

Yoga has been shown to improve overall fitness and school performance, and help with weight loss in obese children (although studies are small with many methodological variations), have a positive effect on ADHD symptoms, including reduction in impulsivity, anxiety, and social difficulties (Cerrillo-Urbina et al. 2015).

Smaller studies have also shown benefit for yoga in asthma, anxiety, and lower cholesterol and triglyceride levels in children. Challenges in interpretation of the yoga literature in children are small study size and lack of randomized controlled trials, although adverse effects are rarely reported. Overall, few adverse effects have been reported with yoga, which can be enjoyed in children as early as preschool (Birdee et al. 2009) (Rosen et al 2015).

Tai Chi

Movements are based on the organic mechanics of the living body. Tai chi forms share five basic characteristics that include: naturalness, harmony, regulation, relaxation, and efficiency. This approach ensures that the practice of tai chi follows normal physiological function and minimizes the potential for injuries. Small studies have indicated the benefit of tai chi in children with asthma and ADHD (Field 2012).

Martial Arts

Martial arts such as kung fu have had good acceptance in overweight adolescents in a randomized controlled trial of sedentary adolescents in weekly sessions over the 6-month study period. Motivation for behavior change and enjoyment of physical activity were positive findings (Tsang et al. 2013).

Exergames: On the Frontier of Fitness?

Virtual technology has provided a creative and enjoyable platform for new generations of exercise games (exergames) through devices such as the Wii and Xbox 360 to deliver a range of interactive games to users in school, at home, or in community settings. Studies show that some of the games such as track and beach volleyball provided moderate to vigorous activity when children were measured for oxygen consumption and heart rate when gaming. This approach can offer important options to children who might not otherwise feel comfortable or be able to join in other activities (Wu, Wu, and Chu 2015; Mills et al. 2013, Murphy et al. 2009).

Changing Behavior

One of the great challenges in adding physical activity to day-to-day life is finding motivation to get started, followed by the challenge of finding the willpower to sustain change. This can be especially challenging if the patient is experiencing depression or fatigue related to a mental or physical challenge, is unsupported by family or school community, or feels overwhelmed by their situation; for example, an obese child who has faced repeated bullying and stigma in PE class.

This is where the art of medicine manifests in the form of compassionate listening, the offering of hope and encouragement, and working with the child or adolescent to find their motivation—the reasons they want to make changes and the first steps they feel they can successfully take to move them forward. Training in the art of motivational interviewing can be extremely helpful in the clinical interaction, and can be briefly described as helping the patient identify their own reasons for wanting to change, encouraging their sense of self-efficacy, and acting as a guide and partner in problem solving (Morton et al. 2015; Borrelli, Tooley, and Scott-Sheldon 2015).

An overview consists of the following steps.

Express Empathy

To increase patient motivation, especially in adolescents, avoid giving advice and instead listen to your patient's experience. This affords the patient the opportunity to experience the discrepancy between their current choices and where they want to be.

Develop Discrepancy

Paraphrasing is a useful technique to develop this discrepancy which can be thought of as the patient's internal discrepancy—the incongruity between what they are doing and the goals or values they aspire to that will harness the patient's own motivation to change behavior.

Avoid Argument

Paradoxically, patients' attachment to their health risk behavior may actually increase as they explain why it is reasonable. Often patients will defend their current behaviors to avoid experiencing ambivalence. In motivational interviewing, the goal is to understand the patient's perspective of their illness/health, which allows the clinician to build rapport and gain insight into which steps may be most successful in partnership with the patient.

Roll with Resistance

Essentially this means being flexible enough in the interview to shift focus away from a point of strong resistance to one about which patients are more amenable to change. This approach emphasizes the patients' personal choice and puts them in control of their behavior and choices. This might entail reflecting back the patient's words in a respectful way so as to highlight the ambivalence they may be feeling.

Affirm Self-Efficacy

Assume the partnership role rather than a directive role and reinforce successful change as it happens.

A Prescription for Exercise

With or without the use of motivational interviewing, some patients respond very well to a written exercise prescription to help reinforce change behavior. Counseling children and families in the details of exercise can be simplified by the use of an exercise prescription, a simple yet powerful way to emphasize the importance of exercise for good health. Although adults often use a structured FITT prescription (Frequency, Intensity, Type, Time) based on percentage heart rate maximum and heart rate reserve, this approach is not generally used in children and adolescents because of the high variation in size and developmental stages. An alternative is a simplified recommendation such as:

Rx

- Enjoyable exercise _____ (*type is patient's choice or clinician's recommendation*)
- 5–6 times a week
- Total of ___ minutes/day (*provide range of minutes to start with depending on the child's baseline starting point*)
- Repeat for one month
- Adjust prn

A simple exercise diary given to the child, perhaps with the promise of a small reward if returned at a follow-up visit, can be a great motivator to help keep the child on track. Just as with adults, it is important to meet the child where they are initially. Some children may need to start very slowly with low-impact activity and build confidence and endurance gradually. Ultimately it is important to include variety in exercise choices to include aerobic, resistance, flexibility, balance and agility, along with endurance elements to avoid injury, boredom, or burnout. Sports-related concussion is an area of active research inquiry that is beyond the scope of this chapter (Purcell, Canadian Paediatric Society, and Sports Medicine 2012, 2014).

Summary

Discussion of enjoyable exercise in the well child visit sends the message to the child and family that you consider exercise an integral part of health. Clinicians who model healthy behaviors, and who are open to discussing their own obstacles and challenges as they relate to exercise, can be wonderful role models to children. Insight into the common barriers to physical activity faced by families and children allows the practitioner be a better guide to help families navigate obstacles, especially if the practitioner is skilled in motivational interviewing. Ultimately physical activity must be promoted and supported at home, school, and within the broader community.

Additional Resources

USDA Lifecycle Nutrition: An extensive site providing links to all of the nutrition and exercise resources below and more.

Let's Move: An extensive exercise and healthy nutrition-based national initiative launched in February 2010.

BAM! Body and Mind: An interactive website for children through the CDC that features educational and interactive games and exercise diaries.

SuperTracker: An online dietary and physical activity assessment tool that provides information on diet quality, physical activity status, related nutrition messages, and links to nutrient and physical activity information.

The Fitness Jumpsite: A website with lots of fitness information including equipment reviews, book review, and an interactive fitness forum.

Nutrition and Physical Activity from the National Center for Chronic Disease Prevention and Health Promotion. This site provides diverse current news and research about nutrition and physical activity.

References

Abbott, G., J. Hnatiuk, A. Timperio, J. Salmon, K. Best, and K. D. Hesketh. 2015. "Cross-sectional and longitudinal associations between parents' and preschoolers' physical activity and TV viewing: the HAPPY Study." *J Phys Act Health*. doi: 10.1123/jpah.2015-0136.

American Academy of Pediatrics Council on Sports, Medicine, Fitness, T. M. McCambridge, and P. R. Stricker. 2008. "Strength training by children and adolescents." *Pediatrics* 121(4): 835–40. doi: 10.1542/peds.2007-3790.

American Academy of Pediatrics. Committee on Public, Education. 2001. "American Academy of Pediatrics: Children, adolescents, and television." *Pediatrics* 107(2): 423–6.

Andrade, L. B., M. C. Britto, N. Lucena-Silva, R. G. Gomes, and J. N. Figueroa. 2014. "The efficacy of aerobic training in improving the inflammatory component of asthmatic children. Randomized trial." *Respir Med* 108(10): 1438–45. doi: 10.1016/j.rmed.2014.07.009.

Beggs, S., Y. C. Foong, H. C. Le, D. Noor, R. Wood-Baker, and J. A. Walters. 2013. "Swimming training for asthma in children and adolescents aged 18 years and under." *Cochrane Database Syst Rev* 4: CD009607. doi: 10.1002/14651858.CD009607.pub2.

Birdee, G. S., G. Y. Yeh, P. M. Wayne, R. S. Phillips, R. B. Davis, and P. Gardiner. 2009. "Clinical applications of yoga for the pediatric population: a systematic review." *Acad Pediatr* 9(4): 212–20 e1–9. doi: 10.1016/j.acap.2009.04.002.

Borrelli, B., E. M. Tooley, and L. A. Scott-Sheldon. 2015. "Motivational interviewing for parent-child health interventions: a systematic review and meta-analysis." *Pediatr Dent* 37(3): 254–65.

Brown, H. E., N. Pearson, R. E. Braithwaite, W. J. Brown, and S. J. Biddle. 2013. "Physical activity interventions and depression in children and adolescents: a systematic review and meta-analysis." *Sports Med* 43(3): 195–206. doi: 10.1007/s40279-012-0015-8.

Carrel, A. L., R. R. Clark, S. E. Peterson, B. A. Nemeth, J. Sullivan, and D. B. Allen. 2005. "Improvement of fitness, body composition, and insulin sensitivity in overweight children in a school-based exercise program: a randomized, controlled study." *Arch Pediatr Adolesc Med* 159(10): 963–8. doi: 10.1001/archpedi.159.10.963.

Carson, V., N. Kuzik, S. Hunter, S. A. Wiebe, J. C. Spence, A. Friedman, M. S. Tremblay, L. G. Slater, and T. Hinkley. 2015. "Systematic review of sedentary behavior and cognitive development in early childhood." *Prev Med*. doi: 10.1016/j.ypmed.2015.07.016.

Centers for Disease Control and Prevention, Division of Nutrition, Physical Activity, and Obesity. "Facts about Physical Activity." http://www.cdc.gov/physicalactivity/data/facts.htm.

Cerrillo-Urbina, A. J., A. Garcia-Hermoso, M. Sanchez-Lopez, M. J. Pardo-Guijarro, J. L. Santos Gomez, and V. Martinez-Vizcaino. 2015. "The effects of physical exercise in children with attention deficit hyperactivity disorder: a systematic review and meta-analysis of randomized control trials." *Child Care Health Dev*. doi: 10.1111/cch.12255.

Clemes, S. A., S. E. Barber, D. D. Bingham, N. D. Ridgers, E. Fletcher, N. Pearson, J. Salmon, and D. W. Dunstan. 2015. "Reducing children's classroom sitting time using sit-to-stand desks: findings from pilot studies in UK and Australian primary schools." *J Public Health (Oxf)*. doi: 10.1093/pubmed/fdv084.

Committee on Environmental, Health, and J. M. Tester. 2009. "The built environment: designing communities to promote physical activity in children." *Pediatrics* 123(6): 1591–8. doi: 10.1542/peds.2009-0750.

Council on Sports, Medicine, Fitness, and Health Council on School. 2006. "Active healthy living: prevention of childhood obesity through increased physical activity." *Pediatrics* 117(5): 1834–42. doi: 10.1542/peds.2006-0472.

Dobbins, M., H. Husson, K. DeCorby, and R. L. LaRocca. 2013. "School-based physical activity programs for promoting physical activity and fitness in children and adolescents aged 6 to 18." *Cochrane Database Syst Rev* 2:CD007651. doi: 10.1002/14651858.CD007651.pub2.

Downing, K. L., J. Hnatiuk, and K. D. Hesketh. 2015. "Prevalence of sedentary behavior in children under 2 years: a systematic review." *Prev Med*. doi: 10.1016/j.ypmed.2015.07.019.

"Exercise is Medicine Canada." http://www.exerciseismedicine.ca/professional-resources/exercise-prescription-referral-tool.

Field, T. 2012. "Exercise research on children and adolescents." *Complement Ther Clin Pract* 18(1): 54–9. doi: 10.1016/j.ctcp.2011.04.002.

Garcia-Calzon, S., A. Moleres, A. Marcos, C. Campoy, L. A. Moreno, M. C. Azcona-Sanjulian, M. A. Martinez-Gonzalez, J. A. Martinez, G. Zalba, A. Marti, and Evasyon Study Group. 2014. "Telomere length as a biomarker for adiposity changes after a multidisciplinary intervention in overweight/obese adolescents: the EVASYON study." *PLoS One* 9(2):e89828. doi: 10.1371/journal.pone.0089828.

Giannini, C., T. de Giorgis, A. Mohn, and F. Chiarelli. 2007. "Role of physical exercise in children and adolescents with diabetes mellitus." *J Pediatr Endocrinol Metab* 20(2): 173–84.

Giannini, C., A. Mohn, and F. Chiarelli. 2006. "Physical exercise and diabetes during childhood." *Acta Biomed* 77(Suppl 1): S18–25.

Ginsburg, K. R., Communications American Academy of Pediatrics Committee on, Child

American Academy of Pediatrics Committee on Psychosocial Aspects of, and Health Family. 2007. "The importance of play in promoting healthy child development and maintaining strong parent-child bonds." *Pediatrics* 119(1): 182–91. doi: 10.1542/peds.2006-2697.

Greenleaf, C., S. B. Martin, and D. Rhea. 2008. "Fighting fat: how do fat stereotypes influence beliefs about physical education?" *Obesity (Silver Spring)* 16(Suppl 2): S53–9. doi: 10.1038/oby.2008.454.

Howe, M., A. Leidel, S. M. Krishnan, A. Weber, M. Rubenfire, and E. A. Jackson. 2010. "Patient-related diet and exercise counseling: do providers' own lifestyle habits matter?" *Prev Cardiol* 13(4): 180–5. doi: 10.1111/j.1751-7141.2010.00079.x.

Hyndman, B. P., A. C. Benson, S. Ullah, and A. Telford. 2014. "Evaluating the effects of the Lunchtime Enjoyment Activity and Play (LEAP) school playground intervention on children's quality of life, enjoyment and participation in physical activity." *BMC Public Health* 14: 164. doi: 10.1186/1471-2458-14-164.

Jerstad, S. J., K. N. Boutelle, K. K. Ness, and E. Stice. 2010. "Prospective reciprocal relations between physical activity and depression in female adolescents." *J Consult Clin Psychol* 78(2): 268–72. doi: 10.1037/a0018793.

Jones, R. A., T. Hinkley, A. D. Okely, and J. Salmon. 2013. "Tracking physical activity and sedentary behavior in childhood: a systematic review." *Am J Prev Med* 44(6): 651–8. doi: 10.1016/j.amepre.2013.03.001.

Kelley, G. A., and K. S. Kelley. 2008. "Effects of aerobic exercise on non-high-density lipoprotein cholesterol in children and adolescents: a meta-analysis of randomized controlled trials." *Prog Cardiovasc Nurs* 23(3): 128–32.

Langford, R., C. Bonell, H. Jones, T. Pouliou, S. Murphy, E. Waters, K. Komro, L. Gibbs, D. Magnus, and R. Campbell. 2015. "The World Health Organization's Health Promoting Schools framework: a Cochrane systematic review and meta-analysis." *BMC Public Health* 15: 130. doi: 10.1186/s12889-015-1360-y.

Latorre-Roman, P. A., A. V. Navarro-Martinez, and F. Garcia-Pinillos. 2014. "The effectiveness of an indoor intermittent training program for improving lung function, physical capacity, body composition and quality of life in children with asthma." *J Asthma* 51(5): 544–51. doi: 10.3109/02770903.2014.888573.

"Lets Move." http://www.letsmove.gov.

Lobelo, F., and I. G. de Quevedo. 2014. "The evidence in support of physicians and health care providers as physical activity role models." *Am J Lifestyle Med* 1.55982761352012E15.

Lynagh, M., K. Cliff, and P. J. Morgan. 2015. "Attitudes and beliefs of nonspecialist and specialist trainee health and physical education teachers toward obese children: evidence for "anti-fat" bias." *J Sch Health* 85(9): 595–603. doi: 10.1111/josh.12287.

Martin, A., D. H. Saunders, S. D. Shenkin, and J. Sproule. 2014. "Lifestyle intervention for improving school achievement in overweight or obese children and adolescents." *Cochrane Database Syst Rev* 3:CD009728. doi: 10.1002/14651858.CD009728.pub2.

Mills, A., M. Rosenberg, G. Stratton, H. H. Carter, A. L. Spence, C. J. Pugh, D. J. Green, and L. H. Naylor. 2013. "The effect of exergaming on vascular function in children." *J Pediatr* 163(3): 806–10. doi: 10.1016/j.jpeds.2013.03.076.

Minges, K. E., N. Owen, J. Salmon, A. Chao, D. W. Dunstan, and R. Whittemore. 2015. "Reducing youth screen time: qualitative metasynthesis of findings on barriers and facilitators." *Health Psychol* 34(4): 381–97. doi: 10.1037/hea0000172.

Morton, K., M. Beauchamp, A. Prothero, L. Joyce, L. Saunders, S. Spencer-Bowdage, B. Dancy, and C. Pedlar. 2015. "The effectiveness of motivational interviewing for health behaviour change in primary care settings: a systematic review." *Health Psychol Rev* 9(2): 205–23. doi: 10.1080/17437199.2014.882006.

Murphy, E. C., L. Carson, W. Neal, C. Baylis, D. Donley, and R. Yeater. 2009. "Effects of an exercise intervention using Dance Dance Revolution on endothelial function and other risk factors in overweight children." *Int J Pediatr Obes* 4(4): 205–14. doi: 10.3109/17477160902846187.

Parrish, A. M., A. D. Okely, M. Batterham, D. Cliff, and C. Magee. 2015. "PACE: A group randomised controlled trial to increase children's break-time playground physical activity." *J Sci Med Sport.* doi: 10.1016/j.jsams.2015.04.017.

Pitukcheewanont, P., N. Punyasavatsut, and M. Feuille. 2010. "Physical activity and bone health in children and adolescents." *Pediatr Endocrinol Rev* 7(3): 275–82.

Purcell, L. K., Healthy Active Living Canadian Paediatric Society, and Committee Sports Medicine. 2012. "Evaluation and management of children and adolescents with sports-related concussion." *Paediatr Child Health* 17(1): 31–4.

Purcell, L. K., Healthy Active Living Canadian Paediatric Society, and Committee Sports Medicine. 2014. "Sport-related concussion: evaluation and management." *Paediatr Child Health* 19(3): 153–65.

Rosen, L., French, A., Sullivan, G. 2015. "Complementary, Holistic, and Integrative Medicine: Yoga." *Pediatr Rev* 36(10): 468–474. doi: 10.1542/pir.36-10-468.

Rothon, C., P. Edwards, K. Bhui, R. M. Viner, S. Taylor, and S. A. Stansfeld. 2010. "Physical activity and depressive symptoms in adolescents: a prospective study." *BMC Med* 8: 32. doi: 10.1186/1741-7015-8-32.

Sallis, J. F., T. L. McKenzie, J. E. Alcaraz, B. Kolody, M. F. Hovell, and P. R. Nader. 1993. "Project SPARK. Effects of physical education on adiposity in children." *Ann N Y Acad Sci* 699: 127–36.

Sallis, R. 2011. "Developing healthcare systems to support exercise: exercise as the fifth vital sign." *Br J Sports Med* 45(6): 473–4. doi: 10.1136/bjsm.2010.083469.

Shai, I., D. Erlich, A. D. Cohen, M. Urbach, N. Yosef, O. Levy, and D. R. Shahar. 2012. "The effect of personal lifestyle intervention among health care providers on their patients and clinics; the Promoting Health by Self Experience (PHASE) randomized controlled intervention trial." *Prev Med* 55(4): 285–91. doi: 10.1016/j.ypmed.2012.08.001.

Soares-Miranda, L., F. Imamura, D. Siscovick, N. S. Jenny, A. L. Fitzpatrick, and D. Mozaffarian. 2015. "Physical activity, physical fitness, and leukocyte telomere length." *Med Sci Sports Exerc.* doi: 10.1249/MSS.0000000000000720.

Toseeb, U., S. Brage, K. Corder, V. J. Dunn, P. B. Jones, M. Owens, M. C. St Clair, E. M. van Sluijs, and I. M. Goodyer. 2014. "Exercise and depressive symptoms in adolescents: a longitudinal cohort study." *JAMA Pediatr* 168(12): 1093–100. doi: 10.1001/jamapediatrics.2014.1794.

Tsang, T. W., M. R. Kohn, C. M. Chow, and M. F. Singh. 2013. "Self-perception and attitude toward physical activity in overweight/obese adolescents: the 'martial fitness' study." *Res Sports Med* 21(1): 37–51. doi: 10.1080/15438627.2012.738444.

Vasconcellos, F., A. Seabra, P. T. Katzmarzyk, L. G. Kraemer-Aguiar, E. Bouskela, and P. Farinatti. 2014. "Physical activity in overweight and obese adolescents: systematic review of the effects on physical fitness components and cardiovascular risk factors." *Sports Med* 44(8): 1139–52. doi: 10.1007/s40279-014-0193-7.

Windt, J., A. Windt, J. Davis, R. Petrella, and K. Khan. 2015. "Can a 3-hour educational workshop and the provision of practical tools encourage family physicians to prescribe physical activity as medicine? A pre-post study." *BMJ Open* 5(7): e007920. doi: 10.1136/bmjopen-2015-007920.

Wu, P. T., W. L. Wu, and I. H. Chu. 2015. "energy expenditure and intensity in healthy young adults during exergaming." *Am J Health Behav* 39(4): 556–61. doi: 10.5993/AJHB.39.4.12.

6 Mind–Body Therapies

Introduction

The use of mind–body therapies reaches back through history in the form of meditation and other spiritual practices focused on health and healing. In the modern medical setting, mind–body therapies are used to harness the connections between emotions and physiology to benefit health with a secular philosophy and intent. Common mind–body therapies include breath work, biofeedback, guided imagery, clinical hypnosis, yoga, tai chi, and mindfulness meditation. Interest in the use of mindfulness in medicine is also increasing as a valuable tool to prevent and address burnout among medical professionals (Fortney et al. 2013; West et al. 2014). Mind–body techniques add an important dimension to the practice of pediatrics by offering powerful, non-invasive and non-pharmacologic treatments applicable in a flexible range of settings. Often called self-regulation skills, the mind–body therapies can be especially helpful when fear, stress, and pain are amplified by a feeling of loss of control and an inability to understand the purpose of the intervention, often the case in pediatrics. Used well, mind–body skills can help a child reframe a painful or difficult experience into one that builds a sense of resiliency, self-control, and confidence (Vohra et al. 2016).

History and Physiology

Mind–body medicine continues to gain acceptance in the mainstream of healthcare in both children and adults based on a wealth of supporting research. Some of the earliest breakthroughs in the field resulted from work by Walter Cannon, MD and his team in the early 1900s exploring the concept of homeostasis and threats to homeostasis. These experiments eventually led to identification of the physiologic cascade involving the hypothalamic-pituitary-adrenal axis catalyzed by intense emotion, which they named the "fight or flight" response (Goldstein 2010; Cannon 1963).

Work by other investigators continued to expand understanding of the field over time. In the early 1970s Hans Selye, MD's team built on Cannon's research and studied the physiology of chronic stress. In 1974 Selye proposed the term "General Adaptation Syndrome" based on a series of experiments showing that while steroids released from the adrenal cortex are useful for adaptation to stress, the prolonged exposure to stress resulted in pathological changes in the animal research subjects (McEwen and Stellar 1993). "Allostasis" was a term used by Sterling and Eyer in the 1980s to define "stability through change," and the term "allostatic load," coined later by McEwen and Stellar, as the accumulated load to assess situations where the demands of adaptation are too much. McEwen and Stellar identified three types of increased allostatic load:

frequent, yet short term stressors; chronic stressors correlated with the inability to turn off the activated stress response; and inadequate response of the adaptation system leading to elevated activity in other systems to accommodate the stress load. Excess allostatic load was subsequently correlated with the development of disease over time (McEwen 1998; Goldstein 2010).

Herbert Benson, MD is widely recognized for his work in the early 1970s exploring the physiologic changes related to triggering what he termed the "relaxation response" with commonly recognized mind–body approaches such as meditation, yoga, and autogenic training. This physiologic response involved reduction in heart rate and respiratory rate, decrease in oxygen consumption, reduction in muscle tone, and an increase in alpha brain waves seen in the wakeful relaxation state (Benson, Beary, and Carol 1974).

As it turns out, the relaxation response is the final common pathway and goal in the mind–body therapies, and can be achieved by individuals in a myriad of ways.

Recent research on the relaxation response indicates cellular level changes that promote mitochondrial energy production, telomere maintenance, and reduction of inflammatory markers (Bhasin et al. 2013).

These accumulated discoveries have led to intense interest in the potential of the various modalities to correlate mind–body intervention with the desired physiologic relaxation response. One of the most successful of these initiatives has been led by Jon Kabat-Zinn, PhD, who introduced mindfulness meditation into a treatment program for chronic pain patients in the early 1980s, and has gone on to develop worldwide training programs in this area for patients, caregivers, and clinicians (Kabat-Zinn 1982; Kabat-Zinn, Lipworth, and Burney 1985).

Modern Relevance

Advances in our ability to measure and modulate physiologic markers, such as telomere length and telomerase levels associated with cellular aging, have reinforced the detrimental impact of stressors on human physiology and subsequently highlighted the protective power of the mind–body therapies (Epel et al. 2009).

For example, early studies have correlated high maternal stress during pregnancy with reduction in leukocyte telomere length in young adults (Entringer et al. 2011).

Shortening of telomere length has also been more recently identified in a prospective study of newborn cord blood of babies born to mothers who had experienced high levels of psychosocial stress during pregnancy. A statistically significant shortening of telomeres was found in offspring of the stressed mothers (Entringer et al. 2013).

Conversely, studies on mindfulness practices have shown positive correlation with increased telomerase levels in a meta-analysis of 190 participants in mindful meditation practice (Schutte and Malouff 2014), and in lengthening of telomeres in breast cancer survivors receiving mindfulness meditation instruction (Carlson et al. 2015).

Other significant advances in mind–body research have been supported by exciting and disruptive research in neuroanatomy, demonstrating the ongoing malleability of the brain throughout life termed neuroplasticity, a term first proposed by William James in his 1890 book *The Principles of Psychology* (Mel 2002; Martin and Morris 2002).

For example, studies have correlated mindfulness-based stress-reduction training with measurable increases in brain gray matter in areas associated with learning and memory, emotional regulation, self-referential processing and perspective taking (Holzel et al. 2011; Fox et al. 2014; Allen et al. 2012).

In addition to the emerging findings in telomere and neuroplasticity research, mind–body therapies can catalyze the healing response, manage a spectrum of autoimmune, cardiovascular, inflammatory, reproductive, neurological, surgical, stress, and pain-related symptoms with versatility, safety, and cost-effectiveness (Bower and Irwin 2015).

Potential Downsides of Mind–Body Medicine

One potential downside of the mind–body therapies is the expectation that people should be able to manage all their conditions or symptoms without the help of conventional therapies or prescription medication. This can place undue pressure on the individual, especially a child, and is not the intent of recommending these therapies. Another important note of caution is the assumption of stress-related symptoms, especially in children. Time must be taken to evaluate symptoms such as sudden onset of behavior changes or regressive behavior, which may relate to a serious issue such as abuse or posttraumatic stress disorder (PTSD) (McClafferty 2011). Other symptoms requiring clarification include: disturbed dreams, night terrors, hypervigilance, social withdrawal, excessive sadness, or irritability. In these cases clinicians should be sure to rule out the threat of serious underlying illness before attributing symptoms to stress, especially in very young and non-verbal children and refer to a pediatric mental health specialist for evaluation as appropriate (Cohen and Mannarino 2015).

PTSD diagnosis includes symptoms in of each of the following four areas for more than 1 month causing significant distress or impairment of functioning. These areas are: re-experiencing, avoidance, negative cognitions and mood, and arousal or hypervigilance (American Psychiatric Association 2013).

Do Children Experience Stress?

Children do experience stress and pain with physiologic changes mirroring those in adults.

Table 6.1 illustrates three levels of stress that have been described by Shonkoff et al.:

In chronic form stress and pain have been shown to have profound and detrimental impact on the developing brain. Research by Shonkoff et al. in children who have

Table 6.1 Three Levels of Stress

Positive stress is within normal range and of limited duration. An example would be the start of a new school year.

Tolerable stress is characterized by an increased level of distress for a longer duration. An important differentiator from toxic stress is the presence of supportive adults who buffer the child from full exposure to the difficult situation.

Toxic stress is the highest level and is characterized by prolonged duration, lack of supportive relationships, and sustained exposures to stress hormones—a combination of events that has been clearly associated with lifelong problems in behavior, learning, and mental and physical health.

Source: Shonkoff, J. P., A. S. Garner, Child Committee on Psychosocial Aspects of, Health Family, Adoption Committee on Early Childhood, Care Dependent, Developmental Section on, and Pediatrics Behavioral. 2012. "The lifelong effects of early childhood adversity and toxic stress." *Pediatrics* 129(1): e232–46.

suffered physical, sexual, or emotional abuse and neglect demonstrates profound dys-regulation of the stress response and association with serious mental and detrimental health effects such as cardiovascular disease, cancer, depression, and asthma in adolescence and adult life (Shonkoff et al. 2012; Johnson et al. 2013).

Signs and Symptoms of Pediatric Stress

Familiarity with signs and symptoms associated with stress in the various age groups can guide early diagnosis and may help with choice of mind–body therapies. Non-judgmental questions about stressors and stress management techniques should be included in routine well visits in the context of anticipatory guidance.

Table 6.2 shows examples of stress symptoms by age as reported by the American Academy of Pediatrics Task Force on the Family (Schor and American Academy of Pediatrics Task Force on the 2003).

Bullying: A Special Topic

Bullying is a complex and common social behavior found from preschool to senior age groups in cultures throughout the world. The bully relationship is characterized by a chronic abuse of power with intent to publicly intimidate and control the victim. A long list of detrimental health effects have been associated with bullying victimization (and bystander and bully roles) in childhood, including increased incidence of somatic problems, anxiety, depression, and significant risk of self-harm and suicide that often extend into adult life, most often seen in the victim (Wolke and Lereya 2015). The topic is covered in more detail in Chapter 19.

Table 6.2 Stress Symptoms by Age as Reported by the American Academy of Pediatrics Task Force on the Family

Age	Stress symptoms
Infants:	Regression and detachment, gaze aversion, flat affect, increased crying, and irritability, sleep disruption, and decrease in appetite, increased startle response.
Children < 12 months:	Exaggerated separation anxiety in addition to the above signs.
Toddlers and preschoolers:	Increase in irritability and negativity, temper tantrums, physicality such as pushing, sleep disruption, night terrors, behavioral and skill regression, clinging, loss of appetite, regression in toilet training, and somatic complaints such as stomachache and headache.
School-age children:	Sleep disruption, regressive behaviors and separation anxiety, somatic complaints (abdominal pain, headache), fatigue, school resistance, bed-wetting, acting out, and increased negativity.
Adolescents:	Increased irritability, anger, verbal outbursts, fatigue, change in sleep patterns (increased sleep or insomnia), nightmares, lightheadedness, dizziness, somatic complaints (migraine, abdominal pain, nausea, chest pain), change in appetite, school avoidance, social withdrawal, depression, conversion reactions, increased risk-taking behaviors such as drug use or sexual activity, and suicidal thoughts or attempts.

Source: Schor, E. L., and American Academy of Pediatrics Task Force on the. 2003. "Family pediatrics: report of the Task Force on the Family." *Pediatrics* 111(6 Pt 2): 1541–71.

It is critically important to inquire about bullying in the pediatric visit, beginning as early as preschool, in order to identify and help families and children avoid or navigate chronic and highly stressful bullying situations that may not be voluntarily disclosed by the child. Mind–body techniques have the potential to serve as tools to help children with stress reduction and self-regulation skills and may assist in the promotion of self-esteem and self-efficacy. More research and advocacy is needed in this important area where pediatricians must take a leadership role (Hemphill, Tollit, and Herrenkohl 2014).

Mind–Body Therapies

Mind–body therapies are diverse and may have considerable overlap, which can make research evaluation challenging. Some of the most common mind–body therapies in children include:

- Breath work
- Autogenics
- Progressive muscle relaxation
- Biofeedback
- Guided imagery
- Clinical hypnosis
- Music therapy
- Yoga
- Tai chi
- Mindfulness meditation
- Compassion based cognitive therapy
- Spirituality and prayer
- Animal-assisted therapy

The following sections will review research in the modalities and provide examples of their use in various medical conditions. It is important to remember that the application of mind–body therapies is highly individualized, so what appeals to one patient may not work in another. It may take a period of trial and error before finding the best fit for the specific need, and preference may change over time.

Conditions

Conditions treated:

- Acute or chronic pain
- Anxiety and stress
- Dysfunctional voiding/enuresis
- Constipation and encopresis
- Sleep disorders
- Habit disorders
- Attention-deficit/hyperactivity disorder
- Asthma
- Obesity
- Diabetes
- Inflammatory bowel disease

- Irritable bowel syndrome
- Cancer treatment side effects

Word Choice Matters

The use of appropriate language is an important nuance when using the mind–body therapies. Tone and pace of the voice are a priority, hopefully modulated to encourage calm confidence in the patient. Word selection is also pivotal, either used to inspire the patient or inadvertently insert doubt and fear into the medical encounter. Children perceive pain and stress in many different ways, therefore skillful use of language can leave the door open for the child to have a successful experience and avoid preconceived expectations of pain or distress.

Breath Work

Breath is a basic, yet powerful function that can be used to positive effect by children as young as preschool age. The use of breath for centering and in calming rituals spans cultures and traditions; for example, the inclusion of breath work as an integral component of yoga, termed "pranayama." Breathing can be done both consciously and unconsciously, and is one of the very few body functions that involve both the voluntary (skeletal muscles) and involuntary (smooth muscles, gastrointestinal tract, heart, blood pressure) nervous systems, allowing regulation of both parasympathetic and sympathetic systems. Young children can enjoy simple breathing exercises such as the "belly breath" where the stomach is relaxed while the lungs are fully filled to a count of four, then the breath released while the stomach is pulled back in to a count of four. This approach to abdominal breathing can help children master diaphragmatic breathing, which is associated with stimulation of the vagal nerve and activation of the parasympathetic nervous system (Stromberg, Russell, and Carlson 2015; Russell et al. 2014).

Breath counting to five and back to one, for example, is another simple exercise to help children focus on the breath. Use of tools such as pinwheel or other simple toy that moves with the exhaled breath may also be used in various clinical settings to help younger children regulate their breathing. Older children may be interested in exploring the various electronic resources and smart phone apps designed to help regulate the breath. Mastery of breath is an important basic skill used to enhance the efficacy of other mind–body therapies.

Progressive Muscle Relaxation

Progressive muscle relaxation consists of isolating a muscle group, deliberately increasing tension in those selected muscles for 8–10 seconds, then deliberately releasing the tension. This process is repeated systematically until all the major muscle groups have been addressed, often moving from the feet to the head. The purpose of the exercise is to develop discrepancy between the tense state and the relaxed state—facilitating recognition and recall of the relaxation response. Even preschool-age children can learn progressive muscle relaxation, which is often accompanied by breathing exercises and music. Progressive muscle relaxation is often used in combination with other mind–body modalities.

Memory and Attention

A study by Hashim of 132 healthy students aged 10–11 years comparing six sessions of 30-minute prerecorded progressive muscle relaxation versus 12 sessions for effect on short-term memory, emotional distress, and sustained attention found that the greatest improvement of short-term memory was seen in the group receiving 12 sessions. No significant differences were seen in reduction of anxiety and attention, both of which improved in each group (Hashim and Zainol 2015).

Headache

Progressive muscle relaxation training facilitated by a school nurse has been shown to be helpful in tension-type headaches in students aged 10–18 years in the school setting in a series of several randomized controlled trials (Larsson et al. 2005).

Asthma

Progressive muscle relaxation training coupled with breathing techniques was shown to improve self-perceived health status, asthma signs and symptoms, peak expiratory flow rate, anxiety, and reliance on asthma medication in the treatment group in a randomized controlled trial of 40 children with asthma (Chiang et al. 2009).

Mental Health and Sleep

Progressive muscle relaxation in combination with massage and yoga was found to be effective in reduction of depressive symptoms and anxiety in a group of adolescent psychiatric patients (Platania-Solazzo et al. 1992).

The use of group sessions in progressive muscle relaxation has also proven useful in children in small studies of children with ADHD to reduce inattentive behavior (Denkowski and Denkowski 1984).

Other small studies have shown the efficacy of progressive muscle relaxation for behavioral conditions such as ADHD and anxiety in the school-based setting (Richter 1984).

Progressive muscle relaxation has been shown to be effective in adult patients with insomnia, although few research studies exist studying progressive muscle relaxation as an isolated therapy in children (Taylor and Roane 2010).

Autogenics

German psychiatrist and neurologist Dr. Johannes Heinrich Schultz is credited with the development of autogenic training, which uses the premise of relaxing the mind in order to relax the body. Autogenic training involves an average of three short daily sessions of 10–15 minutes, during which the individual repeats a set of statements and visualizations designed to induce a state of relaxation. One of the most significant features of autogenics is its simplicity, as it requires no equipment or extensive training. Autogenic training has significant overlap with biofeedback and can be used in combination with it and other mind–body approaches such as breath work and imagery.

The six classic phrases developed by Schultz are designed to address relaxation, vascular dilation, regulation of heartbeat, slowing of respiratory rate, and calming of brain activity (Lehrer 1996; British Autogenic Society).

Each statement is repeated three times by the individual:

- My arms are heavy.
- My arms are warm.
- My heartbeat is calm and strong.
- My breathing is calm and relaxed.
- My abdomen radiates warmth.
- My forehead is pleasantly cool.

Finish with:

- My neck and shoulders are heavy (classically repeated three times).
- I am at peace (repeat three times).

Autogenic training was shown to be effective in reduction of migraine headache pain in a randomized controlled study of 30 children aged 7–18 years (Labbe 1995), and has been used in a randomized controlled trial to evaluate mood regulation in adolescent soccer players, although results for its efficacy were equivocal in this study (Hashim and Hanafi Ahmad Yusof 2011).

Autogenics will be used as part of a randomized controlled trial in addressing approaches to stress management in German medical trainees and may prove to be a valuable tool in programs developed to support physician health and wellness (Kuhlmann et al. 2015).

Biofeedback

Biofeedback is used to train individuals to control normally involuntary functions such as heart rate, blood pressure, muscle tension, and skin temperature. It has been studied in children since the late 1970s and has strong supporting evidence with a low risk–benefit ratio in a range of conditions. Biofeedback has been shown to be a commonly used integrative modality in U.S. pediatric anesthesia programs, where 38 out 43 programs (83%) offered biofeedback in their pain programs (Lin et al. 2005).

Commonly used types of biofeedback in children include:

- Electromyography (measures muscle tension)
- Thermal biofeedback (measures vasodilation)
- Heart rate variability (heart rate regulation)
- Neurofeedback (regulation of slow cortical potentials)

Migraine

Biofeedback has strong supporting evidence in the prevention and treatment of both migraine and tension headache in pediatrics. Both electromyography and thermal biofeedback have shown efficacy in a variety of studies (Parisi et al. 2011; Termine et al. 2011).

Dysfunctional Voiding

Another area with strong supporting evidence for biofeedback in children is dysfunctional voiding, often caused by vesicoureteral reflux and recurrent urinary tract infections. Biofeedback can be used to address symptoms of frequency, urgency, enuresis, and daytime incontinence by allowing the child to gain control of the pelvic floor and urethral sphincter (Tugtepe et al. 2015).

A 2015 retrospective study of 40 pediatric patients with dysfunctional voiding confirmed significant improvement in four biofeedback sessions as compared to the traditional 6–10 sessions, lending yet more support for this approach (Sener et al. 2015).

Positive results were enhanced by the use of animated biofeedback (based on age-appropriate child friendly games) in a study of 120 girls with dysfunctional voiding where treatment in the animation arm reduced number of sessions nearly in half from eight to four as compared to non-animated biofeedback (Kaye and Palmer 2008).

Animated biofeedback has also been shown to be effective in treating encopresis (Kajbafzadeh et al. 2011).

ADHD

EEG neurofeedback has proven to be an effective intervention in children with ADHD. This technique involves learned self-regulation of slow cortical potentials. Research has been very active in this area over the past decade and the accumulating results are encouraging (Lofthouse et al. 2012).

Age-appropriate animated gaming technology programs have also been developed to facilitate ADHD training, which have been associated with improvement in both behavior and attention scores. A 2013 literature review by Mayer et al. showed good efficacy in learned self-regulation with negligible risk in children (Mayer, Wyckoff, and Strehl 2013).

Children who received neurofeedback training in an in-school program sustained faster and more substantial gains in attention and behavior over the control group who received cognitive behavioral therapy in at-school sessions. Findings in the neurofeedback group were sustained 6 months following the 40-session treatment course (Steiner et al. 2014).

Unanswered questions remaining about neurofeedback include the optimal number of sessions and ongoing concerns about insurance reimbursement.

EEG neurofeedback is under study for other conditions such as seizures, symptoms of traumatic brain injury, chronic pain, autistic behaviors, headache, depression, anxiety, addictions, and sleep problems although research is in relatively early stages in many of these areas, especially in children (Fovet, Jardri, and Linden 2015; Friedrich et al. 2014; Friedrich et al. 2015).

Heart Rate Variability

Heart rate variability monitoring is another commonly used type of biofeedback with evidence in children and adolescents. In simplified terms, the goal is increased heart rate variability within specified parameters which is associated with a healthy and optimally functioning heart. Measurement of heart rate variability can be done using a variety of hand-held or desktop software systems available commercially (Shaffer, McCraty, and Zerr 2014).

Emerging research shows regulation of heart rate variability to be quite complex, related to the baroreceptor reflex and vagal nerve stimulation. Existence of an intrinsic cardiac nervous system has also been demonstrated, with various branches responsible for generating heart rhythm and beat variability. This intrinsic cardiac system communicates with the central nervous system, allowing the opportunity for self-regulation through breath, positive thoughts and other mind–body approaches to modulate beat-to-beat variability (McCraty and Shaffer 2015; Lehrer and Gevirtz 2014).

Research is active in the area of the correlation between low heart rate variability and emotional dysregulation, depression, and decreased psychological flexibility (Sgoifo et al. 2015).

For example, self-reported depression in children has been shown to correlate with a decrease in heart rate variability (Blood et al. 2015). Excessive online gaming behavior has also been associated with decrease in heart rate variability in controlled studies of college students (Chang et al. 2015; McCraty and Shaffer 2015).

Guided Imagery

Guided imagery is a somewhat misleading term because the skillful use of imagery deliberately invokes all five senses (sight, sound, taste, touch, smell) to offer tools for those without strong visual imagery skills to benefit from the session. Ideally, the imagery creates a deeply relaxed state and allows vivid sensations and images to arise. The use of guided imagery is found in a wide range of cultures, often involves the use of music and breath work, and may overlap the use of progressive muscle relaxation, hypnosis, meditation and other mind–body therapies. There is no license or regulatory board for guided imagery (Vohra et al. 2016). Training resources are listed at the end of the chapter. Contraindications to the use of imagery include mental illness or a history of PTSD cases in which cases consultation with a trained mental health specialist is indicated.

Physiologic changes associated with guided imagery include measurable changes in immune biomarkers and reduction in salivary cortisol (Astin et al. 2003; Trakhtenberg 2008; Gruzelier 2002).

Positive effects of imagery have been seen in a variety of pediatric conditions, including in lifestyle interventions to assist in weight loss for 29 overweight Latino adolescents where use of scripted guided imagery recordings in a 12-week program in the study group were associated with reduction in sedentary behavior, increase in physical activity, and large reductions in salivary cortisol during the time span of the 45-minute recording. The use of imagery was well tolerated with no adverse effects reported (Weigensberg et al. 2014).

Benefit of guided imagery has also been shown in children with recurrent abdominal pain in a study by van Tilburg et al. of 34 children using a home-based program of audio-recorded guided imagery over a 2-month period. Guided imagery was found to be more effective in reduction of abdominal pain, disability, medical visits, and also improved quality of life. Improvements were sustained in the treatment group over the 6-month study follow-up (van Tilburg et al. 2009).

Guided imagery paired with progressive muscle relaxation was shown to be significantly more effective in reducing days of pain and missed activities in 22 children in a 2-month randomized trial by Weydert et al. Children were seen in weekly sessions for 4 weeks where they received direct instructions from a therapist, and also received take home practice recordings. In this study children were asked to identify and describe an image that represented their pain, and then to identify and describe an image that would cure their pain (Weydert et al. 2006).

Research demonstrating efficacy of guided imagery exists in a variety of other medical conditions including pre-procedural anxiety in a pediatric oncology clinic (combined with progressive muscle relaxation) (Shockey et al. 2013), asthma (Lahmann et al. 2009), and sickle cell disease pain where the use of guided imagery was also seen to reduce use of pain medication and increase sense of self-efficacy in a sample of 20 children 6–11 years of age (Dobson and Byrne 2014).

Conversely, nurse-led imagery to reduce needle stick discomfort was not found to be effective in a randomized crossover trial of 37 girls receiving human papilloma virus immunization (Nilsson et al. 2015).

Hypnosis

Clinical hypnosis has strong support for a variety of medical conditions in children and typically has a strong overlay with imagery (Evans, Tsao, and Zeltzer 2008). A 2005 survey of 43 pediatric anesthesia fellowship programs in the U.S. showed that that 44% of the 38 responding institutions offered hypnosis as a treatment therapy for acute and chronic pain (Lin et al. 2005).

Success of hypnosis can be facilitated by children's openness to storytelling, imagination, and fantasy. Hypnosis used in the medical encounter can be described as a combined state of focused attention, dissociation from the usual state of awareness (like daydreaming), and heightened responsiveness to suggestions (Green et al. 2005).

This state of increased concentration while being deeply relaxed is often called a trance state. Self-hypnosis, where individuals learn to induce the trance state using a simple physical trigger such as a breath or a finger tap, has been shown to be very effective in children even at very young ages (Kohen and Kaiser 2014).

Kohen and Olness et al. reported on 505 hypnotic interventions in children as young as 3 years of age with a variety of conditions including enuresis, pain, asthma, habit disorders (cough, tics), encopresis, and anxiety. A reported 51% of children had complete resolution of the presenting symptom, most often after four or fewer visits. Significant improvement was seen in 32% of the children, some improvement in 9%, and only 7% of children in this report showed no improvement (Kohen et al. 1984).

Other conditions where hypnosis has been shown to be effective include:

- Irritable bowel syndrome in both children and adults where hypnosis has been shown to be highly effective in providing sustained symptom relief in a solid body of randomized controlled trials (Palsson 2015).
- A review by Jensen explored the use of hypnosis for treatment of chronic pain associated with a variety of conditions such as migraine headache, musculoskeletal issues, burn trauma, arthritis and others. Modern imaging studies have demonstrated that pain is not centralized in the brain or nervous system, rather fMRI and PET scan studies show that pain is associated with activity in a range of areas including the prefrontal cortex, thalamus, and anterior cingulate cortex and others. Hypnosis has also been associated with increased alpha brain activity in those experiencing relief of pain. Imaging studies on the impact of hypnosis for pain management have shown that various areas of the brain involved in pain processing respond to hypnosis. Pain intensity, quality, degree of unpleasantness, sense of comfort and the ability to screen out unpleasant sensations and allow in comfortable sensations have each been shown to be modifiable with hypnosis. In

addition to pain reduction, hypnosis was shown to be associated with improved sleep, greater overall wellbeing, and a greater sense of control in many patients (Jensen and Patterson 2014).

- Self-hypnosis was found to be highly effective in the treatment of insomnia based on chart review of 84 children, with 68% of children requiring two or fewer sessions to reduce onset of sleep (Anbar and Slothower 2006).
- In a range of respiratory conditions, including asthma, hypnosis has been shown to improve symptom frequency and severity, reduce medication use, and reduce fear during acute attacks in one small randomized controlled trial (Brown 2007).
- Hypnosis has been shown to help with cystic fibrosis, both physical and psychological issues, such as increased peak expiratory flow rates and reduction of anxiety (McBride, Vlieger, and Anbar 2014).

Another area where hypnosis has been shown to be useful is vocal cord dysfunction, which can mimic asthma in its presentation with associated wheezing and dyspnea (Kaslovsky and Gottsegen 2015). Also, one hour of instruction in self-hypnosis was shown to be highly effective for procedural pain and stress in a randomized controlled trial of 44 children undergoing voiding cystourethography (VCUG) for dysfunctional voiding (Butler et al. 2005).

Hypnosis has also been used in the pediatric office setting to reinforce preventive health counseling and to reduce anxiety for surrounding routine vaccination (Chambers et al. 2009).

Steps in Hypnosis

While there are six classic stages to a hypnosis session (introduction, induction, deepening, therapeutic suggestions, awakening, and debriefing), each session is unique to the individual patient. One of the surprising things about hypnosis in children is that they may continue to play or engage in a creative activity such as drawing while undergoing hypnosis as opposed to adults who may appear extremely drowsy.

Caveats regarding use of hypnosis in children as with other mind–body therapies include referral or consultation with a mental health specialist for any child with a history of abuse or pre-existing mental illness, and the use of only fully trained practitioners. In the U.S. only the American Society of Clinical Hypnosis (ASCH) currently offers a formal certification process for professionals in medicine, psychology, dentistry, social work and nursing. The National Pediatric Hypnosis Training Institute offers ASCH-certified pediatric specialization.

Mindfulness

Mindfulness might be described as the cultivation of awareness in the present moment, regardless of ongoing events. Mindfulness has gained popularity in medicine in part due to its focus on improvement of emotional self-regulation and attention. Jon Kabat-Zinn, PhD has pioneered the use of mindfulness-based stress reduction (MBSR) in the Western medical setting by designing an 8-week program that uses a range of mind–body modalities such as breath work, progressive muscle relaxation, mindful eating, movement, yoga, and meditation to introduce the concept of mindfulness to a broad range of people (Kabat-Zinn 1982).

Although MBSR is not the only approach to mindfulness training, it has gained wide popularity and acceptance. Use of this program in a range of randomized controlled trials has been associated with reduction of emotional reactivity, improvement in quality of life and coping capacity, reduction in anxiety, depression, emotional reactivity, and beneficial modulation of inflammatory markers (Rosenkranz et al. 2013).

Emerging research has also shown MBSR to increase telomere length in healthy adult volunteers (Schutte and Malouff 2014).

Limitations in Mindfulness Research

Some of the recognized limitations in mindfulness research to date include the difficulty in creating randomized controlled trials, risk of bias, use of highly experienced lifelong meditators, and lack of longitudinal studies, especially in children. Another challenge is quantifying the elusive nature of attention, which can be subdivided into three components—alerting, orienting, and conflict monitoring—as well as measuring change over time (Tang, Holzel, and Posner 2015).

Mindfulness in Pediatrics

Despite acknowledged research challenges, the use of mindfulness in children has shown promise with the outcome goals of harnessing relaxation, self-regulation, focus, and creativity. Training in mindfulness was offered by 21% of academic pediatric anesthesia pain management services in the U.S. surveyed for provision of CAM programs at their institutions (Lin et al. 2005). Extensive literature reviews by Gotonk et al. (Gotink et al. 2015) and by Simkin and Black (Simkin and Black 2014) show the application and efficacy in a wide range of pediatric conditions including anxiety, pain, depression, ADHD, school stress, conduct disorder, sleep disorder, and chronic pain.

Systematic review and meta-analysis of other mindfulness-based interventions in a total of 1348 children in treatment groups and 876 controls showed good efficacy overall for improvement in cognitive performance and resilience to stress. Due to the variability in study design, small study size, and differences in measurement tools, concrete recommendations for use are not available, although in general results are encouraging and adverse effects negligible (Zenner, Herrnleben-Kurz, and Walach 2014).

Increase in self-esteem and higher acceptance of self also suggest this approach as a possible tool to help children address peer victimization. Programs in mindfulness are under study in children as young as preschool age; for example, a 12-week curriculum in mindfulness-based kindness in a public school setting involving 68 children demonstrated an increase in prosocial behavior and improvement in self-regulation compared to control group. The curriculum focused on age-appropriate lessons and practice sessions involving mindfulness, empathy, kindness, compassion, gratitude, and sharing with the goal of cultivating attention and emotional regulation. Students received two 20–30-minute lessons weekly for 12 weeks. Students in the treatment group also showed improvements on report cards 3 months after the intervention ended, especially in areas of learning, social-emotional development, and health (Flook et al. 2015).

Mindfulness-based stress reduction training has been found to be beneficial and well accepted in adolescents; for example, in a randomized trial of 102 adolescent psychiatric outpatients with a variety of diagnoses, those in the treatment group (8 weekly 2-hour classes with accompanying manual) had significantly reduced symptoms of anxiety, depression, and somatic complaints. Increased self-esteem and sleep quality were reported as was overall improvement in functioning over the 5-month study period as compared to controls (Biegel et al. 2009).

Adolescents aged 13–21 with high baseline life stressors in a randomized controlled trial in an urban primary care who learned MBSR (8-week traditional program with some modifications for language and class length) also demonstrated improvements in calmness, conflict avoidance, self-awareness and self-regulation over the control group who received a Healthy Topics educational curriculum (Kerrigan et al. 2011). Mindfulness interventions by Perry-Parrish (Perry-Parrish et al. 2016) and Sibinga in the school-based settings (Sibinga et al. 2016) have shown positive outcomes in development of self-regulation skills and stress reduction.

Another important area of research is the use of mindfulness in caretakers of children with significant medical disabilities, who are often at high risk for comorbidities of chronic stress including depression and anxiety (Lee 2013).

For example, a 6-week intervention consisting of 90 minutes of traditional MBSR training in 243 mothers of children with a range of neurodevelopmental disabilities including autism resulted in a significant reduction in stress, depression, and anxiety, and improvement in sleep quality (Dykens et al. 2014).

Compassion-Based Meditation

There is a substantial overlap in the use of mindfulness and meditative practices based on compassion meditation. This is an area of intense research interest examining both psychological and physical effects of compassion-based meditation practice. Effects documented include meditation-dependent cortical plasticity and lengthening of telomeres. Emotional regulation, improved attention and cognition, prosocial behavior and moral decision making are other positive outcomes that have been demonstrated in multiple studies, although these have been done primarily in adults (Sun et al. 2015).

Yoga

Synergy of mindfulness, breath work, and movement is found in yoga, tai chi, and traditional types of physical activity. Yoga especially has a long history of use as a mind–body therapy and is increasing in popularity among Western children in part because of a surge in commercially available DVDs, books, and yoga studios designed specifically towards children. Some schools have also adopted yoga programs as a way to offer low-impact physical activity and for stress reduction (Rosen et al. 2015). Data from the 2102 National Health Interview Survey (NHIS) showed that an estimated 3.1% of children in the U.S. use yoga, an increase from 2.3% in 2007 (Black et al. 2015).

Positive effects of yoga have been documented with fMRI that show a decrease of neurological stimulation to the thalamus consistent with the sense of external stimuli being blocked, leaving the mind clear and focused (Mohandas 2008).

Increases in vagal stimulation and decrease in cortisol, along with increases in serotonin and endorphins, have also been documented, adding to the evolving explanation of yoga's beneficial effects (Newberg and Iversen 2003).

Yoga has shown benefits as early as prenatally, an area where research interest is high. A review of 10 randomized controlled trials found a statistically significant lowering of prenatal disorders, reduced risk of small for gestational age, and reduced levels of pain and stress in mothers, concluding yoga to be both safe and effective during preg-nancy in the groups studied (Jiang et al. 2015). Prenatal yoga has also been shown to be beneficial in treating maternal depression (Kawanishi et al. 2015), which is associated with an increased risk of adverse fetal outcomes, although the direct cause and effect mechanism remain unclear. It has been shown that prenatal stress alters fetal epigenetic regulation (Braithwaite et al. 2015), and has a detrimental effect on the fetal immune system (Veru et al. 2014).

A 10-week school-based yoga program pilot study (Yoga 4 Classrooms 30-minute weekly class) was administered to a class of second and third grade students with sali-vary cortisol measured at time 0 and after week 10 intervention. Improvement was seen in the second grade class, who showed a significant drop in salivary cortisol over the study period which correlated with before and after behavioral assessment survey by a teacher. Perceived improvement was seen in the second grade class but not the third grade class in this study. Lack of control group, number of other variables in the chil-dren's lives over the 10-week study, and small sample size were obvious barriers, but this study did show successful insertion of a class-based yoga program into an elemen-tary school setting (Butzer et al. 2015).

An after-school-based randomized intervention in 32 fourth and fifth grade inner city students compared a 12-week 1-hour per week yoga class to a no-yoga group. Results showed significant improvement in the post-intervention negative behavior scores and improvement in wellbeing (Berger, Silver, and Stein 2009).

A variety of small studies have examined the benefit of yoga in children with autism and found some improvements in maladaptive behavior (Koenig, Buckley-Reen, and Garg 2012; Rosenblatt et al. 2011).

A systematic review was conducted of 34 controlled studies of yoga in children for a variety of conditions including general physical fitness, ADHD, cardiovascular fit-ness, anxiety, IBS, and eating disorder. Most of the interventions included a variety of postures, breathing, and meditation; however, the great variability of study design and quality precluded firm conclusions or specific recommendations about the use of yoga in any specific condition. No adverse effects were reported in the studies and many reported positive effects on behavior and stress levels. Conclusion of the review was positive for yoga having the potential to increase physical activity and offer new approaches to stress management in children (Birdee et al. 2009).

There is no standard credentialing for teaching yoga to children. A minimum of 200 hours is recognized by the U.S. Yoga Alliance (www.yogaalliance.org), but this applies for adult teaching only.

Tai Chi

Tai chi has been shown in small studies to have a beneficial effect on mood in middle school-aged children with no adverse effects reported, but study variability and small number of participants limit conclusions. A randomized controlled trial showed that an intervention with a Chinese Chan-based mind–body exercise Nei Yang Gong was significantly superior to progressive muscle relaxation in improving self-control in a group of 48 autistic children in a twice a week for 4-week trial. Nei Yang Gong is described as similar to tai chi, with a focus on self-awareness and self-control to foster a calm, relaxed state to achieve smooth circulation of Qi and blood (Chan et al. 2013).

Music Therapy

Music therapy, as defined by the American Music Therapy Association, is the clinical and evidence-based use of music interventions to accomplish individualized goals within a therapeutic relationship by a credentialed professional who has completed a music therapy program degree. Music therapists work closely with nursing and other healthcare professionals to best meet the individual needs of the patient, which often include pain control, distraction, and calming (Stouffer, Shirk, and Polomano 2007).

But more than emotional soothing, music therapy has been shown to have a significant role in enhancing neuroplasticity in the brain throughout the lifespan (Stegemoller 2014).

Music therapy has been used successfully in both the neonatal intensive care unit and pediatric intensive care units for pain control and increased coping (Standley 2012).

Music therapy has also been shown to reduce salivary cortisol and increase pumped volume of breast milk in 30 mothers of premature infants in a randomized controlled trial using 4 sessions of 15 minutes of music therapy (Ak et al. 2015).

Procedural pain and chest physiotherapy are other areas where music has been shown to be efficacious in children. Music therapists work with children and families to find music that is soothing to the child within guidelines of pitch, rhythm, harmony, and tempo—are all integral parts of the auditory and neurological processing of the music. Physiological stress markers such as serum cortisol and inflammatory cytokines have also been shown to be modulated by music therapy in various patient groups. Music can be live or recorded and can be used in both acute and ongoing settings (Stouffer, Shirk, and Polomano 2007).

Use of music therapy during IV placement has been successful in the pediatric emergency department setting, where it was found to facilitate procedures and was appreciated by staff and caretakers as well (Hartling et al. 2013).

Music therapy is also becoming widely used and accepted in pediatric oncology to address procedural pain, anxiety, and caretaker stress. Music therapy has been used successfully during radiation therapy, and for depression and anxiety associated with diagnosis and treatment. Music has been found to reduce sense of isolation and enhance quality of life (Tucquet and Leung 2014).

A review of 26 studies involving the perioperative use of music in pediatric surgery demonstrated a statistically significant positive effect in reduction of post-operative pain, anxiety, and distress in children undergoing a variety of invasive and non-invasive surgery (van der Heijden et al. 2015).

Music therapy has also been shown to improve cardiac parameters including heart rate and blood pressure and to blunt rise in serum glucose in a randomized controlled study in the post-operative setting of a pediatric day surgery unit.

A 2014 Cochrane Database Systematic Review found evidence to support the use of a trained music therapist in children in improvement of skills in social interaction, verbal communication, initiating behavior and social–emotional reciprocity. It was also found to have potential to improve quality of child–parent relationships (Geretsegger et al. 2014) (The American Music Therapy Association at www.musictherapy.org).

Animal-Assisted Therapy

Animal-assisted therapy is an important element of mind–body medicine and has been associated with a range of beneficial health effects. Studies are more plentiful in adults, where animal-assisted therapy has been shown to reduce blood pressure, improve markers of cardiovascular disease, and reduce overall mortality as well as significantly increase physical activity (Halm 2008).

A study following the introduction of therapy dogs into a children's hospital in Italy found significant positive response from children, parents, and staff and saw no change in independently monitored infection rates pre versus post dog introduction (Caprilli and Messeri 2006).

A randomized controlled trial of therapy dogs into a post-operative pediatric setting for 20 minutes (40 children aged 3–17 years) was well received by the children and family. Patients were monitored for EEG changes, heart rate, blood pressure, oxygen saturation, cerebral prefrontal oxygenation, salivary cortisol, and Faces Pain Scale. Study results showed that the study group had reduction in salivary cortisol, faster recovery and alertness after anesthesia, reduced pain perception, and induced a positive emotional response as measured by EEG and cerebral oxygenation (Calcaterra et al. 2015).

Research on the effects of equine-assisted therapy for children with autism has shown encouraging benefit in both motor skills and in social functioning in a growing number of studies (Borgi et al. 2015).

A randomized controlled trial of therapeutic riding in 127 autistic children over a 10-week period showed significant improvements in the treatment group in irritability and hyperactivity by the halfway point of the study. Significant improvements were also seen in social cognition, social communication, and number of words and new words spoken (Gabriels et al. 2015).

More research is needed to determine optimal structure and timing of these interventions.

Spirituality

Prayer is one of the most commonly used complementary practices in the U.S. and may serve as a key organizing principle in a patient's life (Barnes et al. 2004), yet few clinicians receive training in spirituality in healthcare and some may be fearful of initiating a conversation they feel is beyond their scope of practice.

A child's sense of spirituality can help them to develop a structure for coping and offer an important connection to family, community, and culture. Common yet intangible elements of pediatric illness such as nightmares, fear, suffering, loss of control, and facing terminal illness require clinicians to have something to offer that can help children and families in their most vulnerable times. Spirituality can offer some a protective effect and provide a way to bring some sense of meaning to the difficult events that may be unfolding. The downsides of spirituality for children are mainly defined by their lack of ability to decide their own beliefs and may be influenced by the possibility of guilt, exposure to religious vendettas or prejudice, for example, if a belief system is unaccepting of other cultures, homosexuality, or gender. Some belief systems may even withhold medical care from a child in certain situations.

The AAP has a structure for approaching religious traditions and spirituality and recommends that: religious beliefs and practices of the family must be respected; parents must be held accountable for withholding medical care that is likely to result in death or suffering; the constitutional guarantees of freedom of religion do not serve as a valid legal defense when a child is harmed (Schor and American Academy of Pediatrics Task Force on the 2003).

The role of spirituality (not necessarily religion) is of critical importance in healthcare, but is rarely addressed in medical training, despite the fact that large systematic literature reviews (n = 12,327) (Best, Butow, and Olver 2015) have shown that a majority of patients express interest in discussing religion and spirituality in the medical visit, although others do not. The difficulty lies in identifying which is which.

Research by Best et al. on patients who are interested in discussing spirituality have identified four overarching themes: desire for a deeper doctor–patient relationship where the doctor knows them as a person; disempowerment on the part of the patient which leads to hesitation in discussing spiritual matters; the question of spiritual guidance—most patients do not want their doctor to preach to them or expect spiritual advice; spirituality and healing—when patients feel valued by their doctor it has been shown to enhance their ability to cope and to find a sense of meaning in the illness. Conversely, patients who did not want spirituality brought into the medical visit felt questions about spirituality were intrusive, or might imply a more serious illness (Best, Butow, and Olver 2015).

Raising the question of spirituality allows the clinician to delve deeper and see what elements of the patient's character and social connections rise to the surface in times of trouble. It is also important for the practitioner to understand what spiritual perspective they themselves are bringing into the patient interactions.

For example, a 2008 survey on the spiritual practices of 208 academic pediatricians found that 67% felt a religious affiliation and the majority felt that their personal spiritual practice and beliefs influenced their interactions with both patients and colleagues, especially if they attended religious services on a regular basis (Catlin et al. 2008).

A survey of academic pediatric oncologists found that 85% considered themselves spiritual, rather than identifying with a specific religion, although one in four reported attending religious services two to three times per month in the year preceding the survey and more than half felt that their spiritual or religious beliefs impacted their interactions with patients and colleagues (Ecklund et al. 2007).

It can be very illuminating for both patient and clinician to reflect on what brings the patient strength, and what strengths the patient brings to a challenging medical situation.

Preferred approaches to spiritual care identified by patients included: individualized, voluntary, inclusive of clergy, and based on assessment and support of the patient's religion or spirituality. Desired approaches included: the doctor initiating asking about spiritual beliefs, offering encouragement and affirmation, providing compassion, encouraging realistic hope, advice on how to best care for oneself while ill, and discussing the impact of religion and spirituality on medical decision making.

Doctor-initiated prayer was favored overall, but patients felt it was important for the doctor to have a sense of them as a person prior to taking that step. Silent prayer was more accepted in this study group. Spiritual inquiry was most welcomed when the illness was serious, which created desire for a connection to allow better discussion of difficult issues. Overall, patients in the study felt that doctors should make efforts to identify which patients would welcome the discussion (Best, Butow, and Olver 2015).

There are some programs that are working to incorporate spirituality training into practice to help bridge the gap between what patients want and need in the clinical visit, and what training doctors receive. For example, a U.S. medical school, Kansas City University of Medicine and Biosciences, has developed an experiential course on spirituality that is embedded in to the third year of training. Elements of the course include learning to take a spiritual history, understand how the patient's spiritual beliefs impact their health, gain insight into their own spiritual beliefs by writing about their own spiritual history, and highlight the value of the chaplain on the healthcare team (Graves, Shue, and Arnold 2002).

Spirituality in Children

There is a wealth of research on spiritual needs of children in healthcare, especially pertaining to oncology and palliative care settings where skillful intervention directed to the needs of the family and the patient can have tremendous importance (Barnes et al. 2000; Moore, Talwar, and Moxley-Haegert 2015).

Efforts led by Christina Puchalski MD, MS, FACP at the George Washington University School of Medicine and Health Sciences have been instrumental in shaping the field and working on a national and international level to bring consensus to the spiritual elements in healthcare (Puchalski, Vitillo et al. 2014; Vitillo and Puchalski 2014; Puchalski, Blatt et al. 2014). One of the instruments she developed is called the FICA Spiritual History Tool for use in the clinical setting (Puchalski 2014). An example of the FICA:

Faith and belief:

* Do you consider yourself spiritual or religious?
* Do you have spiritual beliefs that help you cope with stress?
* What gives your life meaning?

Importance:

* What importance does your faith or belief have in your life?
* Have your beliefs influenced how you take care of yourself in this illness?
* What role do your beliefs play in regaining your health?

Community:

* Are you part of a spiritual or religious community?
* Is this of support to you and how?
* Is there a group of people you really love or who are important to you?

Address in care:

* How would you like me to address these issues in your healthcare?

Summary

The field of mind–body medicine is expansive and includes a range of approaches including breath work, progressive muscle relaxation, autogenics, biofeedback, guided imagery, clinical hypnosis, mindfulness and compassion meditation, yoga, tai chi, music therapy, spirituality and others. Research in the use of mind–body therapies in children is robust and introduces a flexible range of non-pharmacological approaches that can be used alone or in conjunction with conventional therapies. In addition to addressing pain, stress, and fear, the mind–body therapies offer children the opportunity to develop self-regulation skills, sense of self-efficacy, and confidence that they have potential to benefit children and adolescents in multiple areas of their lives.

Resources

Breath Work

- Commercially available CDs and apps.

Biofeedback

- Board certification in biofeedback is available from organizations such as the Biofeedback Certification International Alliance (www.bcia.org), and Biofeedback Foundation of Europe, although professional licensure in a medical field is not required.
- The Association for Applied Psychology and Biofeedback (www.aapb.org).
- Biofeedback Certification International Alliance (www.bcia.org).
- International Society of Neurofeedback and Research (www.isnr.org).

Guided Imagery

- No Board certification exists.
- Many commercially available CDs.
- Free resource through Kaiser Permanente of Health Journeys podcasts created and narrated by Belleruth Naparstak, LISW, BCD on a wide variety of topics (https://healthy.kaiserpermanente.org/).
- The Academy for Guided Imagery: a 150-hour, mentored, distance learning, certificate program for health professionals in one-on-one interactive guided imagery (http://www.academyforguidedimagery.com/certificationtraining/index.html).

Imagery resources for children include:

- *Shambala Calm and Clarity: Guided Meditations for ADHD, Hyperactive or Busy Kids* by Mellisa Dormoy.
- *Shambala Kids, Relaxed and in Control: Guiding my Emotions for Good Self Control* by Mellisa Dormoy.
- *Magic Island: Relaxation for Kids* by Betty Mehling.
- *The Sleep Fairy: Guided Relaxation for Children* by Lisa Malkiewicz.
- *MindWorks for Children*, guided imagery by Roxanne Daleo, PhD.
- *Mindfulness Meditations for Teens* by Bodhipaksa.

- *Starbright—Meditations for Children* by Maureen Garth.
- *Imaginations: Relaxation Stories and Guided Imagery for Kids* by Carolyn Clarke.
- *The Mindful Child* by Susan Kaiser Greenland.
- *The Mindfulness Revolution* edited by Barry Boyce.
- *Train Your Mind, Change Your Brain* by Sharon Begley.
- *The Relaxation and Stress Reduction Workbook for Kids* by Lawrence Shapiro, PhD.

Hypnosis

- The American Society for Clinical Hypnosis (http://www.asch.net), and The Society for Clinical and Experimental Hypnosis (http://www.sceh.us), membership limited to healthcare professionals, are the primary training resources in the United States. The American Society of Clinical Hypnosis offers recognized certification based on the completion of a rigorous standard of training and supervision.
- Books with information on hypnotic scripts and metaphors for use in children.
  - *Hypnosis and Hypnotherapy with Children*. Karen Olness, MD and Daniel Kohen, 1996, The Guilford Press, NY, NY.
  - *Harry the Hypnopotomous: Metaphorical Tales for the Treatment of Children*. Linda Thompson, PhD, MSN, CPNP, 2005, Crown House Publishing, Ltd., Wales, U.K.
  - *Hypnosis and Hypnotherapy With Children, Fourth Edition*, Apr 1, 2011 by Daniel P. Kohen and Karen Olness.
- The National Pediatric Hypnosis Training Institute: NPHTI offers training and workshop specific to the pediatric population (http://www.nphti.net).

Spirituality

- *Nurturing Spirituality in Children: Simple Hands on Activities* by Peggy Joy Jenkins, PhD.
- *Planting Seeds: Practicing Mindfulness with Children* by Thich Nhat Hanh.
- *The Last Great Adventure of Life: Sacred Resources for Living and Dying from a Hospice Counselor* by Maria Dancing Heart Hoagland.
- Stanford Center for Compassion (www.ccare.stanford.edu/compassionweek2014/).
- Emory Tibet Partnership Compassion Based Cognitive Therapy (www.tibet.emory.edu/cognitively-based-compassion-training/index.html).

References

Ak, J., P. B. Lakshmanagowda, C. M. P. G, and J. Goturu. 2015. "Impact of music therapy on breast milk secretion in mothers of premature newborns." *J Clin Diagn Res* 9(4): CC04–6. doi: 10.7860/JCDR/2015/11642.5776.

Allen, M., M. Dietz, K. S. Blair, M. van Beek, G. Rees, P. Vestergaard-Poulsen, A. Lutz, and A. Roepstorff. 2012. "Cognitive-affective neural plasticity following active-controlled mindfulness intervention." *J Neurosci* 32(44): 15601–10. doi: 10.1523/JNEUROSCI.2957-12.2012.

American Psychiatric Association. 2013. *Diagnostic and Statistical Manual of Mental Disorders* (5th ed.). Washington, D.C.

Anbar, R. D., and M. P. Slothower. 2006. "Hypnosis for treatment of insomnia in school-age children: a retrospective chart review." *BMC Pediatr* 6: 23. doi: 10.1186/1471-2431-6-23.

Astin, J. A., S. L. Shapiro, D. M. Eisenberg, and K. L. Forys. 2003. "Mind-body medicine: state of the science, implications for practice." *J Am Board Fam Pract* 16(2): 131–47.

Barnes, L. L., G. A. Plotnikoff, K. Fox, and S. Pendleton. 2000. "Spirituality, religion, and pediatrics: intersecting worlds of healing." *Pediatrics* 106(4 Suppl): 899–908.

Barnes, P. M., E. Powell-Griner, K. McFann, and R. L. Nahin. 2004. "Complementary and alternative medicine use among adults: United States, 2002." *Adv Data* (343): 1–19.

Benson, H., J. F. Beary, and M. P. Carol. 1974. "The relaxation response." *Psychiatry* 37(1): 37–46.

Berger, D. L., E. J. Silver, and R. E. Stein. 2009. "Effects of yoga on inner-city children's well-being: a pilot study." *Altern Ther Health Med* 15(5): 36–42.

Best, M., P. Butow, and I. Olver. 2015. "Do patients want doctors to talk about spirituality? A systematic literature review." *Patient Educ Couns*. doi: 10.1016/j.pec.2015.04.017.

Bhasin, M. K., J. A. Dusek, B. H. Chang, M. G. Joseph, J. W. Denninger, G. L. Fricchione, H. Benson, and T. A. Libermann. 2013. "Relaxation response induces temporal transcriptome changes in energy metabolism, insulin secretion and inflammatory pathways." *PLoS One* 8(5): e62817. doi: 10.1371/journal.pone.0062817.

Biegel, G. M., K. W. Brown, S. L. Shapiro, and C. M. Schubert. 2009. "Mindfulness-based stress reduction for the treatment of adolescent psychiatric outpatients:a randomized clinical trial." *J Consult Clin Psychol* 77(5): 855–66. doi: 10.1037/a0016241.

Birdee, G. S., G. Y. Yeh, P. M. Wayne, R. S. Phillips, R. B. Davis, and P. Gardiner. 2009. "Clinical applications of yoga for the pediatric population: a systematic review." *Acad Pediatr* 9(4): 212–220 e1–9. doi: 10.1016/j.acap.2009.04.002.

Black, L. I., T. C. Clarke, P. M. Barnes, B. J. Stussman, and R. L. Nahin. 2015. "Use of complementary health approaches among children aged 4–17 years in the United States: National Health Interview Survey, 2007–2012." *Natl Health Stat Report* 78: 1–19.

Blood, J. D., J. Wu, T. M. Chaplin, R. Hommer, L. Vazquez, H. J. Rutherford, L. C. Mayes, and M. J. Crowley. 2015. "The variable heart: high frequency and very low frequency correlates of depressive symptoms in children and adolescents." *J Affect Disord* 186: 119–126. doi: 10.1016/j.jad.2015.06.057.

Borgi, M., D. Loliva, S. Cerino, F. Chiarotti, A. Venerosi, M. Bramini, E. Nonnis, M. Marcelli, C. Vinti, C. De Santis, F. Bisacco, M. Fagerlie, M. Frascarelli, and F. Cirulli. 2015. "Effectiveness of a standardized equine-assisted therapy program for children with autism spectrum disorder." *J Autism Dev Disord*. doi: 10.1007/s10803-015-2530-6.

Bower, J. E., and M. R. Irwin. 2015. "Mind-body therapies and control of inflammatory biology: a descriptive review." *Brain Behav Immun*. doi: 10.1016/j.bbi.2015.06.012.

Braithwaite, E. C., M. Kundakovic, P. G. Ramchandani, S. E. Murphy, and F. A. Champagne. 2015. "Maternal prenatal depressive symptoms predict infant NR3C1 1F and BDNF IV DNA methylation." *Epigenetics* 10(5): 408–17. doi: 10.1080/15592294.2015.1039221.

British Autogenic Society. http://www.autogenic-therapy.org.uk/index.htm.

Brown, D. 2007. "Evidence-based hypnotherapy for asthma: a critical review." *Int J Clin Exp Hypn* 55 (2): 220–49. doi: 10.1080/00207140601177947.

Butler, L. D., B. K. Symons, S. L. Henderson, L. D. Shortliffe, and D. Spiegel. 2005. "Hypnosis reduces distress and duration of an invasive medical procedure for children." *Pediatrics* 115(1): e77–85. doi: 10.1542/peds.2004-0818.

Butzer, B., D. Day, A. Potts, C. Ryan, S. Coulombe, B. Davies, K. Weidknecht, M. Ebert, L. Flynn, and S. B. Khalsa. 2015. "Effects of a classroom-based yoga intervention on cortisol and behavior in second- and third-grade students: a pilot study." *J Evid Based Complementary Altern Med* 20(1): 41–9. doi: 10.1177/2156587214557695.

Calcaterra, V., P. Veggiotti, C. Palestrini, V. De Giorgis, R. Raschetti, M. Tumminelli, S. Mencherini, F. Papotti, C. Klersy, R. Albertini, S. Ostuni, and G. Pelizzo. 2015. "Post-operative benefits of animal-assisted therapy in pediatric surgery: a randomised study." *PLoS One* 10(6): e0125813. doi: 10.1371/journal.pone.0125813.

Cannon, Walter B. MD. 1963. *The Wisdom of the Body*. New York: W. W. Norton & Company.

Caprilli, S., and A. Messeri. 2006. "Animal-assisted activity at A. Meyer Children's Hospital: a pilot study." *Evid Based Complement Alternat Med* 3(3): 379–83. doi: 10.1093/ecam/nel029.

Carlson, L. E., T. L. Beattie, J. Giese-Davis, P. Faris, R. Tamagawa, L. J. Fick, E. S. Degelman, and M. Speca. 2015. "Mindfulness-based cancer recovery and supportive-expressive therapy maintain telomere length relative to controls in distressed breast cancer survivors." *Cancer* 121(3): 476–84. doi: 10.1002/cncr.29063.

Catlin, E. A., W. Cadge, E. H. Ecklund, E. A. Gage, and A. A. Zollfrank. 2008. "The spiritual and religious identities, beliefs, and practices of academic pediatricians in the United States." *Acad Med* 83(12): 1146–52. doi: 10.1097/ACM.0b013e31818c64a5.

Chambers, C. T., A. Taddio, L. S. Uman, C. M. McMurtry, and H. ELPinKIDS Team. 2009. "Psychological interventions for reducing pain and distress during routine childhood immunizations: a systematic review." *Clin Ther* 31(Suppl 2): S77–103. doi: 10.1016/j.clinthera.2009.07.023.

Chan, A. S., S. L. Sze, N. Y. Siu, E. M. Lau, and M. C. Cheung. 2013. "A Chinese mind-body exercise improves self-control of children with autism: a randomized controlled trial." *PLoS One* 8(7): e68184. doi: 10.1371/journal.pone.0068184.

Chang, J. S., E. Y. Kim, D. Jung, S. H. Jeong, Y. Kim, M. S. Roh, Y. M. Ahn, and B. J. Hahm. 2015. "Altered cardiorespiratory coupling in young male adults with excessive online gaming." *Biol Psychol*. doi: 10.1016/j.biopsycho.2015.07.016.

Chiang, L. C., W. F. Ma, J. L. Huang, L. F. Tseng, and K. C. Hsueh. 2009. "Effect of relaxation-breathing training on anxiety and asthma signs/symptoms of children with moderate-to-severe asthma: a randomized controlled trial." *Int J Nurs Stud* 46(8): 1061–70. doi: 10.1016/j.ijnurstu.2009.01.013.

Cohen, J. A., and A. P. Mannarino. 2015. "Trauma-focused cognitive behavior therapy for traumatized children and families." *Child Adolesc Psychiatr Clin N Am* 24(3): 557–70. doi: 10.1016/j.chc.2015.02.005.

Denkowski, K. M., and G. C. Denkowski. 1984. "Is group progressive relaxation training as effective with hyperactive children as individual EMG biofeedback treatment?" *Biofeedback Self Regul* 9(3): 353–64.

Dobson, C. E., and M. W. Byrne. 2014. "Original research: using guided imagery to manage pain in young children with sickle cell disease." *Am J Nurs* 114(4): 26–36; test 37, 47. doi: 10.1097/01.NAJ.0000445680.06812.6a.

Dykens, E. M., M. H. Fisher, J. L. Taylor, W. Lambert, and N. Miodrag. 2014. "Reducing distress in mothers of children with autism and other disabilities: a randomized trial." *Pediatrics* 134(2): e454–63. doi: 10.1542/peds.2013–3164.

Ecklund, E. H., W. Cadge, E. A. Gage, and E. A. Catlin. 2007. "The religious and spiritual beliefs and practices of academic pediatric oncologists in the United States." *J Pediatr Hematol Oncol* 29(11): 736–42. doi: 10.1097/MPH.0b013e31815a0e39.

Entringer, S., E. S. Epel, R. Kumsta, J. Lin, D. H. Hellhammer, E. H. Blackburn, S. Wust, and P. D. Wadhwa. 2011. "Stress exposure in intrauterine life is associated with shorter telomere length in young adulthood." *Proc Natl Acad Sci U S A* 108(33): E513–8. doi: 10.1073/pnas.1107759108.

Entringer, S., E. S. Epel, J. Lin, C. Buss, B. Shahbaba, E. H. Blackburn, H. N. Simhan, and P. D. Wadhwa. 2013. "Maternal psychosocial stress during pregnancy is associated with newborn leukocyte telomere length." *Am J Obstet Gynecol* 208(2): 134 e1–7. doi: 10.1016/j.ajog.2012.11.033.

Epel, E., J. Daubenmier, J. T. Moskowitz, S. Folkman, and E. Blackburn. 2009. "Can meditation slow rate of cellular aging? Cognitive stress, mindfulness, and telomeres." *Ann N Y Acad Sci* 1172: 34–53. doi: 10.1111/j.1749-6632.2009.04414.x.

Evans, S., J. C. Tsao, and L. K. Zeltzer. 2008. "Complementary and alternative medicine for acute procedural pain in children." *Altern Ther Health Med* 14(5): 52–6.

Flook, L., S. B. Goldberg, L. Pinger, and R. J. Davidson. 2015. "Promoting prosocial behavior and self-regulatory skills in preschool children through a mindfulness-based Kindness Curriculum." *Dev Psychol* 51(1): 44–51. doi: 10.1037/a0038256.

Fortney, L., C. Luchterhand, L. Zakletskaia, A. Zgierska, and D. Rakel. 2013. "Abbreviated mindfulness intervention for job satisfaction, quality of life, and compassion in primary care clinicians: a pilot study." *Ann Fam Med* 11(5): 412–20. doi: 10.1370/afm.1511.

Fovet, T., R. Jardri, and D. Linden. 2015. "Current issues in the use of fMRI-based neurofeedback to relieve psychiatric symptoms." *Curr Pharm Des* 21(23): 3384–94.

Fox, K. C., S. Nijeboer, M. L. Dixon, J. L. Floman, M. Ellamil, S. P. Rumak, P. Sedlmeier, and K. Christoff. 2014. "Is meditation associated with altered brain structure? A systematic review and meta-analysis of morphometric neuroimaging in meditation practitioners." *Neurosci Biobehav Rev* 43: 48–73. doi: 10.1016/j.neubiorev.2014.03.016.

Friedrich, E. V., A. Sivanathan, T. Lim, N. Suttie, S. Louchart, S. Pillen, and J. A. Pineda. 2015. "An effective neurofeedback intervention to improve social interactions in children with autism spectrum disorder." *J Autism Dev Disord.* doi: 10.1007/s10803-015-2523-5.

Friedrich, E. V., N. Suttie, A. Sivanathan, T. Lim, S. Louchart, and J. A. Pineda. 2014. "Brain-computer interface game applications for combined neurofeedback and biofeedback treatment for children on the autism spectrum." *Front Neuroeng* 7: 21. doi: 10.3389/fneng.2014.00021.

Gabriels, R. L., Z. Pan, B. Dechant, J. A. Agnew, N. Brim, and G. Mesibov. 2015. "Randomized controlled trial of therapeutic horseback riding in children and adolescents with autism spectrum disorder." *J Am Acad Child Adolesc Psychiatry* 54(7): 541–9. doi: 10.1016/j.jaac.2015.04.007.

Geretsegger, M., C. Elefant, K. A. Mossler, and C. Gold. 2014. "Music therapy for people with autism spectrum disorder." *Cochrane Database Syst Rev* 6: CD004381. doi: 10.1002/14651858.CD004381.pub3.

Goldstein, D. S. 2010. "Adrenal responses to stress." *Cell Mol Neurobiol* 30(8): 1433–40. doi: 10.1007/s10571-010-9606-9.

Gotink, R. A., P. Chu, J. J. Busschbach, H. Benson, G. L. Fricchione, and M. G. Hunink. 2015. "Standardised mindfulness-based interventions in healthcare: an overview of systematic reviews and meta-analyses of RCTs." *PLoS One* 10(4): e0124344. doi: 10.1371/journal.pone.0124344.

Graves, D. L., C. K. Shue, and L. Arnold. 2002. "The role of spirituality in patient care: incorporating spirituality training into medical school curriculum." *Acad Med* 77(11): 1167.

Green, J. P., A. F. Barabasz, D. Barrett, and G. H. Montgomery. 2005. "Forging ahead: the 2003 APA Division 30 definition of hypnosis." *Int J Clin Exp Hypn* 53(3): 259–64. doi: 10.1080/00207140590961321.

Gruzelier, J. H. 2002. "A review of the impact of hypnosis, relaxation, guided imagery and individual differences on aspects of immunity and health." *Stress* 5(2): 147–63. doi: 10.1080/10253890290027877.

Halm, M. A. 2008. "The healing power of the human-animal connection." *Am J Crit Care* 17(4): 373–6.

Hartling, L., A. S. Newton, Y. Liang, H. Jou, K. Hewson, T. P. Klassen, and S. Curtis. 2013. "Music to reduce pain and distress in the pediatric emergency department: a randomized clinical trial." *JAMA Pediatr* 167(9): 826–35. doi: 10.1001/jamapediatrics.2013.200.

Hashim, H. A., and H. Hanafi Ahmad Yusof. 2011. "The effects of progressive muscle relaxation and autogenic relaxation on young soccer players' mood states." *Asian J Sports Med* 2(2): 99–105.

Hashim, H. A., and N. A. Zainol. 2015. "Changes in emotional distress, short term memory, and sustained attention following 6 and 12 sessions of progressive muscle relaxation training in 10–11 years old primary school children." *Psychol Health Med* 20(5): 623–8. doi: 10.1080/13548506.2014.1002851.

Hemphill, S. A., M. Tollit, and T. I. Herrenkohl. 2014. "Protective factors against the impact of school bullying perpetration and victimization on young adult externalizing and internalizing problems." *J Sch Violence* 13(1): 125–145. doi: 10.1080/15388220.2013.844072.

Holzel, B. K., J. Carmody, M. Vangel, C. Congleton, S. M. Yerramsetti, T. Gard, and S. W. Lazar. 2011. "Mindfulness practice leads to increases in regional brain gray matter density." *Psychiatry Res* 191(1): 36–43. doi: 10.1016/j.pscychresns.2010.08.006.

Jensen, M. P., and D. R. Patterson. 2014. "Hypnotic approaches for chronic pain management: clinical implications of recent research findings." *Am Psychol* 69(2): 167–77. doi: 10.1037/a0035644.

Jiang, Q., Z. Wu, L. Zhou, J. Dunlop, and P. Chen. 2015. "Effects of yoga intervention during pregnancy: a review for current status." *Am J Perinatol* 32(6): 503–14. doi: 10.1055/s-0034-1396701.

Johnson, S. B., A. W. Riley, D. A. Granger, and J. Riis. 2013. "The science of early life toxic stress for pediatric practice and advocacy." *Pediatrics* 131(2): 319–27. doi: 10.1542/peds.2012-0469.

Kabat-Zinn, J. 1982. "An outpatient program in behavioral medicine for chronic pain patients based on the practice of mindfulness meditation: theoretical considerations and preliminary results." *Gen Hosp Psychiatry* 4(1): 33–47.

Kabat-Zinn, J., L. Lipworth, and R. Burney. 1985. "The clinical use of mindfulness meditation for the self-regulation of chronic pain." *J Behav Med* 8(2): 163–90.

Kajbafzadeh, A. M., L. Sharifi-Rad, S. M. Ghahestani, H. Ahmadi, M. Kajbafzadeh, and A. H. Mahboubi. 2011. "Animated biofeedback: an ideal treatment for children with dysfunctional elimination syndrome." *J Urol* 186(6): 2379–84. doi: 10.1016/j.juro.2011.07.118.

Kaslovsky, R., and D. Gottsegen. 2015. "Hypnosis for asthma and vocal cord dysfunction in a patient with autism." *Am J Clin Hypn* 58(2): 195–203. doi: 10.1080/00029157.2014.989566.

Kawanishi, Y., S. J. Hanley, K. Tabata, Y. Nakagi, T. Ito, E. Yoshioka, T. Yoshida, and Y. Saijo. 2015. "Effects of prenatal yoga: a systematic review of randomized controlled trials." *Nihon Koshu Eisei Zasshi* 62(5): 221–31. doi: 10.11236/jph.62.5_221.

Kaye, J. D., and L. S. Palmer. 2008. "Animated biofeedback yields more rapid results than non-animated biofeedback in the treatment of dysfunctional voiding in girls." *J Urol* 180(1): 300–5. doi: 10.1016/j.juro.2008.03.078.

Kerrigan, D., K. Johnson, M. Stewart, T. Magyari, N. Hutton, J. M. Ellen, and E. M. Sibinga. 2011. "Perceptions, experiences, and shifts in perspective occurring among urban youth participating in a mindfulness-based stress reduction program." *Complement Ther Clin Pract* 17(2): 96–101. doi: 10.1016/j.ctcp.2010.08.003.

Koenig, K. P., A. Buckley-Reen, and S. Garg. 2012. "Efficacy of the Get Ready to Learn yoga program among children with autism spectrum disorders: a pretest-posttest control group design." *Am J Occup Ther* 66(5): 538–46. doi: 10.5014/ajot.2012.004390.

Kohen, D. P., K. N. Olness, S. O. Colwell, and A. Heimel. 1984. "The use of relaxation-mental imagery(self-hypnosis) in the management of 505 pediatric behavioral encounters." *J Dev Behav Pediatr* 5(1): 21–5.

Kohen, D. P., Kaiser, P. 2014. "Clinical hypnosis with children and adolescents—What? Why? How?: origins, applications, and efficacy." *Children.* 74–98.

Kuhlmann, S. M., A. Burger, G. Esser, and F. Hammerle. 2015. "A mindfulness-based stress prevention training for medical students (MediMind): study protocol for a randomized controlled trial." *Trials* 16: 40. doi: 10.1186/s13063-014-0533-9.

Labbe, E. E. 1995. "Treatment of childhood migraine with autogenic training and skin temperature biofeedback: a component analysis." *Headache* 35(1): 10–3.

Lahmann, C., M. Nickel, T. Schuster, N. Sauer, J. Ronel, M. Noll-Hussong, K. Tritt, D. Nowak, F. Rohricht, and T. Loew. 2009. "Functional relaxation and guided imagery as complementary therapy in asthma: a randomized controlled clinical trial." *Psychother Psychosom* 78(4): 233–9. doi: 10.1159/000214445.

Larsson, B., J. Carlsson, A. Fichtel, and L. Melin. 2005. "Relaxation treatment of adolescent headache sufferers: results from a school-based replication series." *Headache* 45(6): 692–704. doi: 10.1111/j.1526-4610.2005.05138.x.

Lee, J. 2013. "Maternal stress, well-being, and impaired sleep in mothers of children with developmental disabilities: a literature review." *Res Dev Disabil* 34(11): 4255–73. doi: 10.1016/j.ridd.2013.09.008.

Lehrer, P. M. 1996. "Varieties of relaxation methods and their unique effects. ." *Int J Stress Manag* 3(1): 1–15.

Lehrer, P. M., and R. Gevirtz. 2014. "Heart rate variability biofeedback: how and why does it work?" *Front Psychol* 5: 756. doi: 10.3389/fpsyg.2014.00756.

Lin, Y. C., A. C. Lee, K. J. Kemper, and C. B. Berde. 2005. "Use of complementary and alternative medicine in pediatric pain management service: a survey." *Pain Med* 6(6): 452–8. doi: 10.1111/j.1526-4637.2005.00071.x.

Lofthouse, N., L. E. Arnold, S. Hersch, E. Hurt, and R. DeBeus. 2012. "A review of neurofeedback treatment for pediatric ADHD." *J Atten Disord* 16(5): 351–72. doi: 10.1177/1087054711427530.

Martin, S. J., and R. G. Morris. 2002. "New life in an old idea: the synaptic plasticity and memory hypothesis revisited." *Hippocampus* 12(5): 609–36. doi: 10.1002/hipo.10107.

Mayer, K., S. N. Wyckoff, and U. Strehl. 2013. "One size fits all? Slow cortical potentials neurofeedback: a review." *J Atten Disord* 17(5): 393–409. doi: 10.1177/1087054712468053.

McBride, J. J., A. M. Vlieger, and R. D. Anbar. 2014. "Hypnosis in paediatric respiratory medicine." *Paediatr Respir Rev* 15(1): 82–5. doi: 10.1016/j.prrv.2013.09.002.

McClafferty, H. 2011. "Complementary, holistic, and integrative medicine:mind-body medicine." *Pediatr Rev* 32(5): 201–3. doi: 10.1542/pir.32-5-201.

McCraty, R., and F. Shaffer. 2015. "Heart Rate variability: new perspectives on physiological mechanisms, assessment of self-regulatory capacity, and health risk." *Glob Adv Health Med* 4(1): 46–61. doi: 10.7453/gahmj.2014.073.

McEwen, B. S. 1998. "Stress, adaptation, and disease. Allostasis and allostatic load." *Ann N Y Acad Sci* 840: 33–44.

McEwen, B. S., and E. Stellar. 1993. "Stress and the individual. Mechanisms leading to disease." *Arch Intern Med* 153(18): 2093–101.

Mel, B. W. 2002. "Have we been hebbing down the wrong path?" *Neuron* 34(2): 175–7.

Mohandas, E. 2008. "Neurobiology of Spirituality." *Mens Sana Monogr* 6(1): 63–80.

Moore, K., V. Talwar, and L. Moxley-Haegert. 2015. "Definitional ceremonies: narrative practices for psychologists to inform interdisciplinary teams' understanding of children's spirituality in pediatric settings." *J Health Psychol* 20(3): 259–72. doi: 10.1177/1359105314566610.

Newberg, A. B., and J. Iversen. 2003. "The neural basis of the complex mental task of meditation: neurotransmitter and neurochemical considerations." *Med Hypotheses* 61(2): 282–91.

Nilsson, S., M. Forsner, B. Finnstrom, and E. Morelius. 2015. "Relaxation and guided imagery do not reduce stress, pain and unpleasantness for 11- to 12-year-old girls during vaccinations." *Acta Paediatr* 104(7): 724–9. doi: 10.1111/apa.13000.

Palsson, O. S. 2015. "Hypnosis treatment of gastrointestinal disorders: a comprehensive review of the empirical evidence." *Am J Clin Hypn* 58(2): 134–58. doi: 10.1080/00029157.2015.1039114.

Parisi, P., L. Papetti, A. Spalice, F. Nicita, F. Ursitti, and M. P. Villa. 2011. "Tension-type headache in paediatric age." *Acta Paediatr* 100(4): 491–5. doi: 10.1111/j.1651-2227.2010.02115.x.

Perry-Parrish, C., Copeland-Linder, N., Webb, L.,Shields, AH., Sibinga, EM. 2016. "Mindfulness-Based Approaches for Children and Youth." *Curr Probl Pediatr Adolesc Health Care* 46(6): 172–8. doi: 10.1016/j.cppeds.2015.12.006. Epub 2016 Mar 8.

Platania-Solazzo, A., T. M. Field, J. Blank, F. Seligman, C. Kuhn, S. Schanberg, and P. Saab. 1992. "Relaxation therapy reduces anxiety in child and adolescent psychiatric patients." *Acta Paedopsychiatr* 55(2): 115–20.

Puchalski, C. M. 2014. "The FICA Spiritual History Tool #274." *J Palliat Med* 17(1): 105–6. doi: 10.1089/jpm.2013.9458.

Puchalski, C. M., B. Blatt, M. Kogan, and A. Butler. 2014. "Spirituality and health: the development of a field." *Acad Med* 89(1): 10–6. doi: 10.1097/ACM.0000000000000083.

Puchalski, C. M., R. Vitillo, S. K. Hull, and N. Reller. 2014. "Improving the spiritual dimension of whole person care: reaching national and international consensus." *J Palliat Med* 17(6): 642–56. doi: 10.1089/jpm.2014.9427.

Richter, N. C. 1984. "The efficacy of relaxation training with children." *J Abnorm Child Psychol* 12(2): 319–44.

Rosen, L., French, A., Sullivan, G. 2015. "Complementary, Holistic, and Integrative Medicine: Yoga." *Pediatr Rev* 36(10): 468–74. doi: 10.1542/pir.36-10-468.

Rosenblatt, L. E., S. Gorantla, J. A. Torres, R. S. Yarmush, S. Rao, E. R. Park, J. W. Denninger, H. Benson, G. L. Fricchione, B. Bernstein, and J. B. Levine. 2011. "Relaxation response-based yoga improves functioning in young children with autism: a pilot study." *J Altern Complement Med* 17(11): 1029–35. doi: 10.1089/acm.2010.0834.

Rosenkranz, M. A., R. J. Davidson, D. G. Maccoon, J. F. Sheridan, N. H. Kalin, and A. Lutz. 2013. "A comparison of mindfulness-based stress reduction and an active control in modulation of neurogenic inflammation." *Brain Behav Immun* 27(1): 174–84. doi: 10.1016/j.bbi.2012.10.013.

Russell, M. E., B. Hoffman, S. Stromberg, and C. R. Carlson. 2014. "Use of controlled diaphragmatic breathing for the management of motion sickness in a virtual reality environment." *Appl Psychophysiol Biofeedback* 39(3–4): 269–77. doi: 10.1007/s10484-014-9265-6.

Schor, E. L., and American Academy of Pediatrics Task Force on the. 2003. "Family pediatrics: report of the Task Force on the Family." *Pediatrics* 111(6 Pt 2): 1541–71.

Schutte, N. S., and J. M. Malouff. 2014. "A meta-analytic review of the effects of mindfulness meditation on telomerase activity." *Psychoneuroendocrinology* 42: 45–8. doi: 10.1016/j.psyneuen.2013.12.017.

Sener, N. C., A. Altunkol, U. Unal, H. Ercil, O. Bas, K. Gumus, H. Ciftci, and E. Yeni. 2015. "Can a four-session biofeedback regimen be used effectively for treating children with dysfunctional voiding?" *Int Urol Nephrol* 47(1): 5–9. doi: 10.1007/s11255-014-0837-4.

Sgoifo, A., L. Carnevali, M. L. Pico Alfonso, and M. Amore. 2015. "Autonomic dysfunction and heart rate variability in depression." *Stress* 18(3): 1–10. doi: 10.3109/10253890.2015.1045868.

Shaffer, F., R. McCraty, and C. L. Zerr. 2014. "A healthy heart is not a metronome: an integrative review of the heart's anatomy and heart rate variability." *Front Psychol* 5: 1040. doi: 10.3389/fpsyg.2014.01040.

Sibinga, EM, Webb L., Ghazarian, SR., Ellen, JM. "School-Based Mindfulness Instruction: an RCT." *Pediatrics* 137(1). doi: 10.1542/peds.2015-2532. Epub 2015 Dec 18.

Shockey, D. P., V. Menzies, D. F. Glick, A. G. Taylor, A. Boitnott, and V. Rovnyak. 2013. "Preprocedural distress in children with cancer: an intervention using biofeedback and relaxation." *J Pediatr Oncol Nurs* 30(3): 129–38. doi: 10.1177/1043454213479035.

Shonkoff, J. P., A. S. Garner, Child Committee on Psychosocial Aspects of, Health Family, Adoption Committee on Early Childhood, Care Dependent, Developmental Section on, and Pediatrics Behavioral. 2012. "The lifelong effects of early childhood adversity and toxic stress." *Pediatrics* 129(1): e232–46. doi: 10.1542/peds.2011-2663.

Simkin, D. R., and N. B. Black. 2014. "Meditation and mindfulness in clinical practice." *Child Adolesc Psychiatr Clin N Am* 23(3): 487–534. doi: 10.1016/j.chc.2014.03.002.

Standley, J. 2012. "Music therapy research in the NICU: an updated meta-analysis." *Neonatal Netw* 31(5): 311–16. doi: 10.1891/0730-0832.31.5.311.

Stegemoller, E. L. 2014. "Exploring a neuroplasticity model of music therapy." *J Music Ther* 51(3): 211–27. doi: 10.1093/jmt/thu023.

Steiner, N. J., E. C. Frenette, K. M. Rene, R. T. Brennan, and E. C. Perrin. 2014. "In-school neurofeedback training for ADHD: sustained improvements from a randomized control trial." *Pediatrics* 133(3): 483–92. doi: 10.1542/peds.2013-2059.

Stouffer, J. W., B. J. Shirk, and R. C. Polomano. 2007. "Practice guidelines for music interventions with hospitalized pediatric patients." *J Pediatr Nurs* 22(6): 448–56. doi: 10.1016/j.pedn.2007.04.011.

Stromberg, S. E., M. E. Russell, and C. R. Carlson. 2015. "Diaphragmatic breathing and its effectiveness for the management of motion sickness." *Aerosp Med Hum Perform* 86(5): 452–7. doi: 10.3357/AMHP.4152.2015.

Sun, S., Z. Yao, J. Wei, and R. Yu. 2015. "Calm and smart? A selective review of meditation effects on decision making." *Front Psychol* 6: 1059. doi: 10.3389/fpsyg.2015.01059.

Tang, Y. Y., B. K. Holzel, and M. I. Posner. 2015. "The neuroscience of mindfulness meditation." *Nat Rev Neurosci* 16(4): 213–25. doi: 10.1038/nrn3916.

Taylor, D. J., and B. M. Roane. 2010. "Treatment of insomnia in adults and children: a practice-friendly review of research." *J Clin Psychol* 66(11): 1137–47. doi: 10.1002/jclp.20733.

Termine, C., A. Ozge, F. Antonaci, S. Natriashvili, V. Guidetti, and C. Wober-Bingol. 2011. "Overview of diagnosis and management of paediatric headache. Part II: therapeutic management." *J Headache Pain* 12(1): 25–34. doi: 10.1007/s10194-010-0256-6.

Trakhtenberg, E. C. 2008. "The effects of guided imagery on the immune system: a critical review." *Int J Neurosci* 118(6): 839–55. doi: 10.1080/00207450701792705.

Tucquet, B., and M. Leung. 2014. "Music therapy services in pediatric oncology: a national clinical practice review." *J Pediatr Oncol Nurs* 31(6): 327–38. doi: 10.1177/1043454214533424.

Tugtepe, H., D. T. Thomas, R. Ergun, T. Abdullayev, C. Kastarli, A. Kaynak, and T. E. Dagli. 2015. "Comparison of biofeedback therapy in children with treatment-refractory dysfunctional voiding and overactive bladder." *Urology* 85(4): 900–4. doi: 10.1016/j.urology.2014.12.031.

van der Heijden, M. J., S. Oliai Araghi, M. van Dijk, J. Jeekel, and M. G. Hunink. 2015. "The effects of perioperative music interventions in pediatric surgery: a systematic review and meta-analysis of randomized controlled trials." *PLoS One* 10(8): e0133608. doi: 10.1371/journal.pone.0133608.

van Tilburg, M. A., D. K. Chitkara, O. S. Palsson, M. Turner, N. Blois-Martin, M. Ulshen, and W. E. Whitehead. 2009. "Audio-recorded guided imagery treatment reduces functional abdominal pain in children: a pilot study." *Pediatrics* 124(5): e890–7. doi: 10.1542/peds.2009-0028.

Veru, F., D. P. Laplante, G. Luheshi, and S. King. 2014. "Prenatal maternal stress exposure and immune function in the offspring." *Stress* 17(2): 133–48. doi: 10.3109/10253890.2013.876404.

Vitillo, R., and C. Puchalski. 2014. "World Health Organization authorities promote greater attention and action on palliative care." *J Palliat Med* 17(9): 988–9. doi: 10.1089/jpm.2014.9411.

Vohra, S., McClafferty, H., et al. 2106. "Mind Body Therapies in Children and Youth." Section on Integrative Medicine. *Pediatrics* 138(3). pii: e20161896. doi: 10.1542/peds.2016-1896. Epub 2016 Aug 22.

Weigensberg, M. J., C. J. Lane, Q. Avila, K. Konersman, E. Ventura, T. Adam, Z. Shoar, M. I. Goran, and D. Spruijt-Metz. 2014. "Imagine HEALTH: results from a randomized pilot lifestyle intervention for obese Latino adolescents using Interactive Guided ImagerySM." *BMC Complement Altern Med* 14: 28. doi: 10.1186/1472-6882-14-28.

West, C. P., L. N. Dyrbye, J. T. Rabatin, T. G. Call, J. H. Davidson, A. Multari, S. A. Romanski, J. M. Hellyer, J. A. Sloan, and T. D. Shanafelt. 2014. "Intervention to promote physician well-being, job satisfaction, and professionalism: a randomized clinical trial." *JAMA Intern Med* 174(4): 527–33. doi: 10.1001/jamainternmed.2013.14387.

Weydert, J. A., D. E. Shapiro, S. A. Acra, C. J. Monheim, A. S. Chambers, and T. M. Ball. 2006. "Evaluation of guided imagery as treatment for recurrent abdominal pain in children: a randomized controlled trial." *BMC Pediatr* 6: 29. doi: 10.1186/1471-2431-6-29.

Wolke, D., and S. T. Lereya. 2015. "Long-term effects of bullying." *Arch Dis Child*. doi: 10.1136/archdischild-2014-306667.

Zenner, C., S. Herrnleben-Kurz, and H. Walach. 2014. "Mindfulness-based interventions in schools-a systematic review and meta-analysis." *Front Psychol* 5: 603. doi: 10.3389/fpsyg.2014.00603.

7 Sleep

Introduction

Emerging science has shown that sleep is a surprisingly complex process. The circadian rhythm is rooted in evolution, exquisitely sensitive to light, and part of an elegant feedback loop that involves endocrine, immune, metabolic, skeletal muscle, and nervous system functions (van Diepen, Foster, and Meijer 2015).

The suprachiasmatic nuclei of the hypothalamus is considered the "master circadian clock" in mammals and is located immediately above the optic nerve. The cells in this area have a unique array of peptides and neurotransmitters that have been shown to regulate gene function throughout the body. It has also been shown that peripheral circadian oscillators are found in most tissues in multicellular organisms, entrained to the suprachiasmatic nuclei through sophisticated neural and hormonal signals (Fonken and Nelson 2014).

It has been hypothesized that these distributed oscillators may play a role in the wide array of metabolic disruptions seen when sleep duration and quality are compromised.

Restorative sleep is a critical element of good health in children and adolescents, although there is evidence suggesting that sleep duration in children and adolescents has declined over time (Matricciani, Olds, and Petkov 2012).

It has been estimated that one in four children experience a significant sleep disturbance at some point in childhood, leading to disruption of parents' sleep, lost work days and substantial healthcare expense (Owens and Dalzell 2005; Mindell et al. 2006).

Rapid Eye Movement (REM) and Slow Wave Sleep

The two broad categories of sleep, slow wave sleep and rapid eye movement sleep, are both necessary in proper proportion for good health. Rapid eye movement (REM) sleep is associated with cognitive functions, memory storage, and growth of the central nervous system. REM sleep decreases from about 50% of total sleep in infancy to about 20% of sleep after the age of 3–5 years. Slow wave sleep is more broadly associated with restoration and cell repair (Bharti, Mehta, and Malhi 2013).

Sleep Disorders in Young Children

Sleep disorders may be categorized as insufficient sleep quantity or poor sleep quality. Sleep disruptions are typical in infants who have unpredictable sleep cycles of wake-sleep episodes throughout the day. Sleep in infants generally organizes by 6 months, a time when many infants sleep through the night in blocks of 6 or more hours (Tikotzky and Sadeh 2010).

Fortunately, a majority of pediatric sleep disorders in younger children are preventable, and many have been shown to be responsive to behavioral interventions. Some of the most common approaches include: unmodified extinction (cry it out); graduated extinction (allow to cry but parents check at extending intervals while child ideally learns self-soothing behaviors); and bedtime fading (progressively adjusting bedtime forward with positive reinforcement). Strongest support exists for extinction, especially when accompanied by parental education (Moore 2010).

Early training of parents to put infants to bed sleepy but awake has shown to help infants develop independent sleep skills most reliably.

Epidemiologic studies show that certain sleep disorders are relatively common in children: for example, insomnia had a prevalence of 20% in a cross-sectional sample of 700 children ages 5–12 years, and increased to 30% in girls aged 11–12 years old (Calhoun et al. 2014).

Obstructive sleep apnea is seen in 1%–5% of children, and parasomnias (sleep walking, night terrors, confusional arousals) range from approximately 5% to 35% depending on the type. Sleep-related movement disorders, for example, restless leg syndrome, affect approximately 2%–8%. The prevalence of narcolepsy is poorly categorized in children (Meltzer et al. 2010).

Medication use is another important consideration. In a survey sample of 154,957 children, potentially sleep-related medications were used in 6% of children (9,441), with antihistamines being the most commonly used, followed by antipsychotic medication, alpha-adrenergic receptor agonists, and selective serotonin reuptake inhibitors (Meltzer et al. 2010).

Diagnosing Sleep Disorder

Many parents fail to report significant sleep concerns to their child's pediatrician. This may be due to a lack of awareness about the health effects of inadequate sleep, or because clinicians are not asking the appropriate questions about sleep quality, duration, habitual snoring, and obstructive sleep apnea (Erichsen et al. 2012) (Table 7.1).

In children with pre-existing sleep disorders it is important to explore the root causes for sleep disturbance, including medical, family, and school influences.

In otherwise healthy children, physiologic and mental health findings associated with reduced sleep include behavioral, cardiovascular, and metabolic changes.

Table 7.1 Estimated Average Normal Sleep Times by Age

Newborn	2 months	10–19 hours per day (average 13–14.5)
Infant	2–12 months	12–13 hrs. per day
Toddler	1–3 yrs.	11–13 hrs. per day
Preschool	3–5 yrs.	9–10 hrs. per day
Child	6–12 yrs.	9–11 hrs. per day
Adolescence	12–18 yrs.	Recommended 9–9.25, average 7–7.5 hrs.

Source: Bharti, B., A. Mehta, and P. Malhi. 2013. "Sleep problems in children: a guide for primary care physicians." *Indian J Pediatr* 80(6): 492–8.

Conditions such as narcolepsy or restless leg syndrome are less commonly seen in children than in adults and require workup by a pediatric sleep specialist. Children living with chronic illness, especially those with respiratory symptoms, pain, those taking stimulant medications, who have serious neurodevelopmental disorders, or who require prolonged hospitalization, for example in the NICU (Daniels and Harrison 2015) and in the pediatric intensive care unit (Kudchadkar, Aljohani, and Punjabi 2014; Kudchadkar, Yaster, and Punjabi 2014) are at special risk for sleep disorders. In children living with chronic illness, sleep deprivation can amplify the experience of chronic pain and be a confounding factor in depression.

An Overlooked Diagnosis

A study by Meltzer found a prevalence of only 3.7% of children who had received a diagnosis of sleep disorder in a large population-based pediatric primary care network involving chart review of 154,957 children. It was determined that the standard review of systems covered in the well child visits did not routinely include an assessment of sleep (Meltzer et al. 2010) (Table 7.2).

Compounding this missing information is a documented lack of education about pediatric sleep medicine for physicians, and a feeling of being inadequately prepared to counsel patients effectively on the topic (Faruqui et al. 2011; Rosen et al. 1998).

Ideally, sleep screening should be included in every well child visit.

One commonly used approach is the BEARS sleep evaluation tool for children 2–18 years. It addresses five major sleep domains:

B   Bedtime problems
E   Excessive daytime sleepiness
A   Awakenings during the night
R   Regularity and duration of sleep
S   Snoring

The screen includes age and developmental stage-appropriate screening questions to help clinicians ask focused questions. Both child and caretaker should be questioned as the parent may be unaware of a child's symptoms (such as difficulty falling asleep), and vice versa; for example, a child may not be aware of their habitual snoring (Owens and Dalzell 2005).

Peer-victimization (bullying), especially relational (social exclusion), reputational, and cyber peer victimization, have all been associated with sleep disorders, somatic complaints, and anxiety and depression in adolescents and school-age children (Herge, La Greca, and Chan 2015).

A study by Tu demonstrated that sleep duration and quality had a moderating effect for internalizing (anxiety, depression) and externalizing (somatic complaints) symptoms in adolescents experiencing peer victimization (Tu, Erath, and El-Sheikh 2015).

Children and adolescents may avoid disclosure of bullying to parents or caretakers for fear of embarrassment or of escalating retaliation. Evaluation of sleep disturbance in any child provides an important opportunity to screen for peer victimization and take appropriate steps to support the child.

A sleep diary can be invaluable in assessing sleep duration and sleep quality and can

Table 7.2 Findings Associated with Reduced Sleep in Children and Adolescents

Daytime sleepiness
Loss of self-regulation skills with resulting irritability and trouble concentrating (Miller et al. 2015)
Decreased in memory, and school performance (Steenari et al. 2003)
Mood disorders, including anxiety (Baum et al. 2014; Weiner et al. 2015)
Hyperactivity (Waldon et al. 2015; Schneider, Lam, and Mahone 2015)

be reassuring to parents who are frustrated about slow change in a behavioral approach to sleep disorders in children of any age.

Obesity

The circadian system plays an integral role in coordinating the processing of nutrients and orchestrates levels of hormones such as glucagon, insulin, ghrelin and others in a closely regulated manner based on the individual's circadian rhythm (Fonken and Nelson 2014). Short sleep duration is a potential risk factor for overweight/obesity in children (Kjeldsen et al. 2014; Magee and Hale 2012) and has been associated with an increase in cardiovascular risk factors including elevated C-reactive protein, increased adipokines and other inflammatory markers as well as central adiposity (Navarro-Solera et al. 2015).

High variability in sleep habits has also been independently associated with increased caloric intake in adolescents (He et al. 2015), hyperlipidemia (Kong et al. 2011), and increased accidents and injuries (Chau 2015).

Emerging insights into the complex science of sleep also demonstrates a link between sleep quality, cellular aging, and telomere length (Tempaku, Mazzotti, and Tufik 2015), even affecting the developing fetus. For example, research has demonstrated that sleep-disordered breathing in pregnant women was correlated with significantly shortened telomere length in cord blood in fetuses of women at high risk for sleep apnea as compared to those at low risk ($p < 0.05$) (Salihu et al. 2015).

A correlation between telomere shortening and poor sleep quality, low perceived sleep quality, and high perceived stress has also been demonstrated in obese adults. Ongoing discoveries in this line of research may help to shed light on the links between obesity and related chronic illnesses (Prather et al. 2014).

Sleep quality in children and adolescents is affected by many factors including the intrusion of technology and social media (Calamaro et al. 2012), limited outdoor time and loss of connection to the rhythm of the natural world, excessive extracurricular activities, and school pressures. Caffeine use is also on the increase in children and adolescents and can have a significant impact on sleep. A survey of 555 seventh and eighth graders showed that nearly a third of those surveyed were unaware that their favorite beverages contained caffeine, and more than half were unable to identify beverages with the highest caffeine content (Thakre et al. 2015).

A sharp increase in consumption of energy drinks in adolescents has also been documented, many of which contain 160–357 mg of caffeine per 16 ounce can, or 115–208 mg caffeine per "shot"—a 1.9 ounce serving (Owens, Mindell, and Baylor 2014).

A 2006 National Sleep Foundation poll found that 35% of high school students consume at least two servings of caffeinated beverages daily (Foundation 2006).

Caffeine

Caffeine intake in adolescents is associated with later bedtimes, more electronic devices in the bedroom, and greater discrepancy between weekday and weekend sleep schedules, increased sleep onset latency, difficulty staying asleep, and shorter sleep duration (Owens, Mindell, and Baylor 2014).

Caffeine intake has also been associated with increased daytime sleepiness (Orbeta et al. 2006; Calamaro et al. 2012) and has been shown to have a negative correlation on academic success, despite expectations to the contrary (James, Kristjansson, and Sigfusdottir 2011).

Light at Night

Another consideration is light at night, especially in adolescents. Both animal and human studies demonstrate that even dim light at night has been shown to disrupt the circadian clock gene leading to metabolic disruption, interference with glucocorticoid and melatonin signaling, and weight gain compared to control subjects (Fonken and Nelson 2014).

Televisions, computer screens, and smart phones are important sources of light at night that have been correlated with insufficient sleep time, and in the case of computers and smart phones the perception of insufficient sleep (Falbe et al. 2015).

Early studies in adult humans show that chronic exposure to light at night has been associated with increase in body-mass-index, as well as increased risk of metabolic syndrome, hypertension, cancer, and abnormal lipid profiles in adult shift workers. These findings may have important implications for adolescents who shift their rhythm to accommodate homework or late night social networking activities (Fonken and Nelson 2014; Fonken et al. 2013; Obayashi et al. 2013).

Caretaker Implications

Lifestyle factors do not impact children in a vacuum. Many parents and caretakers face similar challenges with technology intrusion and limited free time, adding complexity and increasing work–family conflict. This has been shown to impact children and adolescents in important ways, including a negative impact on sleep quality (Davis et al. 2015).

A study by Davis and McHale measured the effect on sleep in children 9–17 years whose parents were given increased control over their schedule, and supervisor support to prioritize work–life balance and reduce work–family conflict. The study included no direct components that were focused on parenting practices. There was no significant difference in total hours worked per week between study and control groups. Parents in the intervention group of the 12-month study spent a statistically greater amount of time per day with children, particularly mothers with adolescent girls. Results in the intervention group showed improvements in youth sleep latency, reduction in night-to-night variability in sleep duration, and improved sleep quality compared to control group (McHale et al. 2015).

Common Sleep Disorders in Children

Insomnia

Insomnia refers to difficulty initiating or maintaining sleep with subsequent impact on daily functioning. This impact might include behavior such as fussiness, irritability, daytime sleepiness, impaired school performance or reduced overall quality of life.

Insomnia in children falls into two main categories; one is behavioral onset of childhood type, most often seen in children who have not acquired self-soothing behaviors. For example, infants or children who are unable to fall asleep without repeated rocking, feeding, or having a caretaker present. Behavioral insomnia of childhood limit-setting type is more commonly seen in preschoolers, toddlers, and school-age children who may resist enforcement of bedtime rules and structured routine. In some cases, this behavior may be driven by an underlying issue such as generalized anxiety disorder or by separation anxiety. In other cases, insomnia presents in conjunction with a more serious condition, for example ADHD, depression, or posttraumatic stress disorder. Children with oppositional behavior disorder can also have difficulty with enforcement of a bedtime routine.

In adolescents, as in adults, a state of high physiologic arousal can be a significant driver of insomnia, and may be worsened by worry about the consequences of not sleeping well on their next day's activities. Screening for stimulant medications (caffeine, decongestants, bronchodilators, ADHD treatments, drugs of abuse, SSRIs, and others) and comorbid conditions such as restless leg syndrome, obstructive sleep apnea, and others is indicated in any child with insomnia.

Evaluation

Evaluation for insomnia lends itself to a comprehensive integrative approach that considers all aspects of the child and family lifestyle including medical history, medications, sleep–wake routine, quality of daytime activities, nutrition, supplements, physical activity, exposure to outdoor light, stressors (home, school, afterschool), noise, and environmental exposures.

Integrative Approach to Treatment

Treatment of pediatric insomnia emphasizes age-appropriate sleep hygiene and preventive lifestyle measures. No long-term studies are available about the use of medications or supplements for pediatric insomnia, making lifestyle approaches a priority. Approaching sleep as a foundation of good health and encouraging children to master self-regulation rather than relying on an external substance (conventional or complementary) offers an important opportunity for children to build a strong sense of self-efficacy.

Lifestyle Approaches: Foundations of Integrative Medicine

Foundations of Healthy Sleep Applicable to all Children and Adolescents

- Maintain a regular sleep–wake schedule, including on weekends.
- Encourage a positive approach to restful sleep.

- Keep television and electronics out of the bedroom.
- Create a sense of 'safe sanctuary' in the bedroom.
- Sleep in a dark, cool room.
- Get consistent exposure to natural outdoor light.
- Daily enjoyable physical activity.
- Avoid caffeine in food and beverages.
- Avoid large amounts of liquid before bedtime.
- Address recurrent stressors at home and in school, including caretakers' stress.
- Create a bedtime routine from preschool age onward using age-appropriate relaxation tools such as breath work, guided imagery, progressive muscle relaxation, yoga, music, aromatherapy, drawing, journaling, reading, and others.

Age-Specific Recommendations

Young children:

- Teach self-soothing sleep skills early through use of transitional objects (blankets, soft toys).
- Practice gradual elimination of feeding or other caretaker support behaviors if young children have become dependent on external support for sleep induction such as feeding and rocking.
- Practice consistent reinforcement of bedtime rules.
- Avoid use of the bedroom for punishment or time-out.
- Learn to sleep with minimal (if any) light in the room. Total darkness and a cool environment are best.

School-age children:

- Avoid going to bed hungry (if possible), although heavy meals before bed should be discouraged.
- Teach a positive approach to restful sleep, encourage creation of personalized bedtime routine.
- Encourage use of a blue blocking tool on computers and phones in the evening.
- Avoid staying up late as a reward for good behavior.

Adolescents:

- Avoid sleeping in on weekends to "catch up on sleep."
- Limit or eliminate naps.
- Prioritize regular physical activity and daily morning outdoor time.
- Use bedroom for sleeping only; limit or eliminate technology use and television in bedroom.
- Use a blue light blocker in the evening (downloadable apps available).
- Develop a bedtime routine to deliberately gear down mind and body.
- Go to bed only when sleepy.
- Do not watch the clock.
- If still awake after 15–20 minutes get up and do restful activity.
- Avoid caffeine in late afternoon and evening.

- Snack, rather than a heavy meal before bed.
- Avoid alcohol and smoking, which can, among other things, interfere with quality of sleep.

Mind–Body Approaches

Mind–body therapies to aid sleep are valuable because they can help avoid medications and are non-habituating. They can encourage self-efficacy in children and adolescents, and can be used in the home or inpatient settings. A range of mind–body approaches are available, from simple breathing techniques, progressive muscle relaxation, biofeedback, journaling, guided imagery, self-hypnosis, to yoga, mindfulness meditation, or cognitive behavior therapy. In general mind–body approaches are low risk, cost effective, and flexible. Appropriate caution is indicated in any child with a history of a difficult experience with mind–body techniques, or any history of emotional, sexual, or physical trauma (McClafferty 2011).

Mindfulness

Mindfulness has been categorized by Shapiro as consisting of three core elements: intention, attention, and attitude allowing an open, non-judgmental awareness (Shapiro et al. 2006).

A wait list control study by Biegel et al. studied mindfulness in 102 children aged 14–18 years with a variety of psychiatric disorders seen in an outpatient setting. Teens in the treatment group reported significantly reduced symptoms of anxiety and depression, and improved sleep quality as well as increased self-esteem, and diagnostic improvement over the 5-month study period that included eight weekly 2-hour sessions. The course was slightly modified from traditional MBSR in that the at-home mindfulness practices were reduced to 20–35 minutes from 45 minutes and no day-long retreat was included. Topics of discussion were tailored to areas relevant to adolescents (Biegel et al. 2009).

A randomized controlled trial of 54 adults using a modified 8-week mindfulness program for chronic insomnia, mindfulness-based therapy for insomnia (MBTI), targeted hyperarousal compared to traditional 8-week MBSR. The MBTI group showed significant decrease in severity of insomnia that lasted until 6-month treatment follow-up (Ong et al. 2014).

Hypnosis

Clinical hypnosis, including self-hypnosis, has a history of successful use in the treatment of insomnia (Becker 2015).

Hypnosis in children with insomnia of an average duration of 3 years proved to be highly effective in a study by Anbar. Insomnia resolved after one to two sessions in the majority of the 75 patients, aged 7–17 years, for an overall success rate of 85% in this study population (Anbar and Slothower 2006).

Cognitive Behavioral Therapy

Age-appropriate cognitive-behavioral therapy has been shown to be effective in children with behavioral insomnia in several studies. The goal is redirection of fears and development of a more effective bedtime routine. One interesting approach includes having the child write a letter to the thing they are afraid of, for example the monster under the bed, stating that they are no longer afraid of it and it can go away (Tikotzky and Sadeh 2010).

Small studies exist on the successful use of guided imagery to improve sleep quality in mothers of preterm infants (Schaffer et al. 2013).

Dietary Supplements

Consider use of dietary supplements only after full evaluation and consultation with primary care clinician.

Melatonin

The body's natural neurohormone melatonin is produced in the pineal gland, synthesized from L-tryptophan, converted to 5-hydroxytryptophan (5-HTP), and then into serotonin, which undergoes two further transformations to become melatonin.

Melatonin has a primary role as mediator of the circadian rhythm and begins to rise in response to dim light in the evening. Levels peak in the middle of the night, then fall gradually through the early morning until being suppressed by sunlight in the morning. Exposure to artificial light at night will also suppress its release (Ferracioli-Oda, Qawasmi, and Bloch 2013).

In addition to regulation of the circadian rhythm, melatonin has an active role in in a variety of metabolic and immune functions through its antioxidant and anti-inflammatory properties (Karaaslan and Suzen 2015), and has been shown to have involvement in regulation of neuronal plasticity (Iyer, Wang, and Gillette 2014).

The primary indication for its use is to advance the timing of sleep onset in the treatment of delayed sleep phase disorder (a clinical diagnosis) to help shift the sleep–wake cycle back into the desired pattern. Some of the benefits of melatonin are its relative lack of association with habituation/dependence and a lack of hangover effects. Melatonin is easily available and widely used in the U.S. where it is classified as a dietary supplement, not regulated by the FDA, although it is regulated in Europe. It is classified as a natural health product in Canada (Bendz and Scates 2010).

Melatonin has been relatively well studied in children, although important questions remain about its long-term impact on puberty and the overall endocrine system. Long-term safety research is needed before conclusive safety recommendations can be made or long-term use is recommended (Rossignol and Frye 2011).

Some of the challenges in interpreting studies on the use of melatonin in children include wide variability of dosing, variation in timing of administration, and the variety of diagnosis treated. No dosing guidelines currently exist in pediatrics in the United States.

MELATONIN IN DELAYED SLEEP ONSET DISORDER

A meta-analysis of five adult studies involving 91 adults and four trials involving 226 children found that melatonin advanced sleep time by an average of 0.67 hours. The most common side effect in the studies reviewed included headache. Dose varied from 0.3 mg to 6 mg in the studies reviewed, leaving many question about optimal doses and timing administration. Conclusions and recommendations included limiting use in patients with identified delayed onset of sleep, use of a small dose, and administration 3–6 hours prior to desired onset of dim-light melatonin onset (van Geijlswijk, Korzilius, and Smits 2010).

Melatonin has been studied in a randomized, double-blind, placebo-controlled trial in 62 children aged 6–12 years old with the diagnosis of idiopathic chronic sleep-onset insomnia, where a dose of 5 mg administered at a consistent time in the early evening advanced sleep time by nearly an hour on average with minimum side effects reported (Smits et al. 2003).

A larger meta-analysis of 19 studies involving 1683 subjects, adults and children found an overall improvement in sleep quality, decrease in sleep latency, and increased overall sleep time compared to placebo in patients with primary sleep disorders (Ferracioli-Oda, Qawasmi, and Bloch 2013).

MELATONIN IN NEURODEVELOPMENTAL DISORDERS

Melatonin has also been found to be effective in addressing sleep disorders in children with various neurodevelopmental disabilities. It should be noted that sleep hygiene including consistent reinforcement of bedtime rules remains a first-line approach. For example, in children with autism spectrum disorders, a systematic review and meta-analysis of 35 studies demonstrated a correlation between below average melatonin levels in those with autism, with abnormalities in melatonin production or receptor functions. Findings overall supported the use of melatonin and reported significantly improved sleep duration and sleep onset latency. Melatonin was also associated with reduction in behavioral problems during daytime in several studies. Minimal side effects were reported in this meta-analysis (Rossignol and Frye 2011).

A 2014 review by Rossignol and Frye concluded similar findings in improvement in sleep quality and decrease in sleep latency onset, and improvement in daytime behavioral issues in some subjects was again observed in multiple randomized controlled trials included in the review (Rossignol and Frye 2011).

Melatonin has been evaluated in some studies in children with ADHD, where insomnia has been shown to affect an estimated 20%–25% of those affected. Some studies have shown efficacy and reported negligible side effects, although a precautionary approach supports the use of melatonin only in children with persistent, severe insomnia who are experiencing difficulty with daily functioning until additional research is available. Dose range is variable in this literature with an average of 3 mg to 5 mg noted administered 1–3 hours before bedtime. No published guidelines currently exist (Cortese et al. 2013; Bendz and Scates 2010; Hvolby 2015).

Herbal Medicine for Sleep

Chamomile (*Matricaria recutita*) is a botanical that has been used in folk medicine for thousands of years for its antioxidant, anti-inflammatory, and antispasmodic gastrointestinal and mild anxiolytic properties (McKay and Blumberg 2006a).

Its mechanism of action is not completely understood, but one pathway is thought to work through apigenin, a flavonoid component of the plant that has been shown to bind to benzodiazepine receptors and influence activity of neurotransmitters including gamma butyric acid (GABA), dopamine, and serotonin (Awad et al. 2007; Sanchez-Ortuno et al. 2009).

Although it is widely used as a sleep aid, particularly in tea form, a paucity of research exists for its use in sleep disorders, especially in children (Zick et al. 2011).

The best-studied species is German chamomile, a member of the Compositae family.

One of the few randomized controlled trials on its efficacy in sleep used 90 mg dry extract of chamomile flowering tops standardized up to 2.5 mg of (-)-α-bisabolol and ≥2.5 mg of apigenin per tablet in a 4-week trial in 34 adults. No significant differences were seen in total sleep time, sleep latency, sleep quality, or number of nighttime awakenings in the study group versus controls. No significant adverse events were reported (Zick et al. 2011).

Based on evidence to date, chamomile, especially in tea form, might be recommended as a soothing addition to the bedtime ritual, but lacks supporting data as a primary treatment for insomnia in children. It appears to have a wide margin of safety, other than in those with potential allergy, especially in those with allergy to other plants in the daisy family (Asteraceae or Compositae) including mugwort and ragweed. Chamomile has been shown to have antiplatelet effects and may theoretically interfere with anticoagulants via inhibition of vitamin K. It may also interfere with other sedative or benzodiazepines factors, which should be considered before recommending its use (McKay and Blumberg 2006b).

VALERIAN (*VALERIANA OFFICINALIS*)

Valerian is another herb widely used to promote and regulate sleep, although a meta-analysis of 24 studies using valerian in adults showed high study design variability, small numbers, and insignificant results compared to placebo. No randomized controlled trials are available in children. Overall no significant adverse effects were seen in this meta-analysis. Valerian is non-addictive and has been reported to require regular use for several weeks for effect to be seen (Leach and Page 2014).

Review of the literature for the efficacy of hops (*Humulus lupulus*), another popular botanical for adult insomnia, sometimes used in combination with valerian, failed to find conclusive evidence for efficacy in primary sleep disorder. No randomized trials are available in children (Salter and Brownie 2010; Koetter et al. 2007).

The German Commission E Monographs list hops as approved for insomnia (Cornu et al. 2010). Lemon balm (*Melissa officinalis*) is another herb with a long history of use as a mild sedative used to promote relaxation prior to sleep. To date there are no randomized controlled trials in children. Lemon balm is often used in combination with other herbs, such as valerian, often in tea form. Adverse events have been rarely reported in the adult literature (Kennedy et al. 2003).

Other Complementary Approaches

A systematic review of 20 studies by Sarris and Byrne of other complementary approaches to insomnia in the adult population found support for the use of acupressure, tai chi, and yoga, mixed support for acupuncture and L-tryptophan, and weak support for the use of herbal medicines. Variability of study design and quality was high (Sarris and Byrne 2011).

Practical Clinical Approach

Although more research is needed, evidence to support an integrative approach to pediatric insomnia incudes institution of an age-approach to sleep hygiene that incudes regular sleep–wake cycle, daily outdoor time (preferably in the morning), regular exercise, healthy nutrition, avoidance of caffeine, mindful use of electronics, effective stress management skills, limiting exposure to electronics in the evenings and at night, a blue blocker on all electronic screens, and a relaxing bedtime ritual that allows for reliable slowing and settling of mind and body to prepare for restful sleep.

Sleep Disordered Breathing

Sleep disordered breathing in children can range from simple recurrent snoring to obstructive sleep apnea (OSA). The risk of sleep disordered breathing is increased by up to fourfold in the presence of obesity, which has been determined to be an independent risk factor for both snoring and for OSA in children. Adolescents who experience sleep disordered breathing have also been shown to have a sevenfold risk of accompanying metabolic syndrome (Redline et al. 2007).

Obstructive sleep apnea is a serious illness in children requiring subspecialty evaluation. Prevalence estimates range of 1%–5% of the pediatric population (Marcus et al. 2012).

The clinical hallmarks of obstructive sleep apnea include repeated episodes of apnea during sleep, followed by loud gasping or choking that repeatedly interrupt the normal sleep cycle. The desaturations caused by the apnea have been associated with both metabolic and behavioral comorbidities. Some of the most serious are cardiovascular effects including elevated autonomic variability, increased mean arterial pressure, tachycardia, arrhythmias, and strain on both right and left ventricular function. Decreased cerebral brain flow has also been documented. Increase in systemic inflammatory markers are seen in children with OSA, thought to be related to the recurring physiologic stress of intermittent hypoxia and reactive sympathetic nervous system activation (Gileles-Hillel et al. 2014).

Behavioral changes associated with OSA are also significant and include hyperactivity, daytime hypersomnolence, depression, aggression, and abnormal social behaviors. The obvious overlap with ADHD makes it critical that children being considered for an ADHD diagnosis have been evaluated for a primary sleep disorder. The American Academy of Pediatrics Clinical Practice Guidelines for Obstructive Sleep Apnea emphasize that all children should be screened for snoring (Marcus et al. 2012).

Nocturnal enuresis is also associated with OSA and should be a trigger to screen for habitual snoring in pediatric patients. Deficits in cognition are widely reported in children with OSA, including poor school performance, reduced executive function, poor impulse control, learning difficulties, and reduction in general intelligence. Fortunately, many behavioral problems have been shown to improve or resolve after definitive treatment (Marcus et al. 2012).

No consensus guidelines for when to evaluate with a sleep study currently exist, although the American Academy of Pediatrics guidelines suggest that children who snore more than 3 nights per week and have signs or symptoms of OSA should be considered for sleep study or referral to an ENT or sleep specialist. OSA is conclusively diagnosed by overnight sleep study. Other tests that could be considered if sleep study is not available include nighttime video recording, nocturnal oximetry, or daytime nap study (Goldbart 2015).

The most common cause of OSA is adenotonsillar hypertrophy, and adenotonsillectomy has traditionally been the recommended treatment (Marcus et al. 2012).

Of interest, a randomized trial published in the *New England Journal of Medicine* on 464 children aged 5–9 years old with confirmed diagnosis of OSA compared adenotonsillectomy to watchful waiting for 6 months. Results showed statistically significant improvements quality of life, improved behavior, and better polysomnograph findings in the surgical group, although attention and cognitive function were not significantly changed. However, 46% of the non-obese, and 65% of those with less severe symptoms, in the watchful waiting group showed normalization of polysomnograph findings and no significant cognitive decline over the 6-month waiting period. Authors concluded "medical management and reassessment after a period of observation may be a valid therapeutic option" (Marcus et al. 2013).

OSA is also highly prevalent in children with poorly controlled asthma who have been shown in a large population-based study to have significant improvement in asthma symptoms after adenotonsillectomy (Bhattacharjee et al. 2014).

In conjunction with sleep specialist evaluation, obesity and other metabolic symptoms associated with sleep disorders can be approached with a comprehensive lifestyle program to address weight that includes age-appropriate, supervised physical activity, nutrition modification, motivational interviewing, family support, and mind–body skills training to address behavior modification and self-efficacy. If the child is scheduled to undergo adenotonsillectomy, use of guided imagery to reduce preoperative and post-operative discomfort may be considered to address pre-operative anxiety and post-operative pain (Sng et al. 2013).

Emerging studies have also shown some benefit of the anti-inflammatory leukotriene receptor antagonists, and of intranasal corticosteroids in mild cases (Goldbart 2015).

Given the emerging research, high association with obesity, and the recommendation for adenotonsillectomy in children with OSA, it is important for caregivers to recognize the importance of implementing an effective, evidence-based approach to healthy lifestyle measures that may allow the child to avoid surgery or prescription medication if OSA symptoms improve with weight loss.

Summary

Sleep is a critical component of health in children and should be addressed routinely as a foundation of preventive health. Several of the common sleep disorders have been shown to respond well to lifestyle measures, such as: limiting caffeine and light at night, maintaining normal weight, stress reduction, normalizing sleep–wake cycles, and regular physical activity. Development of a relaxing bedtime routine can help prepare a child for a restful night. Limiting the intrusion of technology into family and sleep time is another important step to consider, and applies to both child and caretaker.

References

Anbar, R. D., and M. P. Slothower. 2006. "Hypnosis for treatment of insomnia in school-age children: a retrospective chart review." *BMC Pediatr* 6: 23. doi: 10.1186/1471-2431-6-23.

Awad, R., D. Levac, P. Cybulska, Z. Merali, V. L. Trudeau, and J. T. Arnason. 2007. "Effects of traditionally used anxiolytic botanicals on enzymes of the gamma-aminobutyric acid (GABA) system." *Can J Physiol Pharmacol* 85(9): 933–42. doi: 10.1139/Y07-083.

Baum, K. T., A. Desai, J. Field, L. E. Miller, J. Rausch, and D. W. Beebe. 2014. "Sleep restriction worsens mood and emotion regulation in adolescents." *J Child Psychol Psychiatry* 55(2): 180–90. doi: 10.1111/jcpp.12125.

Becker, P. M. 2015. "Hypnosis in the management of sleep disorders." *Sleep Med Clin* 10(1): 85–92. doi: 10.1016/j.jsmc.2014.11.003.

Bendz, L. M., and A. C. Scates. 2010. "Melatonin treatment for insomnia in pediatric patients with attention-deficit/hyperactivity disorder." *Ann Pharmacother* 44(1): 185–91. doi: 10.1345/aph.1M365.

Bharti, B., A. Mehta, and P. Malhi. 2013. "Sleep problems in children: a guide for primary care physicians." *Indian J Pediatr* 80(6): 492–8. doi: 10.1007/s12098-012-0960-0.

Bhattacharjee, R., B. H. Choi, D. Gozal, and B. Mokhlesi. 2014. "Association of adenotonsillectomy with asthma outcomes in children: a longitudinal database analysis." *PLoS Med* 11(11): e1001753. doi: 10.1371/journal.pmed.1001753.

Biegel, G. M., K. W. Brown, S. L. Shapiro, and C. M. Schubert. 2009. "Mindfulness-based stress reduction for the treatment of adolescent psychiatric outpatients: a randomized clinical trial." *J Consult Clin Psychol* 77(5): 855–66. doi: 10.1037/a0016241.

Calamaro, C. J., K. Yang, S. Ratcliffe, and E. R. Chasens. 2012. "Wired at a young age: the effect of caffeine and technology on sleep duration and body mass index in school-aged children." *J Pediatr Health Care* 26(4): 276–82. doi: 10.1016/j.pedhc.2010.12.002.

Calhoun, S. L., J. Fernandez-Mendoza, A. N. Vgontzas, D. Liao, and E. O. Bixler. 2014. "Prevalence of insomnia symptoms in a general population sample of young children and preadolescents: gender effects." *Sleep Med* 15(1): 91–5. doi: 10.1016/j.sleep.2013.08.787.

Chau, K. 2015. "Impact of sleep difficulty on single and repeated injuries in adolescents." *Accid Anal Prev* 81: 86–95. doi: 10.1016/j.aap.2015.04.031.

Cornu, C., L. Remontet, F. Noel-Baron, A. Nicolas, N. Feugier-Favier, P. Roy, B. Claustrat, M. Saadatian-Elahi, and B. Kassai. 2010. "A dietary supplement to improve the quality of sleep: a randomized placebo controlled trial." *BMC Complement Altern Med* 10: 29. doi: 10.1186/1472-6882-10-29.

Cortese, S., T. E. Brown, P. Corkum, R. Gruber, L. M. O'Brien, M. Stein, M. Weiss, and J. Owens. 2013. "Assessment and management of sleep problems in youths with attention-deficit/hyperactivity disorder." *J Am Acad Child Adolesc Psychiatry* 52(8): 784–96. doi: 10.1016/j.jaac.2013.06.001.

Daniels, J. M., and T. M. Harrison. 2015. "A case study of the environmental experience of a hospitalized newborn infant with complex congenital heart disease." *J Cardiovasc Nurs*. doi: 10.1097/JCN.0000000000000273.

Davis, K. D., K. M. Lawson, D. M. Almeida, E. L. Kelly, R. B. King, L. Hammer, L. M. Casper, C. A. Okechukwu, G. Hanson, and S. M. McHale. 2015. "Parents' daily time with their children: a workplace intervention." *Pediatrics* 135(5): 875–82. doi: 10.1542/peds.2014-2057.

Erichsen, D., C. Godoy, F. Granse, J. Axelsson, D. Rubin, and D. Gozal. 2012. "Screening for sleep disorders in pediatric primary care: are we there yet?" *Clin Pediatr (Phila)* 51(12): 1125–9. doi: 10.1177/0009922812464548.

Falbe, J., K. K. Davison, R. L. Franckle, C. Ganter, S. L. Gortmaker, L. Smith, T. Land, and E. M. Taveras. 2015. "Sleep duration, restfulness, and screens in the sleep environment." *Pediatrics* 135(2): e367–75. doi: 10.1542/peds.2014-2306.

Faruqui, F., J. Khubchandani, J. H. Price, D. Bolyard, and R. Reddy. 2011. "Sleep disorders in children: a national assessment of primary care pediatrician practices and perceptions." *Pediatrics* 128(3): 539–46. doi: 10.1542/peds.2011-0344.

Ferracioli-Oda, E., A. Qawasmi, and M. H. Bloch. 2013. "Meta-analysis: melatonin for the treatment of primary sleep disorders." *PLoS One* 8(5): e63773. doi: 10.1371/journal.pone.0063773.

Fonken, L. K., T. G. Aubrecht, O. H. Melendez-Fernandez, Z. M. Weil, and R. J. Nelson. 2013. "Dim light at night disrupts molecular circadian rhythms and increases body weight." *J Biol Rhythms* 28(4): 262–71. doi: 10.1177/0748730413493862.

Fonken, L. K., and R. J. Nelson. 2014. "The effects of light at night on circadian clocks and metabolism." *Endocr Rev* 35(4): 648–70. doi: 10.1210/er.2013-1051.

Foundation., National Sleep. 2006. "National Sleep Foundation: Sleep in America Poll."

Gileles-Hillel, A., M. L. Alonso-Alvarez, L. Kheirandish-Gozal, E. Peris, J. A. Cordero-Guevara, J. Teran-Santos, M. G. Martinez, M. J. Jurado-Luque, J. Corral-Penafiel, J. Duran-Cantolla, and D. Gozal. 2014. "Inflammatory markers and obstructive sleep apnea in obese children: the NANOS study." *Mediators Inflamm* 605280. doi: 10.1155/2014/605280.

Goldbart, A. D. 2015. "Sleep medicine." *Curr Opin Pediatr* 27(3): 329–33. doi: 10.1097/MOP.0000000000000218.

He, F., E. O. Bixler, A. Berg, Y. Imamura Kawasawa, A. N. Vgontzas, J. Fernandez-Mendoza, J. Yanosky, and D. Liao. 2015. "Habitual sleep variability, not sleep duration, is associated with caloric intake in adolescents." *Sleep Med*. doi: 10.1016/j.sleep.2015.03.004.

Herge, W. M., A. M. La Greca, and S. F. Chan. 2015. "Adolescent peer victimization and physical health problems." *J Pediatr Psychol*. doi: 10.1093/jpepsy/jsv050.

Hvolby, A. 2015. "Associations of sleep disturbance with ADHD: implications for treatment." *Atten Defic Hyperact Disord* 7(1): 1–18. doi: 10.1007/s12402-014-0151-0.

Iyer, R., T. A. Wang, and M. U. Gillette. 2014. "Circadian gating of neuronal functionality: a basis for iterative metaplasticity." *Front Syst Neurosci* 8: 164. doi: 10.3389/fnsys.2014.00164.

James, J. E., A. L. Kristjansson, and I. D. Sigfusdottir. 2011. "Adolescent substance use, sleep, and academic achievement: evidence of harm due to caffeine." *J Adolesc* 34(4): 665–73. doi: 10.1016/j.adolescence.2010.09.006.

Karaaslan, C., and S. Suzen. 2015. "Antioxidant properties of melatonin and its potential action in diseases." *Curr Top Med Chem* 15(9): 894–903.

Kennedy, D. O., G. Wake, S. Savelev, N. T. Tildesley, E. K. Perry, K. A. Wesnes, and A. B. Scholey. 2003. "Modulation of mood and cognitive performance following acute administration of single doses of Melissa officinalis (Lemon balm) with human CNS nicotinic and muscarinic receptor-binding properties." *Neuropsychopharmacology* 28(10): 1871–81. doi: 10.1038/sj.npp.1300230.

Kjeldsen, J. S., M. F. Hjorth, R. Andersen, K. F. Michaelsen, I. Tetens, A. Astrup, J. P. Chaput, and A. Sjodin. 2014. "Short sleep duration and large variability in sleep duration are independently associated with dietary risk factors for obesity in Danish school children." *Int J Obes (Lond)* 38(1): 32–9. doi: 10.1038/ijo.2013.147.

Koetter, U., E. Schrader, R. Kaufeler, and A. Brattstrom. 2007. "A randomized, double blind, placebo-controlled, prospective clinical study to demonstrate clinical efficacy of a fixed valerian hops extract combination (Ze 91019) in patients suffering from non-organic sleep disorder." *Phytother Res* 21(9): 847–51. doi: 10.1002/ptr.2167.

Kong, A. P., Y. K. Wing, K. C. Choi, A. M. Li, G. T. Ko, R. C. Ma, P. C. Tong, C. S. Ho, M. H. Chan, M. H. Ng, J. Lau, and J. C. Chan. 2011. "Associations of sleep duration with obesity and serum lipid profile in children and adolescents." *Sleep Med* 12(7): 659–65. doi: 10.1016/j.sleep.2010.12.015.

Kudchadkar, S. R., O. A. Aljohani, and N. M. Punjabi. 2014. "Sleep of critically ill children in the pediatric intensive care unit: a systematic review." *Sleep Med Rev* 18(2): 103–10. doi: 10.1016/j.smrv.2013.02.002.

Kudchadkar, S. R., M. Yaster, and N. M. Punjabi. 2014. "Sedation, sleep promotion, and delirium screening practices in the care of mechanically ventilated children: a wake-up call for the pediatric critical care community." *Crit Care Med* 42(7): 1592–600. doi: 10.1097/CCM.0000000000000326.

Leach, M. J., and A. T. Page. 2014. "Herbal medicine for insomnia: A systematic review and meta-analysis." *Sleep Med Rev* 24C: 1–12. doi: 10.1016/j.smrv.2014.12.003.

Magee, L., and L. Hale. 2012. "Longitudinal associations between sleep duration and subsequent weight gain: a systematic review." *Sleep Med Rev* 16(3): 231–41. doi: 10.1016/j.smrv.2011.05.005.

Marcus, C. L., L. J. Brooks, K. A. Draper, D. Gozal, A. C. Halbower, J. Jones, M. S. Schechter, S. D. Ward, S. H. Sheldon, R. N. Shiffman, C. Lehmann, K. Spruyt, and Pediatrics American Academy of. 2012. "Diagnosis and management of childhood obstructive sleep apnea syndrome." *Pediatrics* 130(3): e714–55. doi: 10.1542/peds.2012-1672.

Marcus, C. L., R. H. Moore, C. L. Rosen, B. Giordani, S. L. Garetz, H. G. Taylor, R. B. Mitchell, R. Amin, E. S. Katz, R. Arens, S. Paruthi, H. Muzumdar, D. Gozal, N. H. Thomas, J. Ware, D. Beebe, K. Snyder, L. Elden, R. C. Sprecher, P. Willging, D. Jones, J. P. Bent, T. Hoban, R. D. Chervin, S. S. Ellenberg, S. Redline, and Trial Childhood Adenotonsillectomy. 2013. "A randomized trial of adenotonsillectomy for childhood sleep apnea." *N Engl J Med* 368(25): 2366–76. doi: 10.1056/NEJMoa1215881.

Matricciani, L., T. Olds, and J. Petkov. 2012. "In search of lost sleep: secular trends in the sleep time of school-aged children and adolescents." *Sleep Med Rev* 16(3): 203–11. doi: 10.1016/j.smrv.2011.03.005.

McClafferty, H. 2011. "Complementary, holistic, and integrative medicine: mind-body medicine." *Pediatr Rev* 32(5): 201–3. doi: 10.1542/pir.32-5-201.

McHale, S. M., K. M. Lawson, K. D. Davis, L. Casper, E. L. Kelly, and O. Buxton. 2015. "Effects of a workplace intervention on sleep in employees' children." *J Adolesc Health* 56(6): 672–7. doi: 10.1016/j.jadohealth.2015.02.014.

McKay, D. L., and J. B. Blumberg. 2006a. "A review of the bioactivity and potential health benefits of chamomile tea (Matricaria recutita L.)." *Phytother Res* 20(7): 519–30. doi: 10.1002/ptr.1900.

McKay, D. L., and J. B. Blumberg. 2006b. "A review of the bioactivity and potential health benefits of peppermint tea (Mentha piperita L.)." *Phytother Res* 20(8): 619–33. doi: 10.1002/ptr.1936.

Meltzer, L. J., C. Johnson, J. Crosette, M. Ramos, and J. A. Mindell. 2010. "Prevalence of diagnosed sleep disorders in pediatric primary care practices." *Pediatrics* 125(6): e1410–8. doi: 10.1542/peds.2009-2725.

Miller, A. L., R. Seifer, R. Crossin, and M. K. Lebourgeois. 2015. "Toddlers' self-regulation strategies in a challenge context are nap-dependent." *J Sleep Res* 24(3): 279–87. doi: 10.1111/jsr.12260.

Mindell, J. A., B. Kuhn, D. S. Lewin, L. J. Meltzer, A. Sadeh, and Medicine American Academy of Sleep. 2006. "Behavioral treatment of bedtime problems and night wakings in infants and young children." *Sleep* 29(10): 1263–76.

Moore, M. 2010. "Bedtime problems and night wakings: treatment of behavioral insomnia of childhood." *J Clin Psychol* 66(11): 1195–204. doi: 10.1002/jclp.20731.

Navarro-Solera, M., J. Carrasco-Luna, G. Pin-Arboledas, R. Gonzalez-Carrascosa, J. M. Soriano, and P. Codoner-Franch. 2015. "Short sleep duration is related to emerging cardiovascular risk factors in obese children." *J Pediatr Gastroenterol Nutr* 61(5): 571–6. doi: 10.1097/MPG.0000000000000868.

Obayashi, K., K. Saeki, J. Iwamoto, N. Okamoto, K. Tomioka, S. Nezu, Y. Ikada, and N. Kurumatani. 2013. "Exposure to light at night, nocturnal urinary melatonin excretion, and obesity/dyslipidemia in the elderly: a cross-sectional analysis of the HEIJO-KYO study." *J Clin Endocrinol Metab* 98(1): 337–44. doi: 10.1210/jc.2012-2874.

Ong, J. C., R. Manber, Z. Segal, Y. Xia, S. Shapiro, and J. K. Wyatt. 2014. "A randomized controlled trial of mindfulness meditation for chronic insomnia." *Sleep* 37(9): 1553–63. doi: 10.5665/sleep.4010.

Orbeta, R. L., M. D. Overpeck, D. Ramcharran, M. D. Kogan, and R. Ledsky. 2006. "High caffeine intake in adolescents: associations with difficulty sleeping and feeling tired in the morning." *J Adolesc Health* 38(4): 451–3. doi: 10.1016/j.jadohealth.2005.05.014.

Owens, J. A., and V. Dalzell. 2005. "Use of the 'BEARS' sleep screening tool in a pediatric residents' continuity clinic: a pilot study." *Sleep Med* 6(1): 63–9. doi: 10.1016/j.sleep.2004.07.015.

Owens, J. A., J. Mindell, and A. Baylor. 2014. "Effect of energy drink and caffeinated beverage consumption on sleep, mood, and performance in children and adolescents." *Nutr Rev* 72(Suppl 1): 65–71. doi: 10.1111/nure.12150.

Prather, A. A., B. Gurfein, P. Moran, J. Daubenmier, M. Acree, P. Bacchetti, E. Sinclair, J. Lin, E. Blackburn, F. M. Hecht, and E. S. Epel. 2014. "Tired telomeres: poor global sleep quality, perceived stress, and telomere length in immune cell subsets in obese men and women." *Brain Behav Immun.* doi: 10.1016/j.bbi.2014.12.011.

Redline, S., A. Storfer-Isser, C. L. Rosen, N. L. Johnson, H. L. Kirchner, J. Emancipator, and A. M. Kibler. 2007. "Association between metabolic syndrome and sleep-disordered breathing in adolescents." *Am J Respir Crit Care Med* 176(4): 401–8. doi: 10.1164/rccm.200703-375OC.

Rosen, R., M. Mahowald, A. Chesson, K. Doghramji, R. Goldberg, M. Moline, R. Millman, G. Zammit, B. Mark, and W. Dement. 1998. "The Taskforce 2000 survey on medical education in sleep and sleep disorders." *Sleep* 21(3): 235–8.

Rossignol, D. A., and R. E. Frye. 2011. "Melatonin in autism spectrum disorders: a systematic review and meta-analysis." *Dev Med Child Neurol* 53(9): 783–92. doi: 10.1111/j.1469-8749.2011.03980.x.

Salihu, H. M., L. King, P. Patel, A. Paothong, A. Pradhan, J. Louis, E. Naik, P. J. Marty, and V. Whiteman. 2015. "Association between maternal symptoms of sleep disordered breathing and fetal telomere length." *Sleep* 38(4): 559–66. doi: 10.5665/sleep.4570.

Salter, S., and S. Brownie. 2010. "Treating primary insomnia—the efficacy of valerian and hops." *Aust Fam Physician* 39(6): 433–7.

Sanchez-Ortuno, M. M., L. Belanger, H. Ivers, M. LeBlanc, and C. M. Morin. 2009. "The use of natural products for sleep: a common practice?" *Sleep Med* 10(9): 982–7. doi: 10.1016/j.sleep.2008.10.009.

Sarris, J., and G. J. Byrne. 2011. "A systematic review of insomnia and complementary medicine." *Sleep Med Rev* 15(2): 99–106. doi: 10.1016/j.smrv.2010.04.001.

Schaffer, L., N. Jallo, L. Howland, K. James, D. Glaser, and K. Arnell. 2013. "Guided imagery: an innovative approach to improving maternal sleep quality." *J Perinat Neonatal Nurs* 27(2): 151–9. doi: 10.1097/JPN.0b013e3182870426.

Schneider, H. E., J. C. Lam, and E. M. Mahone. 2015. "Sleep disturbance and neuropsychological function in young children with ADHD." *Child Neuropsychol* 1–14. doi: 10.1080/09297049.2015.1018153.

Shapiro, S. L., L. E. Carlson, J. A. Astin, and B. Freedman. 2006. "Mechanisms of mindfulness." *J Clin Psychol* 62(3): 373–86. doi: 10.1002/jclp.20237.

Smits, M. G., H. F. van Stel, K. van der Heijden, A. M. Meijer, A. M. Coenen, and G. A. Kerkhof. 2003. "Melatonin improves health status and sleep in children with idiopathic chronic sleep-onset insomnia: a randomized placebo-controlled trial." *J Am Acad Child Adolesc Psychiatry* 42(11): 1286–93. doi: 10.1097/01.chi.0000085756.71002.86.

Sng, Q. W., B. Taylor, J. L. Liam, P. Klainin-Yobas, W. Wang, and H. G. He. 2013. "Postoperative pain management experiences among school-aged children: a qualitative study." *J Clin Nurs* 22(7–8): 958–68. doi: 10.1111/jocn.12052.

Steenari, M. R., V. Vuontela, E. J. Paavonen, S. Carlson, M. Fjallberg, and E. Aronen. 2003. "Working memory and sleep in 6- to 13-year-old schoolchildren." *J Am Acad Child Adolesc Psychiatry* 42(1): 85–92.

Tempaku, P. F., D. R. Mazzotti, and S. Tufik. 2015. "Telomere length as a marker of sleep loss and sleep disturbances: a potential link between sleep and cellular senescence." *Sleep Med* 16(5): 559–563. doi: 10.1016/j.sleep.2015.02.519.

Thakre, T. P., K. Deoras, C. Griffin, A. Vemana, P. Podmore, and J. Krishna. 2015. "Caffeine awareness in children: insights from a pilot study." *J Clin Sleep Med.*

Tikotzky, L., and A. Sadeh. 2010. "The role of cognitive-behavioral therapy in behavioral childhood insomnia." *Sleep Med* 11(7): 686–91. doi: 10.1016/j.sleep.2009.11.017.

Tu, K. M., S. A. Erath, and M. El-Sheikh. 2015. "Peer Victimization and adolescent adjustment: the moderating role of sleep." *J Abnorm Child Psychol*. doi: 10.1007/s10802-015-0035-6.

van Diepen, H. C., R. G. Foster, and J. H. Meijer. 2015. "A colourful clock." *PLoS Biol* 13(5): e1002160. doi: 10.1371/journal.pbio.1002160.

van Geijlswijk, I. M., H. P. Korzilius, and M. G. Smits. 2010. "The use of exogenous melatonin in delayed sleep phase disorder: a meta-analysis." *Sleep* 33(12): 1605–14.

Waldon, J., J. Vriend, F. Davidson, and P. Corkum. 2015. "Sleep and attention in children with ADHD and typically developing peers." *J Atten Disord*. doi: 10.1177/1087054715575064.

Weiner, C. L., R. Meredith Elkins, D. Pincus, and J. Comer. 2015. "Anxiety sensitivity and sleep-related problems in anxious youth." *J Anxiety Disord* 32: 66–72. doi: 10.1016/j.janxdis.2015.03.009.

Zick, S. M., B. D. Wright, A. Sen, and J. T. Arnedt. 2011. "Preliminary examination of the efficacy and safety of a standardized chamomile extract for chronic primary insomnia: a randomized placebo-controlled pilot study." *BMC Complement Altern Med* 11: 78. doi: 10.1186/1472-6882-11-78.

8 Environmental Health

Introduction

Why is environmental health training included in pediatric integrative medicine education? Accruing research on the negative health effects of climate change and environmental exposures points toward a disproportionate burden of harm on the developing fetus, infants, children, and adolescents that cannot be ignored by clinicians caring for children. This poses a significant challenge because few clinicians receive even a minimum of training in environmental health, resulting in multiple missed opportunities for preventive counseling (McClafferty 2016)

What We Know

Research evidence establishing conclusive links between several serious pediatric illnesses and environmental exposures has been widely published through the National Institute of Environmental Science of the National Institutes of Health (National Institutes of Health 2011), while environmental links to other pediatric diseases are the subject of active study (Table 8.1).

Autism, a disease now estimated to affect 1 in 68 U.S. children, is a good example of a disease where environmental links are suspected and under active study; for example, using longitudinal evaluations such as the Childhood Autism Risks from Genetics and Environment (CHARGE) study though the University of California—Davis MIND Institute (Hertz-Picciotto et al. 2006).

Slow Progress

The Institute of Medicine published recommendations about the need for basic clinical

Table 8.1 Serious Pediatric Illness Associated with Environmental Toxins

Asthma
ADHD
Breast and other cancers
Autoimmune diseases
Reproductive health
Endocrine disorders, thyroid, diabetes, obesity, metabolic syndrome

competence in environmental health topics for physicians as far back as 1996 (Schenk et al. 1996), yet relatively little progress has been made in this area in most medical disciplines (Gehle, Crawford, and Hatcher 2011). Kilpatrick surveyed 266 pediatricians and reported fewer than one in five having received training in environmental history, despite 53% reporting caring for a patient seriously affected by an environmental exposure, and a majority of pediatricians expressing high interest in the topic (Kilpatrick et al., 2002). Transande surveyed 301 New York pediatricians (Ma et al. 2012) and found that only one in five respondents had received training in environmental history (Trasande et al. 2006).

Why it Matters

This discrepancy in clinician training is unsustainable, as demonstrated by the mounting public outcry about the health effects of toxicants in our food and water.

Some of the exposures most relevant to children include: bisphenol A (BPA), an endocrine disruptor that has been found in infant formula, baby bottles, and dental sealants (Michalowicz 2014; Fenichel, Chevalier, and Brucker-Davis 2013) and orthodontic polycarbonate brackets (Kloukos, Pandis, and Eliades 2013); in inorganic arsenic found in children's apple juice (Wilson, Hooper, and Shi 2012); in rice (Hojsak et al. 2015), and in infant rice cereal (Jackson, Taylor, Punshon et al. 2012; Jackson, Taylor, Karagas et al. 2012).

Emerging research on the carcinogenic potential of glyphosate, found in Monsanto's ubiquitous herbicide Roundup (Guyton et al. 2015) has heightened public outrage as questions continue to mount regarding the effects of these environmental exposures on developing children.

Children are Vulnerable

Certain patient populations can be more vulnerable to environmental toxicants based on socioeconomic status (Miranda et al. 2009), increased sensitivity, timing of exposure, or increased relative exposure dose.

For example, infants have both increased sensitivity and increased relative exposure to toxicants based on surface area and multiple routes of exposure through placental transfer, breast milk, and indirect exposures after birth. Studies on newborn umbilical cord blood illustrate the issue in a manner that cannot be ignored. One of the earliest examples was a benchmark study of the umbilical cord blood of 10 babies born in 2004 by the Environmental Working Group in collaboration with Commonweal. A total of 287 chemicals were identified in the group, the first reported cord blood tests for 261 of the assayed chemicals. Of the chemicals present, 180 were known carcinogens, 217 were neurotoxins, and 208 were associated with abnormal fetal development in animal studies. Among the chemical classes found were organochlorine pesticides, brominated flame retardants, polyaromatic hydrocarbons, and perfluorinated chemicals (Environmental Working Group 2005).

Since then, numerous studies on human cord blood have been published, demonstrating conclusively that harmful environmental toxicants cross the placenta and are also concentrated in breast milk (Frederiksen et al. 2009).

Placenta transfer is an important concern, especially with substances such as methyl mercury, where the pregnant mother may be unaware of a significant ongoing exposure (Sutton et al. 2012).

Adolescents are at risk for disruption of normal sexual development by endocrine-disrupting chemicals (Diamanti-Kandarakis, Christakou, and Marinakis 2012; Akin et al. 2015), and emerging research also suggests a correlation between endocrine disruptors, obesity, and metabolic syndrome in certain phenotypes (Menale et al. 2015).

These recognized environmental exposure risks in childhood underscore the need for pediatric clinicians to be educated about environmental health so they can maximize preventive counseling opportunities and minimize unwanted exposures in their patients.

Pediatric Progress

Longstanding interest in environmental health among members of the American Academy of Pediatrics is reflected in the ongoing publication of *Pediatric Environmental Health, 3rd Edition*, also known as "The Green Book" (Etzel et al. 2003), and by growth of the AAP Council on Environmental Health, responsible for development of educational programs and policy in environmental health for the Academy (Council on Environmental Health).

Examples of the Committee's work is seen in the 2012 Policy Statement on *Pesticide Exposure in Children* (Council on Environmental Health 2012), and the 2014 Policy Statement on *Iodine Deficiency, Pollutant Chemicals, and the Thyroid: New Information on an Old Problem* (Council on Environmental Health et al. 2014), both of which offer an overview of current data and a call for immediate adoption of a precautionary approach to environmental exposures in children.

The Pediatric Academic Society also has an active Environmental Health Special Interest Group, www.academicpeds.org, that writes and presents on current topics in environmental health.

Progress in pediatric advocacy and research has accelerated dramatically over the past 10 to 15 years, reflected in the following developments:

- Fourteen Centers for Children's Environmental Health and Disease Prevention Research in conjunction with the National Institutes of Health and the U.S. Environmental Protection Agency.
- A global network of Pediatric Environmental Health Specialty Units (PEHSU) in conjunction with the U.S. Centers for Disease Control and Prevention/Agency for Toxic Substances and Disease Registry.
- A Story of Health, an educational program developed by the Agency for Toxic Substances and Disease Registry (ATSDR), the Collaborative on Health and the Environment, the University of California, San Francisco's Pediatric Environmental Health Specialty Unit, the California Environmental Protection Agency's Office of Environmental Health Hazard Assessment, and the Science and Environmental Health Network.

In 2013 the American College of Obstetrics and Gynecologists (ACOG) and the American Society for Reproductive Medicine issued a joint opinion statement urging their members and regulatory organizations such as the U.S. EPA to raise awareness about the reproductive effects of environmental toxins on a broader scale, and to take steps to identify and limit toxic environmental exposures (575 2013).

The Scientific Advisory Committee of the Royal College of Obstetricians and Gynecologists published a Scientific Impact Paper the same year reinforcing ACOG concerns calling for adoption of a precautionary principle approach with regards to environmental exposures in areas where data is lacking (Bellingham and Sharpe 2013).

Challenges identified by clinicians regarding incorporation of environmental health into clinical practice seem to organize around several common themes. These include: low sense of self-efficacy regarding patient education; lack of familiarity with the core topics and reliable resources (Trasande et al. 2010); lack of evidence-based guidelines; need for tools to effectively communicate risks to patients; and fear of causing patients more anxiety about potentially unavoidable exposures (Stotland et al. 2014).

Challenges in Environmental Health Education

Some of the inherent challenges in environmental health education include the broad reach of the field and the fact that it is unfamiliar to many clinicians. Compounding the issue are the 84,000 chemicals used commercially in the U.S., the chemical makeup of about 20% of which are kept secret due to a 33-year-old federal trade secret mandate. About 700 chemicals are introduced yearly in the U.S. and 95% of annual requests received by the government to market new chemicals request some level of secrecy (EPA). Separating media hype from scientific fact can also be difficult, as is interpretation of complex regulations.

An Organized Approach

Despite the challenges, parents, patients, and clinicians need accurate information about prevention to reduce or prevent environmental exposures and a framework with which to sort and process emerging research. One option is to group toxicants based on their primary source: air, land, or water, following the model used by the EPA. This is a useful simplified model as long as the dynamic cycle of toxicants movement from air to water to land is recognized.

Categorizing toxicants in this way (air, land, water) reflects the approach used in this chapter. Rather than attempting to cover an exhaustive list of toxicants in each category, a selection of examples with strongest supporting research in pediatrics will be reviewed. Resources for more detailed study are offered at the end of the chapter.

Due to a lack of training, clinicians may be reluctant to even introduce the subject of environmental exposures in the patient visit for fear of seeming ill prepared to answer patients' questions. However, discussion of the topic sends a powerful message to the patient and family that environmental issues have a significant influence on pediatric health. Resources for obtaining a meaningful environmental health history can be found through a variety of resources such as the Children's Environmental Health Network and the American Academy of Pediatrics Council on Environmental Health Resources.

Partners in Information Access for the Public Health Workforce is another excellent resource.

Air

Children have been shown to be more vulnerable to the effects of air pollution than adults, in part because they may receive higher exposure doses due to increased time spent outdoors participating in free play and recreational activities that increase minute ventilation and time of exposure to harmful pollutants (Li et al. 2012).

These exposures can be especially detrimental in the early stages of lung development where specific windows of vulnerability have been identified (Dietert et al. 2000).

For example, emerging research shows that second trimester prenatal exposure to traffic source air pollution, specifically nitrous dioxide and benzene, is associated with deficits in lung function at preschool age (Morales et al. 2015).

The effects of airborne toxicants have significant impact on children's school attendance, cause increased utilization of healthcare resources, and account for a significant number of parents' missed days of work (Kim and American Academy of Pediatrics Committee on Environmental 2004).

Exposure to exhaust fumes from school buses has also been correlated with asthma and other respiratory illnesses in children (Adar et al. 2015).

Internationally, children in developing countries are exposed to concentrations of air pollutants that far exceed the World Health Organization guidelines for safe air quality (Zar and Ferkol 2014; World Health Organization).

Criteria Pollutants and Hazardous Air Pollutants

Air toxicants are generally divided into two main categories, criteria pollutants and hazardous air pollutants. The criteria pollutants are those that are found so reliably in selected geographic locales that they are used to determine the Air Quality Index. The hazardous air pollutants are primarily from man-made sources. Air pollutants with the strongest correlation to pediatric respiratory disease are regulated by the U.S. Clean Air Act Extension of 1970 (P.L. 91-604), which raises the question of whether the current U.S. standards for air are sufficiently protective of children's health. Standards are reviewed every 5 years, and regulations for ozone and particulate matter were last tightened in 1997. The list of most serious offenders in children includes: particulate matter, ozone, sulfur dioxide, nitrogen dioxide, and carbon monoxide, all of which are considered 'criteria pollutants', described in more detail below (Sheffield et al. 2011).

Hazardous air pollutants, or toxic air contaminants, are a group of 188 pollutants and chemical groups with known or suspected links to serious diseases such as cancer, birth defects, and respiratory and neurologic conditions. These can be found in indoor and outdoor air depending on source. Some of the most toxic in this category include benzenes, formaldehyde, polycyclic aromatic hydrocarbons, hexane, perchloroethylene, asbestos, and metals such as mercury and cadmium (U.S. EPA air toxics http://www.epa.gov/oar/toxicair/newtoxics.html).

Polycyclic aromatic hydrocarbons generated through diesel and gas-powered vehicles, waste incinerators, coal-burning factories, tobacco smoke, and other common sources have been shown to readily cross the placenta and affect the fetal brain. An important cross-sectional MRI imaging study by Peterson in community-based minority youth studied from gestation through school age showed a statistically significant dose response relationship between prenatal polycyclic aromatic hydrocarbon exposure and reduction of brain white matter in childhood. This reduction in left-hemisphere white matter was associated with delayed processing speed on cognitive testing and with behavioral disturbances such as ADHD and conduct disorder (Peterson et al. 2015).

The most recent EPA data on hazardous air toxicants was released in early 2011 and is based on data collected in 2005. It identifies 80 of the studied hazardous air pollutants as carcinogens, 10 as carcinogenic to humans, 53 as likely carcinogenic to humans, and 16 with evidence of carcinogenic potential. One hundred ten of the study chemicals were found to have some type of non-cancer adverse effect, most commonly inflammation of the respiratory tract (U.S. EPA 2011).

Selected air toxicants will be discussed below as they relate to children's health. More detailed information on air toxicants can be found on the EPA website or through resources listed at the end of the chapter.

Routes of Exposure

Common airborne exposure routes in children include:

- Air pollution (mobile—traffic and school buses, stationary—factories, refineries, power plants, and natural sources)
- Tobacco smoke (and second and third-hand smoke)
- Dust (especially in toddlers, in lower socioeconomic groups, and in higher density living situations)
- Natural sources (ash, smoke and particulate matter from forest fires and volcanic eruptions)

Several of the most toxic compounds carried in the air, for example mercury, lead, and arsenic, are then deposited onto soil, surface water, or well water and subsequently cycle through the ecosystem causing repeated exposures through contaminated soil, water, and food. Some pediatric conditions associated with air pollution include (Talbott et al. 2015; Ornoy, Weinstein-Fudim, and Ergaz 2015):

- Asthma
- Bronchiolitis (by provoking ongoing inflammation in the lungs)
- Atopic dermatitis
- Allergies
- Prematurity
- Cancer
- Congenital cardiac conditions
- Possibly autism

The Air Quality Index

The Air Quality Index provides the public access to detailed, real-time air quality forecasts, maps, and health advisories about local air based on levels of the criteria air pollutants. Searches can be done by states, cities, or zip code through the interactive website airnow.gov. The site is provided through collaboration by the U.S. Environmental Protection Agency, National Oceanic and Atmospheric Administration, National Park Service, tribal, state, and local agencies. The AirNow system provides access to national air quality information for cities across the U.S. and parts of Canada and Mexico. An international tool is available at AirNow-International. (EPA)

The Six Criteria Pollutants

- Carbon monoxide
- Sulfur oxides
- Nitrogen oxides
- Ozone (ground level)
- Lead
- Particulate matter (Table 8.2)

Particulate Matter and Children

Particulate matter has been shown to affect both lung function and lung growth (as measured by lung function tests) in a study of 1678 Southern California school children. Larger deficits in lung function growth rate were seen in children who spent more time outside (Gauderman et al. 2015).

Associations have been documented between high ambient particulate matter and infant mortality (from respiratory causes and suspected sudden infant death syndrome) nationally (Woodruff, Darrow, and Parker 2008), and internationally (Zar and Ferkol 2014).

Some positive progress has been seen over the past 13 years during which three large cohorts of children in Southern California were studied as part of the Children's Health Study.

Decrease in air pollution levels has led to statistically significant positive effects on lung function growth in children both with and without asthma. Increases in 4-year growth in both FEV1 and FVC were associated with reduced levels of nitrogen dioxide, PM 10, and PM 2.5 across communities studied (Gauderman et al. 2015).

Mechanisms of Toxicity

The criteria pollutants share similar mechanisms of toxicity, primarily inflammation in the respiratory and cardiovascular systems. These toxins target the very young, the elderly, and people with pre-existing cardiac or respiratory conditions (Kim and American Academy of Pediatrics Committee on Environmental 2004).

What follows are some of the emerging research in how criteria air pollutants impact children's health.

Health Conditions Associated with Criteria Air Pollutants in Pediatrics

Asthma

According to the World Health Organization, up to 44% of the asthma burden can be attributed to modifiable environmental factors such as air pollution (Nishimura et al. 2013; Fingerhut et al. 2006).

Both prenatal and postnatal exposures to criteria pollutants have been associated with development and exacerbations of asthma in children. Research is active examining the specifics of individual phenotype that influences immune response, gene-environment, and epigenetic factors in expression of the clinical symptoms of asthma and atopy (Miller and Peden 2014).

A study by Brandt examining the mechanism of asthma exacerbation in response

Table 8.2 Criteria Air Pollutants, U.S. EPA

Carbon monoxide

Carbon monoxide is mainly produced in the process of combustion from mobile sources such as vehicles. On inhalation it absorbs through the alveoli, combines with hemoglobin and forms carboxyhemoglobin, subsequently displacing oxygen on hemoglobin. The highly inflammatory properties of carbon monoxide have been shown to provoke angina and asthma symptoms.

Sulfur oxides

Sulfur oxides are highly reactive byproducts of fossil fuel combustion. Their primary sources are power plants and other industrial facilities. Research has linked even short-term exposures to sulfur dioxide (5 minutes to 24 hours), to a range of serious respiratory effects including airway inflammation and bronchoconstriction.

Nitrogen oxides

Nitrogen dioxide is a highly reactive gas found mainly from mobile sources, and also a component of ground-level ozone and acid rain. Nitrogen dioxide reacts with ammonia, moisture, and other small compounds in air to form ultrafine particles that can penetrate deep into the lungs and provoke inflammation, vasoconstriction, acute respiratory distress, and cardiovascular events such as ventricular tachycardia. In U.S. EPA studies short exposures (30 minutes) have been shown to provoke airway inflammation in healthy people, and to significantly worsen respiratory symptoms in asthmatics. Depending on traffic volume, air measured near roadways can have a 30%–100% higher concentration of nitrogen dioxide than air distant from roadways. Nitrogen dioxide levels can also be elevated inside vehicles, subjecting infants and children to additional exposures.

Ozone (ground level)

Ozone is created at ground level by a chemical reaction between nitrous oxides and reactive hydrocarbons found in motor vehicle exhaust and industrial emissions. The reaction is catalyzed by sunlight, therefore levels are generally higher on warm, sunny, windless days—often in mid-afternoon when children are likely to be outdoors. Ground-level ozone is the primary ingredient of smog. Inhalation of ground-level ozone has been shown to cause airway inflammation, cough, pain with inhalation, wheezing especially during exercise, worsening of asthma, increased susceptibility to bronchitis, pneumonia, and in some cases permanent lung damage with repeated exposures.

Lead

Lead has a long history of serious toxicity, and is persistent in the environment. A substantial body of research has demonstrated the toxic effects of lead on neurologic and behavioral development in infants and young children, contributing to behavior problems, learning deficits, and lowered IQ (CDC, http://www.atsdr.cdc.gov/csem/csem.asp?csem=7&po=10). Primary sources in air include lead smelters, ore and metal processing, manufacture of lead batteries, and leaded aviation fuel. Lead can contaminate air, soil, and water, and be accidentally ingested in lead-contaminated paint or dust. Once in the body it accumulates in bones. Lead has the potential to affect nearly every organ system in the body, including the nervous system, renal function, immune system, reproductive, and cardiovascular systems. One of the most harmful effects of lead is its interference with the oxygen-carrying capacity of the blood. It can also promote apoptosis (programmed cell death), alter many aspects of neuronal structure and function, and disrupt thyroid hormone transport in the brain. Lead toxicity can also disrupt calcium and zinc physiology, mitochondrial function, anti-oxidative enzyme function, and lipid metabolism.

(continued)

Table 8.2 Criteria Air Pollutants, U.S. EPA (continued)

Particulate matter

Particulate matter (PM) is categorized based on diameter in micrometers. The particles can actually be made up of hundreds of different chemicals and consist of a mixture of solid particles and liquid droplets found in the air. Main sources are burning gasoline, diesel, and other fossil fuels in vehicles, power plants, and other industrial processes. Natural sources are forest fires, volcanic eruptions, and dust storms. The size of the particle is directly related to its health effects. The smallest particles penetrate into alveoli and can pass into the bloodstream. All types of fine particulate matter can cause serious respiratory and cardiovascular inflammation, vasoconstriction, asthma, bronchitis, irregular heart rate, non-fatal heart attacks, and premature death in people with pre-existing heart or lung disease. The mechanism of DNA damage is believed to be via oxidative stress. Note: The EPA accelerated research on fine particulate matter in the late 1990s in response to multiple studies linking fine particle air pollution with thousands of deaths and hospitalizations (Sheffield et al. 2011).

to diesel exhaust particles demonstrated accumulation of allergen specific memory T cells (Th2/Th17) cells in the lungs of children in the Cincinnati Childhood Allergy and Air Pollution Study, stimulating secondary allergy recall responses correlated with the development of allergic asthma. Early life exposure to high diesel exhaust particles was significantly associated with increased asthma prevalence among allergic children as opposed to non-allergic children (Brandt et al. 2015).

Nishimura demonstrated a correlation between early life nitrogen dioxide exposure and development of childhood asthma in Latino and African American children, using residential addresses to determine exposures. Results showed statistically significant correlation between exposures to traffic-related air pollutants and childhood asthma during the first year and in the first three years of life (Nishimura et al. 2013).

Several large population studies have demonstrated correlation between increased levels of ultrafine particles and carbon monoxide concentrations and asthma in preschool and school-aged children, especially those living in urban settings (Evans et al. 2014; Stoner, Anderson, and Buckley 2013; Lee et al. 2011), and emergency room admissions for acute asthma exacerbations, especially in the summer months (Gleason, Bielory, and Fagliano 2014).

OZONE AND ASTHMA IN CHILDREN

Ample evidence exists correlating asthma exacerbations and respiratory distress in children with high ambient ozone levels. In a study by White, evaluating 609 pediatric emergency department visits in Atlanta, Georgia the average number of visits was 37% higher on the 6 days when ozone was at highest levels (equal to or greater than 0.11 ppm) during the study period (White et al. 1994).

A 2009 study by Mar also found a statistically significant association between emergency department visits for pediatric asthma and ambient ozone levels during summer in greater Seattle, Washington (Mar and Koenig 2009).

Another large population study of more than 100,000 children aged 2–16 years in Atlanta, Georgia showed a positive correlation between ambient air pollution, especially ozone, and asthma among children born preterm and in children of African American mothers (Strickland et al. 2014).

Bronchiolitis

Sheffield showed a positive correlation between fine particulate matter pollution and infant hospitalizations for bronchiolitis in multiple large urban areas where an increase in the average exposure to fine particulate matter of an infant over the lifetime was correlated with increased costs for the child's healthcare (Sheffield et al. 2011).

A causal association between ozone exposure and bronchiolitis has also been questioned. A study by Burnett in children younger than 2 years found a 35% increase in daily hospitalization for respiratory problems associated with elevated ambient ozone during summer in Toronto, Canada (Burnett et al. 2001).

Atopic Dermatitis

Although an association between ambient air pollution and atopic dermatitis does not seem intuitive, multiple studies confirm a link. A review by Ahn (Ahn 2014) shows that both genetic predisposition and environmental triggers play a role in disease expression in susceptible individuals. Particulate matter, nitrogen dioxide, tobacco smoke, volatile organic compounds, and formaldehyde have all been associated with atopic dermatitis. Although the exact mechanism is unclear, the postulated mechanism is that dermal exposure leads to oxidative stress in the skin prompting an inflammatory response. Dermal exposure to a number of pollutants, including cigarette smoke, has been strongly liked to atopic dermatitis (Yi et al. 2012).

Exposure to tobacco smoke during pregnancy has been associated with DNA methylation identified in cord blood in a Taiwanese birth panel study, where exposures were significantly linked to development of atopic dermatitis at 2 years of age in exposed offspring (Wang et al. 2013) and a German birth cohort study of 2536 children found that exposure to redecorating involving painting, new floor covering, and furniture before birth and in the first year of life was associated with development of atopic dermatitis within the 6 years of the study period (Herbarth et al. 2006).

The presence of atopic dermatitis is significant in that many children with atopic dermatitis develop asthma and allergic rhinitis in later childhood that often persists into adult life (van der Hulst, Klip, and Brand 2007; Kapoor et al. 2008).

Low Birth Weight

A meta-analysis using information from 14 International Collaboration on Air Pollution and Pregnancy Outcomes centers involving nine countries with more than three million live births found that exposure to particulate matter (PM 10 and 2.5), nitrogen dioxide, and traffic density to nearest road and total traffic load is associated with low birth weight at term, described as fetal weight of less than 2500 grams at birth after 37 weeks' gestation (Dadvand et al. 2013; Pedersen et al. 2013).

Autism

In-utero exposure to air pollution (ozone, PM 2.5, nitric oxide, nitrogen dioxide) has also been associated with an increased risk of autism in multiple large randomized studies, with results consistent with increased susceptibility in the third trimester (Kalkbrenner et al. 2015; Volk et al. 2013).

Data from the Nurses' Health Study suggests that fine particulate matter PM 2.5 exposure throughout pregnancy, especially during the third trimester, was strongly correlated with autism (Raz et al. 2015).

Animal studies with ultrafine particulate matter in mice suggest an inflammatory-mediated mechanism in the central nervous system, although both genetic factors and environmental triggers are thought to be involved and many questions remain about the etiology of this complex illness (Arnold 2015; Becerra et al. 2013).

Cancer

Higher prenatal exposures to components of air pollution (nitric oxide, nitrogen dioxide), based on birthplace geographic location, are associated with an increased risk of childhood acute lymphoblastic leukemia (ALL) and with bilateral retinoblastoma, especially in the first two trimesters of pregnancy (Ghosh et al. 2013).

A 2015 study by Danysh comparing traffic-related air pollutants, including 1,3 butadiene, benzene, and particulate matter, with the incidence of childhood central nervous system cancers from a study period of 2001–2009 (n = 1949) found that census tracts with higher concentrations of these toxicants were associated with astrocytoma, medulloblastoma, and primitive neuroectodermal tumors (PNET) respectively (Danysh et al. 2015).

Potential cancer risk was assessed through measurement of phthalate in indoor dust, and phthalate concentrations in indoor and outdoor air in and around early childhood education facilities in Northern California. Results showed that 82%–89% of children in these childcare centers had exposures that exceeded established risk levels for chemicals known to cause reproductive toxicity, and 8%–11% of children under 2 years of age had phthalate exposure estimates that exceeded established risk levels for cancer benchmarks (Gaspar et al. 2014).

Dust samples taken from older homes in California as part of the California Childhood Leukemia Study (2001–2009) showed that dust concentrations of lead, polychlorinated biphenyls, organochlorine insecticides, and polycyclic aromatic hydrocarbons were closely correlated with home age, suggesting that strategies to reduce chemical exposures for children living in older homes should be a priority (Whitehead et al. 2014).

Lead is a prevalent contaminant in indoor air. It can be inhaled in contaminated dust, aerosolized when removing old paint, or aerosolized from contaminated soil or clothes. Blood levels as low as 10 micrograms per deciliter have been shown to cause harm to humans. Raised awareness and frequent cleaning and dusting are critical, especially in areas where young children play (U.S. EPA 2011).

Congenital Heart Defects

Epidemiological studies suggest associations between gestational particulate matter exposure and congenital heart defects, although further studies are needed to confirm causality. A study by Padula examined association between seven air pollutants and traffic exposures in the first 2 months of pregnancy and prevalence of congenital heart defects in infants. Particulate matter less than 10 microns (PM 10) was associated with pulmonary valve stenosis, and traffic density was associated with ventricular septal defects in this study population (Padula et al. 2013; Peretz et al. 2014).

A multi-state controlled study of 3328 live births showed a positive association between nitrogen dioxide exposure and coarctation of the aorta and pulmonary valve stenosis. Exposure to fine particulate matter was associated with hypoplastic left heart syndrome. Authors suggest potential windows of susceptibility to airborne pollutants during pregnancy (Stingone et al. 2014).

Indoor Air: Hazardous Air Pollutants

Indoor air is often considered under a category known as the 'built environment'; man-made structures and surroundings that provide the setting for human activity. One of the biggest challenges in identifying indoor air pollutants is that they are invisible and come from materials and structures found in our everyday environment. Volatile organic compounds (VOCs), gases emitted by products such as paints, cleaning supplies, pesticides, and office machines are significant contributors to this category of pollutants. Benzene, found in gasoline, and formaldehyde, present in cigarette smoke, manufacturing and adhesives for pressed wood products (cabinets, paneling, flooring) are other examples of common hazardous air pollutants. Tobacco smoke is one of the most common exposures in children. An estimated 40% of children worldwide receive exposure in their own homes. The list of serious illness from second and third-hand tobacco smoke exposure to fetal, infant, child, and adolescent health has been widely reported and ranges from low birth weight and sudden infant death syndrome to lower respiratory illness, asthma, cardiovascular disease and cancer-mirroring adult pathology in older age groups (Oberg et al. 2011).

Tobacco smoke carries hundreds of toxicants, including thiocyanate and perchorate (used in rocket fuels, propellants, and explosives), pollutants that compete with iodide for transport into the thyroid follicular cell where it performs a key step in the synthesis of thyroid hormone (Council on Environmental Health et al. 2014).

Air Summary

Clearly, exposures to indoor and outdoor air toxicants can have serious health consequences for the developing fetus and children, especially those with pre-existing conditions. Many agencies nationally, and internationally, are working to improve air quality and clinicians can advocate for patients and their families by staying up to date on emerging research and reliable resources.

Practical Clinical Strategies

Outdoor Air

- Check the local air quality index at AirNow.gov by zip code and AirNow International.
- Counsel patients to avoid outdoor activities on poor air quality days, or time activities to avoid peak pollution.
- Counsel patients to avoid exercising by busy roads whenever possible.
- Children with pre-existing conditions should limit outdoor time on poor quality air days.
- Be aware of stationary source (industrial) pollutants near home, work, and school and avoid exposures as much as possible.
- Children should avoid exposure to idling cars and school buses.

Indoor Air

- Limit children's exposures to pressed particle board, adhesives, indoor cleaners, pesticides, paints, carpeting, and other flooring unless labeled as "low VOC."
- Avoid tracking in toxic dust and contaminants on soil and clothing.
- Check heating and venting sources carefully.
- Check for radon.
- Avoid second-hand and third-hand smoke. Protect infants, children, and adolescents from all tobacco smoke exposure.
- Use a carbon monoxide monitor in the home or workplace.

Land

Land-based pollutants come from a wide range of sources including manufacturing and agriculture and have been widely studied. Many of these pollutants fall into the category of endocrine-disrupting chemicals, which interfere with the synthesis and action of naturally occurring hormones and neurotransmitter receptors. As a broad class, endocrine-disrupting chemicals have been associated with serious health effects in children. Bisphenol A and phthalates are endocrine-disrupting chemicals commonly used in plastic manufacturing. Pesticides and flame retardants are two other important groups of endocrine-disrupting chemicals known to impact children's health. Some of the most concerning research highlights the susceptibility of the fetus, embryo, and primordial germ cells to the effect of endocrine-disrupting chemicals on gene regulation. Although research is accumulating rapidly on the ubiquitous presence of endocrine-disrupting chemicals in our environment, safe exposure levels for the vast majority of these chemicals have not been established (Diamanti-Kandarakis et al. 2009) (Table 8.3).

Unknowns regarding endocrine-disrupting chemicals (Diamanti-Kandarakis et al. 2009):

- Importance of age at exposure—and connection to development of adult disease
- Latency of clinical disease after exposures
- Additive or synergistic properties
- Non-traditional dose responses, critical developmental windows
- Transgenerational, epigenetic effects; DNA methylation and histone acetylation (heritability of exposures)

Bisphenol A and Phthalates

Bisphenol A (BPA) is a chemical that was initially synthesized in 1891. Its estrogenic properties were recognized in the early 1930s (Dodds 1938). However, its use as a pharmaceutical was precluded by development of a second more estrogenic compound, diethylstilbestrol, DES—which was later linked to reproductive cancers in girls born to mothers who took DES during pregnancy. Subsequently, in the 1940s and 1950s BPA was found to be useful in plastic manufacturing to make a hard polycarbonate and epoxy resins used in linings of cans and in other products. BPA has since become one of the world's most highly produced chemicals, with an estimated 15 billion pounds manufactured annually. It is found in many polycarbonate plastics, thermal receipt

Table 8.3 Health Effects of Endocrine-Disrupting Chemicals

Reproductive and developmental abnormalities
Infertility
Delayed puberty
Decreased sperm count
Cryptorchidism
Abnormal development of sex organs
Hypospadias
Miscarriage
Polycystic ovarian syndrome
Cancer breast, prostate, liver
ADHD
Obesity and comorbidities
Insulin resistance
Metabolic syndrome
Cardiovascular disease
Thyroid dysfunction
Allergies and asthma

Source: U.S. EPA. https://www.epa.gov/chemical-research/research-endocrine-disruptors

paper, some dental sealants, linings of metal food cans, and many other items that are not required to be labeled as BPA containing (Rosenfeld 2015).

In 1976 when U.S. Congress passed the Toxic Substances Control Act, BPA was one of the 62,000 chemicals grandfathered in, presumed safe and never tested. Since that time there have been a number of controversies associated with safety standards and accepted exposure levels for humans in the U.S. (Environmental Working Group 2008).

In 1997, the first of what would eventually come to be hundreds of studies linking compounds with endocrine-disrupting properties to harmful health effects was published by vom Saal in the Proceedings of the National Academy of Sciences (vom Saal et al. 1997). vom Saal's study described the effect of diethylstilbestrol (DES) fed to maternal mice on the prostate size of male offspring, showing a 50% increase in free-serum estradiol and a 40% increase in prostatic androgen receptors, and ultimately a 30% increase in prostate size compared to controls, and raised concerns about the alteration of other estrogen-responsive organs in the body. The study concludes with a warning that human fetal exposure to estrogenic chemicals in pharmaceuticals or those present in food or water and air "from pesticides, components of plastic, detergents, hand creams, and other products." Later that year, U.S. Federal Drug Administration testing found BPA contamination to be commonplace in cans of infant formula through leakage from the resin lining. No regulatory actions were taken, and a long series of delays and conflicting industry-sponsored research and advisory input ultimately led to a 2008 U.S. Congressional investigation of the FDA's findings on BPA. In response to a request from Congressional inquiry for information on BPA in their products, the majority of infant formula manufacturers reported a lack of data on the levels of BPA in their products.

Peer-reviewed scientific research continued to accumulate on the adverse health effects of BPA at extremely low doses (Keri et al. 2007), and ultimately it was Canada that moved first to reduce BPA exposure in infants and children by deeming it a "dangerous substance" listed under Schedule 1 of the Canadian Environmental Protection Act, banning its use in baby bottle manufacturing and restricting use in infant formula packaging. This precipitated large manufacturers of infant products in the U.S. to shift towards BPA-free products, a trend that is ongoing. Members of the European Union published a Commission Directive in the Official Journal of the European Union adopting restrictions on the use of BPA in plastic infant bottle manufacturing in 2010 (2011).

Over time significant research has accrued on the ubiquitous nature of BPA, and its human health effects in children and adults. Lack of consensus regarding "safe dose," exposures, and "low dose" exposure continues to fuel debate. It has been established that BPA binds the membrane-associated estrogen receptor, and also acts through the androgen receptor, thyroid hormone receptor, selected peroxisome proliferator-activated receptors, and other endocrine pathways (Watson, Jeng, and Guptarak 2011).

A 2013 review of low-dose BPA effects by Vandenberg et al. (Vandenberg et al. 2013) details animal and human research in this area. Conclusions of the review include: endocrine-disrupting chemicals, including BPA, have a greater potential for disruption when exposures occur during organogenesis and times of tissue differentiation; consistent reproducible adverse low dose effects have been seen in vitro, in animal studies, and in some human studies; doses shown to produce adverse events in animal studies are one to four magnitudes of order lower than the current lowest observed adverse effect level of 50 mg/kg/day; rodent studies of low-dose BPA exposure show adverse effects on male and female reproductive tract, behavior and brain development, and metabolic markers including insulin regulation; BPA induces neoplastic lesions in the rodent mammary gland. Some of the most concerning animal studies demonstrate interference of BPA with neuronal synapse formation and remodeling (Hajszan and Leranth 2010; Wang et al. 2014).

In humans increased urinary BPA has been associated with higher odds of obesity, insulin resistance, cardiovascular disease, polycystic ovarian disease, and type-2 diabetes (Shankar, Teppala, and Sabanayagam 2012; Teppala, Madhavan, and Shankar 2012).

A cross-sectional analysis of 2838 children 6–19 years of age showed statistically significant association between pediatric and adolescent obesity and urinary BPA independent of race, educational level, caloric intake and television watching time (Teppala, Madhavan, and Shankar 2012; Trasande, Attina, and Blustein 2012).

Prenatal BPA exposure has been associated with decreased thyroid stimulating hormone in male infants—a finding of special concern, as thyroid hormone is integral to normal brain development (Chevrier et al. 2013; Brucker-Davis et al. 2011).

Elevated urinary BPA has also been associated with thyroid dysfunction in adolescents, and adults (Meeker and Ferguson 2011).

Neurobehavioral effects of BPA exposure have been investigated in children, with some studies suggesting adverse effects. For example, in a prospective birth cohort of 224 mother–child pairs, every 10-fold increase in gestational BPA concentration was associated with increased anxious and depressed behavior and poorer emotional control at 3 years of age in offspring, especially in girls (Braun et al. 2011; Rosenfeld 2015; Rochester 2013).

Phthalates

Phthalates refer to a group of chemicals used to make hard plastic more flexible, transparent, and durable. They are often referred to as plasticizers. Phthalates are used in an extensive variety of products, including enteric coating of both prescription and over-the-counter drugs, and dietary supplements (Kelley et al. 2012).

One of their most common industrial uses is to soften polyvinyl chloride. Their use ranges from medical care devices and intravenous tubing and catheters to perfume, nail polish, building materials, toys, food, food containers and wrappers, and pesticides among many others. Approximately 500 million pounds of phthalates are produced in the U.S. each year, and most Americans tested have multiple phthalates in their urine. As with BPA, children and infants have the highest body burdens (Vandenberg et al. 2013).

Phthalates are prevalent in the healthcare industry, and have been identified in high concentrations in some healthcare workers (Wilding, Curtis, and Welker-Hood 2009).

The primary mechanism of concern with phthalates is induced reproductive developmental disorders via suppression of genes for cholesterol transport and steroidogenesis in fetal Leydig cells, which leads to decreased cholesterol transport and decreased testosterone synthesis, which can manifest as cryptorchidism, hypospadias, and undescended testicles. In turn, hypospadias has been associated with lower sperm concentration and motility. There are also cross-sectional studies associating urinary phthalates during pregnancy and neurodevelopmental effects in infancy or childhood, including reduction of IQ at 7 years of age in a prospective birth cohort of 328 inner city children (Facheris et al. 2010).

Of concern, two replacements for one type of phthalate, DHEP, di-isononyl phthalate (DINP) and di-isodecyl phthalate (DIDP), have been linked to rise in blood pressure in children (Trasande and Attina 2015) and have also been associated with insulin resistance in adolescents (Attina and Trasande 2015).

There are many types of phthalates with differing health effects. Exposure routes studied include inhalation, direct and indirect ingestion, and dermal contact (diet, prescription drugs, toys, childcare articles, personal care products, indoor sources, outdoor sources).

Phthalates leach out of plastic products and into food. Fatty foods are most likely to absorb phthalates. Low molecular weight phthalates can be dermally absorbed. They have also been shown to pass into breast milk.

Based on accumulating data on detrimental health effects, the Consumer Product Safety Commission convened a Chronic Hazard Advisory Panel in 2010 on phthalates found in children's toys, childcare products, and in products used by women of child-bearing age (Lioy et al. 2015).

Main sources of phthalate exposure in pregnant women were found to be food, beverages, and drugs, personal products and exposures in the indoor environment. Infants' top exposure was in the diet, and also from teethers and toys that were mouthed as well as through dermal contact with childcare articles. Toddlers' exposures came primarily from food and beverages. Toddler exposures were the highest per body weight compared to infants and adults. In older children exposures were highest in food and beverages, and dust in the indoor environment. Many uncertainties remain regarding phthalate exposures, including safe tolerable limits, and possible cumulative and synergistic effects. Three types of phthalates, DBP, BBP, and DHEP, have been permanently banned in toys and childcare articles at levels over 0.1%. Several others are under interim ban pending further study, but have been shown to have antiandrogenic effects. Conclusive data for the safety of phthalate alternatives is lacking.

Practical Patient Counseling

While some manufacturers are now labeling products that are BPA or phthalate free, clinicians and consumers can benefit from a raised awareness about common sources and take concrete steps to avoid or minimize unnecessary exposures.

*   Plastic recycling codes are voluntary, and many plastics are not labeled. If a recycling code is present, in general a code of 7 indicates polycarbonate, which may contain BPA. A recycling code of 3 is likely to contain phthalate.
*   Avoid purchasing food in plastic containers.
*   Avoid heating food in plastic containers or covered with plastic wraps in the microwave.
*   See the Environmental Working Group Skin Deep Cosmetic Data Base (http://www.ewg.org/skindeep/).
*   See the Good Guide (http://www.goodguide.com).

Pesticides

The American Academy of Pediatrics *Technical Statement on Pesticide Exposure in Children* suggests that based on the weight of scientific evidence children's acute and chronic exposures to pesticides should be as limited as possible. This is challenging, as children can be exposed through a variety of routes, including orally, through inhalation, and by dermal contact. Disproportionate dose exposures can occur in children due to higher metabolic rate, greater intake of food or fluids per pound of body weight, and the frequency of hand-to-mouth contact. Residential exposures are common; for example, with insecticide and herbicide use in gardens and pest control products to protect family pets. It has also been well established that pesticides accumulate in indoor air samples, dust, upholstered furniture, and on soft children's toys, or tracked in from the agricultural workplace by parents or other caretakers (Roberts, Karr, and Council On Environmental Health 2012).

Food consumption is a primary route of pesticide exposure in children. This has been demonstrated through testing of urinary organophosphorus pesticide metabolites in children placed on a 5 consecutive day organic diet where urinary concentrations of pesticide metabolites dropped to undetectable levels immediately after the organic diet was begun, and resumed when a conventional diet was reintroduced (Lu et al. 2006, Lu et al. 2008).

Contamination of drinking water, especially well water, is another significant source of exposure (Roberts, Karr, and Council On Environmental Health 2012).

Chronic health effects of pesticide exposures in children vary by exposure type and are under ongoing study. Some of the most concerning include increased risk of cancer (leukemia and brain tumors) (Jurewicz and Hanke 2006), neurodevelopmental abnormalities, asthma, impaired fetal growth, and disruption of normal endocrine function.

For example, a large U.S. National Health and Nutrition Examination Survey (NHANES) cross-sectional analysis showed that children 8–15 years old with a diagnosis of attention-deficit/hyperactivity disorder had higher urinary concentrations of organophosphate metabolites than those with low levels (Bouchard et al. 2010; Kuehn 2010).

A review of epidemiological studies on prenatal and childhood pesticide exposures show that children exposed either prenatally or during childhood may have pervasive developmental problems, delayed reaction times, impaired mental development, and emotional and mental problems in adolescents. Research remains active in this area, with longitudinal prospective birth-cohort studies ongoing though the National Institutes of Health/Environmental Protection Agency (Jurewicz and Hanke 2008).

Increased risk with pesticide exposure to the developing fetus has also been documented, and includes reports of: intrauterine growth retardation, preterm birth, fetal death, and a range of congenital abnormalities (Stillerman et al. 2008).

Extensive data specific to individual subtypes of pesticides is lacking, although the organochlorine DDT has been extensively studied in relation to birth defects and fetal death. Elevated levels in maternal serum and umbilical cord blood have been associated with preterm birth, low birth weight, and intrauterine growth retardation in some studies (Longnecker et al. 2001; Ribas-Fito et al. 2002).

In two studies from Minnesota, a statistically higher rate of birth defects was recorded in fathers whose occupation was listed as pesticide applicator (Roberts, Karr, and Council On Environmental 2012). Multiple pesticides are under study for their estrogen-mimicking activity, particularly the association with urogenital abnormalities in boys (Rogan and Ragan 2007), and interference with normal timing of puberty in male teens (Zawatski and Lee 2013).

More studies examining unknowns such as timing of exposures, synergistic effects, and windows of vulnerability are needed, as are studies taking into consideration potential genetic polymorphisms affecting pesticide metabolism.

Regulatory Concerns

All pesticides sold in the U.S. must be registered with the EPA, yet up to 99% of the product may not be reported on the product label, including chemicals known to be toxic. This leads to significant difficulty diagnosing both acute and chronic exposures. Initiatives to change policy and raise awareness and education of pediatricians are an urgent priority given the extensive use of pesticides in the U.S. and internationally.

Practical Patient Counseling (Council On Environmental Health 2012; Roberts, Karr, and Council On Environmental Health 2012)

- Consume organic produce if possible.
- See the Environmental Working Group Pesticide Shopping Guide.
- Wash all produce, organic and conventional.
- Peel off leafy outer layers, peel fruit and vegetables.
- Trim fat off meat and fish, avoid skin.
- Limit use of pesticides in and around home, school, and office.
- Use non-chemical pest control whenever possible.

- Raise awareness of pesticide spraying and create spraying buffer zones around areas where children live and play.

Flame Retardants

Brominated flame retardants are another important group of endocrine-disrupting chemicals. They are ubiquitous, lipophilic, and highly pro-inflammatory. Historically they have been used in polyurethane foam, children's sleepwear, and in industrial use in computer casings, monitors, high-impact polystyrenes, automotive industry, and in textiles, and construction and building industries. Several types of first-generation flame retardants have been phased out in the U.S. and in Europe, and second-generation flame retardants have also been banned as a class in the EU since 2008. However, these compounds, categorized as persistent organic pollutants, are ubiquitous in ecosystems around the world (Dishaw et al. 2014).

Levels have consistently found to be the highest in infants and children, with North American children having some of the highest levels in the world (Eskenazi et al. 2013). The primary modes of transfer to children have been determined to be through placental transfer, ingestion of breast milk, and ingestion of contaminated dust particles (Toms et al. 2008; Toms et al. 2009; Johnson-Restrepo and Kannan 2009).

Infants also receive exposures through foam-containing baby products (Stapleton et al. 2011). A 2014 systematic review by Kim of 36 articles (17 pediatric) on the health effects of brominated flame retardants (Kim et al. 2014) identified plausible concerns about associations with diabetes, neurodevelopmental and behavioral disorders including ADHD (Eskenazi et al. 2013), cancer, reproductive health effects, and interference with normal thyroid function known to be intimately associated with normal central nervous system development.

The difficulty in identifying pollutants such as flame retardants, BPA, and phthalates and their ubiquitous presence in our environment is sobering. The knowledge that these compounds are present in the majority of infants, children, adolescents, and adults confirms the need for clinicians to be aware of their systemic health effects and educated advocates for a precautionary approach to environmental exposures.

Water

Water pollution is a complex global issue, and one that the World Health Organization and the U.S. EPA have spent hundreds of millions of dollars addressing. This section will offer a brief overview as an introduction to the topic. In the U.S. progress has been guided by the Clean Water Act of 1978, which mandates regulation of specific water contaminants, although over 200 unregulated water contaminants have been identified across the U.S. (Deblonde, Cossu-Leguille, and Hartemann 2011).

Regulated contaminants include:

- Microorganisms
- Disinfectants and disinfection byproducts
- Inorganic chemicals
- Organic chemicals
- Radionuclides
- Perchlorate (added in 2011)

Concern about unregulated contaminants is growing as studies identifying an alarming range of chemicals accrue, among them a wide range of pharmaceuticals and personal care products including antibiotics, antimicrobials, and various classes of persistent organic pollutants (Rahman, Yanful, and Jasim 2009).

Well water is not subject to EPA regulations and can be at high risk of contamination. Pesticides and nitrates are common contaminants, especially from nearby agricultural or concentrated animal-feeding operations. Volatile organic compounds, arsenic, and industrial pollutants are other common pollutants. The EPA recommends annual monitoring of well water (Padhye et al. 2014).

Although many people may use bottled water in an attempt to ensure good quality, the fact is that bottled water is held to the same standards as tap water under the EPA Clean Water Act, which means that some chemicals are identified and regulated, and others are not (Hu, Morton, and Mahler 2011).

Practical Patient Counseling

- Encourage patents to be familiar with their primary water source.
- Bottled water is not necessarily more pure than tap water.
- Activated charcoal filters can be effective point of source filters.
- Well water should be tested annually.

WATER RESOURCES

- EPA Office of Water
- EWG National Drinking Water Database
- CDC Agency for Toxic Substances and Disease Registry
- National Resource Defense Council: Consumer Guide to Water Filters
- NSF International
- USGS Water-Quality Information Pages

Self-Care Notes for Clinicians

It's important for healthcare providers to know that hospitals have significant sources of toxins in air, ranging from volatile organic chemicals in flooring, cleaning products, and wall coverings to the polyvinyl chlorides used in carpeting, and IV bags and tubing, exposing both patient and provider (Calafat et al. 2009). A 2009 report by Physicians for Social Responsibility, "Hazardous Chemicals in Health Care," offers some sobering insights into the levels of chemicals in healthcare workers of all types (Wilding, Curtis, and Welker-Hood 2009).

Summary

All clinicians caring for children have the potential to be effective advocates to help reduce environmental exposures in children. Advocacy and policy efforts can be directed at the individual, local, state, and national level. Practical steps such as encouraging reduction of unnecessary transportation, and educating families and schools about the links between environmental pollution and health, are important first steps. A simplified approach that breaks toxicant exposure down into the categories of air, land, and water that is tailored towards clinical symptoms may be especially helpful in children living with chronic illness, and the power and potential impact of preventive counseling cannot be underestimated. One of the most concerning issues is the slow rate of change in pollutant levels due to complex regulatory constraints and industry pushback. Meaningful societal change will depend on cooperation and engagement from leaders in industry, agriculture, transportation, healthcare, individuals, and government. Advocacy on the part of clinicians caring for children is critical to this work.

References

575, Acog Committee Opinion No. 2013. "Exposure to toxic environmental agents." *Obstet Gynecol* 122(4): 931–5. doi: 10.1097/01.AOG.0000435416.21944.54.

Adar, S. D., J. D'Souza, L. Sheppard, J. D. Kaufman, T. S. Hallstrand, M. E. Davey, J. R. Sullivan, J. Jahnke, J. Koenig, T. V. Larson, and L. J. Liu. 2015. "Adopting clean fuels and technologies on school buses. pollution and health impacts in children." *Am J Respir Crit Care Med* 191(12): 1413–21. doi: 10.1164/rccm.201410-1924OC.

Ahn, K. 2014. "The role of air pollutants in atopic dermatitis." *J Allergy Clin Immunol* 134(5): 993–9; discussion 1000. doi: 10.1016/j.jaci.2014.09.023.

Akin, L., M. Kendirci, F. Narin, S. Kurtoglu, R. Saraymen, M. Kondolot, S. Kocak, and F. Elmali. 2015. "The endocrine disruptor bisphenol A may play a role in the aetiopathogenesis of polycystic ovary syndrome in adolescent girls." *Acta Paediatr* 104(4): e171–7. doi: 10.1111/apa.12885.

Arnold, C. 2015. "Air pollution and ASDs: homing in on an environmental risk factor." *Environ Health Perspect* 123(3): A68. doi: 10.1289/ehp.123-A68.

Attina, T. M., and L. Trasande. 2015. "Association of exposure to d-2-ethylhexylphthalate replacements with increased insulin resistance in adolescents from NHANES 2009–2012." *J Clin Endocrinol Metab* 100(7): 2640–50. doi: 10.1210/jc.2015-1686.

Becerra, T. A., M. Wilhelm, J. Olsen, M. Cockburn, and B. Ritz. 2013. "Ambient air pollution and autism in Los Angeles county, California." *Environ Health Perspect* 121(3): 380–6. doi: 10.1289/ehp.1205827.

Bellingham, M., and R.M. Sharpe. 2013. Scientific Impact Paper. London: Royal College of Obstetricians and Gynaecologists.

Bouchard, M. F., D. C. Bellinger, R. O. Wright, and M. G. Weisskopf. 2010. "Attention-deficit/hyperactivity disorder and urinary metabolites of organophosphate pesticides." *Pediatrics* 125(6): e1270–7. doi: 10.1542/peds.2009-3058.

Brandt, E. B., J. M. Biagini Myers, T. H. Acciani, P. H. Ryan, U. Sivaprasad, B. Ruff, G. K. LeMasters, D. I. Bernstein, J. E. Lockey, T. D. LeCras, and G. K. Khurana Hershey. 2015. "Exposure to allergen and diesel exhaust particles potentiates secondary allergen-specific memory responses, promoting asthma susceptibility." *J Allergy Clin Immunol.* doi: 10.1016/j.jaci.2014.11.043.

Braun, J. M., A. E. Kalkbrenner, A. M. Calafat, K. Yolton, X. Ye, K. N. Dietrich, and B. P. Lanphear. 2011. "Impact of early-life bisphenol A exposure on behavior and executive function in children." *Pediatrics* 128(5): 873–82. doi: 10.1542/peds.2011-1335.

Brucker-Davis, F., P. Ferrari, M. Boda-Buccino, K. Wagner-Mahler, P. Pacini, J. Gal, P. Azuar, and P. Fenichel. 2011. "Cord blood thyroid tests in boys born with and without cryptorchidism: correlations with birth parameters and in utero xenobiotics exposure." *Thyroid* 21(10): 1133–41. doi: 10.1089/thy.2010.0459.

Burnett, R. T., M. Smith-Doiron, D. Stieb, M. E. Raizenne, J. R. Brook, R. E. Dales, J. A. Leech, S. Cakmak, and D. Krewski. 2001. "Association between ozone and hospitalization for acute respiratory diseases in children less than 2 years of age." *Am J Epidemiol* 153(5): 444–52.

Calafat, A. M., J. Weuve, X. Ye, L. T. Jia, H. Hu, S. Ringer, K. Huttner, and R. Hauser. 2009.

"Exposure to bisphenol A and other phenols in neonatal intensive care unit premature infants." *Environ Health Perspect* 117(4): 639–44. doi: 10.1289/ehp.0800265.

Chevrier, J., R. B. Gunier, A. Bradman, N. T. Holland, A. M. Calafat, B. Eskenazi, and K. G. Harley. 2013. "Maternal urinary bisphenol a during pregnancy and maternal and neonatal thyroid function in the CHAMACOS study." *Environ Health Perspect* 121(1): 138–44. doi: 10.1289/ehp.1205092.

Council on Environmental Health. https://www.aap.org/en-us/about-the-aap/Committees-Councils-Sections/Council-on-Environmental-Health/Pages/Welcome-to-COEH.aspx.

Council on Environmental Health. 2012. "Pesticide exposure in children." *Pediatrics* 130(6): e1757–63. doi: 10.1542/peds.2012-2757.

Council on Environmental Health, W. J. Rogan, J. A. Paulson, C. Baum, A. C. Brock-Utne, H. L. Brumberg, C. C. Campbell, B. P. Lanphear, J. A. Lowry, K. C. Osterhoudt, M. T. Sandel, A. Spanier, and L. Trasande. 2014. "Iodine deficiency, pollutant chemicals, and the thyroid: new information on an old problem." *Pediatrics* 133(6): 1163–6. doi: 10.1542/peds.2014-0900.

Dadvand, P., J. Parker, M. L. Bell, M. Bonzini, M. Brauer, L. A. Darrow, U. Gehring, S. V. Glinianaia, N. Gouveia, E. H. Ha, J. H. Leem, E. H. van den Hooven, B. Jalaludin, B. M. Jesdale, J. Lepeule, R. Morello-Frosch, G. G. Morgan, A. C. Pesatori, F. H. Pierik, T. Pless-Mulloli, D. Q. Rich, S. Sathyanarayana, J. Seo, R. Slama, M. Strickland, L. Tamburic, D. Wartenberg, M. J. Nieuwenhuijsen, and T. J. Woodruff. 2013. "Maternal exposure to particulate air pollution and term birth weight: a multi-country evaluation of effect and heterogeneity." *Environ Health Perspect* 121(3): 267–373. doi: 10.1289/ehp.1205575.

Danysh, H. E., L. E. Mitchell, K. Zhang, M. E. Scheurer, and P. J. Lupo. 2015. "Traffic-related air pollution and the incidence of childhood central nervous system tumors: Texas, 2001–2009." *Pediatr Blood Cancer.* doi: 10.1002/pbc.25549.

Deblonde, T., C. Cossu-Leguille, and P. Hartemann. 2011. "Emerging pollutants in wastewater: a review of the literature." *Int J Hyg Environ Health* 214(6): 442–8. doi: 10.1016/j.ijheh.2011.08.002.

Diamanti-Kandarakis, E., J. P. Bourguignon, L. C. Giudice, R. Hauser, G. S. Prins, A. M. Soto, R. T. Zoeller, and A. C. Gore. 2009. "Endocrine-disrupting chemicals: an Endocrine Society scientific statement." *Endocr Rev* 30(4): 293–342. doi: 10.1210/er.2009-0002.

Diamanti-Kandarakis, E., C. Christakou, and E. Marinakis. 2012. "Phenotypes and enviromental factors: their influence in PCOS." *Curr Pharm Des* 18(3): 270–82.

Dietert, R. R., R. A. Etzel, D. Chen, M. Halonen, S. D. Holladay, A. M. Jarabek, K. Landreth, D. B. Peden, K. Pinkerton, R. J. Smialowicz, and T. Zoetis. 2000. "Workshop to identify critical windows of exposure for children's health: immune and respiratory systems work group summary." *Environ Health Perspect* 108(Suppl 3): 483–90.

Dishaw, L. V., L. J. Macaulay, S. C. Roberts, and H. M. Stapleton. 2014. "Exposures, mechanisms, and impacts of endocrine-active flame retardants." *Curr Opin Pharmacol* 19: 125–33. doi: 10.1016/j.coph.2014.09.018.

Dodds, EC, Lawson W. 1938. "Molecular Structure in Relation to Osestrogenic Activity Compounss withouth a Phenanthrene Nucleus." *Proceedings of the Royal Society of London* 135(839): 222–32.

Environmental Working Group. 2005. "Body Burden: The Pollution in Newborns." http://www.ewg.org/research/body-burden-pollution-newborns

Environmental Working Group. 2008. "Timeline: BPA from Invention to Phase-Out " Accessed April 22. http://www.ewg.org/research/timeline-bpa-invention-phase-out

Eskenazi, B., J. Chevrier, S. A. Rauch, K. Kogut, K. G. Harley, C. Johnson, C. Trujillo, A. Sjodin, and A. Bradman. 2013. "In utero and childhood polybrominated diphenyl ether (PBDE) exposures and neurodevelopment in the CHAMACOS study." *Environ Health Perspect* 121(2): 257–62. doi: 10.1289/ehp.1205597.

Etzel, R. A., S. J. Balk, J. R. Reigart, and P. J. Landrigan. 2003. "Environmental health for practicing pediatricians." *Indian Pediatr* 40(9): 853–60.

European Union. 2011. "COMMISSION DIRECTIVE 2011/8/EU of 28 " *Official Journal of the European Union.*

Evans, K. A., J. S. Halterman, P. K. Hopke, M. Fagnano, and D. Q. Rich. 2014. "Increased ultrafine particles and carbon monoxide concentrations are associated with asthma exacerbation among urban children." *Environ Res* 129: 11–19. doi: 10.1016/j.envres.2013.12.001.

Facheris, M. F., A. A. Hicks, P. P. Pramstaller, and I. Pichler. 2010. "Update on the management of restless legs syndrome: existing and emerging treatment options." *Nat Sci Sleep* 2: 199–212. doi: 10.2147/NSS.S6946.

Fenichel, P., N. Chevalier, and F. Brucker-Davis. 2013. "Bisphenol A: an endocrine and metabolic disruptor." *Ann Endocrinol (Paris)* 74(3): 211–20. doi: 10.1016/j.ando.2013.04.002.

Fingerhut, M., D. I. Nelson, T. Driscoll, M. Concha-Barrientos, K. Steenland, L. Punnett, A. Pruss-Ustun, J. Leigh, C. Corvalan, G. Eijkemans, and J. Takala. 2006. "The contribution of occupational risks to the global burden of disease: summary and next steps." *Med Lav* 97(2): 313–21.

Frederiksen, M., K. Vorkamp, M. Thomsen, and L. E. Knudsen. 2009. "Human internal and external exposure to PBDEs—a review of levels and sources." *Int J Hyg Environ Health* 212(2): 109–34. doi: 10.1016/j.ijheh.2008.04.005.

Gaspar, F. W., R. Castorina, R. L. Maddalena, M. G. Nishioka, T. E. McKone, and A. Bradman. 2014. "Phthalate exposure and risk assessment in California child care facilities." *Environ Sci Technol* 48(13): 7593–601. doi: 10.1021/es501189t.

Gauderman, W. J., R. Urman, E. Avol, K. Berhane, R. McConnell, E. Rappaport, R. Chang, F. Lurmann, and F. Gilliland. 2015. "Association of improved air quality with lung development in children." *N Engl J Med* 372(10): 905–13. doi: 10.1056/NEJMoa1414123.

Gehle, K. S., J. L. Crawford, and M. T. Hatcher. 2011. "Integrating environmental health into medical education." *Am J Prev Med* 41(4 Suppl 3): S296–301. doi: 10.1016/j.amepre.2011.06.007.

Ghosh, J. K., J. E. Heck, M. Cockburn, J. Su, M. Jerrett, and B. Ritz. 2013. "Prenatal exposure to traffic-related air pollution and risk of early childhood cancers." *Am J Epidemiol* 178(8): 1233–9. doi: 10.1093/aje/kwt129.

Gleason, J. A., L. Bielory, and J. A. Fagliano. 2014. "Associations between ozone, PM2.5, and four pollen types on emergency department pediatric asthma events during the warm season in New Jersey: a case-crossover study." *Environ Res* 132: 421–9. doi: 10.1016/j.envres.2014.03.035.

Guyton, K. Z., D. Loomis, Y. Grosse, F. El Ghissassi, L. Benbrahim-Tallaa, N. Guha, C. Scoccianti, H. Mattock, K. Straif, and Iarc Lyon France International Agency for Research on Cancer Monograph Working Group. 2015. "Carcinogenicity of tetrachlorvinphos, parathion, malathion, diazinon, and glyphosate." *Lancet Oncol.* doi: 10.1016/S1470-2045(15)70134-8.

Hajszan, T., and C. Leranth. 2010. "Bisphenol A interferes with synaptic remodeling." *Front Neuroendocrinol* 31(4): 519–30. doi: 10.1016/j.yfrne.2010.06.004.

Herbarth, O., G. J. Fritz, M. Rehwagen, M. Richter, S. Roder, and U. Schlink. 2006. "Association between indoor renovation activities and eczema in early childhood." *Int J Hyg Environ Health* 209(3): 241–7. doi: 10.1016/j.ijheh.2006.01.003.

Hertz-Picciotto, I., L. A. Croen, R. Hansen, C. R. Jones, J. van de Water, and I. N. Pessah. 2006. "The CHARGE study: an epidemiologic investigation of genetic and environmental factors contributing to autism." *Environ Health Perspect* 114(7): 1119–25.

Hojsak, I., C. Braegger, J. Bronsky, C. Campoy, V. Colomb, T. Decsi, M. Domellof, M. Fewtrell, N. F. Mis, W. Mihatsch, C. Molgaard, J. van Goudoever, and Espghan Committee on Nutrition. 2015. "Arsenic in rice: a cause for concern." *J Pediatr Gastroenterol Nutr* 60(1): 142–5. doi: 10.1097/MPG.0000000000000502.

Hu, Z., L. W. Morton, and R. L. Mahler. 2011. "Bottled water: United States consumers and their perceptions of water quality." *Int J Environ Res Public Health* 8(2): 565–78. doi: 10.3390/ijerph8020565.

Jackson, B. P., V. F. Taylor, M. R. Karagas, T. Punshon, and K. L. Cottingham. 2012. "Arsenic, organic foods, and brown rice syrup." *Environ Health Perspect* 120(5): 623–6. doi: 10.1289/ehp.1104619.

Jackson, B. P., V. F. Taylor, T. Punshon, and K. L. Cottingham. 2012. "Arsenic concentration and speciation in infant formulas and first foods." *Pure Appl Chem* 84(2): 215–23. doi: 10.1351/PAC-CON-11-09-17.

Johnson-Restrepo, B., and K. Kannan. 2009. "An assessment of sources and pathways of human exposure to polybrominated diphenyl ethers in the United States." *Chemosphere* 76(4): 542–8. doi: 10.1016/j.chemosphere.2009.02.068.

Jurewicz, J., and W. Hanke. 2006. "Exposure to pesticides and childhood cancer risk: has there been any progress in epidemiological studies?" *Int J Occup Med Environ Health* 19(3): 152–69.

Jurewicz, J., and W. Hanke. 2008. "Prenatal and childhood exposure to pesticides and neurobehavioral development: review of epidemiological studies." *Int J Occup Med Environ Health* 21(2): 121–32. doi: 10.2478/v10001-008-0014-z.

Kalkbrenner, A. E., G. C. Windham, M. L. Serre, Y. Akita, X. Wang, K. Hoffman, B. P. Thayer, and J. L. Daniels. 2015. "Particulate matter exposure, prenatal and postnatal windows of susceptibility, and autism spectrum disorders." *Epidemiology* 26(1): 30–42. doi: 10.1097/EDE.0000000000000173.

Kapoor, R., C. Menon, O. Hoffstad, W. Bilker, P. Leclerc, and D. J. Margolis. 2008. "The prevalence of atopic triad in children with physician-confirmed atopic dermatitis." *J Am Acad Dermatol* 58(1): 68–73. doi: 10.1016/j.jaad.2007.06.041.

Kelley, K. E., S. Hernandez-Diaz, E. L. Chaplin, R. Hauser, and A. A. Mitchell. 2012. "Identification of phthalates in medications and dietary supplement formulations in the United States and Canada." *Environ Health Perspect* 120(3): 379–84. doi: 10.1289/ehp.1103998.

Keri, R. A., S. M. Ho, P. A. Hunt, K. E. Knudsen, A. M. Soto, and G. S. Prins. 2007. "An evaluation of evidence for the carcinogenic activity of bisphenol A." *Reprod Toxicol* 24(2): 240–52. doi: 10.1016/j.reprotox.2007.06.008.

Kilpatrick, N., H. Frumkin, J. Trowbridge, C. Escoffery, R. Geller, L. Rubin, G. Teague, J. Nodvin. 2002. "The environmental history in pediatric practice: a study of pediatricians' attitudes, beliefs, and practices." *Environ Health Perspect* 110(8): 823–7.

Kim, J. J., and American Academy of Pediatrics Committee on Environmental. 2004. "Ambient air pollution: health hazards to children." *Pediatrics* 114(6): 1699–707. doi: 10.1542/peds.2004-2166.

Kim, Y. R., F. A. Harden, L. M. Toms, and R. E. Norman. 2014. "Health consequences of exposure to brominated flame retardants: a systematic review." *Chemosphere* 106: 1–19. doi: 10.1016/j.chemosphere.2013.12.064.

Kloukos, D., N. Pandis, and T. Eliades. 2013. "Bisphenol-A and residual monomer leaching from orthodontic adhesive resins and polycarbonate brackets: a systematic review." *Am J Orthod Dentofacial Orthop* 143(4 Suppl): S104–12. e1–2. doi: 10.1016/j.ajodo.2012.11.015.

Kuehn, B. M. 2010. "Increased risk of ADHD associated with early exposure to pesticides, PCBs." *JAMA* 304(1): 27–8. doi: 10.1001/jama.2010.860.

Lee, Y. L., W. H. Wang, C. W. Lu, Y. H. Lin, and B. F. Hwang. 2011. "Effects of ambient air pollution on pulmonary function among schoolchildren." *Int J Hyg Environ Health* 214(5): 369–75. doi: 10.1016/j.ijheh.2011.05.004.

Li, S., G. Williams, B. Jalaludin, and P. Baker. 2012. "Panel studies of air pollution on children's lung function and respiratory symptoms: a literature review." *J Asthma* 49(9): 895–910. doi: 10.3109/02770903.2012.724129.

Lioy, P. J., R. Hauser, C. Gennings, H. M. Koch, P. E. Mirkes, B. A. Schwetz, and A. Kortenkamp. 2015. "Assessment of phthalates/phthalate alternatives in children's toys and childcare articles: Review of the report including conclusions and recommendation of the Chronic Hazard Advisory Panel of the Consumer Product Safety Commission." *J Expo Sci Environ Epidemiol.* doi: 10.1038/jes.2015.33.

Longnecker, M. P., M. A. Klebanoff, H. Zhou, and J. W. Brock. 2001. "Association between maternal serum concentration of the DDT metabolite DDE and preterm and small-for-gestational-age babies at birth." *Lancet* 358(9276): 110–14. doi: 10.1016/S0140-6736(01)05329-6.

Lu, C., D. B. Barr, M. A. Pearson, and L. A. Waller. 2008. "Dietary intake and its contribution to longitudinal organophosphorus pesticide exposure in urban/suburban children." *Environ Health Perspect* 116(4): 537–42. doi: 10.1289/ehp.10912.

Lu, C., K. Toepel, R. Irish, R. A. Fenske, D. B. Barr, and R. Bravo. 2006. "Organic diets significantly lower children's dietary exposure to organophosphorus pesticides." *Environ Health Perspect* 114(2): 260–3.

Ma, S., Z. Yu, X. Zhang, G. Ren, P. Peng, G. Sheng, and J. Fu. 2012. "Levels and congener profiles of polybrominated diphenyl ethers (PBDEs) in breast milk from Shanghai: implication for exposure route of higher brominated BDEs." *Environ Int* 42: 72–7. doi: 10.1016/j.envint.2011.04.006.

Mar, T. F., and J. Q. Koenig. 2009. "Relationship between visits to emergency departments for asthma and ozone exposure in greater Seattle, Washington." *Ann Allergy Asthma Immunol* 103(6): 474–9. doi: 10.1016/S1081-1206(10)60263-3.

McClafferty, H. 2016. "Environmental Health: Children's Health, a Clinician's Dilemma." *Curr Probl Pediatr Adolesc Health Care* 46(6): 184–9. doi: 10.1016/j.cppeds.2015.12.003. Epub 2016 Feb 1.

Meeker, J. D., and K. K. Ferguson. 2011. "Relationship between urinary phthalate and bisphenol A concentrations and serum thyroid measures in U.S. adults and adolescents from the National Health and Nutrition Examination Survey (NHANES) 2007–2008." *Environ Health Perspect* 119(10): 1396–402. doi: 10.1289/ehp.1103582.

Menale, C., M. T. Piccolo, G. Cirillo, R. A. Calogero, A. Papparella, L. Mita, E. M. Del Giudice, N. Diano, S. Crispi, and D. G. Mita. 2015. "Bisphenol A effects on gene expression in adipocytes from children: association with metabolic disorders." *J Mol Endocrinol* 54(3): 289–303. doi: 10.1530/JME-14-0282.

Michalowicz, J. 2014. "Bisphenol A—sources, toxicity and biotransformation." *Environ Toxicol Pharmacol* 37(2): 738–58. doi: 10.1016/j.etap.2014.02.003.

Miller, R. L., and D. B. Peden. 2014. "Environmental effects on immune responses in patients with atopy and asthma." *J Allergy Clin Immunol* 134(5): 1001–8. doi: 10.1016/j.jaci.2014.07.064.

Miranda, M. L., D. Kim, J. Reiter, M. A. Overstreet Galeano, and P. Maxson. 2009. "Environmental contributors to the achievement gap." *Neurotoxicology* 30(6): 1019–24. doi: 10.1016/j.neuro.2009.07.012.

Morales, E., R. Garcia-Esteban, O. A. de la Cruz, M. Basterrechea, A. Lertxundi, M. D. de Dicastillo, C. Zabaleta, and J. Sunyer. 2015. "Intrauterine and early postnatal exposure to outdoor air pollution and lung function at preschool age." *Thorax* 70(1): 64–73. doi: 10.1136/thoraxjnl-2014-205413.

National Institutes of Health, National Institute of Environmental Health Sciences. 2011.

Nishimura, K. K., J. M. Galanter, L. A. Roth, S. S. Oh, N. Thakur, E. A. Nguyen, S. Thyne, H. J. Farber, D. Serebrisky, R. Kumar, E. Brigino-Buenaventura, A. Davis, M. A. LeNoir, K. Meade, W. Rodriguez-Cintron, P. C. Avila, L. N. Borrell, K. Bibbins-Domingo, J. R. Rodriguez-Santana, S. Sen, F. Lurmann, J. R. Balmes, and E. G. Burchard. 2013. "Early-life air pollution and asthma risk in minority children. The GALA II and SAGE II studies." *Am J Respir Crit Care Med* 188(3): 309–18. doi: 10.1164/rccm.201302-0264OC.

Oberg, M., M. S. Jaakkola, A. Woodward, A. Peruga, and A. Pruss-Ustun. 2011. "Worldwide burden of disease from exposure to second-hand smoke: a retrospective analysis of data from 192 countries." *Lancet* 377(9760): 139–46. doi: 10.1016/S0140-6736(10)61388-8.

Ornoy, A., L. Weinstein-Fudim, and Z. Ergaz. 2015. "Prenatal factors associated with autism spectrum disorder (ASD)." *Reprod Toxicol* 56: 155–69. doi: 10.1016/j.reprotox.2015.05.007.

Padhye, L. P., H. Yao, F. T. Kung'u, and C. H. Huang. 2014. "Year-long evaluation on the occurrence and fate of pharmaceuticals, personal care products, and endocrine disrupting chemicals in an urban drinking water treatment plant." *Water Res* 51: 266–76. doi: 10.1016/j. watres.2013.10.070.

Padula, A. M., I. B. Tager, S. L. Carmichael, S. K. Hammond, W. Yang, F. Lurmann, and G. M. Shaw. 2013. "Ambient air pollution and traffic exposures and congenital heart defects in the San Joaquin Valley of California." *Paediatr Perinat Epidemiol* 27(4): 329–39. doi: 10.1111/ ppe.12055.

"Partners in Information Access for the Public Health Workforce." http://www.phpartners.org/ about.html.

Pedersen, M., L. Giorgis-Allemand, C. Bernard, I. Aguilera, A. M. Andersen, F. Ballester, R. M. Beelen, L. Chatzi, M. Cirach, A. Danileviciute, A. Dedele, Mv Eijsden, M. Estarlich, A. Fernandez-Somoano, M. F. Fernandez, F. Forastiere, U. Gehring, R. Grazuleviciene, O. Gruzieva, B. Heude, G. Hoek, K. de Hoogh, E. H. van den Hooven, S. E. Haberg, V. W. Jaddoe, C. Klumper, M. Korek, U. Kramer, A. Lerchundi, J. Lepeule, P. Nafstad, W. Nystad, E. Patelarou, D. Porta, D. Postma, O. Raaschou-Nielsen, P. Rudnai, J. Sunyer, E. Stephanou, M. Sorensen, E. Thiering, D. Tuffnell, M. J. Varro, T. G. Vrijkotte, A. Wijga, M. Wilhelm, J. Wright, M. J. Nieuwenhuijsen, G. Pershagen, B. Brunekreef, M. Kogevinas, and R. Slama. 2013. "Ambient air pollution and low birthweight: a European cohort study (ESCAPE)." *Lancet Respir Med* 1(9): 695–704. doi: 10.1016/S2213-2600(13)70192-9.

Peretz, J., L. Vrooman, W. A. Ricke, P. A. Hunt, S. Ehrlich, R. Hauser, V. Padmanabhan, H. S. Taylor, S. H. Swan, C. A. VandeVoort, and J. A. Flaws. 2014. "Bisphenol a and reproductive health: update of experimental and human evidence, 2007–2013." *Environ Health Perspect* 122(8): 775–86. doi: 10.1289/ehp.1307728.

Peterson, B. S., V. A. Rauh, R. Bansal, X. Hao, Z. Toth, G. Nati, K. Walsh, R. L. Miller, D. Semanek, and F. Perera. 2015. "Effects of prenatal exposure to air pollutants (polycyclic aromatic hydrocarbons) on the development of brain white matter, cognition, and behavior in later childhood." *JAMA Psychiatry*. doi: 10.1001/jamapsychiatry.2015.57.

Rahman, M. F., E. K. Yanful, and S. Y. Jasim. 2009. "Endocrine disrupting compounds (EDCs) and pharmaceuticals and personal care products (PPCPs) in the aquatic environment: implications for the drinking water industry and global environmental health." *J Water Health* 7(2): 224–43. doi: 10.2166/wh.2009.021.

Raz, R., A. L. Roberts, K. Lyall, J. E. Hart, A. C. Just, F. Laden, and M. G. Weisskopf. 2015. "Autism spectrum disorder and particulate matter air pollution before, during, and after pregnancy: a nested case-control analysis within the Nurses' Health Study II Cohort." *Environ Health Perspect* 123(3): 264–70. doi: 10.1289/ehp.1408133.

Ribas-Fito, N., M. Sala, E. Cardo, C. Mazon, M. E. De Muga, A. Verdu, E. Marco, J. O. Grimalt, and J. Sunyer. 2002. "Association of hexachlorobenzene and other organochlorine compounds with anthropometric measures at birth." *Pediatr Res* 52(2): 163–7. doi: 10.1203/00006450-200208000-00006.

Roberts, J. R., C. J. Karr, and Council On Environmental Health. 2012. "Pesticide exposure in children." *Pediatrics* 130(6): e1765–88. doi: 10.1542/peds.2012-2758.

Rochester, J. R. 2013. "Bisphenol A and human health: a review of the literature." *Reprod Toxicol* 42: 132–55. doi: 10.1016/j.reprotox.2013.08.008.

Rogan, W. J., and N. B. Ragan. 2007. "Some evidence of effects of environmental chemicals on the endocrine system in children." *Int J Hyg Environ Health* 210(5): 659–67. doi: 10.1016/j. ijheh.2007.07.005.

Rosenfeld, C. S. 2015. "Bisphenol A and phthalate endocrine disruption of parental and social behaviors." *Front Neurosci* 9: 57. doi: 10.3389/fnins.2015.00057.

Schenk, M., S. M. Popp, A. V. Neale, and R. Y. Demers. 1996. "Environmental medicine content in medical school curricula." *Acad Med* 71(5): 499–501.

Shankar, A., S. Teppala, and C. Sabanayagam. 2012. "Urinary bisphenol a levels and measures of obesity: results from the national health and nutrition examination survey 2003–2008." *ISRN Endocrinol* 2012: 965243. doi: 10.5402/2012/965243.

Sheffield, P., A. Roy, K. Wong, and L. Trasande. 2011. "Fine particulate matter pollution linked to respiratory illness in infants and increased hospital costs." *Health Aff (Millwood)* 30(5): 871–8. doi: 10.1377/hlthaff.2010.1279.

Stapleton, H. M., S. Klosterhaus, A. Keller, P. L. Ferguson, S. van Bergen, E. Cooper, T. F. Webster, and A. Blum. 2011. "Identification of flame retardants in polyurethane foam collected from baby products." *Environ Sci Technol* 45(12): 5323–31. doi: 10.1021/es2007462.

Stillerman, K. P., D. R. Mattison, L. C. Giudice, and T. J. Woodruff. 2008. "Environmental exposures and adverse pregnancy outcomes: a review of the science." *Reprod Sci* 15(7): 631–50. doi: 10.1177/1933719108322436.

Stingone, J. A., T. J. Luben, J. L. Daniels, M. Fuentes, D. B. Richardson, A. S. Aylsworth, A. H. Herring, M. Anderka, L. Botto, A. Correa, S. M. Gilboa, P. H. Langlois, B. Mosley, G. M. Shaw, C. Siffel, A. F. Olshan, and Study National Birth Defects Prevention. 2014. "Maternal exposure to criteria air pollutants and congenital heart defects in offspring: results from the national birth defects prevention study." *Environ Health Perspect* 122(8): 863–72. doi: 10.1289/ehp.1307289.

Stoner, A. M., S. E. Anderson, and T. J. Buckley. 2013. "Ambient air toxics and asthma prevalence among a representative sample of US kindergarten-age children." *PLoS One* 8(9): e75176. doi: 10.1371/journal.pone.0075176.

Stotland, N. E., P. Sutton, J. Trowbridge, D. S. Atchley, J. Conry, L. Trasande, B. Gerbert, A. Charlesworth, and T. J. Woodruff. 2014. "Counseling patients on preventing prenatal environmental exposures—a mixed-methods study of obstetricians." *PLoS One* 9(6): e98771. doi: 10.1371/journal.pone.0098771.

Strickland, M. J., M. Klein, W. D. Flanders, H. H. Chang, J. A. Mulholland, P. E. Tolbert, and L. A. Darrow. 2014. "Modification of the effect of ambient air pollution on pediatric asthma emergency visits: susceptible subpopulations." *Epidemiology* 25(6): 843–50. doi: 10.1097/EDE.0000000000000170.

Sutton, P., T. J. Woodruff, J. Perron, N. Stotland, J. A. Conry, M. D. Miller, and L. C. Giudice. 2012. "Toxic environmental chemicals: the role of reproductive health professionals in preventing harmful exposures." *Am J Obstet Gynecol* 207(3): 164–73. doi: 10.1016/j.ajog.2012.01.034.

Talbott, E. O., V. C. Arena, J. R. Rager, J. E. Clougherty, D. R. Michanowicz, R. K. Sharma, and S. L. Stacy. 2015. "Fine particulate matter and the risk of autism spectrum disorder." *Environ Res* 140: 414–20. doi: 10.1016/j.envres.2015.04.021.

Teppala, S., S. Madhavan, and A. Shankar. 2012. "Bisphenol A and Metabolic Syndrome: Results from NHANES." *Int J Endocrinol* 2012: 598180. doi: 10.1155/2012/598180.

"The UC Davis MIND Institute (Medical Investigation of Neurodevelopmental Disorders)." http://www.ucdmc.ucdavis.edu/mindinstitute/.

Toms, L. M., F. Harden, O. Paepke, J. Hobson, J. J. Ryan, and J. F. Mueller. 2008. "Higher accumulation of polybrominated diphenyl ethers in infants than in adults." *Environ Sci Technol* 42(19): 7510–15.

Toms, L. M., L. Hearn, K. Kennedy, F. Harden, M. Bartkow, C. Temme, and J. F. Mueller. 2009. "Concentrations of polybrominated diphenyl ethers (PBDEs) in matched samples of human milk, dust and indoor air." *Environ Int* 35(6): 864–9. doi: 10.1016/j.envint.2009.03.001.

Trasande, L., and T. M. Attina. 2015. "Association of Exposure to Di-2-Ethylhexylphthalate Replacements With Increased Blood Pressure in Children and Adolescents." *Hypertension* 66(2): 301–8. doi: 10.1161/HYPERTENSIONAHA.115.05603.

Trasande, L., T. M. Attina, and J. Blustein. 2012. "Association between urinary bisphenol A concentration and obesity prevalence in children and adolescents." *JAMA* 308(11): 1113–21. doi: 10.1001/2012.jama.11461.

Trasande, L., J. Boscarino, N. Graber, R. Falk, C. Schechter, M. Galvez, G. Dunkel, J. Geslani, J. Moline, E. Kaplan-Liss, R. K. Miller, K. Korfmacher, D. Carpenter, J. Forman, S. J. Balk, D. Laraque, H. Frumkin, and P. Landrigan. 2006. "The environment in pediatric practice: a study of New York pediatricians' attitudes, beliefs, and practices towards children's environmental health." *J Urban Health* 83(4): 760–72. doi: 10.1007/s11524-006-9071-4.

Trasande, L., N. Newman, L. Long, G. Howe, B. J. Kerwin, R. J. Martin, S. A. Gahagan, and W. B. Weil. 2010. "Translating knowledge about environmental health to practitioners: are we doing enough?" *Mt Sinai J Med* 77(1): 114–23. doi: 10.1002/msj.20158.

United States Environmental Protection Agency. "Indoor Air Quality (IAQ)." http://www.epa. gov/iaq/lead.html-Lead%20Health%20Effects.

United States Environmental Protection Agency. 2011. "Technology Transfer Network—Air Toxics Web Site."

van der Hulst, A. E., H. Klip, and P. L. Brand. 2007. "Risk of developing asthma in young children with atopic eczema: a systematic review." *J Allergy Clin Immunol* 120(3): 565–9. doi: 10.1016/j.jaci.2007.05.042.

Vandenberg L. N., S. Ehrlich, S. M. Belcher, N. Ben-Jonathan, D. C. Dolinoy, E. S. Hugo, P. A. Hunt, R. R. Newbold, B. S. Rubin, K. S. Saili, A. M. Soto, H. S. Wang, F. S. vom Saal. 2013. "Low dose effects of bisphenol A: an integrated review of in vitro, laboratory animal and epidemiology studies." *Endocr Disruptors* 1: e1–20.

Volk, H. E., F. Lurmann, B. Penfold, I. Hertz-Picciotto, and R. McConnell. 2013. "Traffic-related air pollution, particulate matter, and autism." *JAMA Psychiatry* 70(1): 71–7. doi: 10.1001/jamapsychiatry.2013.266.

vom Saal, F. S., B. G. Timms, M. M. Montano, P. Palanza, K. A. Thayer, S. C. Nagel, M. D. Dhar, V. K. Ganjam, S. Parmigiani, and W. V. Welshons. 1997. "Prostate enlargement in mice due to fetal exposure to low doses of estradiol or diethylstilbestrol and opposite effects at high doses." *Proc Natl Acad Sci U S A* 94(5): 2056–61.

Wang, C., R. Niu, Y. Zhu, H. Han, G. Luo, B. Zhou, and J. Wang. 2014. "Changes in memory and synaptic plasticity induced in male rats after maternal exposure to bisphenol A." *Toxicology* 322: 51–60. doi: 10.1016/j.tox.2014.05.001.

Wang, I. J., S. L. Chen, T. P. Lu, E. Y. Chuang, and P. C. Chen. 2013. "Prenatal smoke exposure, DNA methylation, and childhood atopic dermatitis." *Clin Exp Allergy* 43(5): 535–43. doi: 10.1111/cea.12108.

Watson, C. S., Y. J. Jeng, and J. Guptarak. 2011. "Endocrine disruption via estrogen receptors that participate in nongenomic signaling pathways." *J Steroid Biochem Mol Biol* 127(1–2): 44–50. doi: 10.1016/j.jsbmb.2011.01.015.

White, M. C., R. A. Etzel, W. D. Wilcox, and C. Lloyd. 1994. "Exacerbations of childhood asthma and ozone pollution in Atlanta." *Environ Res* 65(1): 56–68. doi: 10.1006/enrs.1994.1021.

Whitehead, T. P., C. Metayer, M. H. Ward, J. S. Colt, R. B. Gunier, N. C. Deziel, S. M. Rappaport, and P. A. Buffler. 2014. "Persistent organic pollutants in dust from older homes: learning from lead." *Am J Public Health* 104(7): 1320–6. doi: 10.2105/AJPH.2013.301835.

Wilding, B. C., K. Curtis, K. Welker-Hood 2009. "Hazardous Chemicals in Health Care." Physicians for Social Responsibility. http://www.psr.org/assets/pdfs/hazardous-chemicals-in-health-care.pdf.

Wilson, D., C. Hooper, and X. Shi. 2012. "Arsenic and lead in juice: apple, citrus, and applebase." *J Environ Health* 75(5): 14–20; quiz 44.

Woodruff, T. J., L. A. Darrow, and J. D. Parker. 2008. "Air pollution and postneonatal infant mortality in the United States, 1999–2002." *Environ Health Perspect* 116(1): 110–15. doi: 10.1289/ehp.10370.

World Health Organization. "Air Pollution and Health." http://www.who.int/phe/health_topics/outdoorair/en/

Yi, O., H. J. Kwon, H. Kim, M. Ha, S. J. Hong, Y. C. Hong, J. H. Leem, J. Sakong, C. G. Lee, S. Y. Kim, and D. Kang. 2012. "Effect of environmental tobacco smoke on atopic dermatitis among children in Korea." *Environ Res* 113: 40–5. doi: 10.1016/j.envres.2011.12.012.

Zar, H. J., and T. W. Ferkol. 2014. "The global burden of respiratory disease-impact on child health." *Pediatr Pulmonol* 49(5): 430–4. doi: 10.1002/ppul.23030.

Zawatski, W., and M. M. Lee. 2013. "Male pubertal development: are endocrine-disrupting compounds shifting the norms?" *J Endocrinol* 218(2): R1–12. doi: 10.1530/JOE-12-0449.

Zoeller, R. T., T. R. Brown, L. L. Doan, A. C. Gore, N. E. Skakkebaek, A. M. Soto, T. J. Woodruff, and F. S. Vom Saal. 2012. "Endocrine-disrupting chemicals and public health protection: a statement of principles from The Endocrine Society." *Endocrinology* 153(9): 4097–110. doi: 10.1210/en.2012-1422.

Part 3
Complementary Approaches

9 Botanicals and Dietary Supplements

Despite a rich history of use in traditional medicine, evidence for the efficacy and safety of botanicals in children remains relatively sparse. Consistent with 2007 National Health Interview Survey (NHIS) results, data from the 2012 survey shows that non-vitamin, non-mineral dietary supplements are the most commonly used complementary modality in children. More than 1 in 10 children in the U.S. use some type of dietary supplement which can come prepared as tablets or capsules, powders, tinctures, syrups, and brewed teas. In infants, use prevalence was recorded at 9% per data from the Infant Feeding Practices Study II, which uses data collected between 2005 and 2007. Botanical supplements were reported in infants as young as 1 month of age. Most common reasons included fussiness, digestion, colic, and relaxation in the form of gripe water (for colic), chamomile, teething tablets, and unspecified types of teas (Zhang, Fein, and Fein 2011). According to the 2012 NHIS survey, fish oil (discussed in Chapter 4) was the most commonly used dietary supplement, surpassing echinacea as the most commonly used by children in 2007. Probiotics (also discussed in Chapter 4) were among the top three reported supplements used in the 2012 report (Black et al. 2015).

Potential advantages of botanical remedies in general include their generally low risk of reported side effects if the substance is pure and used as directed. Potential disadvantages include their slower onset of action, risk for dose dependent toxicity, potential for herb–drug interaction, immature metabolism in infants and children, and increased susceptibility to adverse effects in infants due to impact of dose per body weight ratio (Zhang, Fein, and Fein 2011). Unintended exposures are also a danger; for example, lead has been shown to pass into breast milk from mothers who regularly use Chinese herbs (Chien et al. 2006).

A further significant complicating factor is that botanical products often include hundreds of individual components, making interactions with other medications both more likely and more challenging to isolate the triggering mechanism. Broad commercial availability, lack of quality control, and lack of standardized dosing for children are other important disadvantages. High variability in case reporting of adverse events in pediatric use of medicinal herbs has also hindered forward progress in establishing standard dosing and safety recommendations (Gardiner et al. 2013). Safety and accurate labeling of herbal and dietary supplements in the U.S. is the responsibility of the manufacturer. The FDA is responsible for post-marketing monitoring of adverse events via voluntary reporting and product information. All of these factors make it important for the clinician to ask about the use of dietary supplements and botanicals in every child at every visit, even in infancy, and to create an open and trusting relationship with parents that encourages full disclosure of all complementary and integrative medicine use. The botanicals and dietary supplements reviewed below include those historically used in the pediatric population that have strongest supporting evidence to date: butterbur, chamomile, curcumin, echinacea, St. John's wort, melatonin, and peppermint.

Butterbur

Butterbur (*Petasites hybridus*) belongs to the family Asteraceae. Also known as common butterbur, it grows in Europe, North America, and in parts of Asia. All its parts including the roots, leaves, and bulb are used in making medicines. Historically it has been used to treat a variety of symptoms, including pain, especially migraine headache, allergies, and asthma (Aydin et al. 2013).

Butterbur has been used topically to promote wound healing and to treat skin irritations. Its generic name is *Petasites*, which comes from the Greek *Petasus*, meaning a broad hat worn by shepherds, thought to resemble the plant's leaves, which are traditionally used to wrap butter.

An important caution with butterbur is that the alkaloid content of the plant's extracts contain pyrrolizidine alkaloids (PAs) which have been shown to be hepatotoxic and carcinogenic. All butterbur products used medicinally must be labeled PA free.

In addition to the harmful pyrrolizidine alkaloids, beneficial pharmacologically active compounds of butterbur include petasin and isopetasin, two sesquiterpenes with antispasmodic and anti-inflammatory actions (Aydin et al. 2013). Butterbur's primary mechanism of action is thought to work through calcium channel regulation and inhibition of leukotriene synthesis (D'Andrea, Cevoli, and Cologno 2014).

Pediatric Research Evidence

The majority of butterbur research has been done with adults; however, some research evidence for its effectiveness in children is available. Some of the most promising research has been done in migraine headache where enough evidence has accumulated for butterbur to receive a 'level A' recommendation for prevention of adult episodic migraine in the 2012 American Headache Society and American Academy of Neurology (Loder, Burch, and Rizzoli 2012).

In children some evidence exists for the use of butterbur in migraine treatment.

One uncontrolled study of 108 children with migraine history examined frequency of migraine attack. Dose was graduated by age, from 50 mg per day in 6–9 year olds to 100 mg daily in older youth. Some non-responders received a 50% higher dose for 2 months.

Overall, 77.2% of children showed reduction in migraine frequency. Monthly migraine attacks decreased by an overall 63% by the end of the 4-month study period. Mild adverse events were recorded in eight patients, primarily belching and other non-serious gastrointestinal symptoms (Pothmann and Danesch 2005).

The need for larger, controlled studies is evident, especially because conventional treatments for migraine prevention in children have not provided encouraging results to date (Shamliyan et al. 2013).

Butterbur has been evaluated in small studies for asthma. For example, a clinical trial by Danesch evaluated the effectiveness of butterbur in treating mild to moderate asthma in children (n = 16) and adults (n = 64). Dosing ranged from 50 to 150 mg per day in children depending on age. Significant improvement in number and duration of asthma attacks was reported in the majority of patients, along with increase in forced expiratory volume and peak flow in both groups. Mild adverse events were reported in seven patients, none serious (Sadler et al. 2007).

No studies have been conducted on children related to allergic rhinitis; however, those conducted on adults show mixed evidence for its effectiveness (Sadler et al. 2007).

Cautions

Butterbur products should be PA free, which means that they do not contain pyrrolizidine alkaloids (PAs) which are both hepatotoxic and carcinogenic. Commercially available butterbur must have lower than 0.08 parts per million of PA. People with allergies to daisies, ragweed, or some other herbs may have cross-sensitivity to butterbur. Butterbur is contraindicated in pregnant or lactating women (Pringsheim et al. 2012).

Drug Interactions

Caution is indicated with CYP3A4 enzyme inducers such as carbamazepine, phenobarbital, phenytoin, and rifampin due to potential increased conversion of pyrrolizidine alkaloids if present (Sadler et al. 2007).

Pediatric Dose

The studies conducted on children have found quite high tolerance for butterbur in doses ranging from 50 mg to 150 mg per day, generally divided into three doses given at evenly spaced intervals.

Adult Dose

For treatment of migraine, the recommended dose for adults ranges from 50 to 200 mg given twice daily.

Chamomile

One of the most favored traditional herbs is chamomile (*Matricaria chamomilla* L.), widely used as a medicinal plant. Recorded use dates back to ancient Egypt, Greece, and Rome. Chamomile is the umbrella name encompassing a wide range of plants similar to daisy, which belong to Asteraceae family. German chamomile and Roman chamomile are two of the many different species of chamomile that have been recognized since ancient times for their anti-inflammatory, antispasmodic, carminative, antiseptic, and mild relaxant characteristics. Most research has been done on German chamomile (Gardiner 2007).

Chamomile is grown commercially in many countries around the world, including those in southern and eastern Europe. Hungary is a main producer of the medicinal plant (Singh et al. 2011).

Internally, chamomile is traditionally used in the form of teas, extracts, or tinctures for fever, stomach illnesses, and as an anti-anxiety remedy. Externally, it has been used in creams and lotions to promote wound healing, and to treat skin infections and irritations. In addition to use in herbal teas, the dried flowers are used in massage oils, aromatherapy, lotions and in a variety of other personal care products.

The chamomile flower contains an incredible array of active compounds, including sesquiterpenes, flavonoids (apigenin and luteolin), coumarins, and polyacetylenes. Eleven bioactive phenols are also present, including flavones and flavonols. More than 120 chemical compounds have been identified as either primary or secondary constituents in this humble flower with a range of antifungal, antiseptic, antimicrobial activity, antispasmodic, and anti-inflammatory properties (Singh et al. 2011).

Pediatric Research Evidence

Two clinical trials have investigated the effectiveness of chamomile as remedy for colic in children, although neither studied chamomile as a single intervention. One prospective, randomized, double-blind, placebo-controlled study by Weizman et al. evaluated 68 term infants between 2 and 8 weeks old with a diagnosis of colic. The treatment group received tea containing German chamomile, vervain, licorice, fennel, and balm mint, while the control group received placebo tea free of herbs. Over a trial period of 7 days, infants received up to 150 mL of either herbal tea or placebo during colic episodes, not exceeding more than three times a day. Parents reported elimination of colic in more than half of the treatment group (57%) versus placebo with 26% improvement (Weizman et al. 1993) ($p < 0.01$).

A second randomized, double-blind, controlled trial of 93 infants with colic used a standardized extract of chamomile, fennel, and lemon balm versus placebo twice a day for 7 days. Total crying time was reported to be reduced in 85% of the treatment group versus 49% of the control group (Savino et al. 2005) ($p < 0.005$).

Chamomile in creams and lotions is used to treat pediatric dermatologic conditions such as atopic dermatitis, although research to support its use in this area is not considered robust due to small studies with highly variable study design. A small number of adverse events have been reported with external use.

The anxiolytic properties of chamomile are also widely recognized, but few studies exist to support pediatric use (Parslow et al. 2008).

One randomized, double-blind, placebo-controlled study has examined the efficacy of chamomile in generalized anxiety disorder in adults. Patients with mild generalized anxiety disorder ($n = 61$) were randomized to chamomile extract (220 mg capsule standardized to 1.2% apigenin, one capsule daily for week 1 with incremental dose increase by one capsule per week up to a maximum of five capsules, 1100 mg daily, for 8 weeks) versus placebo. Hamilton Anxiety Rating scores reflected a significant improvement in symptoms of generalized anxiety disorder in the treatment group at week 8 ($p = 0.047$). Few adverse events were reported in either group (Amsterdam et al. 2009).

Cautions

The major cautions for chamomile are related to its potential for causing allergic side effects, especially in those allergic to other members of the aster family including ragweed, asters, and chrysanthemums. Allergies can be revealed in the form of rashes, edema, allergic conjunctivitis, shortness of breath, and—rarely—anaphylaxis (Gardiner 2007).

Interactions

Chamomile can also interact with other drugs, herbs, and dietary medicines, amplifying their aversive effects. For example, by interacting with some benzodiazepines or barbiturates, it can amplify the side effect of drowsiness caused by these medicines. At least three cases of chamomile interacting with cyclosporine in renal transplant cases have been reported through interference with the cytochrome P450 enzyme. Potential interference with warfarin through a similar mechanism has been postulated (Gardiner 2007).

Pediatric Dose

The recommended dose of chamomile differs considerably for different age ranges.

According to the World Health Organization, adult dosing is generally measured in one cup of tea or measured doses of 1–4 mL tincture (1:1 in 45% alcohol), commonly three times per day. Pediatric dosing in a single dose is suggested as 0.6–2 mL of fluid extract (ethanol 45%–60%), and that of the flower head is 2 grams three times per day (World Health Organization 1999).

In very young infants and toddlers, cooled chamomile tea is often used in small amounts throughout the day to sooth colic or to help slow diarrhea. No studies currently exist on specific dosing guidelines for colic or gastrointestinal upset in pediatrics. Organic chamomile is ideally preferred to reduce pesticide exposure. Dosing volume should not interfere with infant or toddler's daily caloric intake.

Curcumin

Although specific studies in pediatrics are limited, emerging research on curcumin makes it important for pediatricians to be aware of its characteristics and potential health benefits.

Curcumin is a naturally occurring polyphenolic compound that accounts for the yellow pigment in the dried rhizomes of the spice turmeric (*Curcuma longa*), made from a plant in the ginger family, Zingiberaceae. It is considered to be an exceptional spice in many cuisines, including Indian, Chinese, Thai, and Iranian, due to its rich flavor and bright yellow color. It is used in the West to flavor mustard and other foods and is classified by the U.S. FDA as Generally Recognized as Safe (GRAS) (Kocaadam and Sanlier 2015).

Historically curcumin has been valued for its medicinal properties in Chinese and Ayurvedic medicine for a wide range of conditions such as infection, sprains, skin aliments, and digestive issues (Bandyopadhyay 2014).

Modern research has shown curcumin to have over 200 active compounds with potent anti-inflammatory, antioxidant, antibacterial, antiviral, antifungal, and anti-cancer properties (anti-invasive and anti-metastatic). Curcuminoids are considered the most biologically active of the compounds and account for an estimated 3%–5% of turmeric (Bandyopadhyay 2014).

The anti-inflammatory effects of curcumin are mediated through cell signaling pathways by downregulation of a host of proinflammatory cytokines. Curcumin has also been shown to have cardioprotective effects via modulation of oxidative stress and possible lipid-lowering effects, although results with lipid-lowering effects have been equivocal in some studies if curcumin is used without an adjuvant (Aggarwal and Sung 2009; Sahebkar 2014). Curcumin has also been shown to significantly decrease the severity of premenstrual symptoms in a double-blinded randomized controlled trial in 70 women (Khayat et al. 2015).

Recent research also demonstrates the role of curcumin as an epigenetic modulator of certain genes by reversing DNA methylation and altering histone modifications known to impact tumor progression and chemotherapeutic efficacy in a range of diseases such as neurocognitive, inflammatory and some cancers (Boyanapalli and Tony Kong 2015; Teiten, Dicato, and Diederich 2013). Curcumin inhibits a variety of cytokine pathways, including IL-6, and has been shown to be more effective than placebo in randomized controlled studies in patients with ulcerative colitis (Triantafyllidi et al. 2015; Kumar et al. 2012).

Pediatric Research Evidence

One of the few studies to explore curcumin dose in pediatrics was done by Suskind et al. in a small study of 11 patients (11–18 years) with inflammatory bowel disease (either Crohn's disease or ulcerative colitis) in remission or with mild disease. Initially patients continued their standard therapy and added 500 mg curcumin twice a day for 3 weeks. Dose was then increased by 1 gram up to twice per day at week 3 for a total of 3 weeks, then increased again to 2 grams twice per day for another 3 weeks. Measurements of symptoms were done at week 3, 6, and 9. Nine patients completed the study. No adverse events were seen. Three patients had significant lowering of their disease activity index scales at week 9 (Suskind et al. 2013).

An in vitro study on infant myeloid leukemia cell lines also showed that curcumin demonstrated growth inhibition of cancer cells by blocking ion channels in the cancer cell with resulting suppression of proliferation of the cell line (Banderali et al. 2011). Curcumin has also been studied in vitro in pediatric epithelial liver tumor cell lines in conjunction with cisplatin as an expanded treatment approach with promising results (Bortel et al. 2015).

These early studies show the potential of curcumin in serious pediatric diseases and reinforce the reason for active interest in its future applications.

Cautions

Bioavailability of curcumin is low due to its hydrophobic properties, poor adsorption, and rapid elimination which can result in low target organ concentrations. For this reason, curcumin used to target systemic disease is often coupled with piperine as an adjuvant to enhance oral bioavailability. For example, in adults, oral curcumin–piperine has been associated with statistically significant improvement in lipid panels in patients with metabolic syndrome and reduction in C-reactive protein (Panahi et al. 2015). There is some evidence that curcumin increases gallbladder emptying and therefore a theoretical risk exists for aggravation of symptoms in those with existing gallstones (Jurenka 2009). Curcumin–piperine compounds are available commercially, and newer delivery models involving the use of nanotechnology, liposomal curcumin, and other methods for curcumin alone are under active study (Panahi et al. 2014).

Curcumin's primary reported side effect relates to mild gastrointestinal upset. There is no evidence that consumption of curcumin in food as a flavoring is dangerous in pregnancy or lactation; however, data on the use of curcumin supplements in pregnancy and lactation is lacking.

Interactions

Addition of piperine to curcumin may augment the effect of certain medications such as anticoagulants, aspirin, clopidogrel (Plavix), and warfarin (Coumadin) among others. Piperine may also increase the bioavailability and delay elimination of certain drugs such as phenytoin, propranolol, and theophylline. In vitro studies have also shown curcumin to inhibit cell death induced by certain chemotherapeutic agents. Its use in oncology patients should be carefully evaluated (Jurenka 2009).

Adult Dose

The therapeutic dose used in many human studies is between 2 to 3 grams. Dose-limiting toxicity has not been documented in the majority of studies to date. A study in adults with colon cancer found 3.6 grams oral curcumin to be pharmacologically effective in the colorectum. Another randomized study in adult patients with inflammatory bowel disease showed statistically significant improvement in the treatment group with 1 gram twice per day (Aggarwal and Sung 2009).

Serious events have not been reported in human adults taking high doses of curcumin; for example, in one study 12 grams orally was tolerated (Lao et al. 2006).

Pediatric Dose

There is no established dose for the use of curcumin in pediatrics, although its use in food is considered safe for children. The study by Suskind et al. referenced above showed good tolerance at doses of 2 grams twice per day in adolescents 11–18 years of age with inflammatory bowel disease, but study size was small.

Echinacea

Echinacea is native to North America and has a long tradition of use for wound healing and for the prevention and treatment of upper respiratory illness, although over time research results for treatment of colds have shown mixed benefit. Antiviral and anti-anxiety properties have also been reported, although data is again sparse, especially in children. Echinacea is a member of the Asteraceae family and is also known as purple coneflower. It is sold in many forms made with variable plant components (root, herb, flower, whole plant), differing methods of extraction and preparation, and often in combination with other ingredients. The majority of commercial preparations have not been tested in clinical trials (Karsch-Volk et al. 2014).

One of the most commonly studied species is *Echinacea purpurea*. The mechanism of action for the prevention or treatment of upper respiratory infection is unclear, but it is related in part to immunomodulatory activity of specific compounds including: alkamides, glycoproteins, polysaccharides, and caffeic acid derivatives. Many other compounds have been isolated from the plant, including a variety of flavonoids, and phenols. Synergistic interactions are likely, but poorly delineated. A 2014 Cochrane Database Systematic Review examined 24 double-blind studies involving

4631 participants, primarily adults, and found significant variability in study design. No benefit was seen in treatment of the common cold, and an overall relative risk reduction of 10%–20% (positive but non-significant) was found for individual prophylaxis of the common cold. No significant adverse events were recorded (Karsch-Volk et al. 2014).

Pediatric Research Evidence

The efficiency of echinacea in treating or preventing pediatric cold symptoms remains questionable (Charrois, Hrudey, Vohra et al. 2006; Karsch-Volk et al. 2014).

Cautions

Overall safety profile is good. The most common adverse events are related to allergic reactions, which can be severe in rare cases. Caution is advised in patients with pre-existing atopy and asthma, or allergy to Asteraceae or Compositae family (chrysanthemums, marigolds, daisies, ragweed) as cross reactivity may occur. Rash with topical use has been reported (Huntley, Thompson Coon, and Ernst 2005). Data on use in pregnancy and lactation is sparse (Perri et al. 2006).

Interactions

Echinacea is a human cytochrome P450 3A4 inhibitor (Awortwe et al. 2015; Wanwimolruk and Prachayasittikul 2014).

Adult Dose

No standard dosing exists.
Resource: *The Complete German Commission E Monographs: Therapeutic Guide to Herbal Medicines.* M. Blumenthal, W.R. Busse, A. Goldberg, J. Gruenwald, T. Hall, C.W. Riggins, R.S. Rister (eds.) S. Klein and R.S. Rister (trans.). 1998. Austin: American Botanical Council; Boston: Integrative Medicine Communications.

Pediatric Dose

No standard dosing exists.

St. John's Wort

St. John's wort (*Hypericum perforatum*) is a plant from the Hypericaceae family that is native to Europe and also found widely in the United States and Canada. There are more than three hundred species that belong to its genus. Since the Middle Ages this plant has been recognized for its healing and anti-inflammatory properties in burns and wounds as a balm. Modern studies have discovered it to be beneficial for reducing depression. Hypericum extract has multiple components associated with its antidepressant effect, the mechanism of which is not fully understood, but is known to be associated with inhibition of the uptake of noradrenaline, serotonin, and GABA at the synaptic junction (Schmidt and Butterweck 2015).

Increased dopaminergic activity in the prefrontal cortex has also been reported. Hypericum has also been shown to modulate serum and salivary cortisol levels in human volunteer studies (Kasper et al. 2010). Some of the challenges in interpreting studies on St. John's wort stem from differences in extract preparation and content (Linde et al. 2015). Research is also active in animal studies around its potential anti-cancer effects (Kiyan et al. 2014), application in Alzheimer's disease (Kraus et al. 2007), and antibacterial and antiviral properties (Huang et al. 2013; Pia Schiavone et al. 2014). Efficacy for St. John's wort has been shown in randomized controlled trials to be more effective than placebo in the treatment of mild and moderate depression in adults, most commonly 900–1200 mg per day in divided doses. Adverse events are rare. St. John's wort has also been shown in multiple studies to be as effective as early generation tricyclic antidepressants, with fewer side effects (Linde, Berner, and Kriston 2008). St. John's wort has also been shown to be as effective as sertraline and fluoxetine with fewer side effects in patients with mild to moderate depression (Kasper et al. 2010).

In a meta-analysis by Rahimi of 13 randomized, double-blind trials comparing St. John's wort to SSRI, St. John's wort in adults was shown to be at least as effective as SSRI with better tolerance and fewer side effects (Rahimi, Nikfar, and Abdollahi 2009).

Pediatric Research Evidence

Fewer studies have been done with St. John's wort in children. One open label study in 26 adolescents evaluated the efficacy and safety of an 8-week trial of 300 mg standardized dose three times per day. Only 11 patients completed the study, and of those 9 (82%) demonstrated significant clinical improvement. No adverse effects were reported (Simeon et al. 2005).

A second small open label study in 33 children and adolescents 6–16 years old with major depression evaluated the effectiveness of 150 mg St. John's wort three times per day, increasing to 300 mg three times per day if no effect was seen at week 4 of the 8-week study. At week 4, 22 participants had doses increased to 900 mg per day. At week 8, 25 of 33 patients were considered responders to treatment. No significant adverse effects were noted (Findling et al. 2003).

Cautions

St. John's wort is generally well tolerated, with rates of adverse effects lower than common antidepressants. Possible side effects include gastrointestinal symptoms, dry mouth, headache, and fatigue. Hypersensitivity to light and allergic skin rashes have been reported. Few reports of adverse events exist in children, although more studies are needed (Charrois et al. 2007).

Evidence is lacking to support the use of St. John's wort in pregnancy or lactation (Deligiannidis and Freeman 2014).

Interactions

St. John's wort interacts with many medications. The most significant mechanism is induction of the CYP450 3A4 enzyme, which can reduce plasma concentrations of drugs using this pathway for metabolism such as oral contraceptives, carbamazepine, cyclosporine, warfarin, protease inhibitors, and non-nucleoside reverse transcriptase inhibitors. Risk of central serotonin syndrome is also a concern and concomitant use of selective serotonin reuptake inhibitors (SSRIs) and St. John's wort should be avoided (Mills et al. 2005; Charrois et al. 2007).

Adult Dose

The recommended dose for adults with depression is 900 to 1800 mg per day in divided doses. Ideally standardized extract to 0.3% hypericin.

Pediatric Dose

Ideally standardized extract to 0.3% hypericin. Pediatric study doses range from 300 to 900 mg/day in divided doses (Charrois et al. 2007).

Melatonin

(Bruni et al. 2015; Shamseer and Vohra 2009)

Melatonin is primarily produced and secreted by the pineal gland, regulated by the suprachiasmatic nucleus and is the main modulator of the circadian rhythm which regulates the sleep–wake cycle. In melatonin synthesis tryptophan is hydroxylated to 5-hydroxytryptophan, which is then decarboxylated to 5-hydroxytryptamine, which is serotonin. Melatonin has been shown to orchestrate a complex range of physiologic functions on the cellular level, including a role in regulation of insulin growth factor (Sharma et al. 2015).

Emerging research highlights its anti-inflammatory, antioxidant, free radical-scavenging properties and its critical role in early organ and nervous system development (Bruni et al. 2015). Its potential for neuroprotective effect in infants with hypoxic-ischemic encephalopathy is also under study.

In supplement form, melatonin advances sleep onset in patients with delayed sleep phase disorder and has become widely used to decrease sleep latency in children. It is still sold over the counter in the U.S., but regulated in Europe and the U.K. According to the National Health Interview Survey results, use of melatonin has increased significantly from 0.1% of children in 2007 to 0.7% of children in 2012 (Black et al. 2015). Difficulty with sleep initiation and maintenance is a common problem in children, with up to 40% of normally developing children noted to have difficulty with sleep at some point in childhood. Prevalence of sleep disturbance climbs sharply in children with developmental disorders such as ADHD and autism, and in those with depression or anxiety (Heussler et al. 2013; Hochadel et al. 2014).

A survey on management practice of pediatric sleep disturbance in 181 Australian pediatricians showed that melatonin was the most commonly prescribed treatment, recommended by 89.1% of respondents. Respondents indicated that they prescribed melatonin for infants as young as 6 months up through adolescence, with an average patient age of 4 years. Recorded doses ranged from 0.5 mg to 12 mg, and time of treatment also varied widely, reflecting lack of consensus on treatment approaches. Fewer than half of pediatricians were aware of potential side effects of melatonin (Heussler et al. 2013).

A survey study of 1273 child and adolescent psychiatrists indicated that one in three of their patients had sleep disorders. Prescription or over-the-counter medication to treat insomnia was recommended by 96% and 88% of practitioners respectively. Melatonin was recommended to patients by more than one in three of these practitioners (Owens et al. 2010; Bendz and Scates 2010).

Pediatric Research Evidence

A meta-analysis of 1683 patients (van Geijlswijk et al. 2010), (170 children in 3 studies) (Smits et al. 2003; Smits et al. 2001) shows good efficacy of melatonin in advancing dim light melatonin onset and reduction of sleep latency in patients with primary sleep disorder. No significant adverse events were reported (Ferracioli-Oda, Qawasmi, and Bloch 2013).

A retrospective study of melatonin treatment in 33 adolescents with delayed sleep phase syndrome (15 with ADHD) treated with melatonin 3–5 mg per day for an average of 6 months showed advance of sleep onset of more than 2 hours on average, with a corresponding increase in sleep duration. Daytime sleepiness decreased and school performance improved (decreased social difficulties, reduced tardiness, reduced absences) (Szeinberg, Borodkin, and Dagan 2006).

Accumulating studies in children with autism highlight the prevalence of abnormalities in melatonin metabolism and circadian rhythm in this patient population. A review by Rossignol and Frye of an accumulated 20 studies on the use of melatonin in children with autism spectrum disorder conclude strong positive effects with decrease in sleep latency, total sleep duration, and improved daytime behaviors. Adverse events were reported as minimal to none. Questions about optimal dose, timing of dose, and duration of treatment are areas of active study (Rossignol and Frye 2014).

Although use is common in children, few longitudinal studies have been done to assess adverse events or treatment-related morbidity. One study followed 94 children with ADHD and chronic sleep onset insomnia for an average of 3.7 years. Dose was 3 mg for body weight under 40 kg and 6 mg above 40 kg. Two thirds of patients used melatonin daily and the majority had resurgence of delayed sleep onset if melatonin was discontinued. Adverse events were reported in 20% of patients and most frequently included dizziness, bedwetting, and sleep maintenance insomnia (Hoebert et al. 2009).

A second open label longitudinal study of 44 children (5–19 years) with a variety of complex neurodevelopmental diagnosis and treatment-resistant circadian rhythm disorders followed patients for a mean of 4.3 years. Doses were variable, ranging from 5 mg to 15 mg. Positive reports of continued efficacy of treatment were present from 93.2% of families and there were no serious adverse events reported (Carr et al. 2007).

Cautions

The best evidence to date for melatonin use in children is in insomnia caused by circadian rhythm sleep disorders. Other conditions such as poor sleep hygiene, depression, anxiety, or other mental health or social issues should not be treated with melatonin as a primary agent. Lack of clear evidence regarding efficacy, dose, and long-term safety remains a relevant concern. Theoretical risk of hypothalamic-gonadal axis suppression and delayed puberty exists, although this was not shown in a follow-up study of 57 Dutch adolescents who had used melatonin for a mean of 3 years (range 1–4.6 years) at a mean dose of 2.69 mg (0.3–10 mg). Recurring headache was reported in 38% of this study population as a primary adverse effect (van Geijlswijk et al. 2011).

Larger controlled trials are needed to identify the children who will most benefit from melatonin treatment and to determine appropriate doses and duration of treatment.

Interactions

Melatonin is primarily metabolized by CYP1A2 therefore drugs that inhibit this pathway such as tricyclic antidepressants, cimetidine, and fluvoxamine may increase melatonin levels. Melatonin can also decrease blood pressure and serum glucose concentrations.

Pediatric Dose

Lack of sufficient research and controlled trials preclude definitive dosing guidelines.

Timing of the dose of melatonin plays a critical role in treatment outcome. Ideally, maximum effect is seen with administration at 3–5 hours before dim light melatonin onset (DMLO), which occurs with large individual differences. DMLO can be measured in individuals by measurement of melatonin in saliva.

Clinical recommendations published in the *European Journal of Paediatric Neurology* (Bruni et al. 2015) for melatonin use and dosing in children with sleep–wake rhythm disorders or sleep onset insomnia are summarized below.

- Measure dim light melatonin onset (DLMO) if possible to narrow dose timing.
- Minimum age: no studies currently exist on the minimum age for melatonin administration.
- Melatonin is not generally effective for sleep maintenance issues.

  To shift sleep–wake cycle:

- Dose should be delivered 2–3 hours before DLMO if measurable.
- Otherwise melatonin should be given 3–4 hours prior to desired sleep onset.
- Start with low dose of fast release melatonin (0.2–0.5 mg) 3–4 hours before bedtime; increase by 0.2–0.5 mg every week as needed to a maximum of 3 mg in children <40 kg, and 5 mg in children >40 kg.
- In general aim for lowest effective dose.

  For sleep induction:

- Administer 30 minutes before bedtime.
- Start with 1–3 mg 30 minutes before sleep or before procedure (EEG, MRI, etc.).

  Treatment duration:

- Tailor to individual, usually not less than 1 month.
- Consider treatment withdrawal just before puberty or shortly after puberty given theoretical risk of hypothalamic-gonadal axis suppression and delayed puberty.

- In prolonged treatment, stop melatonin once a year for a week, usually during summer, after a normal sleep cycle is established.

If melatonin treatment loses efficacy:

- Check timing of dose.
- In some cases, dose reduction is needed.
- May be result of slow melatonin metabolism.
- Revisit diagnosis for cofounders.
- Check for concurrent medications such as oral contraceptives, cimetidine, fluvoxamine that will slow melatonin metabolism.
- Conversely concurrent medications that will speed metabolism include: carbamazepine, esomeprazole, omeprazole.

Problems with sleep maintenance after start of treatment:

- Dose is likely too high.

Further study is needed in all age groups (Bruni et al. 2015).

Peppermint

The word mint is derived from the Latin *mentha*, and peppermint (*Mentha* x *piperita*) is a perennial herb resulting from cross-fertilization between spearmint and water mint that has been valued for its taste and health benefits dating back to ancient Greece, Egypt, and Rome (Kline et al. 2001).

Peppermint is widely found in North America, and southern and central Europe. Peppermint extracts are commonly used in flavoring foods or personal care products including rubs for muscle pain or to aid in relief of congestion. The leaf has traditionally been chewed to assist in digestion and is often used in tea form (McKay and Blumberg 2006).

Peppermint oil, obtained from the ground and distilled stem, leaves, and flowers of the plant, has multiple pharmacologically active compounds, with menthol being the primary active ingredient. Studies indicate an antispasmodic effect on gastrointestinal smooth muscle thought to be mediated primarily through calcium channel blockade (Kligler and Chaudhary 2007).

It is unclear whether the analgesic effects have a central or local action in patients with irritable bowel syndrome (Kearns et al. 2015).

Enteric-coated peppermint oil is often used as a way to bypass the upper gastrointestinal tract to avoid gastroesophageal reflux related to relaxation of the lower esophageal sphincter. Probably the most common use for oral peppermint oil is to help address symptoms of irritable bowel syndrome with its associated abdominal pain, bloating, and excess flatulence. Enteric-coated peppermint oil capsules were found to be safe and effective in short-term use in adults with irritable bowel syndrome in a systematic review by Khanna (Khanna, MacDonald, and Levesque 2014).

Doses in the reviewed studies varied, although the majority varied between 0.2 and 0.4 mL up to three times per day in adults. Adverse events reported were infrequent, mild, and short lived, including heartburn, belching, or perianal discomfort. Topically, peppermint oil has been reported to reduce symptoms of tension headache in some adult studies. Mechanism appears to be related to reduction of smooth muscle contraction and increased blood flow to the skin of the forehead (Gobel et al. 1995).

There is also evidence to support the use of peppermint oil for reducing colonic spasm associated with barium enema in adult patients (Kligler and Chaudhary 2007).

Pediatrics Research Evidence

Few randomized controlled studies exist on the use of peppermint oil in children. One is a 2-week trial by Kline et al. in which 42 children 8–17 years with irritable bowel syndrome were given enteric-coated peppermint oil. Dose was either 0.1 mL or 0.2 mL three times a day as determined by weight (less than or greater than 45 kg respectively). Results showed a significant reduction in pain episodes in the treatment group, 76% as opposed to 19% receiving placebo. No adverse events were reported in the study group (Kline et al. 2001).

Cautions

Peppermint oil may aggravate gastroesophageal reflux disease and hiatal hernia due to relaxation of the lower esophageal sphincter. It is contraindicated in patients with cholelithiasis or cholecystitis due to its choleretic effect. There are rare reports of newborns with glucose-6-phosphate dehydrogenase deficiency developing jaundice with topical menthol exposure (Olowe and Ransome-Kuti 1980).

In excessive doses peppermint oil has rarely been associated with interstitial nephritis and acute renal failure, and even death. It is contraindicated in pregnancy due to history of use in precipitating menstruation. It is anecdotally associated with reduction in human milk supply, although data is insufficient to determine safety during lactation. The most common adverse effects reported in clinical trials include heartburn, perianal burning, allergic reaction, and nausea. Face and mouth should be avoided in topical application. Dermatitis has also been reported in some patients with topical use (Kearns et al. 2015; McKay and Blumberg 2006; Khanna, MacDonald, and Levesque 2014).

Interactions

Peppermint may inhibit the action of the cytochrome P4503A4, which can be associated with reduced clearance of drugs such as cyclosporine (Dresser et al. 2002). Enteric-coated peppermint oil may dissolve prematurely in the presence of drugs that raise the gastric pH such as antacids, histamine-2 receptor blocker, and proton pump inhibitors (Charrois, Hrudey, Gardiner et al. 2006).

Dose

The dose for children has not been clearly defined, although in clinical practice 0.1–0.2 mL of enteric-coated peppermint oil two to three times per day is a frequent recommendation in children (Charrois, Hrudey, Gardiner et al. 2006).

One pharmacokinetic pilot study in six pediatric patients with irritable bowel syndrome measured plasma menthol concentration at serial intervals after standard 83 mg dose of menthol in delayed-release peppermint oil. Peak plasma concentrations varied in time from 2.5 to 8 hours (average lag time of appearance of plasma menthol 2 hours), prohibiting reliable estimation of elimination rate or elimination half-life (Kearns et al. 2015).

References

Aggarwal, B. B., and B. Sung. 2009. "Pharmacological basis for the role of curcumin in chronic diseases: an age-old spice with modern targets." *Trends Pharmacol Sci* 30(2): 85–94. doi: 10.1016/j.tips.2008.11.002.

Amsterdam, J. D., Y. Li, I. Soeller, K. Rockwell, J. J. Mao, and J. Shults. 2009. "A randomized, double-blind, placebo-controlled trial of oral Matricaria recutita (chamomile) extract therapy for generalized anxiety disorder." *J Clin Psychopharmacol* 29(4): 378–82. doi: 10.1097/JCP.0b013e3181ac935c.

Awortwe, C., V. K. Manda, C. Avonto, S. I. Khan, I. A. Khan, L. A. Walker, P. J. Bouic, and B. Rosenkranz. 2015. "Echinacea purpurea up-regulates CYP1A2, CYP3A4 and MDR1 gene expression by activation of pregnane X receptor pathway." *Xenobiotica* 45(3): 218–29. doi: 10.3109/00498254.2014.973930.

Aydin, A. A., V. Zerbes, H. Parlar, and T. Letzel. 2013. "The medical plant butterbur (Petasites): analytical and physiological (re)view." *J Pharm Biomed Anal* 75: 220–9. doi: 10.1016/j.jpba.2012.11.028.

Banderali, U., D. Belke, A. Singh, A. Jayanthan, W. R. Giles, and A. Narendran. 2011. "Curcumin blocks Kv11.1 (erg) potassium current and slows proliferation in the infant acute monocytic leukemia cell line THP-1." *Cell Physiol Biochem* 28(6): 1169–80. doi: 10.1159/000335850.

Bandyopadhyay, D. 2014. "Farmer to pharmacist: curcumin as an anti-invasive and antimetastatic agent for the treatment of cancer." *Front Chem* 2: 113. doi: 10.3389/fchem.2014.00113.

Bendz, L. M., and A. C. Scates. 2010. "Melatonin treatment for insomnia in pediatric patients with attention-deficit/hyperactivity disorder." *Ann Pharmacother* 44(1): 185–91. doi: 10.1345/aph.1M365.

Black, L. I., T. C. Clarke, P. M. Barnes, B. J. Stussman, and R. L. Nahin. 2015. "Use of complementary health approaches among children aged 4–17 years in the United States: National Health Interview Survey, 2007–2012." *Natl Health Stat Report* (78): 1–19.

Bortel, N., S. Armeanu-Ebinger, E. Schmid, B. Kirchner, J. Frank, A. Kocher, C. Schiborr, S. Warmann, J. Fuchs, and V. Ellerkamp. 2015. "Effects of curcumin in pediatric epithelial liver tumors: inhibition of tumor growth and alpha-fetoprotein in vitro and in vivo involving the NFkappaB- and the beta-catenin pathways." *Oncotarget.* doi: 10.18632/oncotarget.5673.

Boyanapalli, S. S., and A. N. Tony Kong. 2015. "'Curcumin, the king of spices': epigenetic regulatory mechanisms in the prevention of cancer, neurological, and inflammatory diseases." *Curr Pharmacol Rep* 1(2): 129–39. doi: 10.1007/s40495-015-0018-x.

Bruni, O., D. Alonso-Alconada, F. Besag, V. Biran, W. Braam, S. Cortese, R. Moavero, P. Parisi, M. Smits, K. Van der Heijden, and P. Curatolo. 2015. "Current role of melatonin in pediatric neurology: clinical recommendations." *Eur J Paediatr Neurol* 19(2): 122–33. doi: 10.1016/j.ejpn.2014.12.007.

Carr, R., M. B. Wasdell, D. Hamilton, M. D. Weiss, R. D. Freeman, J. Tai, W. J. Rietveld, and J. E. Jan. 2007. "Long-term effectiveness outcome of melatonin therapy in children with treatment-resistant circadian rhythm sleep disorders." *J Pineal Res* 43 (4): 351–9. doi: 10.1111/j.1600-079X.2007.00485.x.

Charrois, T. L., J. Hrudey, P. Gardiner, S. Vohra, Holistic American Academy of Pediatrics Provisional Section on Complementary, and Medicine Integrative. 2006. "Peppermint oil." *Pediatr Rev* 27(7): e49–51.

Charrois, T. L., J. Hrudey, S. Vohra, Holistic American Academy of Pediatrics Provisional Section on Complementary, and Medicine Integrative. 2006. "Echinacea." *Pediatr Rev* 27(10): 385–7.

Charrois, T. L., C. Sadler, S. Vohra, Holistic American Academy of Pediatrics Provisional Section on Complementary, and Medicine Integrative. 2007. "Complementary, holistic, and integrative medicine: St. John's wort." *Pediatr Rev* 28(2): 69–72.

Chien, L. C., C. Y. Yeh, H. C. Lee, H. Jasmine Chao, M. J. Shieh, and B. C. Han. 2006. "Effect of the mother's consumption of traditional Chinese herbs on estimated infant daily intake of lead from breast milk." *Sci Total Environ* 354(2–3): 120–6. doi: 10.1016/j.scitotenv.2005.01.033.

D'Andrea, G., S. Cevoli, and D. Cologno. 2014. "Herbal therapy in migraine." *Neurol Sci* 35(Suppl 1): 135–40. doi: 10.1007/s10072-014-1757-x.

Deligiannidis, K. M., and M. P. Freeman. 2014. "Complementary and alternative medicine therapies for perinatal depression." *Best Pract Res Clin Obstet Gynaecol* 28(1): 85–95. doi: 10.1016/j.bpobgyn.2013.08.007.

Dresser, G. K., V. Wacher, S. Wong, H. T. Wong, and D. G. Bailey. 2002. "Evaluation of peppermint oil and ascorbyl palmitate as inhibitors of cytochrome P4503A4 activity in vitro and in vivo." *Clin Pharmacol Ther* 72(3): 247–55. doi: 10.1067/mcp.2002.126409.

Ferracioli-Oda, E., A. Qawasmi, and M. H. Bloch. 2013. "Meta-analysis: melatonin for the treatment of primary sleep disorders." *PLoS One* 8(5): e63773. doi: 10.1371/journal.pone.0063773.

Findling, R. L., N. K. McNamara, M. A. O'Riordan, M. D. Reed, C. A. Demeter, L. A. Branicky, and J. L. Blumer. 2003. "An open-label pilot study of St. John's wort in juvenile depression." *J Am Acad Child Adolesc Psychiatry* 42(8): 908–14. doi: 10.1097/01.CHI.0000046900.27264.2A.

Gardiner, P. 2007. "Complementary, holistic, and integrative medicine: chamomile." *Pediatr Rev* 28 (4): e16–8.

Gardiner, P., D. Adams, A. C. Filippelli, H. Nasser, R. Saper, L. White, and S. Vohra. 2013. "A systematic review of the reporting of adverse events associated with medical herb use among children." *Glob Adv Health Med* 2(2): 46–55. doi: 10.7453/gahmj.2012.071.

Gobel, H., G. Schmidt, M. Dworschak, H. Stolze, and D. Heuss. 1995. "Essential plant oils and headache mechanisms." *Phytomedicine* 2(2): 93–102. doi: 10.1016/S0944-7113(11)80053-X.

Heussler, H., P. Chan, A. M. Price, K. Waters, M. J. Davey, and H. Hiscock. 2013. "Pharmacological and non-pharmacological management of sleep disturbance in children: an Australian Paediatric Research Network survey." *Sleep Med* 14(2): 189–94. doi: 10.1016/j.sleep.2012.09.023.

Hochadel, J., J. Frolich, A. Wiater, G. Lehmkuhl, and L. Fricke-Oerkermann. 2014. "Prevalence of sleep problems and relationship between sleep problems and school refusal behavior in school-aged children in children's and parents' ratings." *Psychopathology* 47(2): 119–26. doi: 10.1159/000345403.

Hoebert, M., K. B. van der Heijden, I. M. van Geijlswijk, and M. G. Smits. 2009. "Long-term follow-up of melatonin treatment in children with ADHD and chronic sleep onset insomnia." *J Pineal Res* 47(1): 1–7. doi: 10.1111/j.1600-079X.2009.00681.x.

Huang, N., N. Singh, K. Yoon, C. M. Loiacono, M. L. Kohut, and D. F. Birt. 2013. "The immuno-regulatory impact of orally-administered Hypericum perforatum extract on Balb/C mice inoculated with H1n1 influenza A virus." *PLoS One* 8 (9): e76491. doi: 10.1371/journal.pone.0076491.

Huntley, A. L., J. Thompson Coon, and E. Ernst. 2005. "The safety of herbal medicinal products derived from Echinacea species: a systematic review." *Drug Saf* 28(5): 387–400.

Jurenka, J. S. 2009. "Anti-inflammatory properties of curcumin, a major constituent of Curcuma longa: a review of preclinical and clinical research." *Altern Med Rev* 14(2): 141–53.

Karsch-Volk, M., B. Barrett, D. Kiefer, R. Bauer, K. Ardjomand-Woelkart, and K. Linde. 2014. "Echinacea for preventing and treating the common cold." *Cochrane Database Syst Rev* 2: CD000530. doi: 10.1002/14651858.CD000530.pub3.

Kasper, S., F. Caraci, B. Forti, F. Drago, and E. Aguglia. 2010. "Efficacy and tolerability of Hypericum extract for the treatment of mild to moderate depression." *Eur Neuropsychopharmacol* 20(11): 747–65. doi: 10.1016/j.euroneuro.2010.07.005.

Kearns, G. L., B. P. Chumpitazi, S. M. Abdel-Rahman, U. Garg, and R. J. Shulman. 2015.

"Systemic exposure to menthol following administration of peppermint oil to paediatric patients." *BMJ Open* 5 (8): e008375. doi: 10.1136/bmjopen-2015-008375.

Khanna, R., J. K. MacDonald, and B. G. Levesque. 2014. "Peppermint oil for the treatment of irritable bowel syndrome: a systematic review and meta-analysis." *J Clin Gastroenterol* 48(6): 505–12. doi: 10.1097/MCG.0b013e3182a88357.

Khayat, S., H. Fanaei, M. Kheirkhah, Z. B. Moghadam, A. Kasaeian, and M. Javadimehr. 2015. "Curcumin attenuates severity of premenstrual syndrome symptoms: a randomized, double-blind, placebo-controlled trial." *Complement Ther Med* 23(3): 318–24. doi: 10.1016/j.ctim.2015.04.001.

Kiyan, H. T., B. Demirci, K. H. Baser, and F. Demirci. 2014. "The in vivo evaluation of anti-angiogenic effects of Hypericum essential oils using the chorioallantoic membrane assay." *Pharm Biol* 52(1): 44–50. doi: 10.3109/13880209.2013.810647.

Kligler, B., and S. Chaudhary. 2007. "Peppermint oil." *Am Fam Physician* 75(7): 1027–30.

Kline, R. M., J. J. Kline, J. Di Palma, and G. J. Barbero. 2001. "Enteric-coated, pH-dependent peppermint oil capsules for the treatment of irritable bowel syndrome in children." *J Pediatr* 138(1): 125–8.

Kocaadam, B., and N. Sanlier. 2015. "Curcumin, an active component of turmeric (Curcuma longa), and its effects on health." *Crit Rev Food Sci Nutr* 0. doi: 10.1080/10408398.2015.1077195.

Kraus, B., H. Wolff, J. Heilmann, and E. F. Elstner. 2007. "Influence of Hypericum perforatum extract and its single compounds on amyloid-beta mediated toxicity in microglial cells." *Life Sci* 81(11): 884–94. doi: 10.1016/j.lfs.2007.07.020.

Kumar, S., V. Ahuja, M. J. Sankar, A. Kumar, and A. C. Moss. 2012. "Curcumin for maintenance of remission in ulcerative colitis." *Cochrane Database Syst Rev* 10: CD008424. doi: 10.1002/14651858.CD008424.pub2.

Lao, C. D., M. T. th Ruffin, D. Normolle, D. D. Heath, S. I. Murray, J. M. Bailey, M. E. Boggs, J. Crowell, C. L. Rock, and D. E. Brenner. 2006. "Dose escalation of a curcuminoid formulation." *BMC Complement Altern Med* 6: 10. doi: 10.1186/1472-6882-6-10.

Linde, K., M. M. Berner, and L. Kriston. 2008. "St John's wort for major depression." *Cochrane Database Syst Rev* 4: CD000448. doi: 10.1002/14651858.CD000448.pub3.

Linde, K., L. Kriston, G. Rucker, S. Jamil, I. Schumann, K. Meissner, K. Sigterman, and A. Schneider. 2015. "Efficacy and acceptability of pharmacological treatments for depressive disorders in primary care: systematic review and network meta-analysis." *Ann Fam Med* 13(1): 69–79. doi: 10.1370/afm.1687.

Loder, E., R. Burch, and P. Rizzoli. 2012. "The 2012 AHS/AAN guidelines for prevention of episodic migraine: a summary and comparison with other recent clinical practice guidelines." *Headache* 52(6): 930–45. doi: 10.1111/j.1526-4610.2012.02185.x.

McKay, D. L., and J. B. Blumberg. 2006. "A review of the bioactivity and potential health benefits of chamomile tea (Matricaria recutita L.)." *Phytother Res* 20(7): 519–30. doi: 10.1002/ptr.1900.

Mills, E., P. Wu, B. C. Johnston, K. Gallicano, M. Clarke, and G. Guyatt. 2005. "Natural health product-drug interactions: a systematic review of clinical trials." *Ther Drug Monit* 27(5): 549–57.

Olowe, S. A., and O. Ransome-Kuti. 1980. "The risk of jaundice in glucose-6-phosphate dehydrogenase deficient babies exposed to menthol." *Acta Paediatr Scand* 69(3): 341–5.

Owens, J. A., C. L. Rosen, J. A. Mindell, and H. L. Kirchner. 2010. "Use of pharmacotherapy for insomnia in child psychiatry practice: a national survey." *Sleep Med* 11(7): 692–700. doi: 10.1016/j.sleep.2009.11.015.

Panahi, Y., M. S. Hosseini, N. Khalili, E. Naimi, M. Majeed, and A. Sahebkar. 2015. "Antioxidant and anti-inflammatory effects of curcuminoid-piperine combination in subjects with metabolic syndrome: a randomized controlled trial and an updated meta-analysis." *Clin Nutr*. doi: 10.1016/j.clnu.2014.12.019.

Panahi, Y., N. Khalili, M. S. Hosseini, M. Abbasinazari, and A. Sahebkar. 2014. "Lipid-modifying effects of adjunctive therapy with curcuminoids-piperine combination in patients with metabolic syndrome: results of a randomized controlled trial." *Complement Ther Med* 22(5): 851–7. doi: 10.1016/j.ctim.2014.07.006.

Parslow, R., A. J. Morgan, N. B. Allen, A. F. Jorm, C. P. O'Donnell, and R. Purcell. 2008. "Effectiveness of complementary and self-help treatments for anxiety in children and adolescents." *Med J Aust* 188(6): 355–9.

Perri, D., J. J. Dugoua, E. Mills, and G. Koren. 2006. "Safety and efficacy of echinacea (Echinacea angustafolia, e. purpurea and e. pallida) during pregnancy and lactation." *Can J Clin Pharmacol* 13(3): e262–7.

Pia Schiavone, B. I., L. Verotta, A. Rosato, M. Marilena, S. Gibbons, E. Bombardelli, C. Franchini, and F. Corbo. 2014. "Anticancer and antibacterial activity of hyperforin and its derivatives." *Anticancer Agents Med Chem* 14(10): 1397–1401.

Pothmann, R., and U. Danesch. 2005. "Migraine prevention in children and adolescents: results of an open study with a special butterbur root extract." *Headache* 45(3): 196–203. doi: 10.1111/j.1526-4610.2005.05044.x.

Pringsheim, T., W. Davenport, G. Mackie, I. Worthington, M. Aube, S. N. Christie, J. Gladstone, W. J. Becker, and Group Canadian Headache Society Prophylactic Guidelines Development. 2012. "Canadian Headache Society guideline for migraine prophylaxis." *Can J Neurol Sci* 39(2 Suppl 2): S1–59.

Rahimi, R., S. Nikfar, and M. Abdollahi. 2009. "Efficacy and tolerability of Hypericum perforatum in major depressive disorder in comparison with selective serotonin reuptake inhibitors: a meta-analysis." *Prog Neuropsychopharmacol Biol Psychiatry* 33(1): 118–27. doi: 10.1016/j.pnpbp.2008.10.018.

Rossignol, D. A., and R. E. Frye. 2014. "Melatonin in autism spectrum disorders." *Curr Clin Pharmacol* 9(4): 326–34.

Sadler, C., L. Vanderjagt, S. Vohra, Holistic American Academy of Pediatrics Provisional Section on Complementary, and Medicine Integrative. 2007. "Complementary, holistic, and integrative medicine: butterbur." *Pediatr Rev* 28(6): 235–8.

Sahebkar, A. 2014. "A systematic review and meta-analysis of randomized controlled trials investigating the effects of curcumin on blood lipid levels." *Clin Nutr* 33(3): 406–14. doi: 10.1016/j.clnu.2013.09.012.

Savino, F., F. Cresi, E. Castagno, L. Silvestro, and R. Oggero. 2005. "A randomized double-blind placebo-controlled trial of a standardized extract of Matricariae recutita, Foeniculum vulgare and Melissa officinalis (ColiMil) in the treatment of breastfed colicky infants." *Phytother Res* 19(4): 335–40. doi: 10.1002/ptr.1668.

Schmidt, M., and V. Butterweck. 2015. "The mechanisms of action of St. John's wort: an update." *Wien Med Wochenschr* 165(11–12): 229–35. doi: 10.1007/s10354-015-0372-7.

Shamliyan, T. A., R. L. Kane, R. Ramakrishnan, and F. R. Taylor. 2013. "Episodic migraines in children: limited evidence on preventive pharmacological treatments." *J Child Neurol* 28(10): 1320–41. doi: 10.1177/0883073813488659.

Shamseer, L., and S. Vohra. 2009. "Complementary, holistic, and integrative medicine: melatonin." *Pediatr Rev* 30(6): 223–8. doi: 10.1542/pir.30-6-223.

Sharma, S., H. Singh, N. Ahmad, P. Mishra, and A. Tiwari. 2015. "The role of melatonin in diabetes: therapeutic implications." *Arch Endocrinol Metab* 59(5): 391–9. doi: 10.1590/2359-3997000000098.

Simeon, J., M. K. Nixon, R. Milin, R. Jovanovic, and S. Walker. 2005. "Open-label pilot study of St. John's wort in adolescent depression." *J Child Adolesc Psychopharmacol* 15(2): 293–301. doi: 10.1089/cap.2005.15.293.

Singh, O., Z. Khanam, N. Misra, and M. K. Srivastava. 2011. "Chamomile (Matricaria chamomilla L.): an overview." *Pharmacogn Rev* 5(9): 82–95. doi: 10.4103/0973-7847.79103.

Smits, M. G., E. E. Nagtegaal, J. van der Heijden, A. M. Coenen, and G. A. Kerkhof. 2001.

"Melatonin for chronic sleep onset insomnia in children: a randomized placebo-controlled trial." *J Child Neurol* 16(2): 86–92.

Smits, M. G., H. F. van Stel, K. van der Heijden, A. M. Meijer, A. M. Coenen, and G. A. Kerkhof. 2003. "Melatonin improves health status and sleep in children with idiopathic chronic sleep-onset insomnia: a randomized placebo-controlled trial." *J Am Acad Child Adolesc Psychiatry* 42(11): 1286–93. doi: 10.1097/01.chi.0000085756.71002.86.

Suskind, D. L., G. Wahbeh, T. Burpee, M. Cohen, D. Christie, and W. Weber. 2013. "Tolerability of curcumin in pediatric inflammatory bowel disease: a forced-dose titration study." *J Pediatr Gastroenterol Nutr* 56(3): 277–9. doi: 10.1097/MPG.0b013e318276977d.

Szeinberg, A., K. Borodkin, and Y. Dagan. 2006. "Melatonin treatment in adolescents with delayed sleep phase syndrome." *Clin Pediatr (Phila)* 45(9): 809–18. doi: 10.1177/0009922806294218.

Teiten, M. H., M. Dicato, and M. Diederich. 2013. "Curcumin as a regulator of epigenetic events." *Mol Nutr Food Res* 57(9): 1619–29. doi: 10.1002/mnfr.201300201.

Triantafyllidi, A., T. Xanthos, A. Papalois, and J. K. Triantafillidis. 2015. "Herbal and plant therapy in patients with inflammatory bowel disease." *Ann Gastroenterol* 28(2): 210–20.

van Geijlswijk, I. M., R. H. Mol, T. C. Egberts, and M. G. Smits. 2011. "Evaluation of sleep, puberty and mental health in children with long-term melatonin treatment for chronic idiopathic childhood sleep onset insomnia." *Psychopharmacology (Berl)* 216(1): 111–20. doi: 10.1007/s00213-011-2202-y.

van Geijlswijk, I. M., K. B. van der Heijden, A. C. Egberts, H. P. Korzilius, and M. G. Smits. 2010. "Dose finding of melatonin for chronic idiopathic childhood sleep onset insomnia: an RCT." *Psychopharmacology (Berl)* 212(3): 379–91. doi: 10.1007/s00213-010-1962-0.

Wanwimolruk, S., and V. Prachayasittikul. 2014. "Cytochrome P450 enzyme mediated herbal drug interactions (Part 1)." *EXCLI J* 13: 347–91.

Weizman, Z., S. Alkrinawi, D. Goldfarb, and C. Bitran. 1993. "Efficacy of herbal tea preparation in infantile colic." *J Pediatr* 122(4): 650–2.

World Health Organization. 1999. "WHO Monographs on Selected Medicinal Plants."

Zhang, Y., E. B. Fein, and S. B. Fein. 2011. "Feeding of dietary botanical supplements and teas to infants in the United States." *Pediatrics* 127(6): 1060–6. doi: 10.1542/peds.2010-2294.

10 Manual Medicine

Manual medicine is a broad term that includes osteopathy, craniosacral therapy, therapeutic massage, and chiropractic among other therapies. In some instances, there is significant overlap between the practices despite different training approaches. The overarching goal of the manual medicine therapies is to balance the musculoskeletal system within the context of whole body health by using a hands-on approach for diagnosis and treatment. Many of the manual medicine practices are based upon the belief that self-healing is supported by pain-free movement of the musculoskeletal system. Use of manual medicine dates back thousands of years and has been recorded in early civilizations around the world including those in Indonesia, Egypt, China, Japan, and India. Practitioners have also been recorded as "bone setters" in many cultures. Hippocrates and Galen both recorded manipulative treatments for scoliosis in early works. Historically, manual therapies have been the source of great controversy in the evolution of modern medical practice. Manipulative therapies had largely fallen out of favor by the 18th century, then resurfaced in medical societies and writings in the 19th century, accompanied by continuing controversy and dissent within the medical profession (Pettman 2007).

In many cases manual medicine research specific to pediatrics is sparse, yet the prevalence of use of the manual medicine therapies in pediatrics requires clinicians to be familiar with these therapies in terms of philosophy, training requirements, scope of practice, and potential benefits and risks. In fact, statistics from the 2012 National Health Interview Survey based on data from 2007 to 2012 showed that prevalence of use of complementary therapies held steady in children at an estimated 12% with non-vitamin, non-mineral dietary supplements and osteopathic or chiropractic manipulation continuing as the most commonly used complementary health approaches in 2012, consistent with 2007 survey results (Black et al. 2015).

An overarching concern in the use of manual medicine in children is that of safety. A 2014 literature review of cases involving serious events in children treated with manual therapies found that 12 articles identified 15 serious adverse events, including three deaths (two in previously healthy infants under 3 months of age) and 12 serious injuries. The most common intervention associated with harm was high-velocity, extension, and rotational spinal manipulation. An underlying undiagnosed and pre-existing pathology was identified in the majority of these cases. In addition to the serious events noted, 775 mild to moderate events were recorded, including: crying, soreness, transient headache, syncope, transient apnea, and self-limited bradycardia (Todd et al. 2014).

Given the high prevalence of pediatric visits to manual medicine practitioners, especially chiropractic, these numbers reflect a low rate of overall complications. However, it is difficult to overemphasize the importance of a detailed history and exam and the importance of in-depth and appropriate pediatric training prior to considering use of a manual medicine technique in any infant or child (Hestbaek and Stochkendahl 2010).

Osteopathy

Background Information

Andrew Still founded the field of osteopathy and established the American Osteopathic College in 1892. His initial theories of manipulation were based on the "Law of the Artery," a theory of dysfunction of blood flow leading to deformity or disease. His work emphasized the body's intrinsic self-healing ability, and the connection between each body part and its optimal physiologic functioning. Still postulated that every disease resulted from some anatomical deviation of the body from its normal position and shape. The American Association of Colleges of Osteopathic Medicine describes the core philosophy of osteopathy such that *all parts of a body are interrelated and each one of them represents a functional unit which, when disturbed, can often be fixed with a particular set of hands-on approach known as osteopathic manipulation. Simply stated, structure influences function.* The concept is based upon *four principles* in which the *first* principle states that functions and structure of each body part are interrelated like a machine in which all parts work in their places and fixed time and energy. The *second* principle states that a human body is a single dynamic unit of function; although all are interrelated, each one of them has different functions but they focus on one main task at the end. The *third* principle states that the human body possesses self-healing and self-regulatory mechanisms and the osteopaths are taught in a way so that they are trained to augment the intrinsic mechanism. The *fourth* one is that the rational treatment is based upon applying these principles (Parker 2014).

Mechanism of Action

Osteopathic treatments are generally very safe and gentle, based on basic principles of physiology and anatomy to treat disorders. Work is focused on the core areas of the joints, nervous system, and muscle in order to release tension in the body and provide benefit to the patient. Modern osteopathic training emphasizes primary care and preventive health.

The osteopathic practitioner takes a history by asking detailed questions and studies the patient's physical appearance including the posture, muscles, joints and ligaments, as the premise is that the external appearance is a mirror of internal problems. Once a physical examination has been done, a diagnosis is made and treatment plan decided. Some osteopathic physicians have moved away from including manipulation in their practices, but those that do select the desired osteopathic manipulative techniques best tailored to the individual. These are generally performed in the office, or at times prescribed for home. Although training varies, some of the more common techniques include: myofascial release, articulation, facilitated positional release, strain-counterstrain, osteopathy in the cranial field (also known as craniosacral technique, discussed further below) and thrust-high velocity low amplitude. Others techniques include the soft tissue technique where pressure is applied to the patient's trigger points. The muscles fibers are stretched so that the pain can be released. Direct pressure can be temporarily painful, but can be effective in resolving pain. Articulation is used by the practitioners to improve the joint movement. Under this method, the practitioner improves the rhythm of the patient's joints and muscles through a to-and-fro movement so that blood can be supplied to all parts of joints, which is associated with improved blood supply which will lead to pain reduction. Manipulation through strain-counterstrain is also a technique used to improve muscle and joint mobility and to relieve pain. The aim is to restore the motion of the joints so that the body can move freely and without any tension. Through this technique, the practitioners target the nerve endings so that blood flow can be improved and muscular relaxation can be achieved. If the osteopathic treatment fails to yield results, the patient may be referred for further workup.

Pediatric Evidence

Although interest in the use of osteopathy in children is growing, few randomized controlled trials exist. A 2013 systematic review by Posadzki et al. included 17 randomized controlled trials from around the world encompassing 887 pediatric patients. Conditions included in the studies were: cerebral palsy, respiratory conditions, otitis media, musculoskeletal function, attention-deficit/hyperactivity disorder, length of stay in preterm infants, congenital nasolacrimal duct obstruction, and dysfunctional voiding. Seven of the trials were found to favor osteopathic manipulation, seven showed no effect, and three did not report between treatment and control group findings. Control interventions, primary outcome measures, osteopathic manipulation techniques, frequency of interventions, and duration of interventions were highly variable. Reviewers found high study variability and serious methodological limitations in the majority of studies. Most sample sizes were insufficient to draw conclusion or derive recommendations. Reporting of presence or absence of adverse events was variable, although overall no adverse events were noted (Posadzki, Lee, and Ernst 2013).

A 2012 Cochrane Database Systematic Review of manipulative therapies for infant colic identified six studies involving a total of 325 infants. In the majority of studies primary outcome measure was daily hours of crying which was found to be reduced by a mean of 1 hour and 12 minutes. However, reviewers found the majority of trials were not blinded and therefore biased, leaving insufficient data to offer definitive recommendation (Dobson et al. 2012).

Cautions and Possible Side Effects

The process of osteopathy has few reported side effects in the generally healthy patient. Osteoporosis is a potential contraindication, as are certain skin conditions that may be exacerbated. Similarly, work with a patient with a history of acute infection may be contraindicated because manipulation could theoretically increase the flow of infected fluid within the body. Craniosacral technique, discussed below, should be used with due caution in the very young, the very old, or in those with history of head or neck trauma.

Training and Licensing Required for Providers (Gevitz 2009)

It is estimated that by 2019, more than 25% of U.S. medical school graduates will be from osteopathic programs. This is a significant shift after a long history of marginalization of osteopathy by the mainstream medical community. By the late 1890s Still's graduate trainees had opened several osteopathic schools around the U.S., eventually called the Associated Colleges of Osteopathy. An American Osteopathic Association was formed not long after, and the desire for accreditation led to a greater uniformity in training and a mandatory 3-year curriculum. Licensing eventually followed, but training was still considered inferior to MD school per the Flexner report of 1910 (Flexner 1910).

Many challenges followed as changes were implemented to expand osteopathic curriculum and training against strong resistance of the medical community. After World War II, osteopathic colleges began to receive federal funding, which allowed upgrading of faculty and facilities and resulted in an increase of new osteopathic hospitals across the country. Private insurers began to cover patient costs, and residency programs then began to increase in number.

By the early 1960s the American Osteopathic Association had a total of 11 specialty boards in areas such as: radiology, surgery, pediatrics, anesthesia, and others. By 1995 approximately 60% of Doctors of Osteopathic Medicine (DOs) in training were doing so in ACGME-accredited residencies.

By the end of the 20th century, state licensure for osteopathy was available through the standard national osteopathic licensing, National Board of Osteopathic Medical Examiners Comprehensive Osteopathic Medical Licensing Examination (NBOME/COMLEX) and/or the standard National Medical Licensing Examination (NBME). In 2015 there were 30 accredited 4-year osteopathic medical schools in the U.S. where students earn the Degree of Doctor of Osteopathic Medicine (DO).

DOs are licensed by individual states in the U.S., similar to physicians with an MD degree, and go on to complete residency training in their chosen area.

Craniosacral Therapy

Background Information

Craniosacral technique (osteopathy in the cranial field) was developed by W. G. Sutherland in the late 1890s based on his perception of the articular mobility of the cranial bones, mobility of the intracranial and intra-spinal membranes, fluctuation of the cerebral spinal fluid, and involuntary mobility of the sacrum between the ilium (Bordoni and Zanier 2015).

The technique became the basis for skull palpation based on the idea that the craniosacral system includes neurocranial and viscerocranial sutures, cerebrospinal fluid, and the fascia of the brain and spinal cord, intricately connected to the musculoskeletal and nervous systems. Fascia restrictions are thought to lead to abnormal movement of the cerebrospinal fluid, which has been measured by palpation, and by modern tools such as magnetic resonance imaging, and myelogram. It has been shown that restricted connective tissue can have increased pain receptors, and demonstrate fibrosis and increased inflammation related to stiffness, muscle tension, and pain (Haller et al. 2015).

Mechanism of Action

In simplified terms, the technique involves gentle manual palpation techniques to release fascial restrictions between the cranium and the sacrum to reduce pain. An important component of craniosacral treatment is called the primary respiration, which is reflected in the motion of the cranial bones, sacrum, dural membranes, central nervous system, and cerebrospinal fluid. The primary respiratory mechanism is described as a two-phase rhythmic impulse, and the goal of the craniosacral practitioner is to treat the patient through manipulation of this primary respiratory mechanism (Jakel and von Hauenschild 2011, 2012).

In one of few longitudinal randomized controlled trials in this area, 54 adult patients with chronic neck pain showed significant improvement in pain intensity with craniosacral treatment (weekly 45-minute treatment for 8 weeks) versus sham treatment. Improvements in functional disability and in overall quality of life were also seen in the treatment group. Results were maintained up to 3 months post intervention. No serious adverse events were reported (Haller et al. 2015).

Pediatric Evidence

A 2011 literature review of adult and pediatric patients found significant study variability and insufficient data to draw definitive conclusions about the safety or efficacy of craniosacral treatment, especially in children. More research is needed (Jakel and von Hauenschild 2011).

Cautions and Possible Side Effects

At present, there is very limited research available on craniosacral therapy, particularly in children. Appropriate caution is indicated in any patient with history of head or neck injury and in the very young.

Training and Licensing Required for Providers

The Craniosacral Therapy Association of North America is a non-profit organization founded in the late 1990s to help bring organization and more standardized training to the field with the goal of establishing a curriculum of study, a system of teacher approval, and develop a registry of teachers. Before practicing craniosacral therapy, practitioners typically acquire approximately 700 hours of training in craniosacral therapy school. At present there is no regulation of craniosacral therapy training in the U.S. Internationally the field is at a similar state of development (Jakel and von Hauenschild 2012).

Therapeutic Massage

Background Information

The history of massage shows its long use as a healing modality based on ancient Chinese medical texts and in India within the Ayurvedic tradition. Massage has also been recorded in Egypt and Japan around 2500 BC as part of the range of therapies including acupuncture, acupressure, amno and tui na. In Greece, massage was historically recorded as being used by athletes in conjunction with essential oils. Hippocrates also included massage in his writings (Sherman et al. 2005).

A systematic review of massage research in Europe, America, Australia, Singapore, and South Korea suggests that massage therapy is a common complementary healing therapy in modern medicine (Harris et al. 2014).

Massage is a broad term that encompasses a variety of techniques that involve deliberate stroking and stretching of the muscles and connective tissue with the use of moderate hand pressure to release tension and pain. Stimulation of pressure receptors that activate the vagus nerve trigger the relaxation response which is accompanied by enhancement of blood flow and stimulation of lymph drainage in the targeted area (Field 2014).

Massage has been widely studied in both children and adults and has been shown to be effective in the management of acute and chronic pain, anxiety, depression, and overall quality of life (Post-White et al. 2003; Field 2014).

A variety of massage styles and techniques exist, including trigger point therapy that is focused on a tight area or knot within muscle tissue associated with referred pain patterns. Trigger point therapy uses cycles of isolated pressure and release in order to loosen the muscle and reduce pain. Another common approach is known as Swedish massage. This technique starts with light pressure and builds to medium pressure, especially in areas of specific pain and discomfort. Similar to Swedish massage is the deep tissue massage, which addresses deep tissues of the body to treat pain and tension. Sports massage is yet another technique designed for athletes that may focus on a specific painful area associated with overuse or injury (Post-White et al. 2003).

Specially tailored massage techniques have been shown to be effective and well tolerated in the prenatal population (Field et al. 2012), in preterm infants (Beachy 2003), in the geriatric population (Borsheski and Johnson 2014), as well as for in those in critical care settings (Vahedian-Azimi et al. 2014).

Mechanism of Action

A 2014 review by Field presents a range of studies that link massage to stimulation of the vagus nerve with resulting triggering of the relaxation response associated with decreased heart rate, blood pressure, and respiratory rate. Studies on infant massage have also been shown to increase gastric motility and increase insulin and insulin growth factor-1. Decrease in cortisol and substance-P has been reported, as has increase in natural killer cells associated with enhanced immune function. Functional MRI has shown that massage can increase cerebral blood flow to areas of the brain associated with stress, fear, and depression (Field 2014).

Pediatric Evidence

While a 2013 Cochrane Systematic Database Review of 34 studies on the use of healthy infants under 6 months found high heterogenicity and generally low quality of study design (Bennett, Underdown, and Barlow 2013), a more recent study has shown benefit in term infants including more rapid weight gain, improvement in sleep times, and reduced irritability (Field 2014).

The beneficial use of massage in certain higher risk pediatric populations continues to accrue. Some of the most compelling studies demonstrate its effectiveness in the neonatal intensive care unit in reduction of heart rate variability, reduction in cortisol, and increase in oxygen saturation and body temperature in preterm infants (Field, Diego, and Hernandez-Reif 2010).

Of note, studies on the use of massage in pregnant women who are depressed have shown a decrease in the prevalence of premature birth and an improvement in birth weight (Field et al. 2009).

Pediatric oncology patients are another special group that may benefit from massage. For example, four weekly massage sessions as compared to four quiet-time control sessions was correlated with reduced heart rate and decreased anxiety in a pilot study of 17 children with cancer. No significant adverse events were reported (Post-White et al. 2009).

A survey in 129 pediatric oncology patients in academic centers in Canada showed that nearly one in two used massage in conjunction with their conventional therapy (Valji et al. 2013). Massage was also used in approximately one third of pediatric oncology patients in a survey of 169 families in Scotland (Revuelta-Iniesta et al. 2014).

A survey of 110 juvenile onset fibromyalgia patients showed that 10% used massage in their treatment with greater than 90% of these patients finding it useful (Verkamp et al. 2013).

A review of studies examining complementary and alternative medicine in pediatric rheumatology patients with a variety of diagnoses such as juvenile onset arthritis, systemic lupus erythematosus, scleroderma and others found that 64% used some type of complementary medicine for pain and overall wellbeing. Massage was consistently among the most frequently used therapies reported in this survey (April and Walji 2011).

Asthmatic children have also been shown to experience benefit from massage in the form of improvement in forced expiratory flow in the first second (FEV1) in a controlled study of 60 children. Treatment group received a 20-minute massage by parents at bedtime every night for 5 weeks in addition to regular treatment suggesting benefit ($p = 0.04$). FEV1/FVC (forced vital capacity) was significantly improved $p < 0.01$. Again, no adverse events were reported (Fattah and Hamdy 2011).

Some infant massage studies also demonstrate benefit to the caregiver. For example, a randomized controlled trial of 17 infant–mother pairs with HIV positive mothers and nine control group participants reported that mothers in the treatment group had increased confidence in reading infant cues, reduction in depression, reduction in parental distress, and improved infant linear growth and weight gain (Oswalt and Biasini 2011).

Cautions and Possible Side Effects

Data on serious adverse events from the use of massage in children is scarce. Potential side effects could include soreness, transient decreases in blood pressure, bruising, and even fracture in rare cases involving cancer, osteogenesis imperfecta, or severe osteoporosis.

Training and Licensing Required for Providers

In the U.S. a national certification credential was created in the 1990s to help standardize education and testing procedures and to provide the basis for a minimum practice requirement. Broadly, there are three types of credential available to massage therapists: a certificate from a specific training school; membership in the national American Massage Therapy Association which requires a minimum of 500 hours of education; and national certification which requires a minimum 750 hours of education at an accredited school, 250 hours of hands-on experience, background check, and cardiopulmonary resuscitation training. The U.S. national certifying body is the

National Certification Board for Therapeutic Massage and Bodywork (NCBTMB), established in 1992.

Licensing for massage therapists, which differs from credentialing, varies state to state. A licensed massage therapist (LMT) credential reflects that an individual has acquired the minimum number of training hours and has passed a competency exam such as the National Certification Exam. Most, but not all, states in the U.S. regulate massage training and require a minimum number of training hours, successful exam result, and ongoing continuing medical education. Updated information may be found through the American Massage Therapy Association (AMTA).

Pediatric massage training in the U.S. is highly variable; for example, one credential as a Certified Pediatric Massage Therapist is available after attendance of a 2-day training course that is open to healthcare professionals, professional massage therapists, parents, and caregivers. Given the high variability in training, due diligence in training, credentialing, and experience with a variety of pediatric conditions are indicated for all practitioners of pediatric massage therapy which appears to be a promising therapy for reduction of pediatric pain and stress.

Chiropractic

(Pettman 2007; Hestbaek and Stochkendahl 2010)

Background Information

Despite a lack of compelling evidence supporting its use in children, it is important for clinicians caring for children to be well informed about chiropractic due to the prevalence of its use in children and adolescents. Results from the National Health Interview Survey, 2007–2012, show that use of chiropractic or osteopathic manipulation remained the second most commonly used type of complementary medicine after natural products, representing an estimated 3.3% (more than 2 million children). This aligns with the conditions identified as the most common reasons for the use of complementary therapies including back or neck pain at 8.9%, and other musculoskeletal at 6% of those surveyed (Black et al. 2015).

Daniel David Palmer is credited with the development of the field of chiropractic, derived from the Greek *cheiros* (hand) and *praktos* (done by). He reportedly began as a "natural healer," and in 1897 opened his first college, The Palmer College of Cure, now in operation as the Palmer College of Chiropractic in Davenport, Iowa. Use of x-rays was introduced into chiropractic practice by Palmer's son Bartlett Joshua Palmer, "B.J.," in 1910. Introduction of the neurocalometer, a device to locate out of position vertebrae, rolled out in the early 1920s, a source of great controversy in the field at the time (Moore 1995).

Currently, the most commonly used chiropractic treatment is known as adjustment or spinal manipulation, especially related to cervical spinal manipulation. This typically consists of controlled manually applied force and torque with the goal of restoring joint mobility and alignment. This technique is often referred to as high-velocity low-amplitude (HVLA) thrust and usually characterized as the Diversified technique (Huggins et al. 2012).

Chiropractic practitioners may also employ the use of an Activator Adjusting Instrument, a tool estimated to be used by 51.2% of American Chiropractors in a 2005

National Board of Chiropractic Examiner's Job Analysis survey. (National Board of Chiropractic Examiners. Job Analysis of Chiropractic: a project report, survey analysis and summary of the practice of chiropractic within the United States. Greeley, Colorado, U.S.A.: National Board of Chiropractic Examiners; 2005.)

Despite the tool's high use in the chiropractic community, no high-quality randomized controlled trials to support the efficacy or safety of the Activator Adjusting Instrument were found in a review of the chiropractic literature by Huggins (Huggins et al. 2012).

Current controversies within the chiropractic field include scope of practice, especially expansion with specialized training to include prescribing medications, desire to serve as primary care providers, and anti-vaccination stance.

A survey of 1247 North American chiropractic students found that 52% agreed that chiropractors should be trained in evidence-based practice, and a majority agreed that the emphasis of chiropractic practice is to address vertebral subluxation. More than half of respondents (55%) did not support expansion of scope of practice to include prescribing medications after appropriate advanced training. More than two thirds (69%) believed that chiropractors should be considered mainstream health practitioners (Gliedt et al. 2015).

Chiropractic is widely used in children and adolescents in Europe. A survey of 956 chiropractors found that approximately 8% of patients seen were children. Conditions treated included skeletal (57%), neurologic (24%), gastrointestinal (12%), infectious (3.5%), genitourinary (1.5%), immune (1.4%), and other miscellaneous conditions. An aggregate of 557 adverse events were reported, including 534 mild, 23 moderate, and no severe events (Marchand 2012).

Mechanism of Action

In a chiropractic adjustment the practitioners typically apply pressure to the joints in a particular direction so that the joints can stretch and separate and their position can be restored. At times, due to the pressure, the patient may experience a popping sound ("cavitation") thought possibly related to the shifting liquids in the spinal vertebrae. The ultimate goal of the chiropractic therapy is purportedly to ease pain. The therapy is also thought to reduce the pressure on the spinal disc, although this is not reliably supported by current evidence (Erwin and Hood 2014).

Pediatric Evidence

Despite its prevalence of use, a paucity of research is available on the safety and efficacy of chiropractic in children (Hestbaek and Stochkendahl 2010; Alcantara, Ohm, and Kunz 2009) including its use in otitis media (Pohlman and Holton-Brown 2012), and in colic, asthma, enuresis, musculoskeletal pain, or autism (Gleberzon et al. 2012).

A survey of 135 doctors of chiropractic with a pediatric diplomate indicated that 24% of pediatric patients seen were less than 5 years old, and 15% were between 5 and 18 years. A majority of patients had parents or caretakers under chiropractic care.

The most common technique was "Diversified," used by 59%. This is described as a full spine technique that employs high-velocity low-amplitude force. The Activator, a mechanically assisted treatment device, was used by 63% of respondents. Additional techniques used by respondents included myofascial work, muscle testing (applied kinesiology), infant toggle (upper cervical technique), "Bio-Geometric Integration" (includes a geometric model of the body, biodynamics, force dynamics), and neuro-emotional techniques. Health promotion included breastfeeding recommendations and disease prevention, and screening advice. Nutrition and dietary counseling, physical fitness and exercise recommendation, stress reduction, and self-care advice were also offered. Trigger point therapy, electrical stimulation therapy, foot orthotics, homeo-pathic remedies, massage, laser light therapy, allergy testing, brain balance therapy, and neuromuscular re-education were also mentioned as techniques in use (Pohlman et al. 2010).

Cautions and Possible Side Effects

One of the most challenging aspects in evaluating the safety and efficacy of chiropractic treatment is the heterogenicity and quality of published studies. A confounding factor is the lack of a uniform approach to description and reporting of adverse events (Todd et al. 2014).

The adverse events of highest concern in chiropractic treatment are associated with the rotational component of high-velocity low-amplitude cervical spine adjustment, and accompanying risk of cerebrovascular accident. Risk of diagnostic error or inad-equate patient assessment are important concerns in pediatric care, as are damage due to immature development of the spine, and possible dislocation of the first cervical vertebrae. A 2007 comprehensive systematic review of the literature on adverse events in pediatric chiropractic identified 13 reports of harm, nine were considered serious, one moderate, and one minor. Several of these cases had underlying pathology, includ-ing spinal cord astrocytoma, osteogenesis imperfecta, and congenital occipitalization (Vohra et al. 2007).

A study of 90 chiropractors in Boston by Lee and Kemper found that 17% would treat a hypothetical neonate with a fever themselves rather than immediately refer to an MD, DO, or an emergency facility, a practice at odds with recommended pediatric guidelines (Lee, Li, and Kemper 2000).

A clear need continues for prospective population-based studies to accurately iden-tify the incidence of serious adverse events related to chiropractic practice in pediatrics (Humphreys 2010).

Barriers to development of a reporting and learning system to monitor and report adverse events have been identified as time pressure, patient-related concerns, and fear of blame (Pohlman et al. 2015).

Training and Licensing Required for Providers

Training

In 2105 there were 19 accredited North American chiropractic colleges offering a 4–5-year Doctor of Chiropractic degree. The curriculum generally includes 2 years' education on basic science and then 2–3 years of chiropractic-specific education with a mixture of class work, laboratory, and clinical experience. A clinical internship is a more recent addition to training. Trainees must pass three national board exams prior to completion of their 4-year degree. Each accredited school offers at least one pedi-atric course. Some questions on pediatrics are included on the national chiropractic board exam. Opportunities exist to pursue a clinical specialty, known as a diplomate certification, in topics including: clinical neurology, sports chiropractic, nutrition, orthopedics, radiology, rehabilitation, and pediatrics. Specialization is offered either through part-time post-graduate continuing medical education courses or in residency training. The pediatric post-graduate diplomate program was established in 1993 and consists of 180–360 hours of weekend courses over a 2–3-year period (Pohlman et al. 2010).

In the U.S., accreditation of chiropractic colleges is offered through the Council on Chiropractic Education through the Department of Health and Human Services in the Department of Health, Education, and Welfare. Prerequisite training for admission to chiropractic college has historically included 2 years of undergraduate study with an emphasis on basic science, although some programs may require completion of an undergraduate degree. There is no residency requirement after graduation.

A cross-sectional survey of 135 chiropractors found that approximately 31% of patients seen were younger than 18 years. The health conditions in children treated by chiropractors in this survey included back or neck pain, asthma, birth trauma, colic, constipation, ear infection, and upper respiratory infection (Pohlman et al. 2010).

Licensing

License to practice chiropractic is offered on a by-state level in the U.S. Licensure laws exist in all 50 U.S. states, and all states require a passing score on the National Board of Chiropractic Examiners. Scope of practice can vary by state, with some limiting practice to the neuromusculoskeletal system, and others allowing assessment of conditions beyond the musculoskeletal system and recommendation of vitamins.

References

Alcantara, J., J. Ohm, and D. Kunz. 2009. "The safety and effectiveness of pediatric chiropractic: a survey of chiropractors and parents in a practice-based research network." *Explore (NY)* 5(5): 290–5. doi: 10.1016/j.explore.2009.06.002.

April, K. T., and R. Walji. 2011. "The state of research on complementary and alternative medicine in pediatric rheumatology." *Rheum Dis Clin North Am* 37(1): 85–94. doi: 10.1016/j.rdc.2010.11.011.

Beachy, J. M. 2003. "Premature infant massage in the NICU." *Neonatal Netw* 22(3): 39–45. doi: 10.1891/0730-0832.22.3.39.

Bennett, C., A. Underdown, and J. Barlow. 2013. "Massage for promoting mental and physical health in typically developing infants under the age of six months." *Cochrane Database Syst Rev* 4: CD005038. doi: 10.1002/14651858.CD005038.pub3.

Black, L. I., T. C. Clarke, P. M. Barnes, B. J. Stussman, and R. L. Nahin. 2015. "Use of complementary health approaches among children aged 4–17 years in the United States: National Health Interview Survey, 2007–2012." *Natl Health Stat Report* 78: 1–19.

Bordoni, B., and E. Zanier. 2015. "Sutherland's legacy in the new millennium: the osteopathic cranial model and modern osteopathy." *Adv Mind Body Med* 29(2): 15–21.

Borsheski, R., and Q. L. Johnson. 2014. "Pain management in the geriatric population." *Mo Med* 111(6): 508–11.

Dobson, D., P. L. Lucassen, J. J. Miller, A. M. Vlieger, P. Prescott, and G. Lewith. 2012. "Manipulative therapies for infantile colic." *Cochrane Database Syst Rev* 12: CD004796. doi: 10.1002/14651858.CD004796.pub2.

Erwin, W. M., and K. E. Hood. 2014. "The cellular and molecular biology of the intervertebral disc: a clinician's primer." *J Can Chiropr Assoc* 58(3): 246–57.

Fattah, M. A., and B. Hamdy. 2011. "Pulmonary functions of children with asthma improve following massage therapy." *J Altern Complement Med* 17(11): 1065–8. doi: 10.1089/acm.2010.0758.

Field, T. 2014. "Massage therapy research review." *Complement Ther Clin Pract* 20(4): 224–9. doi: 10.1016/j.ctcp.2014.07.002.

Field, T., M. Diego, and M. Hernandez-Reif. 2010. "Preterm infant massage therapy research: a review." *Infant Behav Dev* 33(2): 115–24. doi: 10.1016/j.infbeh.2009.12.004.

Field, T., M. Diego, M. Hernandez-Reif, O. Deeds, and B. Figueiredo. 2009. "Pregnancy massage reduces prematurity, low birthweight and postpartum depression." *Infant Behav Dev* 32(4): 454–60. doi: 10.1016/j.infbeh.2009.07.001.

Field, T., M. Diego, M. Hernandez-Reif, L. Medina, J. Delgado, and A. Hernandez. 2012. "Yoga and massage therapy reduce prenatal depression and prematurity." *J Bodyw Mov Ther* 16(2): 204–9. doi: 10.1016/j.jbmt.2011.08.002.

Flexner A. 1910. *Medical Education in the United States and Canada. A Report to the Carnegie Foundation for the Advancement of Teaching.* Edited by D. B. Updike. Boston, Mass: The Merrymount Press.

Gevitz, N. 2009. "The transformation of osteopathic medical education." *Acad Med* 84(6): 701–6. doi: 10.1097/ACM.0b013e3181a4049e.

Gleberzon, B. J., J. Arts, A. Mei, and E. L. McManus. 2012. "The use of spinal manipulative therapy for pediatric health conditions: a systematic review of the literature." *J Can Chiropr Assoc* 56(2): 128–41.

Gliedt, J. A., C. Hawk, M. Anderson, K. Ahmad, D. Bunn, J. Cambron, B. Gleberzon, J. Hart, A. Kizhakkeveettil, S. M. Perle, M. Ramcharan, S. Sullivan, and L. Zhang. 2015. "Chiropractic identity, role and future: a survey of North American chiropractic students." *Chiropr Man Therap* 23(1): 4. doi: 10.1186/s12998-014-0048-1.

Haller, H., R. Lauche, H. Cramer, T. Rampp, F. J. Saha, T. Ostermann, and G. Dobos. 2015. "Craniosacral therapy for the treatment of chronic neck pain: a randomized sham-controlled trial." *Clin J Pain*. doi: 10.1097/AJP.0000000000000290.

Harris, P. E., K. L. Cooper, C. Relton, and K. J. Thomas. 2014. "Prevalence of visits to massage therapists by the general population: a systematic review." *Complement Ther Clin Pract* 20(1): 16–20. doi: 10.1016/j.ctcp.2013.11.001.

Hestbaek, L., and M. J. Stochkendahl. 2010. "The evidence base for chiropractic treatment of musculoskeletal conditions in children and adolescents: the emperor's new suit?" *Chiropr Osteopat* 18: 15. doi: 10.1186/1746-1340-18-15.

Huggins, T., A. L. Boras, B. J. Gleberzon, M. Popescu, and L. A. Bahry. 2012. "Clinical effectiveness of the activator adjusting instrument in the management of musculoskeletal disorders: a systematic review of the literature." *J Can Chiropr Assoc* 56(1): 49–57.

Humphreys, B. K. 2010. "Possible adverse events in children treated by manual therapy: a review." *Chiropr Osteopat* 18: 12. doi: 10.1186/1746-1340-18-12.

Jakel, A., and P. von Hauenschild. 2011. "Therapeutic effects of cranial osteopathic manipulative medicine: a systematic review." *J Am Osteopath Assoc* 111(12): 685–93.

Jakel, A., and P. von Hauenschild. 2012. "A systematic review to evaluate the clinical benefits of craniosacral therapy." *Complement Ther Med* 20(6): 456–65. doi: 10.1016/j.ctim.2012.07.009.

Lee, A. C., D. H. Li, and K. J. Kemper. 2000. "Chiropractic care for children." *Arch Pediatr Adolesc Med* 154(4): 401–7.

Marchand, A. M. 2012. "Chiropractic care of children from birth to adolescence and classification of reported conditions: an internet cross-sectional survey of 956 European chiropractors." *J Manipulative Physiol Ther* 35(5): 372–80. doi: 10.1016/j.jmpt.2012.04.008.

Moore, J. S. 1995. "The neurocalometer: watershed in the evolution of a new profession." *Chiropr Hist* 15(2): 51–4.

Oswalt, K., and F. Biasini. 2011. "Effects of infant massage on HIV-infected mothers and their infants." *J Spec Pediatr Nurs* 16(3): 169–78. doi: 10.1111/j.1744-6155.2011.00291.x.

Parker, J. D. 2014. "Reversing the paradox: evidence-based medicine and osteopathic medicine." *J Am Osteopath Assoc* 114(11): 826–7. doi: 10.7556/jaoa.2014.166.

Pettman, E. 2007. "A history of manipulative therapy." *J Man Manip Ther* 15(3): 165–74.

Pohlman, K. A., L. Carroll, L. Hartling, R. T. Tsuyuki, and S. Vohra. 2015. "Barriers to implementing a reporting and learning patient safety system: pediatric chiropractic perspective." *J Evid Based Complementary Altern Med.* doi: 10.1177/2156587215609191.

Pohlman, K. A., and M. S. Holton-Brown. 2012. "Otitis media and spinal manipulative therapy: a literature review." *J Chiropr Med* 11(3): 160–9. doi: 10.1016/j.jcm.2012.05.006.

Pohlman, K. A., M. A. Hondras, C. R. Long, and A. G. Haan. 2010. "Practice patterns of doctors of chiropractic with a pediatric diplomate: a cross-sectional survey." *BMC Complement Altern Med* 10: 26. doi: 10.1186/1472-6882-10-26.

Posadzki, P., M. S. Lee, and E. Ernst. 2013. "Osteopathic manipulative treatment for pediatric conditions: a systematic review." *Pediatrics* 132(1): 140–52. doi: 10.1542/peds.2012-3959.

Post-White, J., M. Fitzgerald, K. Savik, M. C. Hooke, A. B. Hannahan, and S. F. Sencer. 2009. "Massage therapy for children with cancer." *J Pediatr Oncol Nurs* 26(1): 16–28. doi: 10.1177/1043454208323295.

Post-White, J., M. E. Kinney, K. Savik, J. B. Gau, C. Wilcox, and I. Lerner. 2003. "Therapeutic massage and healing touch improve symptoms in cancer." *Integr Cancer Ther* 2(4): 332–44. doi: 10.1177/1534735403259064.

Revuelta-Iniesta, R., M. L. Wilson, K. White, L. Stewart, J. M. McKenzie, and D. C. Wilson. 2014. "Complementary and alternative medicine usage in Scottish children and adolescents during cancer treatment." *Complement Ther Clin Pract* 20(4): 197–202. doi: 10.1016/j.ctcp.2014.05.003.

Sherman, K. J., D. C. Cherkin, J. Kahn, J. Erro, A. Hrbek, R. A. Deyo, and D. M. Eisenberg. 2005. "A survey of training and practice patterns of massage therapists in two US states." *BMC Complement Altern Med* 5: 13. doi: 10.1186/1472-6882-5-13.

Todd, A. J., M. T. Carroll, A. Robinson, and E. K. Mitchell. 2014. "Adverse events due to chiropractic and other manual therapies for infants and children: a review of the literature." *J Manipulative Physiol Ther.* doi: 10.1016/j.jmpt.2014.09.008.

Vahedian-Azimi, A., A. Ebadi, M. Asghari Jafarabadi, S. Saadat, and F. Ahmadi. 2014. "Effect of massage therapy on vital signs and GCS scores of ICU patients: a randomized controlled clinical trial." *Trauma Mon* 19(3): e17031. doi: 10.5812/traumamon.17031.

Valji, R., D. Adams, S. Dagenais, T. Clifford, L. Baydala, W. J. King, and S. Vohra. 2013. "Complementary and alternative medicine: a survey of its use in pediatric oncology." *Evid Based Complement Alternat Med* 2013: 527163. doi: 10.1155/2013/527163.

Verkamp, E. K., S. R. Flowers, A. M. Lynch-Jordan, J. Taylor, T. V. Ting, and S. Kashikar-Zuck. 2013. "A survey of conventional and complementary therapies used by youth with juvenile-onset fibromyalgia." *Pain Manag Nurs* 14(4): e244–50. doi: 10.1016/j.pmn.2012.02.002.

Vohra, S., B. C. Johnston, K. Cramer, and K. Humphreys. 2007. "Adverse events associated with pediatric spinal manipulation: a systematic review." *Pediatrics* 119(1): e275–83. doi: 10.1542/peds.2006-1392.

11 Aromatherapy

Aromatherapy is the therapeutic use of volatile plant oils to address physical and psychological disorders. Volatile plant oils, also known as essential oils, are extracted from aromatic plants by steam distillation or mechanical pressing, processes which do not, by definition, involve the use of chemical solvents. The volatile oils consist of a range of chemical groups such as esters, terpenes, phenols, and aldehydes, which produce their characteristic odors and therapeutic properties. One of the challenges in their use is the high variability of composition, even of the same plants from different geographical locations. Although use of essential oils is recorded throughout history, by report the actual term was not coined until a French chemist, Rene Gattefosse, proposed the use of essential oils as "aromatherapy" in a book published in 1937 (PDQ 2002).

The field was furthered by a French physician, Jean Valnet, who published *The Practice of Aromatherapy* in 1990, thereby introducing the field to a broader audience of healthcare practitioners (Valnet 1990).

Aromatherapy is now widely used in the U.S., Canada, U.K., and Europe. One survey study by Adams et al. on a total of 926 children at two children's hospitals in Canada found aromatherapy was used by 16.1% of children, most often in conjunction with conventional care (Adams et al. 2013).

In a subset of the above-mentioned Canadian study, of the 202 patients seen in the respiratory clinics of either hospital, 37.1% indicated current use of aromatherapy (Richmond et al. 2014).

The U.S. Food and Drug Administration classifies most essential oils as generally recognized as safe (GRAS) when used at normally recognized concentration levels. Essential oils are highly concentrated and are therefore always diluted for dermal use. They may be diluted in water, oils, ointments, or creams. Typical dilution strengths include a 2% dilution for massage oils or lotions (10 drops essential oil to 1 ounce of carrier oil), a 1% solution is suggested for children or people with skin sensitivity (5 drops essential oil to 1 ounce of carrier oil or lotion), or a 0.5% dilution for use on the face or with high skin sensitivity (2–3 drops to 1 ounce of carrier oil or lotion).

Nonmedical use of essential oils, for example peppermint oil, is common in the food and perfume industries. Although essential oils are used orally in certain European countries including France and Germany, where they are recognized as medical aromatherapy, discussion here will be limited to external use, which is more typical in the U.S. and U.K.

Overview

Interest in the use of aromatherapy in healthcare is supported by emerging studies using functional MRI that correlate the aroma with specific stimulation in the brain, particularly of the ventral striatum, also referred to as the limbic striatum, which has been associated with positive emotions, memories, and reward (Villemure, Laferriere, and Bushnell 2012).

Olfaction has also been shown to influence neural reorganization in studies on neuroplasticity and loss of sense of smell (Kollndorfer et al. 2014). Despite some intriguing studies, many questions remain about aromatherapy's specific mechanisms of action.

Some of the most common documented uses of aromatherapy are for stress relief and anxiety (Cooke and Ernst 2000), although clinical studies on the use of aromatherapy run the gamut of conditions and show high study variability, making definitive recommendations difficult (Wilcock et al. 2004).

In external use, essential oils can be used in direct and indirect inhalation, or as part of an oil or cream. An example of direct inhalation would be the use of drops of oil placed into hot water or a bath, allowing the aerosolized vapors to be inhaled by the individual. Indirect aromatherapy is seen when essential oils are used in a room diffuser or when drops of essential oil are placed on a tissue or pillow. Aromatherapy massage is a third common approach where the essential oil is diluted into a neutral carrier cream or oil. In addition to their use in aromatherapy, essential oils have been widely used topically for their antimicrobial, antiviral, and antifungal effects (Aridogan et al. 2002).

A benefit of aromatherapy is the ability to tailor individual treatments, yet the high variability inherent in this approach has also resulted in a lack of consistency in research and evaluation of the individual essential oils.

Possible risks include dermatitis due to allergy in some patients. Phototoxicity is a second risk, sometimes seen with citrus oils in particular. In some patients, certain odors might trigger an unpleasant or traumatic memory. There has been a report of repeated exposure to lavender and tea tree oil causing reversible gynecomastia in three prepubertal boys due to the estrogenic and antiandrogenic properties of these essential oils (Henley et al. 2007). However, this theory has been challenged in the medical literature and more study is needed (Carson, Tisserand, and Larkman 2014).

Essential Oils Overview

Lavender

Background

Lavender oil from the flowers of *Lavandula angustifolia* contains primarily linalyl acetate and linalool, as determined by gas chromatography and mass spectrometry, and these are considered the most active components (Carrasco et al. 2015). Lavender or *Lavare* (Latin meaning to wash) has a history dating back thousands of years and was used by Egyptians and Romans for mummification processes, and for bathing and perfuming. Lavender has been shown to have antimicrobial activity against many bacteria, including pseudomonas (Vegh et al. 2012).

Lavender is primarily known for its anxiolytic properties and usefulness in reducing procedural pain in a variety of settings, although variable study design and size preclude definitive recommendations in both children and adults (Kim et al. 2011).

Pediatric Evidence

Inhalation of lavender essential oil was found to reduce amount of pain medication needed in a randomized controlled study of 48 post-tonsillectomy patients ages 6–12 years in a 3-day post-operative observation period (Soltani et al. 2013).

There is some evidence to suggest benefit of inhaled lavender in aiding sleep in children (Lillehei and Halcon 2014).

And a small randomized study showed benefit of lavender aromatherapy massage in 40 full-term infants with colic. Infants in the treatment group received abdominal massage from their mothers using lavender essential oil. Crying time was reduced in the treatment group (Cetinkaya and Basbakkal 2012).

Lavender essential oil in the infant bath was also found to reduce stress and saliva cortisol levels in mothers, and to decrease crying time and improve sleep in a small study of 30 infant–mother pairs (Field et al. 2008).

Lavender aromatherapy has also been used in a variety of hospice and palliative care settings in children and adults with mixed results, possibly due to methodological issues.

Possible Side Effects and Cautions

Lavender oil is used for children through topical use or diffusion only; for example, in a room diffuser or in drops of essential oil in a bathtub or in a cream or oil. It is not advised for prepubertal children to use lavender oil topically because of remaining questions about links to gynecomastia (Diaz et al. 2015).

Drops are concentrated and should be kept away from children and avoided in those known to be allergic to lavender. It is sun-sensitive oil and may predispose to sunburn if used topically.

Tea Tree Oil

Background

Tea tree oil is obtained from the leaves of *Melaleuca alternifolia*, a tree indigenous to Australia. It has a long history of use for treating wounds, cuts, and burns. Early use included crushing and soaking of the leaves to make poultices and steaming leaves for use in treating coughs and sore throats. Tea tree oil was developed in the 1920s and 1930s, when awareness of its antibacterial properties became recognized (Carson, Hammer, and Riley 2006).

Tea tree oil has been extensively studied and is widely used as a topical agent for its anti-inflammatory, antifungal, antibacterial, antiprotozoal, and antiviral properties. A variety of in vitro and in vivo studies show benefit in treatment of a range of illnesses from foot fungus to methicillin-resistant *Staphylococcus aureus* (Terzi et al. 2007; Caelli et al. 2000; Hammer, Carson, and Riley 1998). It has also been shown to be an effective treatment for head lice in children (Di Campli et al. 2012).

A 2015 Cochrane Database Systematic Review found some supportive research for its use in mild-to-moderate acne (Cao et al. 2015), although symptoms of pruritus, burning, redness, and excessive dryness have been reported with its use (Bagherani and Smoller 2015).

A wide variety of commercial products are available over the counter in multiple countries around the world. No standardized recommendations exist for the use of tea tree oil in children.

Possible Side Effects and Cautions

Studies from Australia where tea tree oil is commonly used show a higher prevalence of reported allergic reactions as compared to other essential oils (de Groot and Schmidt 2015). As with any essential oil, aspiration is a risk in young children and can lead to serious consequences due of the presence of aromatic hydrocarbons and other volatile compounds (Richards, Wang, and Buchanan 2015; Morris et al. 2003).

Bergamot

Background (Navarra et al. 2015)

Citrus bergamia Risso, known as bergamot, is a hybrid of bitter orange and lemon. It is endemic to the Calabria region of Italy. The oil of Bergamot is produced from the peel of the citrus fruit bergamot. Its primary commercial use is as an essential oil in the fragrance industry, although the bitter juice has been shown to have anti-inflammatory, anti-cancer, and hypo-lipid and hypoglycemic properties. Primary components of bergamot include limonene (25%–53%), linalool (2%–20%), linalyly acetate (15%–40%), and other volatile and non-volatile compounds. Phototoxicity is a common concern unless the essential oil is free of furocoumarins. Bergamot essential oil is used in many perfumes, as well as in the pharmaceutical and food industries for its distinctive aroma and flavor; for example, bergamot is what lends the distinctive flavor to Earl Grey tea. Historical use includes use in wound care due to its antimicrobial properties (Navarra et al. 2015).

When used in aromatherapy it has been shown in several small studies to improve mood, depression, and anxiety, at times in conjunction with lavender or other essential oils (Navarra et al. 2015).

Possible Side Effects and Cautions

Phototoxicity, as mentioned previously. It has also been reported in one case that over-consumption of bergamot-flavored tea led to blurred vision, twitches, cramps, and abnormal sensations when consumed in high doses (Finsterer 2002).

Peppermint

Background (Herro and Jacob 2010, Dagli et al. 2015)

Peppermint *(Mentha piperita)* is covered in detail in Chapter 9, Botanicals. It is one of the most widely used botanicals in aromatherapy, flavoring, fragrance, pharmaceuticals, and foods (Charrois et al. 2006).

Peppermint has been shown to have antibacterial and antifungal properties. When used in aromatherapy, peppermint has historically been used to target headache and upper respiratory congestion; for example, as used in menthol chest rubs (Dagli et al. 2015). Peppermint has also been studied in aromatherapy for post-operative nausea and vomiting, although results have been inconclusive in randomized controlled studies (Hines et al. 2012).

Possible Side Effects and Cautions

Peppermint can cause skin irritation in sensitive individuals; it can also cause heartburn and perianal burning when taken internally. It should also not be used internally or near children's faces because it may induce tongue spasms, bronchospasm, and respiratory arrest (Kligler and Chaudhary 2007).

Training and Licensing

Historically, training and certification in aromatherapy was only available for lay practitioners, resulting in a lack of professional standardization of training for medical professionals and absence of a licensing process in the U.S. or U.K. This lack of standardized training resulted in a wide variety of individual approaches and a lack of consistency in research. The National Association for Holistic Aromatherapy (www.naha.org) and the Alliance of International Aromatherapists (www.alliance-aromatherapists.org) are moving to standardize aromatherapy certification in the U.S. In addition, the Aromatherapy Registration Council, an independent non-profit organization, founded in 1997, offers voluntary exams to establish and test a core base of knowledge, earn a certificate of recognition, and become a registered aromatherapist. Recertification through the Aromatherapy Registration Council is required every 5 years. The Canadian Federation of Aromatherapists also has standards for certification. (www.cfacanada.com). An international resource is the International Federation of Aromatherapists (www.ifaroma.org)

Summary

Aromatherapy when individualized and used appropriately in children can provide a safe, complementary approach to a number of conditions, including stress and pain.

References

Adams, D., S. Dagenais, T. Clifford, L. Baydala, W. J. King, M. Hervas-Malo, D. Moher, and S. Vohra. 2013. "Complementary and alternative medicine use by pediatric specialty outpatients." *Pediatrics* 131(2): 225–32. doi: 10.1542/peds.2012-1220.

Aridogan, B. C., H. Baydar, S. Kaya, M. Demirci, D. Ozbasar, and E. Mumcu. 2002. "Antimicrobial activity and chemical composition of some essential oils." *Arch Pharm Res* 25(6): 860–4.

Bagherani, N., and B. R. Smoller. 2015. "Role of tea tree oil in treatment of acne." *Dermatol Ther*. doi: 10.1111/dth.12235.

Caelli, M., J. Porteous, C. F. Carson, R. Heller, and T. V. Riley. 2000. "Tea tree oil as an alternative topical decolonization agent for methicillin-resistant Staphylococcus aureus." *J Hosp Infect* 46(3): 236–7. doi: 10.1053/jhin.2000.0830.

Cao, H., G. Yang, Y. Wang, J. P. Liu, C. A. Smith, H. Luo, and Y. Liu. 2015. "Complementary therapies for acne vulgaris." *Cochrane Database Syst Rev* 1:CD009436. doi: 10.1002/14651858. CD009436.pub2.

Carrasco, A., R. Martinez-Gutierrez, V. Tomas, and J. Tudela. 2015. "Lavandula angustifolia and Lavandula latifolia essential oils from Spain: aromatic profile and bioactivities." *Planta Med*. doi: 10.1055/s-0035-1558095.

Carson, C. F., K. A. Hammer, and T. V. Riley. 2006. "Melaleuca alternifolia (Tea Tree) oil: a review of antimicrobial and other medicinal properties." *Clin Microbiol Rev* 19(1): 50–62. doi: 10.1128/CMR.19.1.50-62.2006.

Carson, C. F., R. Tisserand, and T. Larkman. 2014. "Lack of evidence that essential oils affect puberty." *Reprod Toxicol* 44: 50–1. doi: 10.1016/j.reprotox.2013.09.010.

Cetinkaya, B., and Z. Basbakkal. 2012. "The effectiveness of aromatherapy massage using lavender oil as a treatment for infantile colic." *Int J Nurs Pract* 18(2): 164–9. doi: 10.1111/j.1440-172X.2012.02015.x.

Charrois, T. L., J. Hrudey, P. Gardiner, S. Vohra, Holistic American Academy of Pediatrics Provisional Section on Complementary, and Medicine Integrative. 2006. "Peppermint oil." *Pediatr Rev* 27(7): e49–51.

Cooke, B., and E. Ernst. 2000. "Aromatherapy: a systematic review." *Br J Gen Pract* 50(455): 493–6.

Dagli, N., R. Dagli, R. S. Mahmoud, and K. Baroudi. 2015. "Essential oils, their therapeutic properties, and implication in dentistry: A review." *J Int Soc Prev Community Dent* 5(5): 335–40. doi: 10.4103/2231-0762.165933.

de Groot, A. C., and E. Schmidt. 2015. "Eucalyptus oil and tea tree oil." *Contact Dermatitis*. doi: 10.1111/cod.12450.

Di Campli, E., S. Di Bartolomeo, P. Delli Pizzi, M. Di Giulio, R. Grande, A. Nostro, and L. Cellini. 2012. "Activity of tea tree oil and nerolidol alone or in combination against Pediculus capitis (head lice) and its eggs." *Parasitol Res* 111(5): 1985–92. doi: 10.1007/s00436-012-3045-0.

Diaz, A., L. Luque, Z. Badar, S. Kornic, and M. Danon. 2015. "Prepubertal gynecomastia and chronic lavender exposure: report of three cases." *J Pediatr Endocrinol Metab*. doi: 10.1515/jpem-2015-0248.

Field, T., T. Field, C. Cullen, S. Largie, M. Diego, S. Schanberg, and C. Kuhn. 2008. "Lavender bath oil reduces stress and crying and enhances sleep in very young infants." *Early Hum Dev* 84(6): 399–401. doi: 10.1016/j.earlhumdev.2007.10.008.

Finsterer, J. 2002. "Earl Grey tea intoxication." *Lancet* 359(9316): 1484. doi: 10.1016/S0140-6736(02)08436-2.

Hammer, K. A., C. F. Carson, and T. V. Riley. 1998. "In-vitro activity of essential oils, in particular Melaleuca alternifolia (tea tree) oil and tea tree oil products, against Candida spp." *J Antimicrob Chemother* 42(5): 591–5.

Henley, D. V., N. Lipson, K. S. Korach, and C. A. Bloch. 2007. "Prepubertal gynecomastia linked to lavender and tea tree oils." *N Engl J Med* 356(5): 479–85. doi: 10.1056/NEJMoa064725.

Herro, E., and S. E. Jacob. 2010. "Mentha piperita (peppermint)." *Dermatitis* 21(6): 327–9.

Hines, S., E. Steels, A. Chang, and K. Gibbons. 2012. "Aromatherapy for treatment of postoperative nausea and vomiting." *Cochrane Database Syst Rev* 4: CD007598. doi: 10.1002/14651858.CD007598.pub2.

Kim, S., H. J. Kim, J. S. Yeo, S. J. Hong, J. M. Lee, and Y. Jeon. 2011. "The effect of lavender oil on stress, bispectral index values, and needle insertion pain in volunteers." *J Altern Complement Med* 17(9): 823–6. doi: 10.1089/acm.2010.0644.

Kligler, B., and S. Chaudhary. 2007. "Peppermint oil." *Am Fam Physician* 75(7): 1027–30.

Kollndorfer, K., K. Kowalczyk, E. Hoche, C. A. Mueller, M. Pollak, S. Trattnig, and V. Schopf. 2014. "Recovery of olfactory function induces neuroplasticity effects in patients with smell loss." *Neural Plast* 2014: 140419. doi: 10.1155/2014/140419.

Lillehei, A. S., and L. L. Halcon. 2014. "A systematic review of the effect of inhaled essential oils on sleep." *J Altern Complement Med* 20(6): 441–51. doi: 10.1089/acm.2013.0311.

Morris, M. C., A. Donoghue, J. A. Markowitz, and K. C. Osterhoudt. 2003. "Ingestion of tea tree oil (Melaleuca oil) by a 4-year-old boy." *Pediatr Emerg Care* 19(3): 169–71. doi: 10.1097/01.pec.0000081241.98249.7b.

Navarra, M., C. Mannucci, M. Delbo, and G. Calapai. 2015. "Citrus bergamia essential oil: from basic research to clinical application." *Front Pharmacol* 6: 36. doi: 10.3389/fphar.2015.00036.

PDQ. 2002. "Aromatherapy and Essential Oils (PDQ®): Health Professional Version." In *PDQ Cancer Information Summaries*. Bethesda, MD.

Richards, D. B., G. S. Wang, and J. A. Buchanan. 2015. "Pediatric tea tree oil aspiration treated with surfactant in the emergency department." *Pediatr Emerg Care* 31(4): 279–80. doi: 10.1097/PEC.0000000000000234.

Richmond, E., D. Adams, S. Dagenais, T. Clifford, L. Baydala, W. J. King, and S. Vohra. 2014. "Complementary and alternative medicine: A survey of its use in children with chronic respiratory illness." *Can J Respir Ther* 50(1): 27–32.

Soltani, R., S. Soheilipour, V. Hajhashemi, G. Asghari, M. Bagheri, and M. Molavi. 2013. "Evaluation of the effect of aromatherapy with lavender essential oil on post-tonsillectomy pain in pediatric patients: a randomized controlled trial." *Int J Pediatr Otorhinolaryngol* 77(9): 1579–81. doi: 10.1016/j.ijporl.2013.07.014.

Terzi, V., C. Morcia, P. Faccioli, G. Vale, G. Tacconi, and M. Malnati. 2007. "In vitro antifungal activity of the tea tree (Melaleuca alternifolia) essential oil and its major components against plant pathogens." *Lett Appl Microbiol* 44(6): 613–8. doi: 10.1111/j.1472-765X.2007.02128.x.

Valnet, J. 1990. *The Practice of Aromatherapy: A Classic Compendium of Plant Medicines & Their Healing Properties*. Rochester, NY: Healing Arts Press.

Vegh, A., T. Bencsik, P. Molnar, A. Boszormenyi, E. Lemberkovics, K. Kovacs, B. Kocsis, and G. Horvath. 2012. "Composition and antipseudomonal effect of essential oils isolated from different lavender species." *Nat Prod Commun* 7(10): 1393–6.

Villemure, C., A. C. Laferriere, and M. C. Bushnell. 2012. "The ventral striatum is implicated in the analgesic effect of mood changes." *Pain Res Manag* 17(2): 69–74.

Wilcock, A., C. Manderson, R. Weller, G. Walker, D. Carr, A. M. Carey, D. Broadhurst, J. Mew, and E. Ernst. 2004. "Does aromatherapy massage benefit patients with cancer attending a specialist palliative care day centre?" *Palliat Med* 18(4): 287–90.

12 Whole Medical Systems

"Whole medical system" refers to a complete approach to diagnosis and practice of healthcare. Some examples of whole medical systems include traditional Chinese medicine, homeopathy, and Ayurveda. These systems reflect traditional and customary medical procedures practiced in various cultures around the world. A selection of the better-studied whole medical systems will be covered here, including those with some supporting evidence in pediatrics, although in many cases evidence for the use of many traditional whole medical systems remains relatively scant in the U.S. (Romeyke and Stummer 2015; Edwards et al. 2013).

Homeopathy

Overview

Homeopathy is a 200-year-old science that developed in part as a reaction to concerns about the harsh treatment in use in medical treatments of the day (Bell and Boyer 2013). It was introduced in Germany during the 18th century and is now a widely practiced healing method, especially in European countries, England, Pakistan, and India (Spigelblatt 2005).

Any homeopathy use by children in the U.S. was estimated at 1.8% of children in 2012, with practitioner-based homeopathy used by 0.2% of children, demonstrating a high use of self-directed family care (Black et al. 2015).

This is line with statistics that reflect that the majority of homeopathic sales in the U.S. occur over the counter at commercial retailers such as drugstores, grocery stores, and large wholesale retailers, a route that has far less oversight by the U.S. FDA than prescription pharmaceuticals despite being a multi-billion-dollar market in the U.S. alone. The federal Food, Drug, and Cosmetic Act, originally passed in 1938, covered homeopathic remedies and recognized the Homeopathic Pharmacopeia of the United States as an official compendium with clear standards and expectations. However, due to presumption of low risk to consumers because of the small levels of active ingredients in homeopathic products, the FDA does not require pre-market approval on homeopathic products that meet the FDA requirements for labeling and manufacture. One of the loopholes in the current regulations is oversight of combination products that contain some homeopathic and other nonhomeopathic ingredients. These receive less scrutiny because they are not considered homeopathic remedies. Oversight of homeopathic remedies has been controversial and concerns have been raised about lack of active ingredients, delay in diagnosis and effective treatment if consumers are self-treating, and lack of full awareness of active ingredients, evidence of efficacy, or potential side effects (Kuehn 2009). For example an FDA warning about safety concerns related to over-the-counter homeopathic teething tablets and gels was issued in Fall of 2016 due to reports of adverse events in infants and children including seizures.

Reasons associated with the use of homeopathy in the pediatric population include a desire to relieve suffering associated with symptoms such as runny nose, cough, and sore throat in children without the overuse of prescription drugs or over-the-counter drugs that have been associated with serious side effects in children, including intentional and non-intentional overdose of acetaminophen, nonsteroidal anti-inflammatories, antihistamines, or decongestants (Bell and Boyer 2013).

The use of homeopathy in children has been associated with fewer and less severe side effects than over-the-counter drugs, earlier resolution of symptoms, and lower cost than conventional care (2005; Bell and Boyer 2013).

A core belief in homeopathy is that the body functions on principle of cures, meaning that the illness in question can be cured from the things that caused it in the first place, i.e., "like cures like." Homeopathic remedies are found in the form of liquids or pills that are manufactured from natural animal, mineral, and plant substances prepared in a highly specific way that involves a series of dilutions, which has been a source of great controversy in medical circles as the mechanism of its action remains poorly understood (Bell and Boyer 2013).

One of the most challenging aspects of integrating homeopathy into practice is its highly individualized nature. There are no set protocols to follow. Many studies have shown variable results, and randomized controlled trials have been hard to interpret due to small sample size, methodological variability, and lack of validated outcome measures. These issues are compounded by a lack of research funding and a lack of practitioners participating in research (Merrell and Shalts 2002).

Brief History

Homeopathy was initially named by a German physician, Samuel Hahnemann (1755–1843), based on the work of scientists who preceded him. Hahnemann refined his approach and recorded his work in multiple editions of his historical book *Organon of Rational Medicine* (1810), later known as simply Organon (Schmidt 2010). Hahnemann taught that the homeopathic procedure to prepare remedies had two elements: dilution and succussion/trituration (vigorous shaking or agitation). He believed that succussion released the dynamic powers of the medicines based on his interpretation of the emerging theories of energy, force, and friction at the time. Hahnemann also wrote extensively about the dynamic forces of the particles of the remedies being "potentiated" to release their internal medicinal forces (Waisse 2012).

Typical dilution patterns still in use include repeated series of dilutions followed by successions. For example, the X series of dilutions is a 1:10-dilution ratio, and the C series refers to a 1:100-dilution ratio. For example, a 30 C potency means that the solution has been diluted over 30 consecutive steps, with each dilution using a ratio of 1 part diluted material to 100 parts solvent. Succussion accompanies each dilution step, typically 20 times per step. Modern measurement methods have shown that homeopathic solutions prepared in this manner have unique characteristics as compared to placebo. Many questions remain about the specific mechanism of action of homeopathy and lines of research inquiry are active involving theories based on quantum electrodynamics and nanoparticle technology which rely on the body as a complex system, rather than the medicine, to do the work of healing (Bellavite et al. 2014; Bell and Boyer 2013; Bell et al. 2013).

Type of Assessments

Initially, the patient planning to undergo homeopathy treatment has a detailed interview that includes a medical history and in-depth evaluation of lifestyle and other habits. The interview is a very important part of the assessment as it provides a foundation for diagnosis and paves the path for self-discovery and healing. Open-ended questions are usually asked to best understand the patient's unique characteristics and help establish an accurate diagnosis. There are more than 100 remedies used by the homeopaths to treat illnesses, but the selection of the remedies depends on the needs of the patient based on the intake interview (Merrell and Shalts 2002; Colas et al. 2015).

Evidence in Pediatrics

Evaluation of the use of homeopathy in children has concentrated on a few conditions, including: acute upper respiratory illness, otitis media (Bell and Boyer 2013), ADHD, and headache.

Otitis

An early trial of homeopathic remedy sought to examine efficacy of homeopathic treatment in pain relief in 230 children with acute otitis. The initial homeopathic dose was given in the office visit; if pain was not resolved in 6 hours a second type of homeopathic remedy was given. Six hours later if pain was not resolved antibiotics were begun. In this study 39% of children achieved pain control in the first 6 hours, another 33% had pain relief after 12 hours. This was found to be 2.4 times faster than placebo controls. No adverse events were seen and cost savings was estimated at 14% (Frei and Thurneysen 2001).

A randomized double blind placebo-controlled trial of 75 children received an individualized homeopathic medicine versus placebo orally three times a day for 5 days or until symptoms resolved—whichever came first. Results showed fewer treatment failures in the homeopathic group, although results were not statistically significant. Rate of symptom improvement was significantly faster in the treatment group (p < 0.05). The most commonly prescribed homeopathic remedies included Pulsatilla nigricans, Chamomilla, Sulphur, and Calcarea carbonica (Jacobs, Springer, and Crothers 2001).

A multicenter cohort of 1577 patients compared conventional, mixed, or homeopathic treatment in patients with acute respiratory illness, sore throat, ear pain, cough, or sinus pain. The 857 patients treated with homeopathy alone showed more rapid onset of improvement in the treatment group in children, (p = 0.0488). Overall study conclusions were limited to "homeopathic treatment for acute respiratory and ear complaints was not inferior to conventional treatment." In addition to more rapid onset of improvement, a second benefit to homeopathic treatment was a lower rate of adverse events as compared to conventional treatment groups in both children and adults (Haidvogl et al. 2007).

A 2011 study of 120 children with acute otitis randomized patients to receive either a commercial combination homeopathic eardrop or standard therapy. The combination drops were given every 4 hours until improvement of symptoms. This study also documented a more rapid rate of symptom improvement compared to standard therapy (Taylor and Jacobs 2011).

A further double-blinded placebo-controlled trial of individualized homeopathic remedies versus conventional treatment (analgesics, antipyretics, anti-inflammatories) was conducted in 81 children with acute otitis media. Non-responders in either group were prescribed antibiotics on day 3 of illness. Antibiotics were prescribed in 97.5% of the conventional group versus no antibiotics in the homeopathic group. A majority of those in the homeopathic group, > 85%, received six homeopathic medications in combination. The rate of symptomatic improvement was faster in the homeopathic group on average. Most frequently used remedies included Pulsatilla nigricans, Mercurius solubilis, Silicea, Chamomilla, Lycopodium clavatum, and Sulphur (Sinha et al. 2012).

Upper Respiratory Infections (URI)

A 6-month prospective study of 499 French children with acute upper respiratory illness showed that homeopathic treatment significantly reduced both number of episodes of upper respiratory illness ($p < 0.001$) and the number of complications children experienced ($p < 0.001$) in addition to reduced direct medical costs including medical visit, prescriptions, and further testing ($p < 0.05$). Parents of the patients treated with homeopathic remedies also needed to take significantly less sick leave from work ($p < 0.001$) in this study population (Trichard, Chaufferin, and Nicoloyannis 2005).

A small pilot study of 30 patients under the age of 5 years examined the number of upper respiratory infections in a 6-month period prior to beginning homeopathic treatment versus the number of recorded upper respiratory illnesses after beginning homeopathic care. Results favored the homeopathic treatment approach ($p < 0.001$) (Ramchandani 2010).

Arguments favoring homeopathic treatment for acute otitis media and upper respiratory infection in children include: evidence of more rapid symptom improvement, lower fill rates in a watchful waiting approach to antibiotic prescriptions, reduction in frequency and severity of side effects of treatment, reduced cost of homeopathic treatment, and reduced parental leave from work. While results appear promising, concerns include need for individualization of treatment by a practitioner trained in homeopathy and a need for more carefully designed randomized controlled trials (Bukutu, Deol, and Vohra 2008).

ADHD

Although interest is high in non-pharmacologic treatment of ADHD, studies on the use of homeopathic remedies have not shown conclusive benefits to date (Coulter and Dean 2007; Frei et al. 2007).

More studies are underway (Catala-Lopez et al. 2015).

Asthma

One prospective observational longitudinal study of individualized oral homeopathic treatments in 30 children with asthma compared its use in conjunction with conventional measures by measuring frequency of acute exacerbations, medication use, and spirometry. Improvements in the treatment group were seen at both 3 months and 6 months in symptom frequency, night awakening, inhaler use, and oral corticosteroid use. Spirometry was significantly improved at month six of treatment. This study showed positive effect of individualized homeopathic remedy used in conjunction with conventional medicine, although lack of control group and small study size were limiting factors (Shafei, AbdelDayem, and Mohamed 2012).

Atopic Dermatitis

An observational longitudinal study on 213 children with atopic diseases included 76 with atopic dermatitis. Eight-year follow-up on 40 of those patients with atopic dermatitis who had started homeopathic treatment before 5 years of age showed that 70% had complete resolution of the disease (Rossi et al. 2012).

Migraine

A multi-national study of 168 children and adolescents investigated the use of individualized homeopathic remedies for migraine headache over a 6-month time period. Results showed a significant reduction in time off school ($p < 0.001$) and statistically significant reduction in frequency, severity, and duration of migraine episodes during the 3-month follow-up period. Preventive remedies most commonly used included Ignatia amara, Lycopodium clavatum, Natrum muriaticum, Gelsemium, and Pulsatilla. Remedies most used in the treatment of acute attacks included Belladonna, Ignatia amara, and Iris versicolor. Although results are encouraging, limitations of the study included funding by the manufacturer of the homeopathic remedies, symptoms based on parental recall, lack of control group, and possibility of placebo effect (Danno et al. 2013).

A prospective 2-year multicenter study in 212 adults with migraine showed significant benefit to the majority of patients treated with individualized homeopathic remedies. Migraine severity, frequency, and reduction in use of conventional health services were all significantly reduced and sustained over the 2-year follow-up period (Witt, Ludtke, and Willich 2010).

Homeopathic remedies have been used successfully in a randomized controlled trial of 32 immunocompromised children and young adults undergoing stem cell transplant for the treatment of stomatitis. Patients in the treatment group had a significantly lower incidence and severity of stomatitis associated with chemotherapy with no adverse effects noted (Oberbaum et al. 2001). Of note, this result was not found to be reproducible in a second trial other than a trend toward reduced use of pain medication (Sencer et al. 2012).

Cautions and Possible Side Effects

In general homeopathy is considered low risk, although in some cases self-limited aggravation of symptoms has been reported in some cases, which paradoxically is considered a positive response. Extreme sensitivity or allergy to the homeopathic compound would be one of the few direct contraindications to its use. In addition to the 2016 FDA warning about adverse events related to teething tablets and gels for infants, a negative report does exist in relation to Zicam intranasal products, zinc-containing remedies for colds and upper respiratory illness in both children and adults, which have been associated with anosmia, and several products were pulled off the market based on FDA warnings. In 2006 the manufacturer of Zicam products settled 340 lawsuits filed by consumers based on loss of sense of smell for $12 million (Kuehn 2009).

A 2009 Cochrane Database Systematic Review showed that homeopathic remedies have shown promise in some studies in immunocompromised cancer patients with no serious adverse events reported even in this highly vulnerable population (Kassab et al. 2009). There is no body of evidence to support its safe use in pregnant or nursing women and therefore its use is not recommended.

Training and Licensing in U.S. and Internationally

Training in homeopathy is very variable and can be obtained through programs nationally and internationally. The North American Society of Homeopaths was created in 1990 to set standards of competency in classical homeopathy through standardized training and the Council for Homeopathic Certification (CHC) examination process. Generally, homeopathy can be used legally by those who can practice medicine in their states, including MD, DO, ND, DDS, and DVM. Three states in the U.S. have homeopathic licensing laws, including Arizona, Connecticut, and Nevada, meaning that MDs and DOs in these states must be licensed by their state homeopathic licensing board. Other healthcare practitioners may be able to prescribe based on specific state laws. For example, homeopathy is included in the scope of practice in states that license naturopathic physicians. The Homeopathic Academy of Naturopathic Physicians also offers a certifying exam. There is no specific licensing for the practice of homeopathy in pediatrics.

Naturopathy

Summary and Overview

The system of naturopathy is similar to Ayurveda and other complementary methods of healing as it is based on the fact that the body can heal itself by restoring its natural balance. This approach to health includes considering the whole person (mental, emotional, and social), elimination of unhealthy lifestyle habits, and introduction of healthy practices. Acupuncture, chiropractic, and homeopathy are often included in naturopathic practice to encourage the body's natural healing response. Key principles that have been widely recognized in naturopathy include: the healing power of nature, identify and treat the cause rather than the symptoms, first do no harm, doctor as teacher, treat the whole person, and focus on prevention. The National Center for Complementary and Integrative Health lists some of the approaches used in naturopathy and they include homeopathy, hydrotherapy, nutrition as therapy, botanicals, exercise therapy, practitioner-guided detoxification, physiotherapy, psychotherapy, and counseling (National Center for Complementary and Integrative Health [a]).

The 2007 U.S. National Health Statistics Report by Barnes et al. showed increase in use of naturopathy in children in the U.S. from 2002 to 2007 to include an estimated 237,000 children (Barnes, Bloom, and Nahin 2008). Naturopathy is practiced widely in various countries, each with differing training requirements (Braun et al. 2013, Cottingham et al. 2015; Klein et al. 2015).

In the U.S. there are three main pathways followed by naturopathic practitioners: *naturopathic physicians* who have completed a 4-year graduate level degree at an accredited school with oversight by the Council on Naturopathic Medical Education recognized by the U.S. Department of Education; *traditional naturopaths* who have received training through non-accredited programs; *other healthcare providers* who may offer some types of naturopathic therapies from a range of non-accredited programs. These might include physicians, osteopaths, chiropractic, dentists, nurses, or other practitioners who have taken training in the context of their own practices. In the U.S. there is state-to-state variation for licensing requirements for naturopathic physicians. In the states requiring a license to practice, naturopathic physicians must complete a 4-year degree, pass a licensing exam, and maintain continuing education requirements. There is no requirement for residency after graduation, although some postdoctoral training is available. Traditional naturopaths are not eligible for licensing in the U.S. (National Center for Complementary and Integrative Health [a]).

Brief History

The history of naturopathy can be traced back to 19th century Europe. Dr. Benedict Lust, a German physician, introduced naturopathy in North America in 1892. He established the American Institute of Naturopathy in New York City.

Type of Assessment

The main types of assessment used are detailed health history, nutritional analysis, pulse diagnosis, previous medical reports, and lab testing. The interview includes all important lifestyle elements such as stress level, daily lifestyle, family health history, food pattern and intake, and diet, and includes a physical examination.

Evidence in Pediatrics

While some elements of naturopathy such as healthy nutrition, physical activity, and stress management are familiar, other elements of naturopathic practice such as hydrotherapy, colonic irrigation, fasting, and use of herbal or nutritional supplements have not been investigated in the pediatric population (Lee and Kemper 2000).

One of the few areas with current supporting evidence for the use of naturopathy in pediatrics is the use of a naturopathic eardrop to treat pain in acute otitis media. A double-blind randomized controlled study by Sarrell et al. in 171 children with acute otitis demonstrated efficacy of a naturopathic herbal extract eardrop in reducing otalgia over a 3-day watch and wait period (Sarrell, Cohen, and Kahan 2003).

One concern in pediatrics is the increased risk of vaccine-preventable illnesses in children who receive primary care from a naturopath opposed to routine vaccination. A study of 213,884 children in Washington State showed that use of naturopathy was associated with significantly more vaccine-preventable disease diagnosis (Downey et al. 2010).

Cautions and Possible Side Effects

Concerns related to children and adolescents using naturopathy include excessive use of fasts, enema usage, diet restrictions, and possibility of allergic reaction or cross-reaction to untested natural products. Insufficient data is available for its use in pregnant and breastfeeding women.

Training and Licensing in U.S. and Internationally

In 2012 there were seven accredited training programs for naturopathic doctors in North America, five in the U.S. and two in Canada. At present, about 17 U.S. states and 18% of Canadian provinces provide license to naturopathic doctors, who must pass the naturopathic physicians licensing examination in order to practice in U.S. (Association of Accredited Naturopathic Medical Colleges).

Ayurveda

Background and Overview

Ayurveda is a whole medical system that originated in India approximately 5000 years ago. The word Ayurveda is Sanskrit for "life knowledge." Ayurveda comprises the full scope of health, including mind, body, spirit, and consciousness. Some of its basic principles include elimination of the causes of illness, treatment of the condition, rebuilding and rebalancing of the body, and ongoing support for longevity and rejuvenation. Ayurvedic practitioners believe that the diseases are the outcome of the pathologic and psychophysiological changes, which are caused due to imbalance in the components of the body (Gadgil 2010).

In Ayurveda these components include some form of the three doshas: vata (energy of movement—wind), pitta (energy of metabolism—fire), and kapha (lubrication and structure—earth) and their complex subgroups, including the seven dhatus (seven bodily tissues), the three malas (waste products—urine, stool, sweat), the agni (metabolic energy of digestion), and the swastha (senses, mind, and spirit) (Mukherjee et al. 2012).

Treatment in Ayurveda is highly individualized and dependent on the constitution of the patient. Recommendations vary based on the seasons and may consist of treatment with herbs and spices for rejuvenation and to promote longevity, purification to remove toxins from the body, and a focus on preventive health. Pediatrics has a special branch of Ayurveda, called Bala Tantra or Kaumarabhritya, which covers the span from newborn through 16 years. It is believed that one's constitution, or prakruti, is determined at the time of conception and is determined by the constitution of the parents (Mukherjee et al. 2012).

Type of Assessments

The ultimate aim of the Ayurveda therapy is to restore the body system's harmony and balance. Prior to receiving a prescription for herbal medicines, the patient usually undergoes body cleansing and detoxification because it is believed that the body must be cleansed so that the herbs or compounds can do their job properly. Detoxification is done through various techniques including laxatives, fasting, sinuses cleansing, vomiting and medicated enemas. This process of detoxification is usually called panchakarma by the practitioners. The process of panchakarma is very intensive and may last for weeks in order to make the body ready for Ayurveda treatment. During this treatment the patient is also given heat treatments and massages to relax their nervous system. Once the purification is done, different herbal remedies are used alternately with mineral remedies to restore the body balance (Mukherjee et al. 2012).

In addition to that, the Ayurveda practitioner gives lifestyle recommendations to the patient to encourage a peaceful life and a simple routine of individualized diet and rest. Yoga, meditation, and massage are recommended to Ayurveda patients to help develop internal peace and achieve mental equilibrium (Mukherjee et al. 2012).

Evidence in Pediatrics

Challenges in Ayurvedic research include the need for highly individualized treatment, its principle of "whole person care," making the study of isolated treatments impractical, quality control over herbal remedies, and the use of multiple botanicals in one remedy to promote their synergism. Presence of heavy metal contamination in some Ayurvedic remedies has also been an issue, especially in children.

One area of study that has shown some promise is in ADHD where the use of *Bacopa monnieri* has been investigated. Bacopa has a long history of use in Ayurvedic practice for improving memory and intellect, and to treat anxiety. In vivo animal studies have shown positive benefit for learning and memory. Bacosides A and B are thought to be the active compounds and have been associated with anxiolytic effects, beta-amyloid scavenging, and modulation of acetylcholine levels. Single-extract studies of bacopa, particularly (Central Drug Research Institute) CDRI 08, which is standardized to not less than 55% bacosides, have been associated with improvement in ADHD symptoms in children and adolescents in some studies (Dave et al. 2014), although randomized placebo-controlled trials using CDRI 08 are needed to further establish efficacy and optimal dosing (Kean et al. 2015).

Cautions and Possible Side Effects

The United States is one of the largest markets for Indian botanical exports, accounting for approximately 50% of the market in 2005 (Patwardhan et al. 2005). The individual must ensure that the practitioner prescribing Ayurveda remedies is properly qualified and that quality control is high if herbal preparations are used (Patwardhan et al. 2005). As noted above, heavy metal contamination of Indian-manufactured traditional Ayurvedic medicines has been a serious concern, especially in children (Saper et al. 2008).

Training and Licensing in U.S. and Internationally

At present, there is no accreditation standard to approve the Ayurveda curriculum in U.S. Existing programs can range from 500 to 800 hours on average. The National Ayurvedic Medical Association represents the Ayurvedic profession in the U.S. and serves as a useful resource for learning about U.S. training programs. This is in high contrast to Ayurvedic medical training in India where students undertake 4–6 years of intensive training to master this complex medical system (National Ayurvedic Medical Association).

Traditional Chinese Medicine

Summary and Overview

Traditional Chinese medicine (TCM) is one of the oldest healing systems known and refers to the non-medical Chinese procedures used for healing the body, including consumption of Chinese herbal medicine, dietary therapy, moxibustion, acupuncture, qi gong, and tai chi. TCM is fully incorporated into the Chinese healthcare systems, commonly in conjunction with Western medicine (Tang, Liu, and Ma 2008).

Taoism and Confucianism are the principal components of the traditional Chinese medicine philosophy. Historical texts document the eight chief principles that must be considered for all natural phenomena, including physical symptoms and conditions based on a system of yin and yang (opposite, complementary, interdependent, exchangeable). These principles include: yin/yang, cold/heat, excess/deficiency, and interior/exterior. Furthermore, TCM uses the five basic elements to study the body, organ and tissues functions in the body: wood, water, metal, earth, and fire. Like other whole medicine systems, TCM uses a very individualized approach. In TCM circulation of qi, or energy, and blood are considered as two entities. The organs work in concert to circulate, regulate, and conserve both through specific channels or meridians in the body. Disruption or blockage of these channels can be caused by disease, emotional upset, and factors such as heat, damp, and cold. Acupuncture and the use of herbal therapies are mainstays of TCM. The diagnosis that is used to guide treatments is called Zheng, essentially a state determined by the patient's signs and symptoms at the time (Tang, Liu, and Ma 2008).

Statistics from the U.S. 2007 National Health Interview Survey show that more than 3 million adults had used acupuncture in the previous year.

Brief History

TCM dates back many thousands of years as recorded in ancient texts such as the *Huang Di Nei Jing*, the *Inner Canon of the Yellow Emperor*, considered the highest authority on traditional Chinese medicine. Influence of TCM can be seen in traditional healing systems in Southern Asia and throughout Europe (National Center for Complementary and Integrative Health [b]; Patwardhan et al. 2005).

Types of Assessments

There are four methods of diagnosis of traditional Chinese medicine including observation, interrogation, auscultation, and olfaction, along with pulse taking and palpation. Under observation, the traditional Chinese medicine practitioner observes the patient's outward appearance in order to judge the patient's condition and then make a diagnosis. The belief behind this technique is that the human body's outward appearance, including tongue texture and color, and skin pallor, in part predict the internal condition of the body (Nestler 2002). Through these four techniques, the practitioners prescribe herbal medicines and other TCM treatments to promote healing.

Evidence in Pediatrics

Relatively limited research on safety of traditional Chinese medicines exists, making conclusive recommendations impossible. Challenges in TCM research mirror obstacles faced in other whole medical systems, including the difficulty of studying complex whole person approaches to treatment, lack of full scientific understanding of treatments, uneven quality of studies, and lack of standardization of herbs, and lack of adequate controls.

Despite recognized challenges, use of TCM is widely prevalent in pediatrics; for example, a survey study of 97,401 Taiwanese school children with allergic rhinitis showed that 63.11% had used TCM for symptom treatment, which is fully reimbursed by National Health Insurance in Taiwan (Yen et al. 2015).

A second large population-based survey of TCM use in 45,833 Taiwanese children newly diagnosed with asthma showed that 58% had used TCM. The most common therapy used was an herbal remedy known as Ding-chuan-tang (Huang et al. 2013).

Some recent studies in children show promise. For example, a 12-week randomized trial of the Chinese herbal formula Pei Tu Qing Xin Tang (PTQXT) given orally for 12 weeks in the treatment group of 275 patients aged 5–25 years with moderate to severe atopic dermatitis was associated with significant improvement in standardized disease severity score and in quality of life at 36 months ($p < 0.001$) (Liu et al. 2015).

Research is active in the use of acupuncture in pediatrics as evidenced by a systematic review by Yang et al. of 142 randomized controlled trials involving 12,787 children. Encouraging findings were seen in treatment of nocturnal enuresis, pain, tic disorders, and cerebral palsy, although authors note that larger high-quality studies are needed before definitive recommendations can be given. Adverse events were rare and non-serious in sessions with trained practitioners (Yang et al. 2015).

A 2011 Cochrane Database Systematic Review of 10 randomized and non-randomized controlled trials involving 390 children with autism did not support the use of acupuncture for treatment of autism spectrum disorder (Cheuk, Wong, and Chen 2011).

Cautions and Possible Side Effects

Most TCM medicines are sold in the form of dietary supplements distributed worldwide. These are considered dietary supplements in the U.S., and subsequently subject to less stringent regulations than over-the-counter medications. Reports of contamination with heavy metals and other toxins or drugs have caused significant concerns. For example, in 2004 the FDA banned sales of ephedra (ma haung) due to reports of serious cardiovascular and neurological complications (Haller and Benowitz 2000; Bent et al. 2003).

Chinese herbs may also react with other allopathic medications. In experienced hands acupuncture is considered low risk if the needles used are sterile. Qi gong and tai chi are considered practical and safe techniques with few associated side effects. Reports of allergies, infections, burns, and other more serious outcomes such as pneumothorax exist, but are rare (National Center for Complementary and Integrative Health [b]).

Training and Licensing in U.S. and Internationally

In many states individuals who do not have an MD or DO degree must be certified by the National Certification Commission for Acupuncture and Oriental Medicine (NCCAOM) in order to practice acupuncture. This requires a minimum of 3 years of full-time education before eligibility for national certification. State-to-state variations exist regarding scope of practice for physicians incorporating acupuncture in their medical practice. The American Academy of Medical Acupuncture (AAMA) was founded in 1987 and is a professional society for physicians (MD and DO) in North America who integrate acupuncture into their medical practices (American Academy of Medical Acupuncture).

Requirements for other healthcare professionals vary widely and may include as few as 100 hours of acupuncture training. A clearinghouse for by-state laws on the requirements can be found at acupuncture.com, although individuals should check for updates (Acupuncture.Com).

References

Acupuncture.Com. "State Laws."

American Academy of Medical Acupuncture. http://www.medicalacupuncture.orgAm.

Association of Accredited Naturopathic Medical Colleges. https://aanmc.org/.

Barnes, P. M., B. Bloom, and R. L. Nahin. 2008. "Complementary and alternative medicine use among adults and children: United States, 2007." *Natl Health Stat Report* 12: 1–23.

Bell, I. R., and N. N. Boyer. 2013. "Homeopathic medications as clinical alternatives for symptomatic care of acute otitis media and upper respiratory infections in children." *Glob Adv Health Med* 2(1): 32–43. doi: 10.7453/gahmj.2013.2.1.007.

Bell, I. R., G. E. Schwartz, N. N. Boyer, M. Koithan, and A. J. Brooks. 2013. "Advances in integrative nanomedicine for improving infectious disease treatment in public health." *Eur J Integr Med* 5(2): 126–40. doi: 10.1016/j.eujim.2012.11.002.

Bellavite, P., M. Marzotto, D. Olioso, E. Moratti, and A. Conforti. 2014. "High-dilution effects revisited. 1. Physicochemical aspects." *Homeopathy* 103(1): 4–21. doi: 10.1016/j.homp.2013.08.003.

Bent, S., T. N. Tiedt, M. C. Odden, and M. G. Shlipak. 2003. "The relative safety of ephedra compared with other herbal products." *Ann Intern Med* 138(6): 468–71.

Black, L. I., T. C. Clarke, P. M. Barnes, B. J. Stussman, and R. L. Nahin. 2015. "Use of complementary health approaches among children aged 4–17 years in the United States: National Health Interview Survey, 2007–2012." *Natl Health Stat Report* 78: 1–19.

Braun, L. A., O. Spitzer, E. Tiralongo, J. M. Wilkinson, M. Bailey, S. G. Poole, and M. Dooley. 2013. "Naturopaths and Western herbalists' attitudes to evidence, regulation, information sources and knowledge about popular complementary medicines." *Complement Ther Med* 21(1): 58–64. doi: 10.1016/j.ctim.2012.11.008.

Bukutu, C., J. Deol, and S. Vohra. 2008. "Complementary, holistic, and integrative medicine: therapies for acute otitis media." *Pediatr Rev* 29(6): 193–9. doi: 10.1542/pir.29-6-193.

Catala-Lopez, F., B. Hutton, A. Nunez-Beltran, A. D. Mayhew, M. J. Page, M. Ridao, A. Tobias, M. A. Catala, R. Tabares-Seisdedos, and D. Moher. 2015. "The pharmacological and non-pharmacological treatment of attention deficit hyperactivity disorder in children and adolescents: protocol for a systematic review and network meta-analysis of randomized controlled trials." *Syst Rev* 4: 19. doi: 10.1186/s13643-015-0005-7.

Cheuk, D. K., V. Wong, and W. X. Chen. 2011. "Acupuncture for autism spectrum disorders (ASD)." *Cochrane Database Syst Rev* 9: CD007849. doi: 10.1002/14651858.CD007849.pub2.

Colas, A., K. Danno, C. Tabar, J. Ehreth, and G. Duru. 2015. "Economic impact of homeopathic practice in general medicine in France." *Health Econ Rev* 5(1): 55. doi: 10.1186/s13561-015-0055-5.

Cottingham, P., J. Adams, R. Vempati, J. Dunn, and D. Sibbritt. 2015. "The characteristics, experiences and perceptions of naturopathic and herbal medicine practitioners: results from a national survey in New Zealand." *BMC Complement Altern Med* 15: 114. doi: 10.1186/s12906-015-0616-5.

Coulter, M. K., and M. E. Dean. 2007. "Homeopathy for attention deficit/hyperactivity disorder or hyperkinetic disorder." *Cochrane Database Syst Rev* 4: CD005648. doi: 10.1002/14651858. CD005648.pub2.

Danno, K., A. Colas, J. L. Masson, and M. F. Bordet. 2013. "Homeopathic treatment of migraine in children: results of a prospective, multicenter, observational study." *J Altern Complement Med* 19(2): 119–23. doi: 10.1089/acm.2011.0821.

Dave, U. P., S. R. Dingankar, V. S. Saxena, J. A. Joseph, B. Bethapudi, A. Agarwal, and V. Kudiganti. 2014. "An open-label study to elucidate the effects of standardized Bacopa monnieri extract in the management of symptoms of attention-deficit hyperactivity disorder in children." *Adv Mind Body Med* 28(2): 10–15.

Downey, L., P. T. Tyree, C. E. Huebner, and W. E. Lafferty. 2010. "Pediatric vaccination and vaccine-preventable disease acquisition: associations with care by complementary and alternative medicine providers." *Matern Child Health J* 14(6): 922–30. doi: 10.1007/s10995-009-0519-5.

Edwards, E., D. Mischoulon, M. Rapaport, B. Stussman, and W. Weber. 2013. "Building an evidence base in complementary and integrative healthcare for child and adolescent psychiatry." *Child Adolesc Psychiatr Clin N Am* 22(3): 509–29, vii. doi: 10.1016/j.chc.2013.03.007.

Frei, H., R. Everts, K. von Ammon, F. Kaufmann, D. Walther, S. F. Schmitz, M. Collenberg, M. Steinlin, C. Lim, and A. Thurneysen. 2007. "Randomised controlled trials of homeopathy in hyperactive children: treatment procedure leads to an unconventional study design. Experience with open-label homeopathic treatment preceding the Swiss ADHD placebo controlled, randomised, double-blind, cross-over trial." *Homeopathy* 96(1): 35–41. doi: 10.1016/j.homp.2006.11.004.

Frei, H., and A. Thurneysen. 2001. "Homeopathy in acute otitis media in children: treatment effect or spontaneous resolution?" *Br Homeopath J* 90(4): 180–2.

Gadgil, V. D. 2010. "Understanding ayurveda." *J Ayurveda Integr Med* 1(1): 77–80. doi: 10.4103/0975-9476.59836.

Haidvogl, M., D. S. Riley, M. Heger, S. Brien, M. Jong, M. Fischer, G. T. Lewith, G. Jansen, and A. E. Thurneysen. 2007. "Homeopathic and conventional treatment for acute respiratory and ear complaints: a comparative study on outcome in the primary care setting." *BMC Complement Altern Med* 7: 7. doi: 10.1186/1472-6882-7-7.

Haller, C. A., and N. L. Benowitz. 2000. "Adverse cardiovascular and central nervous system events associated with dietary supplements containing ephedra alkaloids." *N Engl J Med* 343(25): 1833–8. doi: 10.1056/NEJM200012213432502.

Huang, T. P., P. H. Liu, A. S. Lien, S. L. Yang, H. H. Chang, and H. R. Yen. 2013. "Characteristics of traditional Chinese medicine use in children with asthma: a nationwide population-based study." *Allergy* 68(12): 1610–13. doi: 10.1111/all.12273.

Jacobs, J., D. A. Springer, and D. Crothers. 2001. "Homeopathic treatment of acute otitis media in children: a preliminary randomized placebo-controlled trial." *Pediatr Infect Dis J* 20(2): 177–83.

Kassab, S., M. Cummings, S. Berkovitz, R. van Haselen, and P. Fisher. 2009. "Homeopathic medicines for adverse effects of cancer treatments." *Cochrane Database Syst Rev* 2: CD004845. doi: 10.1002/14651858.CD004845.pub2.

Kean, J. D., J. Kaufman, J. Lomas, A. Goh, D. White, D. Simpson, A. Scholey, H. Singh, J. Sarris, A. Zangara, and C. Stough. 2015. "A randomized controlled trial investigating the effects of a special extract of Bacopa monnieri (CDRI 08) on hyperactivity and inattention in male children and adolescents: BACHI Study Protocol (ANZCTRN12612000827831)." *Nutrients* 7(12): 9931–45. doi: 10.3390/nu7125507.

Klein, S. D., L. Torchetti, M. Frei-Erb, and U. Wolf. 2015. "Usage of complementary medicine in Switzerland: results of the Swiss Health Survey 2012 and development since 2007." *PLoS One* 10(10): e0141985. doi: 10.1371/journal.pone.0141985.

Kuehn, B. M. 2009. "Despite health claims by manufacturers, little oversight for homeopathic products." *JAMA* 302(15): 1631–2, 1634. doi: 10.1001/jama.2009.1476.

Lee, A. C., and K. J. Kemper. 2000. "Homeopathy and naturopathy: practice characteristics and pediatric care." *Arch Pediatr Adolesc Med* 154(1): 75–80.

Liu, J., X. Mo, D. Wu, A. Ou, S. Xue, C. Liu, H. Li, Z. Wen, and D. Chen. 2015. "Efficacy of a Chinese herbal medicine for the treatment of atopic dermatitis: a randomised controlled study." *Complement Ther Med* 23(5): 644–51. doi: 10.1016/j.ctim.2015.07.006.

Merrell, W. C., and E. Shalts. 2002. "Homeopathy." *Med Clin North Am* 86(1): 47–62.

Mukherjee, P. K., N. K. Nema, P. Venkatesh, and P. K. Debnath. 2012. "Changing scenario for promotion and development of Ayurveda—way forward." *J Ethnopharmacol* 143(2): 424–34. doi: 10.1016/j.jep.2012.07.036.

National Ayurvedic Medical Association. http://www.ayurvedanama.org/.

National Center for Complementary and Integrative Health [a]. "Naturopathy." https://nccih.nih.gov/health/naturopathy.

National Center for Complementary and Integrative Health [b]. "Traditional Chinese Medicine." https://nccih.nih.gov/health/whatiscam/chinesemed.htm.

Nestler, G. 2002. "Traditional Chinese medicine." *Med Clin North Am* 86(1): 63–73.

Oberbaum, M., I. Yaniv, Y. Ben-Gal, J. Stein, N. Ben-Zvi, L. S. Freedman, and D. Branski. 2001. "A randomized, controlled clinical trial of the homeopathic medication TRAUMEEL S in the treatment of chemotherapy-induced stomatitis in children undergoing stem cell transplantation." *Cancer* 92(3): 684–90.

Patwardhan, B., D. Warude, P. Pushpangadan, and N. Bhatt. 2005. "Ayurveda and traditional Chinese medicine: a comparative overview." *Evid Based Complement Alternat Med* 2(4): 465–73. doi: 10.1093/ecam/neh140.

Ramchandani, N. M. 2010. "Homoeopathic treatment of upper respiratory tract infections in children: evaluation of thirty case series." *Complement Ther Clin Pract* 16(2): 101–8. doi: 10.1016/j.ctcp.2009.09.008.

Romeyke, T., and H. Stummer. 2015. "Evidence-based complementary and alternative medicine in inpatient care: take a look at Europe." *J Evid Based Complementary Altern Med* 20(2): 87–93. doi: 10.1177/2156587214555714.

Rossi, E., P. Bartoli, A. Bianchi, and M. Da Fre. 2012. "Homeopathy in paediatric atopic diseases: long-term results in children with atopic dermatitis." *Homeopathy* 101(1): 13–20. doi: 10.1016/j.homp.2011.09.003.

Saper, R. B., R. S. Phillips, A. Sehgal, N. Khouri, R. B. Davis, J. Paquin, V. Thuppil, and S. N. Kales. 2008. "Lead, mercury, and arsenic in US- and Indian-manufactured Ayurvedic medicines sold via the Internet." *JAMA* 300(8): 915–23. doi: 10.1001/jama.300.8.915.

Sarrell, E. M., H. A. Cohen, and E. Kahan. 2003. "Naturopathic treatment for ear pain in children." *Pediatrics* 111(5 Pt 1): e574–9.

Schmidt, J. M. 2010. "200 years Organon of Medicine: a comparative review of its six editions (1810–1842)." *Homeopathy* 99(4): 271–7. doi: 10.1016/j.homp.2010.08.004.

Sencer, S. F., T. Zhou, L. S. Freedman, J. A. Ives, Z. Chen, D. Wall, M. L. Nieder, S. A. Grupp, L. C. Yu, I. Sahdev, W. B. Jonas, J. D. Wallace, and M. Oberbaum. 2012. "Traumeel S in preventing and treating mucositis in young patients undergoing SCT: a report of the Children's Oncology Group." *Bone Marrow Transplant* 47(11): 1409–14. doi: 10.1038/bmt.2012.30.

Shafei, H. F., S. M. AbdelDayem, and N. H. Mohamed. 2012. "Individualized homeopathy in a group of Egyptian asthmatic children." *Homeopathy* 101(4): 224–30. doi: 10.1016/j.homp.2012.08.006.

Sinha, M. N., V. A. Siddiqui, C. Nayak, V. Singh, R. Dixit, D. Dewan, and A. Mishra. 2012. "Randomized controlled pilot study to compare homeopathy and conventional therapy in acute otitis media." *Homeopathy* 101(1): 5–12. doi: 10.1016/j.homp.2011.08.003.

Spigelblatt, L. 2005. "Homeopathy in the paediatric population." *Paediatr Child Health* 10(3): 173–7.

Tang, J. L., B. Y. Liu, and K. W. Ma. 2008. "Traditional Chinese medicine." *Lancet* 372(9654): 1938–40. doi: 10.1016/S0140-6736(08)61354-9.

Taylor, J. A., and J. Jacobs. 2011. "Homeopathic ear drops as an adjunct to standard therapy in children with acute otitis media." *Homeopathy* 100(3): 109–15. doi: 10.1016/j.homp.2011.03.002.

Trichard, M., G. Chaufferin, and N. Nicoloyannis. 2005. "Pharmacoeconomic comparison between homeopathic and antibiotic treatment strategies in recurrent acute rhinopharyngitis in children." *Homeopathy* 94(1): 3–9.

Waisse, S. 2012. "The science of high dilutions in historical context." *Homeopathy* 101(2): 129–37. doi: 10.1016/j.homp.2012.01.001.

Witt, C. M., R. Ludtke, and S. N. Willich. 2010. "Homeopathic treatment of patients with migraine: a prospective observational study with a 2-year follow-up period." *J Altern Complement Med* 16(4): 347–55. doi: 10.1089/acm.2009.0376.

Yang, C., Z. Hao, L. L. Zhang, and Q. Guo. 2015. "Efficacy and safety of acupuncture in children: an overview of systematic reviews." *Pediatr Res* 78(2): 112–19. doi: 10.1038/pr.2015.91.

Yen, H. R., K. L. Liang, T. P. Huang, J. Y. Fan, T. T. Chang, and M. F. Sun. 2015. "Characteristics of traditional Chinese medicine use for children with allergic rhinitis: a nationwide population-based study." *Int J Pediatr Otorhinolaryngol* 79(4): 591–7. doi: 10.1016/j.ijporl.2015.02.002.

13 Bioenergetic Therapies

Bioenergetic therapies have come to attention in modern medicine as non-invasive therapies that are low cost, technology free, and useful in offering comfort and reducing pain and anxiety in patients with a wide variety of conditions. Some of the oldest types of bioenergetic therapies are shamanism and spiritual healing, which reach dimensions far beyond the boundaries of the typical biopsychosocial healthcare model, causing many to view them with skepticism. The underlying premise in the bioenergetic therapies is that a healthy individual is considered to have an energy field that supports balanced and unobstructed flow, whereas a patient with an imbalanced or obstructed energy field may present with physical or emotional symptoms. The common goal of the bioenergetic therapies is opening of the mind, body, and spirit to encourage the potential for deep healing to occur (Engebretson and Wardell 2012).

Newer iterations of the bioenergetic therapies include reiki, which originated in Japan, and therapeutic touch and healing touch, both originating from the nursing domain. Other bioenergetic therapies include acupuncture, qi gong, tai chi, and homeopathy, all thought to work by harnessing the energetic power of the body. The mechanisms of actions of the bioenergetic therapies as a group have not been fully elucidated, which has naturally slowed their acceptance into mainstream medicine. The bioenergetic therapies may be unfamiliar to some practitioners but are frequently used by patients. An estimated 23,300 adults reported use of some type of bioenergetic therapy in the 2007 NHIS survey (Barnes, Bloom, and Nahin 2008).

More recently, therapeutic touch and healing touch have been growing in popularity with hospital programs in the U.S. in both acute and non-acute settings as a non-pharmaceutical approach to complement conventional care, thereby serving as an important conduit for introduction to a broader medical audience (Rindfleisch 2010; Dufresne et al. 2015).

One of the main cautions noted by the National Center for Complementary and Integrative Health Care is that bioenergetic therapies are not recommended as a substitute for conventional care, and individuals should not postpone seeing a healthcare provider about a health condition, especially one that is chronic or severe.

Background

It is widely recognized that the body has sophisticated electrical pathways, commonly measured by electrocardiogram, electroencephalogram, and electromyography, but discussion of bioenergetic therapies pushes into territory where identification of subtle energies that may surround and move through the body have not been definitely measured or recorded. Theories based in quantum physics and wave theory exist, although to date no consensus has been reached and measurement tools for the bioenergetics therapies remain areas of active study. Despite these challenges, some positive clinical results have been reported. One example shows measurable effects of non-local healing energy. In an experiment by Achterberg et al., 22 recipients placed in fMRI scanners distant from experienced energy healers showed measurable changes in brain activity when the healers sent non-local energy healing. Correlation of brain changes with a randomized "on-off" sequence by the healers was found to be highly significant ($p < 0.000127$) (Achterberg et al. 2005).

Acupuncture point stimulation has also been associated with measurable change in brain function based on fMRI imaging (Chae et al. 2013). Some large reviews of healing therapies have shown modest positive effects in adults; for example, a 2008 Cochrane review of touch therapies for pain included 24 studies involving 1153 adult patients who experienced therapeutic touch, healing touch, or reiki and concluded that touch therapies "may have a modest effect on pain relief." No significant placebo effect was seen in this systematic review (So, Jiang, and Qin 2008).

A second large review of 66 studies on biofield therapies including therapeutic touch, healing touch, or reiki in adults found supporting evidence for the reduction of pain in certain patient populations, reduction of anxiety in hospitalized patients, and reduction of agitated behavior in dementia patients in the study population (Jain and Mills 2010). Studies on the use of biofield therapies in children remain sparse, although interest and demand for them have been shown to increase in families where children have a new cancer diagnosis (McLean and Kemper 2006).

Research on these therapies remains active and guidelines have been established for ongoing research (Jonas and Chez 2004; Feinstein and Eden 2008).

Therapeutic Touch

Summary and Overview

Therapeutic touch is a technique that has become more widely recognized in the last 25 years. It has been used to promote physical healing, management of pain, and for reduction of anxiety, depression, and other stressors. By definition therapeutic touch involves the assimilation of energies, which are transferred by means of the healer's hands, purportedly establishing a kind of association between the healer and patient (Mulloney and Wells-Federman 1996).

Brief History

Therapeutic touch (often abbreviated as TT) in its current form originated in the 1970s from a collaboration between Dr. Dolores Krieger, Ph.D., R.N., Professor Emeritus at New York University, and associate Dora Kunz, an intuitive healer who together established a healing procedure directed towards those with difficult to treat medical problems. The technique is based on the theory that humans are comprised of complex and multidimensional energy systems that are in constant flux with others and their surroundings. This complex interactivity creates potential for one to modulate the energy field of another as seen in the study of the universal life force found in many Eastern cultures and religions (Mulloney and Wells-Federman 1996).

Types of Assessments Offered

Therapeutic touch helps the individual to attain a sense of natural healing and calmness. The basic approach includes the therapist centering their awareness while generating a compassionate intention to promote the patient's innate potential for self-healing. Physical contact is not required. The therapist is trained to perceive the human energy field by sense of touch, and uses hands approximately 2–6 inches above the body to modulate the flow of energy around the patient. There are five phases of therapeutic touch, taught as: centering, assessment, clearing or unruffling, treatment, and evaluation. One of the goals of the procedure is to facilitate the relaxation response in the patient, which in turn facilitates the healing response. Therapists may perceive sensations such as warmth, coolness, static, and tingling (Mulloney and Wells-Federman 1996). Therapeutic touch has been evaluated in adults for a variety of conditions including: pain, wound healing, disability associated with arthritis, tension headache, burn-related pain and anxiety, and post-operative pain, although studies have been hampered by variable quality of design and small sample size (Fazzino et al. 2010).

Evidence in Pediatrics

Pediatric studies are relatively sparse. An early randomized pilot study in 20 HIV-positive children aged 6–12 years demonstrated the effectiveness of therapeutic touch in reduction of anxiety as compared to controls (Ireland 1998).

A review by Ireland and Olson of 14 massage studies and five therapeutic touch studies in a broad range of children showed that both modalities reliably triggered the relaxation response. However, the massage studies overall had better quality of design and more consistent positive results. Insufficient evidence was found to recommend therapeutic touch without further study in this review. No adverse events were reported (Ireland and Olson 2000).

A randomized trial of 78 premature infants evaluated weight, length of hospital stay, medical complications, and parental satisfaction with care in infants receiving therapeutic touch. Results showed a significant reduction in length of stay and rate of medical complication in the treatment group (Dominguez Rosales et al. 2009). Another small study of 40 infants hospitalized in the NICU showed reduction of perceived pain after procedure in infants receiving therapeutic touch as measured by statistically significant reductions in heart rate, respiratory rate, and pain score (Ramada, Almeida Fde, and Cunha 2013).

A study of 10 hospitalized premature infants demonstrated that therapeutic touch was effective in reducing neural activation in response to stimulation mimicking a heel stick as measured by non-invasive near-infrared spectroscopy measuring cerebral oxygenation in sleeping infants undergoing a controlled sensory stimulus. Therapeutic touch was delivered by a trained nurse holding the baby in both hands from 1 minute before stimulus to 30 seconds after stimulus. Although study size was small, these findings add to the growing number of studies searching for non-pharmacologic approaches to pain management in vulnerable infants (Honda et al. 2013).

Cautions and Possible Side Effects

In general, therapeutic touch is considered a safe, gentle treatment. No reports exist of serious adverse events in generally healthy individuals. Reports of fatigue, lightheadedness, or emotional release during therapy exist. Appropriate caution or avoidance should be considered in any patient with psychosis or other serious mental illness, or in those with a history of physical, sexual, or emotional abuse. Bioenergetic therapies should not replace conventional workup if diagnosis is uncertain or in cases where acute care is indicated. It is generally recommended that children, elderly people, or those in poor health should be treated for a very short span of time.

Training and Licensing in the U.S. and Internationally

Credentialing is available through the Therapeutic Touch International Association (http://therapeutic-touch.org). No specific background requirements or licensing exist. Training to become a qualified therapeutic touch practitioner typically consists of a minimum of 12 hours of basic training and 14 hours of intermediate training taught by a qualified practitioner. A 1-year mentorship is also required which includes documentation of case studies and practice sessions.

Healing Touch

Summary and Overview

Healing touch is another bioenergetic therapy that comes out of the nursing domain, with roots in ancient shamanic and aboriginal healing traditions. The technique may involve both physical touch and noncontact touch above the body. It purportedly initiates a flow of energy, establishing a connection between therapist and patient with the goal of facilitating a sense of peace and healing in the recipient. Similar to therapeutic touch, the premise is to restore and balance the energy of the patient's body and spirit.

Brief History and Types of Assessments Offered

The Healing Touch program was founded by Janet Mentgen, R.N., BSN in 1980, with sponsorship of the American Holistic Nurses Association (AHNA). It is based in part on the work done in therapeutic touch and incorporates ancient healing practices from cultures around the world. The practice involves the therapist setting an intention for the highest good of the patient and placement of hands in a certain pattern on or just above the patient's body. The originally developed standardized curriculum is taught through the Healing Touch Program (HTP) (http://www.healingtouchprogram.com) still offered through the Mentgen family. Classes progress from beginning to advanced practice.

The initial step in the process involves the preparation of the healer to summon their own energies to provide assistance in healing. The treatment process begins with a scan of the patient's energy field by placement of the therapist's hand over the body of the client, concentrating on the affected areas. The healer then decides which healing touch techniques should be used. It is used in outpatient, inpatient, and office settings and has also been used in the operating suite and for pre- and post-operative care. It has been introduced into several academic medical centers in the U.S. Healing touch has been evaluated in adults for a variety of conditions including: chronic pain, fibromyalgia, anxiety, post-operative pain, and nausea with mixed positive effects reported. Serious adverse events have not been reported (Anderson and Taylor 2011).

Evidence in Pediatrics

A small pilot study by Kemper et al. evaluated the use of healing touch in pediatric oncology patients and found a statistically significant reduction in stress and decrease in sympathetic activation as measured by heart rate variability (Kemper et al. 2009).

Healing touch has also been used successfully in preterm infants in the NICU in reducing perceived pain as measured by heart rate, oxygenation saturation, and observed pain in a retrospective study of 186 hospitalized neonates when used alone or in conjunction with massage (Hathaway et al. 2015).

Cautions and Possible Side Effects

Healing touch is generally considered a gentle and safe therapy. No serious adverse events have been reported. Like the other bioenergetics therapies, it does not replace conventional care, and people suffering from an ongoing disease should consult with their doctors before treatment. The standard cautions regarding treatment of those with any prior history of trauma (physical, sexual, emotional) or mental illness apply.

Training and Licensing in the U.S. and Internationally

A standardized curriculum covering five levels is available through the Healing Touch Program (http://www.healingtouchprogram.com). Levels 1, 2, and 3 consist of a minimum of 16 hours of course work. Levels 4 and 5 require 30 hours per level. Students who complete each level become eligible for certification. A 1-year mentorship is an integral part of the program. There are no restrictions as to who may take the training. The Healing Touch certification program is currently offered in over 30 countries.

Reiki

Summary and Overview

Reiki is a Japanese term equated with universal life energy, "rei" (universal energy), and "ki" (life energy of all living creatures), introduced as a healing therapy by Dr. Mikao Usui in Japan in the 1840s. It is used to purportedly channel the universal life force to the recipient with the intent for strength, balance, and physical and mental healing. Technically, reiki can be performed with or without direct touch similar to therapeutic and healing touch therapies. Reiki has been studied in adults in a variety of conditions including: musculoskeletal pain, wound healing, stress, post-operative pain, and anxiety. Results are mixed and again limited by study design and small sample sizes as those in the other bioenergetic therapies (Hammerschlag, Marx, and Aickin 2014).

One randomized controlled study done in 49 hospitalized cardiac patients at Yale-New Haven Hospital showed that those receiving reiki treatment by trained nurses had a more beneficial effect on heart rate variability and emotional state than those experiencing music therapy or quiet resting as a control (Friedman et al. 2010).

Reiki is also being explored as a therapy with potential to benefit caregivers (Kundu et al. 2013), and as a supportive therapy for healthcare professionals (Tarantino et al. 2013; Rosada et al. 2015).

Brief History and Assessments

The practitioner begins the treatment with either a hands-on or hands-off technique and sessions vary in length. Training can be undertaken by anyone, and no prior training is required. Reiki training consists of two levels and is received in sessions called attunements provided by a reiki master. Training is variable and there is no national certifying body.

Additional training is needed to progress to the level of reiki master.

Evidence in Pediatrics

Evidence to support the efficacy of reiki in pediatrics remains sparse. In one study, an in-hospital reiki training program offered to 18 families of children admitted to either medical or oncology services was found by 65% of families to enhance relaxation and improve comfort in their hospitalized child. Pain relief was experienced by 41% of participating children. Additional benefits were the family's sense of active participation in the child's care (Kundu et al. 2013).

Cautions and Possible Side Effects

Due caution is indicated with any patient with history of mental illness, or history of physical, sexual, or emotional abuse. Vulnerable patients such as those undergoing treatment for cancer or other serious illness or the very young or old are recommended to receive short treatments in proportion to their tolerance.

Training and Licensing in the U.S. and Internationally

Courses of different varieties are offered around the world to obtain professional qualifications and training to become a reiki practitioner. No national or international standardized certification process exists (Cohen 2004).

When discussing bioenergetic therapies with a patient it is important to keep an open mind so as to invite a full discussion of all therapies in use. Familiarity with the basic bioenergetic therapies can help the practitioner be ready to address questions or provide resources to patients and families. It is important to fully understand the background and training of any complementary practitioner and their experience treating children of various ages. This holds especially true with the bioenergetic therapies where training is less standardized and no licensing or minimum standards for education exist.

Rindfleisch, MD, MPhil provides an excellent overview of an expanded range of bioenergetic therapies applied in primary care in a 2010 article in the journal *Primary Care* (Rindfleisch 2010).

In general, the bioenergetic therapies can be viewed as gentle, non-invasive therapies that can offer comfort to patients and their caregivers with a wide range of medical issues.

They should be provided by a trained individual and are not intended to take the place of conventional care as needed. Family members have also been taught how to administer these therapies to their own children to good effect, which has resulted in a feeling of greater connection and involvement in the child's treatment.

References

Achterberg, J., K. Cooke, T. Richards, L. J. Standish, L. Kozak, and J. Lake. 2005. "Evidence for correlations between distant intentionality and brain function in recipients: a functional magnetic resonance imaging analysis." *J Altern Complement Med* 11(6): 965–71. doi: 10.1089/acm.2005.11.965.

Anderson, J. G., and A. G. Taylor. 2011. "Effects of healing touch in clinical practice: a systematic review of randomized clinical trials." *J Holist Nurs* 29(3): 221–8. doi: 10.1177/0898010110393353.

Barnes, P. M., B. Bloom, and R. L. Nahin. 2008. "Complementary and alternative medicine use among adults and children: United States, 2007." *Natl Health Stat Report* 12: 1–23.

Chae, Y., D. S. Chang, S. H. Lee, W. M. Jung, I. S. Lee, S. Jackson, J. Kong, H. Lee, H. J. Park, H. Lee, and C. Wallraven. 2013. "Inserting needles into the body: a meta-analysis of brain activity associated with acupuncture needle stimulation." *J Pain* 14(3): 215–22. doi: 10.1016/j.jpain.2012.11.011.

Cohen, M. H. 2004. "Legal and ethical issues in complementary medicine: a United States perspective." *Med J Aust* 181(3): 168–9.

Dominguez Rosales, R., M. J. Albar Marin, B. Tena Garcia, M. T. Ruiz Perez, M. J. Garzon Real, M. A. Rosado Poveda, and E. Gonzalez Caro. 2009. "[Effectiveness of the application of therapeutic touch on weight, complications, and length of hospital stay in preterm newborns attended in a neonatal unit]." *Enferm Clin* 19(1): 11–5. doi: 10.1016/j.enfcli.2008.07.001.

Dufresne, F., B. Simmons, P. J. Vlachostergios, Z. Fleischner, R. Joudeh, J. Blakeway, and K. Julliard. 2015. "Feasibility of energy medicine in a community teaching hospital: an exploratory case series." *J Altern Complement Med* 21(6): 339–49. doi: 10.1089/acm.2014.0157.

Engebretson, J., and D. W. Wardell. 2012. "Energy therapies: focus on spirituality." *Explore (NY)* 8(6): 353–9. doi: 10.1016/j.explore.2012.08.004.

Fazzino, D. L., M. T. Griffin, R. S. McNulty, and J. J. Fitzpatrick. 2010. "Energy healing and pain: a review of the literature." *Holist Nurs Pract* 24(2): 79–88. doi: 10.1097/HNP.0b013e3181d39718.

Feinstein, D., and D. Eden. 2008. "Six pillars of energy medicine: clinical strengths of a complementary paradigm." *Altern Ther Health Med* 14(1): 44–54.

Friedman, R. S., M. M. Burg, P. Miles, F. Lee, and R. Lampert. 2010. "Effects of reiki on autonomic activity early after acute coronary syndrome." *J Am Coll Cardiol* 56(12): 995–6. doi: 10.1016/j.jacc.2010.03.082.

Hammerschlag, R., B. L. Marx, and M. Aickin. 2014. "Nontouch biofield therapy: a systematic review of human randomized controlled trials reporting use of only nonphysical contact treatment." *J Altern Complement Med* 20(12): 881–92. doi: 10.1089/acm.2014.0017.

Hathaway, E. E., C. M. Luberto, L. H. Bogenschutz, S. Geiss, R. S. Wasson, and S. Cotton. 2015. "Integrative care therapies and physiological and pain-related outcomes in hospitalized infants." *Glob Adv Health Med* 4(4): 32–7. doi: 10.7453/gahmj.2015.029.

Honda, N., S. Ohgi, N. Wada, K. K. Loo, Y. Higashimoto, and K. Fukuda. 2013. "Effect of therapeutic touch on brain activation of preterm infants in response to sensory punctate stimulus: a near-infrared spectroscopy-based study." *Arch Dis Child Fetal Neonatal Ed* 98(3): F244–8. doi: 10.1136/archdischild-2011-301469.

Ireland, M. 1998. "Therapeutic touch with HIV-infected children: a pilot study." *J Assoc Nurses AIDS Care* 9(4): 68–77. doi: 10.1016/S1055-3290(98)80046-0.

Ireland, M., and M. Olson. 2000. "Massage therapy and therapeutic touch in children: state of the science." *Altern Ther Health Med* 6(5): 54–63.

Jain, S., and P. J. Mills. 2010. "Biofield therapies: helpful or full of hype? A best evidence synthesis." *Int J Behav Med* 17(1): 1–16. doi: 10.1007/s12529-009-9062-4.

Jonas, W. B., and R. A. Chez. 2004. "Recommendations regarding definitions and standards in healing research." *J Altern Complement Med* 10(1): 171–81. doi: 10.1089/107555304322849101.

Kemper, K. J., N. B. Fletcher, C. A. Hamilton, and T. W. McLean. 2009. "Impact of healing touch on pediatric oncology outpatients: pilot study." *J Soc Integr Oncol* 7(1): 12–8.

Kundu, A., R. Dolan-Oves, M. A. Dimmers, C. B. Towle, and A. Z. Doorenbos. 2013. "Reiki training for caregivers of hospitalized pediatric patients: a pilot program." *Complement Ther Clin Pract* 19(1): 50–4. doi: 10.1016/j.ctcp.2012.08.001.

McLean, T. W., and K. J. Kemper. 2006. "Complementary and alternative medicine therapies in pediatric oncology patients." *J Soc Integr Oncol* 4(1): 40–5.

Mulloney, S. S., and C. Wells-Federman. 1996. "Therapeutic touch: a healing modality." *J Cardiovasc Nurs* 10(3): 27–49.

Ramada, N. C., A. Almeida Fde, and M. L. Cunha. 2013. "Therapeutic touch: influence on vital signs of newborns." *Einstein (Sao Paulo)* 11(4): 421–5.

Rindfleisch, J. A. 2010. "Biofield therapies: energy medicine and primary care." *Prim Care* 37(1): 165–79. doi: 10.1016/j.pop.2009.09.012.

Rosada, R. M., B. Rubik, B. Mainguy, J. Plummer, and L. Mehl-Madrona. 2015. "Reiki reduces burnout among community mental health clinicians." *J Altern Complement Med* 21(8): 489–95. doi: 10.1089/acm.2014.0403.

So, P. S., Y. Jiang, and Y. Qin. 2008. "Touch therapies for pain relief in adults." *Cochrane Database Syst Rev* 4: CD006535. doi: 10.1002/14651858.CD006535.pub2.

Tarantino, B., M. Earley, D. Audia, C. D'Adamo, and B. Berman. 2013. "Qualitative and quantitative evaluation of a pilot integrative coping and resiliency program for healthcare professionals." *Explore (NY)* 9(1): 44–7. doi: 10.1016/j.explore.2012.10.002.

Part 4

Clinical Application

14 An Integrative Approach to Preventive Health

Time available for pediatric preventive care in clinical visits has become more and more constricted in the tightly controlled insurance reimbursement climate in the U.S. However, despite the challenges, preventive care remains a major focus in pediatric integrative medicine.

In the U.S. there are typically 32 well child visits, including the prenatal visit, with the majority occurring before the age of 5 years. These offer an important opportunity to reinforce a lifelong foundation of health. The integrative medicine model can be used to enrich these visits by introducing more detailed information on nutrition, selected dietary supplements, stress management tools, physical activity, and sleep counseling and to harness emerging data on topics such as environmental health and the microbiome to maximize children's wellbeing.

Once past the infant stage, an estimated 20% of pediatric office visits are due to behavioral or mental issues, highlighting the importance of addressing nurturing relationships, family and peer connections, self-regulation skills, self-efficacy, effective behavior change, and development of empathy and compassion for others—skills that are routinely taught in integrative medicine.

The Bright Futures resources through the American Academy of Pediatrics provides a foundation of rich resources on traditional pediatric health and health screening, and continues to serve as a classic blueprint for those caring for children and adolescents. The Bright Futures guidelines were updated in 2014, with some of the biggest changes including recommendation for depression screening annually from age 11–21. Screening for dyslipidemia is now recommended for patients between 9 and 11 years old, screening for HIV between 16 and 18 years old (Geoffrey et al. 2014).

This chapter includes a discussion and checklist of proposed integrative anticipatory guidance suggestions by age. Ideally these guidelines would be introduced and consistently reinforced in an integrative medical home that supports child, family, and clinician health. Some opportunities to influence the health of the newborn begin long before birth. As in any practice of medicine, cultural considerations should be respected, and thoughtful assessment of the risk–benefit ratio of any therapy done prior to its use.

Immunizations

The integrative approach in the model presented here fully supports the use of routine immunizations. Despite historic and ongoing controversy, the protective benefits are enormous against illnesses that continue to be prevalent around the world. Although a polarizing topic, no child is well served when adults take extreme positions in this debate. No family should be dismissed from a practice for refusing to vaccinate, just as no family should be encouraged to rely on "herd immunity," relying on high vaccination rates on other children as a protective mechanism for their own children. This places children who are too young to be vaccinated, those without access to medical care or unable to be vaccinated for medical reasons, or children who did not get a full immunologic response at real risk of exposure to serious illnesses (Buttenheim 2012).

Some parents resist vaccinations on moral or religious grounds, or due to underestimation of real risk to their children. Others fear triggering of autism or other serious neurological disease, or have deep skepticism that vaccines can actually prevent illnesses. Of concern, vaccine refusal rates are increasing in the U.S. which tracks with increasing prevalence of outbreaks of measles and pertussis (Omer et al. 2009).

One of the early spikes in anti-vaccination sentiment was caused by a now infamous article by Andrew Wakefield erroneously linking the measles-mumps-rubella (MMR) vaccine to autism. The article was published in *Lancet* in 1998 and later retracted (Editors of The Lancet 2010).

Author Wakefield and his two co-authors were charged with professional misconduct and falsifying research. Wakefield was eventually banned from the practice of medicine. Despite the serious professional fallout to Wakefield, the ripple effect from his erroneous work has been far reaching. Rates of immunization remain impacted in the U.S. and in other developed countries despite a range of large well-designed studies disproving the association between vaccines and any pattern of serious neurodevelopmental disease (Gilmour et al. 2011; Demicheli et al. 2012).

Additional parental concerns involve the number and pacing of vaccines in the current schedule in the first 24 months of life. Again, no established correlation between this schedule and serious neurodevelopmental or immunological outcome has been reported. The American Academy of Pediatrics encourages practitioners to encourage open and respectful dialogue with parents about vaccines, and to work with the parents to be sure every child is fully vaccinated (Gilmour et al. 2011).

Although the term "alternate vaccine schedule" is popular, studies show that the majority of families using this approach are following informal recommendations from family, or picking and choosing vaccines based on input from friends. A minority of 748 families in a study by Dempsey were working with their child's medical provider to formulate a vaccine schedule (Dempsey et al. 2011).

Ideally, striking a balance between mutual respect, trust, flexibility, and collaboration and using evidence-based educational tools will help the parent–clinician team provide the best protection from what in many cases are 100% vaccine-preventable illnesses (Glanz, Kraus, and Daley 2015).

Studies have shown that clinicians who are willing to listen, and who manifest openness with eye contact, receptive body language, and mindful presence in the room are most likely to connect successfully with parents and be able to fully understand their fears and concerns (Leask et al. 2012).

A newer term emerging in the global public health literature is vaccine hesitancy, described by the World Health Organization Strategic Advisory Group of Experts as being influenced by "complacency, convenience, and confidence." Efforts are underway to improve educational approaches and resources and to support global efforts to best protect children from preventable illness (Kumar et al. 2016).

Lifestyle Foundations: Maternal Health

Nutrition

Maternal diet is important to fetal health, and accruing research offers more details on best approaches. A "prudent" diet inclusive of vegetables, fruits, oils, whole grains, water as primary beverage, and fiber rich bread was shown to be associated with statistically significant reduced risk of preterm delivery in a population study of 66,000 pregnant women in Norway as compared to a "Western" diet that included salty and sweet snack foods, white bread, processed meats, and desserts. The traditional diet in this study consisted of potatoes and fish and was also associated with reduction in risk of preterm delivery compared to a "Western" diet (Englund-Ogge et al. 2014).

Weight Management: Obesity Risks

Maintenance of healthy weight throughout pregnancy has long-term implications for fetal and infant health. The 2013 American College of Obstetricians and Gynecologists Committee Opinion No. 549 on Obesity in Pregnancy recommends that preconception counseling should review the fetal risks of obesity in pregnancy which include: gestational diabetes, hypertension, preeclampsia, increased rate of cesarean delivery, and post-partum weight retention. Fetal complications have also been widely reported and include: prematurity, stillbirth, higher rate of congenital anomalies—including neural tube defect, and large for gestational age which predisposes to childhood and adolescent obesity. The report recommends that nutrition counseling and encouragement to begin an exercise program should be offered to all overweight or obese women. Maternal obesity has also been shown to reduce initiation and success at breastfeeding (American College of Obstetricians and Gynecologists 2013).

Dietary Supplements

Similar to folate, docosahexaenoic acid (DHA) has an important role in fetal development. DHA is integral in formation of the fetal brain and nervous system, especially during the third trimester when the fetal brain approximately doubles in size (Makrides 2013).

DHA is also needed for development of the rods and cones of the retina, sperm, and testicles (De Giuseppe, Roggi, and Cena 2014). Adequate DHA has also shown a significant association with prolonging gestation and reducing the risk of preterm delivery at less than 34 weeks gestation in both low-risk and in high-risk pregnancies (Mozurkewich and Klemens 2012).

Maternal consumption of omega-3 fatty acids during and post-pregnancy may also confer a protective effect against allergy by lowering allergen specific Th2 responses and elevated Th1 responses (D'Vaz et al. 2012).

Maternal DHA has also been shown to affect DNA methylation patterns, and research is active examining how this may impact fetal lipid metabolism and future development of lipid disorders (Khaire, Kale, and Joshi 2015).

Although the optimal maternal level is not known, metabolic stores of DHA have been shown to reduce by half during pregnancy and may not return to pre-pregnancy levels until 6 months postpartum. Adequate levels of DHA can be attained through food, especially fish, but mercury contamination can be a concern, especially in pregnancy.

The U.S. EPA is one organization that provides useful resources on this issue (United States Environmental Protection Agency [a]; National Resources Defense Council).

The recommended minimum DHA supplement dose for pregnant and lactating women is 200 mg per day according to the International Society for the Study of Fatty Acids and Lipids. This dose can be reached with 1–2 portions of oily sea fish (such as herring, mackerel, salmon) per week. Although environmental contamination pollutants remain an active concern as noted, the consensus statement reinforces the critical role of DHA in neural development and encourages intake of a variety of fish species and avoidance of regular intake of large predatory fish that have higher levels of contaminants (Koletzko et al. 2007).

Dietary supplements of DHA are a second option. Products labeled "molecularly distilled" are presumed to be toxin free.

Physical Activity

Aerobic exercise is accepted as safe and effective throughout pregnancy (depending on individual restrictions); for example, the fetal heart has been shown to adapt to exercise with positive changes in heart rate and heart rate variability and reduction in body fat (Domingues et al. 2015).

The effects of other types of maternal physical activity on fetal development and neonatal health is not well understood. Studies are underway examining the effects of circuit training, resistance training, and aerobic training on maternal and fetal health, specifically on cardiovascular development and function (Moyer et al. 2015).

Sleep

Sleep disturbance during pregnancy has been associated with stress and depression, and shown to upregulate the inflammatory cascade and negatively impact immune functioning. Maternal sleep disturbance has been associated with increased risk for preterm birth and low birth weight (Okun et al. 2013; Okun et al. 2011).

Sleep disordered breathing in pregnancy has also been associated with shortened fetal leukocyte telomere length as measured in cord blood (Salihu et al. 2015).

These studies highlight the importance of reinforcing the value of regular restorative maternal sleep in the prenatal period as a protective factor in fetal health.

Maternal Stress and Mind–Body Therapies

Emerging studies on the effects of toxic maternal stress, also recognized as unremitting chronic stress, have shown a range of effects on the fetus, including upregulation of the inflammatory cascade, dysregulation of the hypothalamic-pituitary-adrenal axis, and imbalance of the immune system (Avitsur et al. 2015).

Epigenetic effects are also under active study. Work by Shonkoff and colleagues has highlighted the negative effects of intergenerational stressors, and the need to buffer the unborn child from its effects (Shonkoff et al. 2012).

Although a 2011 Cochrane review noted that small study size and design variability limited broad recommendations for mind–body interventions for pregnant women (Marc et al. 2011), a growing body of studies point to benefit with low risk to both mother and growing fetus. Yoga and mindfulness are among the practices that have shown benefit in maternal stress reduction (Sheffield and Woods-Giscombe 2016).

One randomized control trial of 64 Chinese maternal–fetal pairs also noted a statistically significant decrease in cord blood cortisol and infant salivary cortisol in infants of mothers who participated in six structured meditation sessions (Chan 2014).

Both yoga and therapeutic massage were shown to decrease depressive symptoms in women with prenatal depression, and was also correlated with greater birth weight and longer gestational term than control group (Field et al. 2012).

Sufficient research exists to support the recommendation for discussion and intervention of chronic stressors in pregnancy and to encourage expectant mothers to take steps to address stress using non-pharmacologic evidence-based mind–body therapies that have a low incidence of adverse effects.

Environmental Health

A wealth of information exists on the importance of minimizing or preventing exposures to all categories of pollutants and toxicants prenatally and after birth. These topics are reviewed in more detail in Chapter 8, Environmental Health. Accruing literature in the obstetrics-gynecology literature reinforces these concerns and highlights the educational programs for clinicians and patients that are under development in this area (Crighton et al. 2016).

Perinatal Health: Vaginal Versus Cesarean Delivery and the Role of the Microbiome

Accruing research shows that the maternal microbiome, in both uterus and in breast milk, influences the fetal immune and inflammatory systems. Although in the best-case scenario infants would be born vaginally with no exposure to unnecessary antibiotics and exclusively breastfed, in reality this is often not the case. A caution with elective cesarean delivery is that the infant misses exposure to the rich microbiome of the birth canal and is colonized with the bacteria they are exposed to at birth; for example, microbes present in the operating room. A decision to formula feed results in the infant missing the rich microbiota and prebiotics delivered in the breast milk, delaying normal colonization of the gut (Arrieta et al. 2014).

Consequences to these important decisions, vaginal versus cesarean delivery and breast versus bottle feeding, are areas of intense study. Until more is known, clinicians who encourage expectant mothers to plan for a vaginal delivery and help set them up for a successful breastfeeding experience are taking important steps to support the infant's health and wellbeing. While legitimately needed in many cases, exposure to antibiotics peri- and postnatally also interrupt normal microbiome development in the newborn, possibly predisposing to future allergic, inflammatory, and atopic illnesses and their use should be limited whenever safely possible (Romano-Keeler and Weitkamp 2015).

Summary: Maternal Lifestyle Foundations to Promote Fetal Health

- Emphasize a varied, "prudent" whole food diet rich in vegetables and fruits, whole grains, olive oil, and lean proteins. Encourage organic foods when available.
- Maintain a healthy weight.
- Ensure a daily minimum of 200 mg DHA to support fetal neural development.

- Normalize vitamin D levels.
- Encourage enjoyable physical activity.
- Emphasize the importance of restorative sleep.
- Address chronic stress with non-pharmacologic approaches.
- Explore mind–body techniques to encourage relaxation and self-regulation skills.
- Support the choice of vaginal delivery if possible to promote healthy microbiome.
- Support and encourage exclusive breastfeeding for first 6 months of life.
- Raise awareness about preventable environmental exposures pre- and postnatally.

Lifestyle Foundations: Newborn and Infant

Nutrition

Breastfeeding for the first 6 months of life is the recommendation of both the World Health Organization and the American Academy of Pediatrics as the optimal nutrition for newborns and infants (Eidelman 2012), yet the 2014 CDC Breastfeeding Report Card shows that only about 19% of U.S. babies breast feed exclusively at 6 months and many women face significant obstacles to successful breastfeeding at home, on the job, and in the public domain (Centers for Disease Control and Prevention).

Research on breast milk shows that it contains a rich reservoir of changing nutrients for the baby, including an important variety of immunoglobulins, leukocytes, a wide range of proteins, micronutrients, and peptides, fats, and fatty acids, including the anti-inflammatory omega-3 and the proinflammatory omega-6 fatty acids, another important reason to encourage lactating mothers to have adequate DHA intake either from diet or high-quality dietary supplement. Bioactive components in the breast milk are highly varied and an area of active study. They include substances such as stem cells, macrophages, cytokines, chemokines, growth factors including brain-derived neurotrophic factor and insulin-like growth factor, growth regulating hormones, adiponectin, oligosaccharides, and glycans. The human milk oligosaccharides (HMOS) are large non-nutritive sugars—but serve as prebiotics to encourage the growth of beneficial probiotic organisms in the infant gut. It has been shown that these remarkable compounds can also act as receptors of harmful pathogens, another area of active study (Ballard and Morrow 2013).

Breastfeeding has been associated with a wide range of benefits to infant and child, including development of a healthy immune system, optimal gut microbiota, increased intelligence quotient (Smithers, Kramer, and Lynch 2015) and healthy body weight (Hunsberger et al. 2013).

A longitudinal study examining the impact of breast versus formula feeding in 8030 infants showed that infants who were primarily bottle fed for the first 6 months of life were more than twice as likely to be obese at 2 years of age compared to breast-fed babies. In this study population, early introduction of solids at 4 months or earlier and putting the infant to bed with a bottle were also risk factors for obesity at 2 years (Gibbs and Forste 2014).

A source of ongoing controversy in the U.S. is the distribution of infant formula discharge packs to new parents that typically contain samples, coupons, and a variety of marketing and advertising materials. Advocacy efforts, especially renewed focus on the World Health Organization's 1981 International Code of Marketing of Breast-milk Substitutes (World Health Organization), the Joint Commission Perinatal

Core Measures that measure exclusive breastfeeding during perinatal hospitalization (Commission Specifications Manual for Joint Commission National Quality Measures (v2015A1)) and the Healthy People 2020 Maternal, Infant, and Child Health objectives (U.S. Department of Health and Human Services) have helped reduce the prevalence of this practice from more than 70% of hospitals in 2007 to 32% in 2013. This downward trend is encouraging; however, the average of one in three hospitals per state continuing to distribute these marketing materials remains significant. Artificial infant formula is a multimillion dollar industry in the U.S. and a large part of the multibillion dollar global baby food market. U.S. retail sales for baby food, including infant formula, were nearly U.S.$37 billion in 2010 with estimated growth to U.S.$55 billion by 2015, often making unsubstantiated health claims (Belamarich, Bochner, and Racine 2015; Nelson, Li, and Perrine 2015).

For mothers unable to nurse, or who choose not to nurse for personal reasons, an option to consider is pasteurized human donor milk from a highly reputable source, a growing trend globally (Williams et al. 2016).

AAP recommendations include exclusive breastfeeding until ~age 6 months with introduction of complementary solid foods accompanied by continued breastfeeding until 12 months (Klag et al. 2015).

Introduction of solid food types varies widely by culture and family traditions. Longitudinal studies are lacking as to the optimal pediatric diet predictive of adult health; however, accruing evidence suggests health benefits of the Mediterranean type diet as a protective factor against overweight and obesity in children (Kaikkonen, Mikkila, and Raitakari 2014) and daily childhood consumption of fruits and vegetables has been independently associated with improved measures of cardiovascular fitness in adulthood (Aatola et al. 2010; Kaikkonen et al. 2013).

Newborn: Dietary Supplements

Docosahexaenoic Acid (DHA)

Docosahexaenoic acid is passed from mother to infant in the breast milk, with DHA levels in breast milk showing good correlation with maternal DHA stores (Meldrum et al. 2012).

Postnatal supplementation of omega-3 fatty acids has been shown to increase infant omega-3 fatty acid levels and to balance the immune inflammatory response in randomized controlled studies (D'Vaz et al. 2012).

Although improvements in allergic response and in development of asthma have been demonstrated in some studies, conclusive recommendations do not currently exist for infant DHA supplementation (Miles and Calder 2014).

The Institute of Medicine (IOM) has set an acceptable macronutrient distribution range for total omega-3 fatty acid intake at 0.6–1.2 grams per day for ages 1 and up pending further studies to determine conclusive recommendations (Minns et al. 2010).

Synthetic DHA has become an integral ingredient in many infant formulas to promote healthy brain development. Despite marketing claims promising cognitive benefit, studies are lacking supporting the promise of improved cognition in children (Drover et al. 2012).

Newborn Vitamin D

Vitamin D is important in newborns as it has an array of important physiologic roles in addition to regulating calcium and phosphorus metabolism in bone health. Reported associations include roles in autoimmune, inflammatory, cardiovascular, metabolic, and infectious diseases. A 2015 expert position paper by Saggese and colleagues provides an excellent and detailed overview of the subject (Saggese et al. 2015).

Exclusively breastfed infants not receiving vitamin D supplementation are at high risk of vitamin D deficiency. The 2012 American Academy of Pediatrics Breastfeeding Policy Statement recommends that all infants that are not consuming at least 500 mL (16 ounces) of vitamin D-fortified formula or milk be given a vitamin D supplement of 400 IU/day which should be started in the first few days of life. The exact duration of vitamin D supplementation has not been determined (Mansbach, Ginde, and Camargo 2009).

Newborn Toxic Stress

As detailed in Chapter 19, Mental Health, the pattern of toxic stress often starts prenatally and has been shown to have lasting detrimental effect on a child's health. Exposure to stressors such as neglect, abuse, violence, poverty, and to chronic high caretaker stress has been shown to result in "biological embedding" with negative impact on the neuroendocrine-immune-inflammatory systems. The lack of buffering from chronic stressors has been clearly associated with decreased immunity, and reduced resistance to disease as well as a predisposition to pro-inflammatory illnesses such as asthma, metabolic syndrome, obesity, and cardiovascular disease in children. High-level chronic stressors are not limited to low socioeconomic groups. All families should be screened for stressors at well child visits and referred accordingly. Importantly, the presence of a stable source of a nurturing adult can mitigate the effects of chronic stress. Significant work is ongoing in this area in the American Academy of Pediatrics and other national organizations dedicated to raise awareness and encourage clinicians caring for children to intervene and educate individuals, family members, and community organizations to help protect children from the long-term effects of chronic stressors. In infants this involves creating a stable, nurturing environment that provides ample, on-demand nutrition, an organized sleep–wake cycle, and regular access to healthcare. In families in need this may involve home visits and expanded social support (Johnson et al. 2013; Garner 2013).

Newborn Microbiome

Research on the evolution and importance of the newborn gut microbiota is evolving rapidly and evidence is correlating a healthy gut microbiome with a protective effect against acute and chronic illness. Contrary to traditional teaching, the uterus, amniotic fluid, and placenta have all been shown to contain bacteria in normal healthy pregnant women (Arrieta et al. 2014).

In newborns, early gut colonization is generally seen with strict anaerobes such as *Bifidobacterium*, *Clostridium*, and *Bacteroides* (Matamoros et al. 2013) then begins to mimic maternal skin bacteria and vaginal microbiome (if not delivered by cesarean). Breast milk has also been shown to have a unique microbiota that plays a role in conjunction with human milk oligosaccharides to catalyze development of other microbes. *Bifidobacterium* species are most prevalent during the next months of exclusive milk feeding and play the role of fermenting milk oligosaccharides. The introduction of solid foods precipitates a change in the gut microbes and a decrease in *Bifidobacterium* and Enterobacteriaceae and over the first 3 years of life the microbiome aligns with adult species. The microbiome patterns of infants have been shown to vary by geographic location and by diet and have also been shown to be significantly affected by antibiotic exposure (Arrieta et al. 2014).

Conditions that have been associated with an altered microbiome that are under active study include: necrotizing enterocolitis, inflammatory bowel disease, obesity, malnutrition, asthma and atopy, and autism spectrum disorders (Cortese et al. 2016).

No current recommendations exist for pediatric probiotic supplementation; however, there is a growing literature suggesting a protective benefit to early exposure to a wide variety of bacteria in the natural environment. One frequently cited example is the lower incidence of asthma seen in children raised on farms (Ege et al. 2011).

A counterargument to the push for increased time spent in nature is the concern about exposures to environmental toxicants, a real issue in many areas of the world. The topic is complex and evolving and is covered in more detail in Chapter 8, Environmental Health. In addition, large population studies are underway in protected rural living societies such as the Amish in the hope of better understanding the protective factors at play (von Mutius 2016).

Treatment with probiotics is also an area of active study in some newborn conditions; for example, in acute gastroenteritis, where certain strains have been shown to reduce duration of diarrhea. Both *Lactobacillus rhamnosus* GG and *Saccharomyces boulardii* have reduced duration of diarrhea, but have not been shown to consistently shorten hospital stay (Guarino et al. 2014).

Other strains have shown promise in studies in children with rotavirus including *Bifidobacterium longum* and *Lactobacillus acidophilus* (Lee do et al. 2015).

Treatment of infant colic with specific strains of *Lactobacillus reuteri* has been evaluated in randomized controlled trials with mixed results (Lee do et al. 2015).

A study by Sung and colleagues of 167 infants with colic who were either breast or bottle fed failed to find benefit of probiotic treatment and did not result in changes to infant gut microbiome diversity, *E. coli* colonization, or calprotectin levels in this study population, although several variables were identified such as inclusion of infants on proton pump inhibitors and variability of formula in the bottle-fed group. In contrast, a randomized controlled double-blind trial of the same strain of *Lactobacillus reuteri* (DSM 17938) by Chau and colleagues of 52 breastfed infants with colic showed a greater than 50% reduction in daily crying time and fussiness over control group with significance manifesting as early as 1 week into treatment (Chau et al. 2015).

Large randomized trials are ongoing. In the meantime standard recommendations for the use of probiotics in infant colic do not exist (Sung et al. 2014).

Newborn Sleep

Any new parent understands the importance of sleep in newborns. Emerging research using electroencephalogram on healthy newborns shows that a well-developed sleep–wake cycle is present in the first 36 hours or sooner after birth and has an approximate ratio of 51% active sleep and 38% quiet sleep. In infants delivered by elective cesarean section, active sleep was longer and quiet sleep reduced in a study of 80 term infants. This was hypothesized to reflect a lower level of stress than that experienced by infants delivered by vaginal delivery or by emergency cesarean, which may correlate with a lower level of "priming" of the stress response than that typically seen during the normal process of labor if the child is delivered emergently due to fetal distress. Research is active in the study of newborn sleep architecture and its relation to cardiorespiratory markers that may be predictive of sudden infant death syndrome (SIDS) and other neurodevelopmental conditions (Korotchikova et al. 2015).

Chamomile tea (manzanilla) has historically been used to settle restless infants and to help colic as further discussed in Chapter 9, Botanicals. While no published guidelines exist, a widely used practice of 2–3 ounces of cooled tea has been used in many countries throughout the world to soothe infants. Daily volumes should not replace needed calories through breast milk or formula (Gardiner 2007).

Infant Massage

Infant massage is a non-pharmacological tool that may help infants equilibrate sympathetic and parasympathetic nervous systems. Research has shown reduction in stress hormone secretion, decrease in heart rate variability, improved bone density, improved gastric motility, and increased overall weight gain in both preterm and term neonates receiving massage. The mechanism for increased weight gain is not fully understood, but may be related to stimulation of the vagal nerve and increased release of insulin growth factor-1, an area of active study (Field, Diego, and Hernandez-Reif 2011).

Other infant massage studies show how the modality may benefit the caregiver. For example, in a small randomized controlled trial of 17 HIV-positive mother–infant pairs, mothers in the massage group reported increased confidence in reading their infant's cues, and reduction in depression and feelings of parental distress. Infants in the treatment group showed improved infant linear growth and weight gain in this pilot study (Oswalt and Biasini 2011).

Aromatherapy

Aromatherapy can be used in infant massage in the form of adding essential oils such as lavender to massage oil. This has shown benefit in a small study on infant colic (Cetinkaya and Basbakkal 2012).

Aromatherapy can also be used in aerosolized form to promote relaxation, or a few drops of essential oil placed on an infant's blanket for the same reason. A more detailed description of aromatherapy is covered in Chapter 11, Aromatherapy. Essential oils should never be applied near an infants face or taken internally due to risk of aspiration.

Newborn Mind–Body and Bioenergetic Therapies

The use of music therapy is one of the best studied mind–body therapies in infants. For example, in NICU babies, music has been shown to be effective in calming behavior, stabilizing vital signs, and increasing weight gain (Standley 2012, Kemper and Hamilton 2008).

The use of therapeutic touch has been evaluated in a small pilot study in preterm infants to see if it can buffer the stress of a simulated needle stick. Infants who received the treatment arm had a decrease in brain activation as measured by cerebral blood flow (Honda et al. 2013).

Although research is early in these areas, protecting newborns from unnecessary stressors is important and correlated with the emerging research on the detrimental effects of prenatal and early life toxic stress and its impact on physiology.

Newborn Environmental Medicine

Research interest in the effect of environmental toxicants in the prenatal and postnatal environments is high based on the numerous toxicants that cross the placental barrier; for example, perfluorocarboxylic acids (PFCAs) used in production of Teflon, now considered a persistent organic pollutant (Wang et al. 2016).

A wide range of exposures have been documented, from nearly every category of environmental toxin, by research teams around the world (Xu et al. 2016; Metzdorff et al. 1986; Gundacker and Hengstschlager 2012).

The topic is discussed in more detail in Chapter 8, Environmental Health, and is very active in the OB/Gyn literature. Ideally parental education in the preconception time period would offer concrete steps to parents so that they might decrease risk to the fetus. This is a global issue of urgent priority that will require concerted efforts to address (Crighton et al. 2016).

Summary: Newborn and Infant Foundations of Health

- Support and encourage parents to prioritize vaginal delivery if possible.
- Exclusive breastfeeding for the first 6 months, if possible.
- Maternal supplement with DHA if breastfeeding, or use of DHA-containing formula.
- Vitamin D supplementation beginning in first few days of life, especially if breastfed.
- Address or reduce acute and chronic maternal and caretaker stress and stress in the infant's external environment.
- Screen for maternal postnatal depression.
- Support and protect infant's regular sleep–wake cycle.
- Consider use of infant massage to aid sleep.
- Consider use of mind–body therapies such as music therapy to promote relaxation.

Toddler and Preschooler

Lifestyle Foundations

Lifestyle habits are laid down early and often patterned from parents and other caretakers. Prevention is the key to healthy weight in this age group, and relatively few lifestyle interventions exist or have been studied in overweight children in the preschool years. One interesting controlled study evaluated evidence-based behavior change in low-income children who were overweight or obese. Pediatricians targeted four behaviors: milk consumption, juice and sweet beverage consumption, television or screen time, and physical activity using a program called Steps to Growing Up Healthy. The program used a brief motivational interviewing framework that included positive affirmation, open-ended questions, reflective listening, collaborative goal setting, and contracting.

One behavior was chosen to work on by the mother, and a plan of action specific to the child was created in the form of a behavioral contract. Educational material was provided with suggestions for implementation, and a self-monitoring calendar was provided to track goal progress. A toolkit included a child's cup, a measuring cup to show portion size, a portion size placemat, a foam ball, and a pedometer for the mother. Each office visit was followed up 5–7 days later by a call to review the visit and reinforce behavior change. The mean number of interventions over the 12-month study period was 2.7, with more significant results seen in children with 2.0 or more interventions. Results of the study were positive in reduction of weight in the intervention group— by 0.33 percentile with greatest effect in children of normal weight. BMI increased as a whole in the control group with a mean increase of 8.75 ($p < 0.001$) (Cloutier et al. 2015).

Another large study in early phases involves 300 healthy Swedish 4-year-old children and is designed to use a personalized web-based application to promote healthy eating and physical activity over a 6-month trial period (Delisle et al. 2015).

Toddler and Preschooler Nutrition

Preschoolers often experience nutritional gaps that occur for a variety of socioeconomic reasons and cultivated taste preferences (Decsi and Lohner 2014).

Longitudinal studies are lacking as to the optimal pediatric diet predictive of adult health; however, accruing evidence suggests the benefits of the Mediterranean type diet as a protective factor against overweight and obesity in children (Kaikkonen, Mikkila, and Raitakari 2014).

Daily childhood consumption of fruits and vegetables has been independently associated with improved measures of cardiovascular fitness in adulthood (Aatola et al. 2010).

Mothers' quality of diet has been shown to have a measurable effect on that of preschoolers' diet. For example, a longitudinal cohort study of 1640 children 3 years old examined the influence of maternal and family factors on the quality of children's diets and found that mothers who had better quality diets with high intakes of fruit, vegetables, and wholemeal bread and low intakes of less healthy foods had children with best dietary quality, after adjusting for all other factors studied, including maternal education, BMI, smoking, child's birth order, and time spent watching television (Fisk et al. 2011).

Eating behaviors, including a tendency to overeat, seem to be established and stable throughout childhood as demonstrated by a study of 428 twin children studied initially at age 4 and followed up at age 10 in which correlations between the two time points were highly significant ($p < 0.001$) for satiety responsiveness, slowness in eating, and emotional overeating (Ashcroft et al. 2008).

A larger longitudinal study of 6177 children showed high correlation in dietary patterns using questionnaires completed by their mothers when children were 3, 4, 7, and 9 years old. Three patterns were consistently identified through time, "processed," "traditional," and "health conscious," with closest (virtually identical) dietary correlation seen between ages 4 and 7 years. Studies such as these highlight the critical opportunity present to imprint healthy eating habits early in life (Northstone and Emmett 2008). Avoidance of excessive television time in this age group is important, not only to reduce sedentary behavior, but also to limit the number of fast food commercials targeted to young children.

Toddler and Preschooler Dietary Supplements

Vitamin D

Many preschool-age children are vitamin D deficient (Decsi and Lohner 2014). Pediatric vitamin D supplementation recommendations from the AAP and Institute of Medicine are similar and include 400 IU per day for healthy infants younger than 12 months and 600 IU for children 1–18 years. The duration of supplementation has not been established—and levels should be monitored to guide supplementation if deficiency is established (Saggese et al. 2015; Mansbach, Ginde, and Camargo 2009).

Omega-3 Fatty Acids

The preferred choice for adequate omega-3 fatty acid in the pediatric diet is through whole foods. Good sources include fatty fish such as wild caught salmon, sardines, and herring. In reality, however, children in many Western cultures do not receive early taste exposures to fish, which have the highest natural concentrations of EPA/DHA. Environmental toxins such as mercury in fish also remain a concern for children. Many useful resources are available to help families follow local safety guidelines; for example, through the U.S. EPA (United States Environmental Protection Agency [b]).

In general, two age-appropriate portions of fish per week are considered safe, although local conditions may vary and should be followed carefully.

Plant-based sources of omega-3 fatty acids occur primarily in the form of alpha-linolenic acid (ALA), which is the precursor to eicosapentaenoic acid and docosahexaenoic acid (EPA + DHA). Flax seed is the richest natural resource of ALA. However, less than 1% of the original ALA is converted into EPA and DHA, making it an inefficient source relative to fish or other marine foods (Calder and Yaqoob 2009).The Institute of Medicine has set an acceptable macronutrient distribution range for total omega-3 fatty acid intake at 0.6–1.2 g per day for ages 1 year and up.

Physical Activity

Ideally physical activity would be taught through regular patterning of enjoyable activity in parents, siblings, and caretakers. Regular active free play in a safe and stimulating environment, preferably outdoors, should be part of every toddler's day. To date, few studies have assessed physical activity interventions for preschool-age children and efforts are underway to develop tools that will help reliably measure and track physical fitness in the preschool population (Ortega et al. 2015).

Media Time

The 2011 AAP Policy Statement on Media Use in Children Younger than 2 Years concludes that there are few benefits and serious concerns regarding media exposure in young children. If media exposure is to occur, the time should be limited and supervised by a parent or caretaker. Specific concerns include (Media Council on Communications and Brown 2011):

- Direct-to-child fast food advertising
- Correlation with obesity, sedentary behaviors, snacking

- Exposure to violence
- Exposure to adult content
- Delayed language development
- Attention problems
- Reduced interaction with parents
- Missed opportunities for creative free play
- Sleep disruption if television is placed in child's room

Sleep

On average a toddler requires 11–13 hours of sleep per day, while a preschooler requires 9–10 hours per day. Regular sleep–wake cycles are necessary for good health and normal development and should be prioritized in this age group. Large population surveys show that low maternal education, larger household size, and poverty all significantly reduced average sleep times and presence of a regular sleep–wake routine (Hale et al. 2009).

A consistent bedtime routine is also important and in a large population survey (n = 10,085) by Mindell and colleagues was shown to be significantly associated with better sleep outcomes, earlier bedtime, shorter sleep onset latency, reduced night awakenings, and improved daytime behavior (Mindell et al. 2015).

Minimizing light at night and limiting screen time are themes that run through all age groups (Parent, Sanders, and Forehand 2016).

Mind–Body

Preschool age is an important time to be introduced to self-regulation skills. Children in this age group can learn simple breathing exercises, progressive muscle relaxation, simple yoga, guided imagery, and age-appropriate clinical hypnosis (McClafferty 2011) (Vohra et al. 2016).

Research on empathy and learning social acceptance is also active in young children and will hopefully address some of the cultural changes required to help stem the bullying epidemic seen from preschool ages onward (Malti et al. 2012).

Environmental Health

Prevention from environmental exposure continues to be very important in preschool children where early exposures to endocrine-disrupting chemicals and persistent organic pollutants have been associated with a range of reproductive and metabolic conditions (Li et al. 2015).

Primary lines of exposures in young children are food, personal care products such as soaps and shampoos, and plastics often used in food and beverage preparation and storage (Myridakis et al. 2016).

Exposure to particulate matter in outdoor air has also been associated with the development of eczema and asthma in preschool children (Shah et al. 2016).

And second- and third-hand smoke has also been associated with a range of negative effects, including neurocognitive conditions (De Alwis et al. 2015).

Further discussion of environmental exposures can be found in Chapter 8, Environmental Health.

Summary: Toddler and Preschooler Foundations of Health

- Maintain a healthy weight.
- Encourage a varied diet of healthy whole foods.
- Normalize and maintain normal vitamin D levels.
- Ensure adequate omega-3 fatty acids.
- Daily active free play.
- Limit screen time.
- Establish a regular wake–sleep cycle and consistent bedtime routine.
- Address and reduce maternal and caretaker stress.
- Introduce age-appropriate self-regulation skills.
- Minimize environmental exposures, especially to endocrine-disrupting chemicals.

Foundations of Health: School-Age Children

Lifestyle foundations in school-aged children build on those established in early life.

Nutrition

Encouraging a varied healthy whole food diet with an emphasis on whole grains, fruits, vegetables, lean proteins, fish, low-fat dairy, nuts, and legumes is associated with healthy body weight and reduction in future health risks (Martin et al. 2014).

A large European survey of 16,220 children aged 2–9 years showed that higher adherence to a Mediterranean diet pattern was inversely correlated with overweight and obesity (Tognon et al. 2014).

Work is ongoing in school-based programs to improve food quality, especially for those children in lower socioeconomic groups who traditionally have lower overall quality of food intake (Kastorini et al. 2016) and in rural low-income children in the U.S. where rates of obesity are high (Cohen et al. 2014).

Dietary Supplements

As in preschoolers, vitamin D should be normalized and maintained, and adequate omega-3 fatty acids should be encouraged either in whole foods such as fish twice a week, or in supplement form. The Institute of Medicine has set an acceptable macronutrient distribution range for total omega-3 fatty acid intake at 0.6–1.2 g per day for ages 1 year and up.

Physical Activity

Sedentary television-viewing behavior in a large population survey of European children has been correlated with increased prevalence of overweight, and passive overconsumption of high-fat and high-sugar foods (Lissner et al. 2012).

The American Academy of Pediatrics guidelines recommend a minimum of 60 minutes of vigorous activity daily in this age group.

Sleep

School-age children should get on average 9–11 hours of sleep per day, but often fall short. A survey by Buxton and colleagues of 1103 families of children 6–17 years of age showed that 90% of children received less sleep than widely recommended. Factors associated with more sleep included parental education and rules setting, regular sleep–wake routine, regular enforcement of caffeine restriction, and no technology on or in the bedroom overnight (Buxton et al. 2015; Parent, Sanders, and Forehand 2016).

Mind–Body

Introduction or further refinement of self-regulation skills such as mindfulness is important to help school-aged children learn to modulate stressful situations and have been shown to help decrease negative affect in a study of 71 children aged 7–9 years old in a controlled study of an 8-week in-school program in mindfulness that was taught by the children's teachers as part of the regular school curriculum (Vickery and Dorjee 2015).

A second randomized study of 99 fourth and fifth graders who underwent a social–emotional training called MindUP (Hawn Foundation 2008), a 12-lesson course on mindfulness, were shown to have improved emotional control, less depression, and less self-reported peer aggression. Students were also more positively rated by peers as being more prosocial after the course (Schonert-Reichl et al. 2015).

Ideally these types of program will also contribute to ongoing shifts in the pervasive culture of bullying behavior seen in schoolchildren around the world.

Environmental Health

School-aged children continue to be at risk from exposures to a wide range of environmental toxicants, including endocrine-disrupting chemicals, persistent organic pollutants, and fine particulate matter from air pollution and also from school bus diesel exhaust. Time outdoors in green space has also been shown to correlate with improved air quality and a beneficial effect on cognitive development in 2593 school children participating in a 12-month study of its effects in Barcelona, Spain (Schonert-Reichl et al. 2015).

Summary: School-Aged Children Foundations of Health

- Encourage varied intake of healthy whole foods in a Mediterranean diet pattern.
- Normalize and maintain vitamin D status.
- Encourage regular intake of omega-3 fatty acids.
- Encourage a minimum of 60 minutes of active play daily.
- Minimize sedentary technology time.
- Develop regular sleep–wake cycle.
- Address stressors in the home and school setting.
- Continue to introduce and refine mind–body and self-regulation skills.
- Encourage mastery of prosocial behavior.
- Minimize environmental exposures, especially to endocrine-disrupting chemicals.

Lifestyle Foundations: Adolescent Health

Preventive care in adolescence is a chance to reinforce important messages of self-care, resilience, and self-efficacy. These life skills are needed to handle the work of achieving independence and developing healthy habits into adulthood. Clinicians' insight into the adolescent's socioeconomic stressors and other potential sources of toxic stress is important in order to encourage resilience and grit needed to achieve long-term goals. Many adolescents live with chronic illness, particularly overweight and obesity, and this should not preclude a comprehensive preventive wellness approach with the goal of maximizing every element of their health and wellbeing.

Emphasis on adolescent preventive health faces stiff competition in the form of irregular meals, erratic sleep patterns, reproductive health concerns, sexually transmitted diseases, or unplanned pregnancy, accidental injuries, substance abuse, sedentary lifestyle, or serious mental health issues. Aggressive marketing and advertising campaigns pushed out directly to youth via internet, text, and the range of social media platforms add negative pressure by promoting junk food, energy drinks, tobacco, e-cigarettes, fashion, sports and cosmetic companies.

Exposure to substance abuse in the family or in peer groups also poses a significant risk for adolescents initiating drug or substance use. Clinicians can serve as invaluable resources to developing young adults if they are well versed in modern preventive wellness approaches and able to establish a relationship based on trust and mutual respect (Chen et al. 2014).

Mastery of topics such as nutrition, physical activity, stress management, sleep, sexual health, social relationships, managing technology, and balancing academic achievement with a healthy lifestyle can be critically important to lifelong wellbeing.

Nutrition

In addition to promoting health and preventing future disease, one of the most compelling reasons for adolescents to maintain a healthy weight is the challenge of weight loss and the lack of effective programs in this area (Martin et al. 2014).

Overweight and obesity are very likely to track into adult life and carry major social, health, and economic burdens. As with school-aged children, the benefits of the Mediterranean style diet pattern are many, and can have a protective effect against long-term chronic diseases, although it is not followed in a high percentage of adolescents, even in Mediterranean countries. Modeling by parents, encouragement on the part of the clinicians, and additional support in the form of a registered dietician or health coach may be needed (Garcia Cabrera et al. 2015).

Encouragement to eat breakfast daily, to learn about appropriate portion size, and to begin to take responsibility for the quality of their nutrition are good starting points.

Adolescence is also an age where eating disorders can develop, so cultivation of healthy meal habits and a healthy body image are of critical importance.

Dietary Supplements

Adolescents (12–17 years) are more likely to use dietary supplements than younger children according to the 2012 National Health Statistics Report. Adolescents may use dietary supplements for a variety of reasons, among them weight loss, upper respiratory infections, mood disorders, sleep, or to enhance test or athletic performances. Stimulants such as caffeine, ginseng, and yerba mate may be present in unlabeled amounts in energy drinks (Black et al. 2015). The use of dietary supplements should be discussed at every medical visit.

Physical Activity

Many adolescents follow a sedentary lifestyle, and may get minimal or no regular exercise in the course of a normal school day. Cultural and gender differences may present obstacles even if the adolescent is interested in participating. The American Academy of Pediatrics recommends a goal of 60 minutes of vigorous activity daily for adolescents. In children with disabilities or in those who are overweight or obese, starting slowly and gradually building tolerance and endurance is recommended to avoid injury and discouragement.

Sleep

Average sleep requirements for adolescents are approximately 9 hours, although an average of 7 hours is more commonly reported. Sleep in adolescents is associated with a variety of cognitive and behavioral factors that can have significant effect on a teen's quality of life and academic success.

Mind–Body

Mind–body approaches are being explored in adolescent youth to address stress and negative mood, and to improve coping skills. Similar to the emerging studies in school-aged children, early results are positive for therapies such as mindfulness (Sibinga et al. 2016) and yoga in both school and community settings (Khalsa and Butzer 2016).

Mind–body skills can also help adolescents living with chronic illness develop increased resilience and reduce chronic stress (McClafferty 2011).

Adolescence is a time of life when social stressors often peak and mental health issues such as anxiety and depression may surface. Mind–body skills can be of significant benefit in helping adolescents cope in healthier ways, and offer non-pharmaceutical options that may complement other treatments in those living with chronic illness.

Environmental Health

Adolescence is an especially important time to be aware of potential environmental exposures, especially those that may impact reproductive health. For example, exposure to endocrine-disrupting chemicals such as bisphenol A used in plastic manufacturing has been linked to development of polycystic ovarian syndrome (Palioura and Diamanti-Kandarakis 2016).

Summary: Adolescent Foundations of Health

- Encourage a healthy whole food diet.
- Limit sugary beverages.
- Normalize and maintain vitamin D level.

- Encourage daily intake of omega-3 fatty acids.
- Encourage daily enjoyable physical activity.
- Encourage a regular sleep–wake cycle.
- Address toxic stress in the home and school setting.
- Encourage mastery of self-regulation skills.
- Avoid environmental exposures, especially from endocrine-disrupting chemicals.

References

Aatola, H., T. Koivistoinen, N. Hutri-Kahonen, M. Juonala, V. Mikkila, T. Lehtimaki, J. S. Viikari, O. T. Raitakari, and M. Kahonen. 2010. "Lifetime fruit and vegetable consumption and arterial pulse wave velocity in adulthood: the Cardiovascular Risk in Young Finns Study." *Circulation* 122(24): 2521–8. doi: 10.1161/CIRCULATIONAHA.110.969279.

American College of Obstetricians and Gynecologists. 2013. "ACOG Committee opinion no. 549: obesity in pregnancy." *Obstet Gynecol* 121(1): 213–7. doi: http://10.1097/01.AOG.0000425667.10377.60.

Arrieta, M. C., L. T. Stiemsma, N. Amenyogbe, E. M. Brown, and B. Finlay. 2014. "The intestinal microbiome in early life: health and disease." *Front Immunol* 5: 427. doi: 10.3389/fimmu.2014.00427.

Ashcroft, J., C. Semmler, S. Carnell, C. H. van Jaarsveld, and J. Wardle. 2008. "Continuity and stability of eating behaviour traits in children." *Eur J Clin Nutr* 62(8): 985–90. doi: 10.1038/sj.ejcn.1602855.

Avitsur, R., S. Levy, N. Goren, and R. Grinshpahet. 2015. "Early adversity, immunity and infectious disease." *Stress* 18(3): 289–96. doi: 10.3109/10253890.2015.1017464.

Ballard, O., and A. L. Morrow. 2013. "Human milk composition: nutrients and bioactive factors." *Pediatr Clin North Am* 60(1): 49–74. doi: 10.1016/j.pcl.2012.10.002.

Belamarich, P. F., R. E. Bochner, and A. D. Racine. 2015. "A critical review of the marketing claims of infant formula products in the United States." *Clin Pediatr (Phila)*. doi: 10.1177/0009922815589913.

Black, L. I., T. C. Clarke, P. M. Barnes, B. J. Stussman, and R. L. Nahin. 2015. "Use of complementary health approaches among children aged 4–17 years in the United States: National Health Interview Survey, 2007–2012." *Natl Health Stat Report* (78): 1–19.

Buttenheim, A. 2012. "Exposure and vulnerability of California kindergarteners to intentionally unvaccinated children." *LDI Issue Brief* 18(1): 1–4.

Buxton, O. M., A. M. Chang, J. C. Spilsbury, T. Bos, H. Emsellem, and K. L. Knutson. 2015. "Sleep in the modern family: protective family routines for child and adolescent sleep." *Sleep Health* 1(1): 15–27.

Calder, P. C., and P. Yaqoob. 2009. "Omega-3 polyunsaturated fatty acids and human health outcomes." *Biofactors* 35(3): 266–72. doi: 10.1002/biof.42.

Centers for Disease Control and Prevention, Division of Nutrition, Physical Activity, and Obesity. "Breastfeeding Report Cards." http://www.cdc.gov.ezproxy1.library.arizona.edu/breastfeeding/data/reportcard.htm.

Cetinkaya, B., and Z. Basbakkal. 2012. "The effectiveness of aromatherapy massage using lavender oil as a treatment for infantile colic." *Int J Nurs Pract* 18(2): 164–9. doi: 10.1111/j.1440-172X.2012.02015.x.

Chan, K. P. 2014. "Prenatal meditation influences infant behaviors." *Infant Behav Dev* 37(4): 556–61. doi: 10.1016/j.infbeh.2014.06.011.

Chau, K., E. Lau, S. Greenberg, S. Jacobson, P. Yazdani-Brojeni, N. Verma, and G. Koren. 2015. "Probiotics for infantile colic: a randomized, double-blind, placebo-controlled trial investigating Lactobacillus reuteri DSM 17938." *J Pediatr* 166(1): 74–8. doi: 10.1016/j.jpeds.2014.09.020.

Chen, M. Y., L. J. Lai, H. C. Chen, and J. Gaete. 2014. "Development and validation of the short-form Adolescent Health Promotion Scale." *BMC Public Health* 14: 1106. doi: 10.1186/1471-2458-14-1106.

Cloutier, M. M., J. Wiley, T. Huedo-Medina, C. M. Ohannessian, A. Grant, D. Hernandez, and A. A. Gorin. 2015. "Outcomes from a pediatric primary care weight management program: steps to growing up healthy." *J Pediatr* 167(2): 372–7 e1. doi: 10.1016/j.jpeds.2015.05.028.

Cohen, J. F., V. I. Kraak, S. F. Choumenkovitch, R. R. Hyatt, and C. D. Economos. 2014. "The CHANGE study: a healthy-lifestyles intervention to improve rural children's diet quality." *J Acad Nutr Diet* 114(1): 48–53. doi: 10.1016/j.jand.2013.08.014.

Commission, The Joint. Specifications Manual for Joint Commission National Quality Measures (v2015A1). https://manual.jointcommission.org/releases/TJC2015A1/MIF0170.html.

Cortese, R., L. Lu, Y. Yu, D. Ruden, and E. C. Claud. 2016. "Epigenome-Microbiome crosstalk: A potential new paradigm influencing neonatal susceptibility to disease." *Epigenetics*: 0. doi: 10.1080/15592294.2016.1155011.

Crighton, E., A. Abelsohn, J. Blake, J. Enders, K. Kilroy, B. Lanphear, L. Marshall, E. Phipps, and G. Smith. 2016. "Beyond alcohol and tobacco smoke: are we doing enough to reduce fetal toxicant exposure?" *J Obstet Gynaecol Can* 38(1): 56–9. doi: 10.1016/j.jogc.2015.10.009.

D'Vaz, N., S. J. Meldrum, J. A. Dunstan, T. F. Lee-Pullen, J. Metcalfe, B. J. Holt, M. Serralha, M. K. Tulic, T. A. Mori, and S. L. Prescott. 2012. "Fish oil supplementation in early infancy modulates developing infant immune responses." *Clin Exp Allergy* 42(8): 1206–16. doi: 10.1111/j.1365-2222.2012.04031.x.

De Alwis, D., M. Tandon, R. Tillman, and J. Luby. 2015. "Nonverbal reasoning in preschool children: investigating the putative risk of secondhand smoke exposure and attention-deficit/hyperactivity disorder as a mediator." *Scand J Child Adolesc Psychiatr Psychol* 3(2): 115–125.

De Giuseppe, R., C. Roggi, and H. Cena. 2014. "n-3 LC-PUFA supplementation: effects on infant and maternal outcomes." *Eur J Nutr* 53(5): 1147–54. doi: 10.1007/s00394-014-0660-9.

Decsi, T., and S. Lohner. 2014. "Gaps in meeting nutrient needs in healthy toddlers." *Ann Nutr Metab* 65(1): 22–8. doi: 10.1159/000365795.

Delisle, C., S. Sandin, E. Forsum, H. Henriksson, Y. Trolle-Lagerros, C. Larsson, R. Maddison, F. B. Ortega, J. R. Ruiz, K. Silfvernagel, T. Timpka, and M. Lof. 2015. "A web- and mobile phone-based intervention to prevent obesity in 4-year-olds (MINISTOP): a population-based randomized controlled trial." *BMC Public Health* 15: 95. doi: 10.1186/s12889-015-1444-8.

Demicheli, V., A. Rivetti, M. G. Debalini, and C. Di Pietrantonj. 2012. "Vaccines for measles, mumps and rubella in children." *Cochrane Database Syst Rev* 2: CD004407. doi: 10.1002/14651858.CD004407.pub3.

Dempsey, A. F., S. Schaffer, D. Singer, A. Butchart, M. Davis, and G. L. Freed. 2011. "Alternative vaccination schedule preferences among parents of young children." *Pediatrics* 128(5): 848–56. doi: 10.1542/peds.2011-0400.

Domingues, M. R., D. G. Bassani, S. G. da Silva, V. Coll Cde, B. G. da Silva, and P. C. Hallal. 2015. "Physical activity during pregnancy and maternal-child health (PAMELA): study protocol for a randomized controlled trial." *Trials* 16: 227. doi: 10.1186/s13063-015-0749-3.

Drover, J. R., J. Felius, D. R. Hoffman, Y. S. Castaneda, S. Garfield, D. H. Wheaton, and E. E. Birch. 2012. "A randomized trial of DHA intake during infancy: school readiness and receptive vocabulary at 2–3.5 years of age." *Early Hum Dev* 88(11): 885–91. doi: 10.1016/j.earlhumdev.2012.07.007.

Editors of The Lancet. 2010. "Retraction—Ileal-lymphoid-nodular hyperplasia, non-specific colitis, and pervasive developmental disorder in children." *Lancet* 375(9713): 445. doi: 10.1016/S0140-6736(10)60175-4.

Ege, M. J., M. Mayer, A. C. Normand, J. Genuneit, W. O. Cookson, C. Braun-Fahrlander, D. Heederik, R. Piarroux, E. von Mutius, and Gabriela Transregio 22 Study Group. 2011. "Exposure to environmental microorganisms and childhood asthma." *N Engl J Med* 364(8): 701–9. doi: 10.1056/NEJMoa1007302.

Eidelman, A. I. 2012. "Breastfeeding and the use of human milk: an analysis of the American

Academy of Pediatrics 2012 Breastfeeding Policy Statement." *Breastfeed Med* 7(5): 323–4. doi: 10.1089/bfm.2012.0067.

Englund-Ogge, L., A. L. Brantsaeter, V. Sengpiel, M. Haugen, B. E. Birgisdottir, R. Myhre, H. M. Meltzer, and B. Jacobsson. 2014. "Maternal dietary patterns and preterm delivery: results from large prospective cohort study." *BMJ* 348: g1446. doi: 10.1136/bmj.g1446.

Field, T., M. Diego, and M. Hernandez-Reif. 2011. "Potential underlying mechanisms for greater weight gain in massaged preterm infants." *Infant Behav Dev* 34(3): 383–9. doi: 10.1016/j.infbeh.2010.12.001.

Field, T., M. Diego, M. Hernandez-Reif, L. Medina, J. Delgado, and A. Hernandez. 2012. "Yoga and massage therapy reduce prenatal depression and prematurity." *J Bodyw Mov Ther* 16(2): 204–9. doi: 10.1016/j.jbmt.2011.08.002.

Fisk, C. M., S. R. Crozier, H. M. Inskip, K. M. Godfrey, C. Cooper, S. M. Robinson, and Group Southampton Women's Survey Study. 2011. "Influences on the quality of young children's diets: the importance of maternal food choices." *Br J Nutr* 105(2): 287–96. doi: 10.1017/S0007114510003302.

Garcia Cabrera, S., N. Herrera Fernandez, C. Rodriguez Hernandez, M. Nissensohn, B. Roman-Vinas, and L. Serra-Majem. 2015. "Kidmed Test; prevalence of low adherence to the Mediterranean diet in children and young; a systematic review." *Nutr Hosp* 32(n06): 2390–2399. doi: 10.3305/nh.2015.32.6.9828.

Gardiner, P. 2007. "Complementary, holistic, and integrative medicine: chamomile." *Pediatr Rev* 28(4): e16–8.

Garner, A. S. 2013. "Home visiting and the biology of toxic stress: opportunities to address early childhood adversity." *Pediatrics* 132(Suppl 2): S65–73. doi: 10.1542/peds.2013-1021D.

Geoffrey, R. Simon, Baker Cynthia, A. Barden Graham, 3rd, O. W. Brown, A. Hardin, H. R. Lessin, K. Meade, S. Moore, C. T. Rodgers, Practice Committee on, Medicine Ambulatory, E. S. Curry, P. M. Dunca, J. F. Hagan, Jr., A. R. Kemper, J. S. Shaw, J. T. Swanson, and Workgroup Bright Futures Periodicity Schedule. 2014. "2014 recommendations for pediatric preventive health care." *Pediatrics* 133(3): 568–70. doi: 10.1542/peds.2013-4096.

Gibbs, B. G., and R. Forste. 2014. "Socioeconomic status, infant feeding practices and early childhood obesity." *Pediatr Obes* 9(2): 135–46. doi: 10.1111/j.2047-6310.2013.00155.x.

Gilmour, J., C. Harrison, L. Asadi, M. H. Cohen, and S. Vohra. 2011. "Childhood immunization: when physicians and parents disagree." *Pediatrics* 128(Suppl 4): S167–74. doi: 10.1542/peds.2010-2720E.

Glanz, J. M., C. R. Kraus, and M. F. Daley. 2015. "Addressing parental vaccine concerns: engagement, balance, and timing." *PLoS Biol* 13(8): e1002227. doi: 10.1371/journal.pbio.1002227.

Guarino, A., S. Ashkenazi, D. Gendrel, A. Lo Vecchio, R. Shamir, H. Szajewska, Hepatology European Society for Pediatric Gastroenterology, Nutrition, and Diseases European Society for Pediatric Infectious. 2014. "European Society for Pediatric Gastroenterology, Hepatology, and Nutrition/European Society for Pediatric Infectious Diseases evidence-based guidelines for the management of acute gastroenteritis in children in Europe: update 2014." *J Pediatr Gastroenterol Nutr* 59(1): 132–52. doi: 10.1097/MPG.0000000000000375.

Gundacker, C., and M. Hengstschlager. 2012. "The role of the placenta in fetal exposure to heavy metals." *Wien Med Wochenschr* 162(9–10): 201–6. doi: 10.1007/s10354-012-0074-3.

Hale, L., L. M. Berger, M. K. LeBourgeois, and J. Brooks-Gunn. 2009. "Social and demographic predictors of preschoolers' bedtime routines." *J Dev Behav Pediatr* 30(5): 394–402. doi: 10.1097/DBP.0b013e3181ba0e64.

Honda, N., S. Ohgi, N. Wada, K. K. Loo, Y. Higashimoto, and K. Fukuda. 2013. "Effect of therapeutic touch on brain activation of preterm infants in response to sensory punctate stimulus: a near-infrared spectroscopy-based study." *Arch Dis Child Fetal Neonatal Ed* 98(3): F244–8. doi: 10.1136/archdischild-2011-301469.

Hunsberger, M., A. Lanfer, A. Reeske, T. Veidebaum, P. Russo, C. Hadjigeorgiou, L. A. Moreno, D. Molnar, S. De Henauw, L. Lissner, and G. Eiben. 2013. "Infant feeding practices and prevalence of obesity in eight European countries—the IDEFICS study." *Public Health Nutr* 16(2): 219–27. doi: 10.1017/S1368980012003850.

Johnson, S. B., A. W. Riley, D. A. Granger, and J. Riis. 2013. "The science of early life toxic stress for pediatric practice and advocacy." *Pediatrics* 131(2): 319–27. doi: 10.1542/peds.2012-0469.

Kaikkonen, J. E., V. Mikkila, C. G. Magnussen, M. Juonala, J. S. Viikari, and O. T. Raitakari. 2013. "Does childhood nutrition influence adult cardiovascular disease risk? Insights from the Young Finns Study." *Ann Med* 45(2): 120–8. doi: 10.3109/07853890.2012.671537.

Kaikkonen, J. E., V. Mikkila, and O. T. Raitakari. 2014. "Role of childhood food patterns on adult cardiovascular disease risk." *Curr Atheroscler Rep* 16(10): 443. doi: 10.1007/s11883-014-0443-z.

Kastorini, C. M., A. Lykou, M. Yannakoulia, A. Petralias, E. Riza, A. Linos, and Diatrofi Program Research Team. 2016. "The influence of a school-based intervention programme regarding adherence to a healthy diet in children and adolescents from disadvantaged areas in Greece: the DIATROFI study." *J Epidemiol Community Health*. doi: 10.1136/jech-2015-205680.

Kemper, K. J., and C. Hamilton. 2008. "Live harp music reduces activity and increases weight gain in stable premature infants." *J Altern Complement Med* 14(10): 1185–6. doi: 10.1089/acm.2008.0283.

Khaire, A. A., A. A. Kale, and S. R. Joshi. 2015. "Maternal omega-3 fatty acids and micronutrients modulate fetal lipid metabolism: a review." *Prostaglandins Leukot Essent Fatty Acids* 98: 49–55. doi: 10.1016/j.plefa.2015.04.007.

Khalsa, S. B., and B. Butzer. 2016. "Yoga in school settings: a research review." *Ann N Y Acad Sci*. doi: 10.1111/nyas.13025.

Klag, E. A., K. McNamara, S. R. Geraghty, and S. A. Keim. 2015. "Associations between breast milk feeding, introduction of solid foods, and weight gain in the first 12 months of life." *Clin Pediatr (Phila)* 54(11): 1059–67. doi: 10.1177/0009922815569202.

Koletzko, B., I. Cetin, J. T. Brenna, Group Perinatal Lipid Intake Working, Foundation Child Health, Group Diabetic Pregnancy Study, Medicine European Association of Perinatal, Medicine European Association of Perinatal, Nutrition European Society for Clinical, Metabolism, Hepatology European Society for Paediatric Gastroenterology, Committee on Nutrition Nutrition, Associations International Federation of Placenta, Acids International Society for the Study of Fatty, and Lipids. 2007. "Dietary fat intakes for pregnant and lactating women." *Br J Nutr* 98(5): 873–7. doi: 10.1017/S0007114507764747.

Korotchikova, I., N. J. Stevenson, V. Livingstone, C. A. Ryan, and G. B. Boylan. 2015. "Sleep-wake cycle of the healthy term newborn infant in the immediate postnatal period." *Clin Neurophysiol*. doi: 10.1016/j.clinph.2015.12.015.

Kumar, D., R. Chandra, M. Mathur, S. Samdariya, and N. Kapoor. 2016. "Vaccine hesitancy: understanding better to address better." *Isr J Health Policy Res* 5: 2. doi: 10.1186/s13584-016-0062-y.

Leask, J., P. Kinnersley, C. Jackson, F. Cheater, H. Bedford, and G. Rowles. 2012. "Communicating with parents about vaccination: a framework for health professionals." *BMC Pediatr* 12: 154. doi: 10.1186/1471-2431-12-154.

Lee do, K., J. E. Park, M. J. Kim, J. G. Seo, J. H. Lee, and N. J. Ha. 2015. "Probiotic bacteria, B. longum and L. acidophilus inhibit infection by rotavirus in vitro and decrease the duration of diarrhea in pediatric patients." *Clin Res Hepatol Gastroenterol* 39(2): 237–44. doi: 10.1016/j.clinre.2014.09.006.

Li, J., S. Lu, G. Liu, Y. Zhou, Y. Lv, J. She, and R. Fan. 2015. "Co-exposure to polycyclic aromatic hydrocarbons, benzene and toluene and their dose-effects on oxidative stress damage in kindergarten-aged children in Guangzhou, China." *Sci Total Environ* 524–5: 74–80. doi: 10.1016/j.scitotenv.2015.04.020.

Lissner, L., A. Lanfer, W. Gwozdz, G. Olafsdottir, G. Eiben, L. A. Moreno, A. M. Santaliestra-Pasias, E. Kovacs, G. Barba, H. M. Loit, Y. Kourides, V. Pala, H. Pohlabeln, S. De Henauw, K. Buchecker, W. Ahrens, and L. Reisch. 2012. "Television habits in relation to overweight, diet and taste preferences in European children: the IDEFICS study." *Eur J Epidemiol* 27(9): 705–15. doi: 10.1007/s10654-012-9718-2.

Makrides, M. 2013. "DHA supplementation during the perinatal period and neurodevelopment: do some babies benefit more than others?" *Prostaglandins Leukot Essent Fatty Acids* 88(1): 87–90. doi: 10.1016/j.plefa.2012.05.004.

Malti, T., M. Gummerum, M. Keller, M. P. Chaparro, and M. Buchmann. 2012. "Early sympathy and social acceptance predict the development of sharing in children." *PLoS One* 7(12): e52017. doi: 10.1371/journal.pone.0052017.

Mansbach, J. M., A. A. Ginde, and C. A. Camargo, Jr. 2009. "Serum 25-hydroxyvitamin D levels among US children aged 1 to 11 years: do children need more vitamin D?" *Pediatrics* 124(5): 1404–10. doi: 10.1542/peds.2008-2041.

Marc, I., N. Toureche, E. Ernst, E. D. Hodnett, C. Blanchet, S. Dodin, and M. M. Njoya. 2011. "Mind-body interventions during pregnancy for preventing or treating women's anxiety." *Cochrane Database Syst Rev* 7: CD007559. doi: 10.1002/14651858.CD007559.pub2.

Martin, A., D. H. Saunders, S. D. Shenkin, and J. Sproule. 2014. "Lifestyle intervention for improving school achievement in overweight or obese children and adolescents." *Cochrane Database Syst Rev* 3: CD009728. doi: 10.1002/14651858.CD009728.pub2.

Matamoros, S., C. Gras-Leguen, F. Le Vacon, G. Potel, and M. F. de La Cochetiere. 2013. "Development of intestinal microbiota in infants and its impact on health." *Trends Microbiol* 21(4): 167–73. doi: 10.1016/j.tim.2012.12.001.

McClafferty, H. 2011. "Complementary, holistic, and integrative medicine: mind-body medicine." *Pediatr Rev* 32(5): 201–3. doi: 10.1542/pir.32-5-201.

Media Council on Communications, and A. Brown. 2011. "Media use by children younger than 2 years." *Pediatrics* 128(5): 1040–5. doi: 10.1542/peds.2011–1753.

Meldrum, S. J., N. D'Vaz, Y. Casadio, J. A. Dunstan, N. Niels Krogsgaard-Larsen, K. Simmer, and S. L. Prescott. 2012. "Determinants of DHA levels in early infancy: differential effects of breast milk and direct fish oil supplementation." *Prostaglandins Leukot Essent Fatty Acids* 86(6): 233–9. doi: 10.1016/j.plefa.2012.03.006.

Metzdorff, M. T., J. Hill, A. F. Matar, M. G. Strom, A. S. Goldstein, and B. C. Esrig. 1986. "Use of sutureless intraluminal aortic prostheses in traumatic rupture of the aorta." *J Trauma* 26(8): 691–4.

Miles, E. A., and P. C. Calder. 2014. "Omega-6 and omega-3 polyunsaturated fatty acids and allergic diseases in infancy and childhood." *Curr Pharm Des* 20(6): 946–53.

Mindell, J. A., A. M. Li, A. Sadeh, R. Kwon, and D. Y. Goh. 2015. "Bedtime routines for young children: a dose-dependent association with sleep outcomes." *Sleep* 38(5): 717–22. doi: 10.5665/sleep.4662.

Minns, L. M., E. H. Kerling, M. R. Neely, D. K. Sullivan, J. L. Wampler, C. L. Harris, C. L. Berseth, and S. E. Carlson. 2010. "Toddler formula supplemented with docosahexaenoic acid (DHA) improves DHA status and respiratory health in a randomized, double-blind, controlled trial of US children less than 3 years of age." *Prostaglandins Leukot Essent Fatty Acids* 82(4–6): 287–93. doi: 10.1016/j.plefa.2010.02.009.

Moyer, C., J. Livingston, X. Fang, and L. E. May. 2015. "Influence of exercise mode on pregnancy outcomes: ENHANCED by Mom project." *BMC Pregnancy Childbirth* 15: 133. doi: 10.1186/s12884-015-0556-6.

Mozurkewich, E. L., and C. Klemens. 2012. "Omega-3 fatty acids and pregnancy: current implications for practice." *Curr Opin Obstet Gynecol* 24(2): 72–7. doi: 10.1097/GCO.0b013e328350fd34.

Myridakis, A., G. Chalkiadaki, M. Fotou, M. Kogevinas, L. Chatzi, and E. G. Stephanou. 2016. "Exposure of preschool-age Greek children (RHEA Cohort) to bisphenol A, parabens, phthalates, and organophosphates." *Environ Sci Technol* 50(2): 932–41. doi: 10.1021/acs.est.5b03736.

National Resources Defense Council. "Mercury Contamination in Fish, A Guide to Staying Healthy and FIghting Back." http://www.nrdc.org/health/effects/mercury/guide.asp.

Nelson, J. M., R. Li, and C. G. Perrine. 2015. "Trends of US hospitals distributing infant formula packs to breastfeeding mothers, 2007 to 2013." *Pediatrics* 135(6): 1051–6. doi: 10.1542/peds.2015-0093.

Northstone, K., and P. M. Emmett. 2008. "Are dietary patterns stable throughout early and mid-childhood? A birth cohort study." *Br J Nutr* 100(5): 1069–76. doi: 10.1017/S0007114508968264.

Okun, M. L., K. Kiewra, J. F. Luther, S. R. Wisniewski, and K. L. Wisner. 2011. "Sleep disturbances in depressed and nondepressed pregnant women." *Depress Anxiety* 28(8): 676–85. doi: 10.1002/da.20828.

Okun, M. L., C. E. Kline, J. M. Roberts, B. Wettlaufer, K. Glover, and M. Hall. 2013. "Prevalence of sleep deficiency in early gestation and its associations with stress and depressive symptoms." *J Womens Health (Larchmt)* 22(12): 1028–37. doi: 10.1089/jwh.2013.4331.

Omer, S. B., D. A. Salmon, W. A. Orenstein, M. P. deHart, and N. Halsey. 2009. "Vaccine refusal, mandatory immunization, and the risks of vaccine-preventable diseases." *N Engl J Med* 360(19): 1981–8. doi: 10.1056/NEJMsa0806477.

Ortega, F. B., C. Cadenas-Sanchez, G. Sanchez-Delgado, J. Mora-Gonzalez, B. Martinez-Tellez, E. G. Artero, J. Castro-Pinero, I. Labayen, P. Chillon, M. Lof, and J. R. Ruiz. 2015. "Systematic review and proposal of a field-based physical fitness-test battery in preschool children: the PREFIT battery." *Sports Med* 45(4): 533–55. doi: 10.1007/s40279-014-0281-8.

Oswalt, K., and F. Biasini. 2011. "Effects of infant massage on HIV-infected mothers and their infants." *J Spec Pediatr Nurs* 16(3): 169–78. doi: 10.1111/j.1744-6155.2011.00291.x.

Palioura, E., and E. Diamanti-Kandarakis. 2016. "Polycystic ovary syndrome (PCOS) and endocrine disrupting chemicals (EDCs)." *Rev Endocr Metab Disord.* doi: 10.1007/s11154-016-9326-7.

Parent, J., W. Sanders, and R. Forehand. 2016. "Youth screen time and behavioral health problems: the role of sleep duration and disturbances." *J Dev Behav Pediatr.* doi: 10.1097/DBP.0000000000000272.

Romano-Keeler, J., and J. H. Weitkamp. 2015. "Maternal influences on fetal microbial colonization and immune development." *Pediatr Res* 77(1–2): 189–95. doi: 10.1038/pr.2014.163.

Saggese, G., F. Vierucci, A. M. Boot, J. Czech-Kowalska, G. Weber, C. A. Camargo, Jr., E. Mallet, M. Fanos, N. J. Shaw, and M. F. Holick. 2015. "Vitamin D in childhood and adolescence: an expert position statement." *Eur J Pediatr* 174(5): 565–76. doi: 10.1007/s00431-015-2524-6.

Salihu, H. M., L. King, P. Patel, A. Paothong, A. Pradhan, J. Louis, E. Naik, P. J. Marty, and V. Whiteman. 2015. "Association between maternal symptoms of sleep disordered breathing and fetal telomere length." *Sleep* 38(4): 559–66. doi: 10.5665/sleep.4570.

Schonert-Reichl, K. A., E. Oberle, M. S. Lawlor, D. Abbott, K. Thomson, T. F. Oberlander, and A. Diamond. 2015. "Enhancing cognitive and social-emotional development through a simple-to-administer mindfulness-based school program for elementary school children: a randomized controlled trial." *Dev Psychol* 51(1): 52–66. doi: 10.1037/a0038454.

Shah, L., G. Mainelis, M. Ramagopal, K. Black, and S. L. Shalat. 2016. "Use of a robotic sampler (PIPER) for evaluation of particulate matter exposure and eczema in preschoolers." *Int J Environ Res Public Health* 13(2). doi: 10.3390/ijerph13020242.

Sheffield, K. M., and C. L. Woods-Giscombe. 2016. "Efficacy, feasibility, and acceptability of perinatal yoga on women's mental health and well-being: a systematic literature review." *J Holist Nurs* 34(1): 64–79. doi: 10.1177/0898010115577976.

Shonkoff, J. P., A. S. Garner, Child Committee on Psychosocial Aspects of, Health Family, Adoption Committee on Early Childhood, Care Dependent, Developmental Section on, and Pediatrics Behavioral. 2012. "The lifelong effects of early childhood adversity and toxic stress." *Pediatrics* 129(1): e232–46. doi: 10.1542/peds.2011-2663.

Sibinga, E. M., L. Webb, S. R. Ghazarian, and J. M. Ellen. 2016. "School-based mindfulness instruction: an RCT." *Pediatrics* 137(1): 1–8. doi: 10.1542/peds.2015-2532.

Smithers, L. G., M. S. Kramer, and J. W. Lynch. 2015. "Effects of breastfeeding on obesity and intelligence: causal insights from different study designs." *JAMA Pediatr* 169(8): 707–8. doi: 10.1001/jamapediatrics.2015.0175.

Standley, J. 2012. "Music therapy research in the NICU: an updated meta-analysis." *Neonatal Netw* 31(5): 311–6. doi: 10.1891/0730-0832.31.5.311.

Sung, V., H. Hiscock, M. L. Tang, F. K. Mensah, M. L. Nation, C. Satzke, R. G. Heine, A. Stock, R. G. Barr, and M. Wake. 2014. "Treating infant colic with the probiotic Lactobacillus reuteri: double blind, placebo controlled randomised trial." *BMJ* 348: g2107. doi: 10.1136/bmj.g2107.

Tognon, G., A. Hebestreit, A. Lanfer, L. A. Moreno, V. Pala, A. Siani, M. Tornaritis, S. De Henauw, T. Veidebaum, D. Molnar, W. Ahrens, and L. Lissner. 2014. "Mediterranean diet, overweight and body composition in children from eight European countries: cross-sectional and prospective results from the IDEFICS study." *Nutr Metab Cardiovasc Dis* 24(2): 205–13. doi: 10.1016/j.numecd.2013.04.013.

United States Environmental Protection Agency [a]. "Advisories and Technical Resources for Fish and Shellfish Consumption." http://water.epa.gov/scitech/swguidance/fishshellfish/fish-advisories/index.cfm

United States Environmental Protection Agency [b]. "Human Health Water Quality Criteria." http://water.epa.gov/scitech/swguidance/standards/criteria/health/methylmercury.cfm

U.S. Department of Health and Human Services. "Healthy People 2020: maternal, infant, and child health." http://www.healthypeople.gov/2020/topicsobjectives2020/objectiveslist.aspx?topicId=2.

Vickery, C. E., and D. Dorjee. 2015. "Mindfulness training in primary schools decreases negative affect and increases meta-cognition in children." *Front Psychol* 6: 2025. doi: 10.3389/fpsyg.2015.02025.

Vohra, S., McClafferty, H., et al. 2016. "Mind-Body Therapies in Children and Youth." Section on Integrative Medicine. *Pediatrics* 138(3). pii: e20161896. doi: 10.1542/peds.2016-1896. Epub 2016 Aug 22.

von Mutius, E. 2016. "The microbial environment and its influence on asthma prevention in early life." *J Allergy Clin Immunol*. doi: 10.1016/j.jaci.2015.12.1301.

Wang, Y., M. Adgent, P. H. Su, H. Y. Chen, P. C. Chen, C. A. Hsiung, and S. L. Wang. 2016. "Prenatal exposure to perfluorocarboxylic acids (PFCAs) and fetal and postnatal growth in the Taiwan Maternal and Infant Cohort Study." *Environ Health Perspect*. doi: 10.1289/ehp.1509998.

Williams, T., H. Nair, J. Simpson, and N. Embleton. 2016. "Use of donor human milk and maternal breastfeeding rates: a systematic review." *J Hum Lact*. doi: 10.1177/0890334416632203.

World Health Organization. "International Code of Marketing of Breast-milk Substitutes." http://www.who.int/nutrition/publications/code_english.pdf.

Xu, L., J. Ge, X. Huo, Y. Zhang, A. T. Lau, and X. Xu. 2016. "Differential proteomic expression of human placenta and fetal development following e-waste lead and cadmium exposure in utero." *Sci Total Environ* 550: 1163–70. doi: 10.1016/j.scitotenv.2015.11.084.

15 Allergy and Asthma

Allergy

Overview

Allergies and asthma have become the most commonly reported chronic conditions in children globally, taking a huge emotional, physical, and financial toll on children and their families (Schroder et al. 2015).

The worldwide prevalence and complexity of allergic diseases is increasing, prompting calls for new partnerships to address this global burden of disease. The World Health Organization White Book on Allergy highlights theories on the increasing prevalence, including the impact of climate change, environmental pollutants, reduced biodiversity, and changing weather patterns. Inflammatory-driven comorbid illnesses including obesity, cardiovascular disease, depression and anxiety, and gastrointestinal illnesses add to the complexity of treatment and contribute to increased risk of work and school absence, and high healthcare costs (Pawankar 2014).

Data from the U.S. 2007 National Health Interview Survey demonstrates that allergies and asthma are among the top 15 most common medical conditions in which integrative therapies are used, making it important for clinicians to have familiarity with these approaches (Barnes, Bloom, and Nahin 2008).

Among the many types of allergies, the most common ones include (Pawankar 2014):

- Atopic dermatitis and contact dermatitis.
- Seasonal allergic rhinitis.
- Allergic conjunctivitis.
- Allergen-triggered asthma.
- Food allergy.
- Insect sting/bite allergy.
- Protein-based latex allergy.
- Hives known as urticaria.
- Eosinophilic disorders.
- The most severe form of allergy to food or drug is classified as *anaphylaxis*.

In response to the increased prevalence, general recommendations call for more comprehensive global epidemiologic studies, reduction of indoor and outdoor pollutants on an international scale, better training programs for healthcare providers, and effective public educational programs in prevention. An international coalition of top scientists called the International Collaboration in Asthma, Allergy, and Immunology has formed to help address these urgent issues (Pawankar 2014).

Etiology

In simplified terms, when a person sensitive to certain allergens contacts them through inhalation or dermal exposure, IgE antibodies are released which combine in an intricate cascade to mount an inflammatory-driven allergic reaction. Many allergies are transferred genetically and can manifest in those predisposed to atopy, an inherited predisposition to overenthusiastic production of IgE to small amounts of proteins commonly found in the environment. This has been demonstrated in maternal exposure to cigarette smoke and home renovation where cord blood has been shown to have elevated IgE levels (Boyce et al. 2012; Yu et al. 2016).

This predisposition puts affected individuals at risk for developing more than one type of allergic disorder. The atopic or allergic march theory refers to the development of atopic dermatitis and subsequent sensitization to aerosolized and food allergens in childhood that can progress to allergic rhinitis and asthma later in life (Spergel 2010).

In many children the allergic process starts in infancy with atopic dermatitis, discussed in detail in the Chapter 16, Dermatology, then progresses with sensitization to cow's milk, peanuts, egg, or other foods introduced after age 6 months. This break in the skin's barrier predisposes to sensitization and hyperreactivity to indoor allergens such as dust mites and common house pets such as dogs and cats. Upper respiratory viral illness, such as respiratory syncytial virus and influenza, are common precipitants of infections in childhood that may predispose a sensitized child to wheezing. Recurrent wheezing episodes can lead to an eventual diagnosis of asthma. Later exposure to outdoor allergens from trees, grass and a variety of pollens creates symptoms of allergic rhinitis and conjunctivitis. Cross reactivity to other allergens can also develop such as to nuts, and certain fruits and vegetables. Food allergy in the U.S. alone has been found to affect an estimated 8% of children, with nearly 40% having a history of severe reactions and another 30% with multiple food allergies. Peanut, milk, and shellfish are the most common allergens in children (Pawankar 2014).

Later in life sensitization can reappear, triggered by environmental exposures at work or through exposure to tobacco smoke, leading to further difficulties with asthma or manifesting as chronic obstructive pulmonary disease in some patients (Thomsen 2015).

New onset of symptoms such as asthma related to sensitizations can present in the elderly (Gillman and Douglass 2012). Wide variability exists in the manifestation of symptoms of the atopic march. Some children may not have full clinical expression of illness, or may present with asthma as a primary illness. Active study in filaggrin gene mutations associated with atopy has helped to link these illnesses in a more coherent manner, although many questions remain to be answered (Osawa, Akiyama, and Shimizu 2011). Low vitamin D has also been associated with increased allergy risk and prevalence and severity of asthma (Allen and Koplin 2016; Bener et al. 2014).

The role of epigenetics (heritable changes in gene activity independent of DNA sequence) is under active study as an etiologic factor in allergy and asthma prevalence. Although many questions remain to be answered definitely, DNA methylation of specific genes has been associated with persistent atopic asthma in inner city children. DNA methylation has also been shown to be more predictive of food allergy than IgE in a study of 48 children, and has also been shown to be associated with risk of eczema.

Infant cord blood with specific DNA methylation signatures has also been shown to be predictive of later asthma risk (DeVries and Vercelli 2015).

Diet is a complex topic in allergy, and includes active questions about optimal timing of introduction of foods in infancy, the need for dietary diversity in early life, adequate fiber intake which impacts microbiome diversity, and the value of home cooked over fast and processed foods (Thorburn, Macia, and Mackay 2014; Tilg and Moschen 2015).

Some protective effects against allergy have been identified. These include what was originally termed the "hygiene hypothesis," a protective effect against allergic rhinitis noted in those growing up with multiple siblings (Strachan 1989); childhood exposure to a farming environment (Von Ehrenstein et al. 2000); breastfeeding has also been shown to have some protective effect in asthma, eczema, and allergic rhinitis; and diversity of the microbiome is a fourth area of active inquiry that shows promise of a protective effect against allergies (Allen and Koplin 2016).

Prevalence

The prevalence of allergic diseases overall has increased steadily over the past five decades, and may be difficult to quantify accurately due to the presence of multiple types of allergies in the same individual. Globally the WHO gives estimates that approximately 300 million people live with asthma, with the prevalence predicted to increase to 400 million in 2025. Another 200–500 million people are estimated to have food allergies. One in every 10 people is estimated to have drug allergy, most commonly to penicillin. Rhinitis is found in an estimated 400 million people globally (Pawankar 2014).

In the U.S., allergic rhinitis is the fifth most common adult disease overall, and the most common chronic illness in children with an estimated 30%–40% experiencing symptoms (Jackson, Howie, and Akinbami 2013). Allergic rhinitis is estimated to impact nearly one in every six people in the U.S. and accounts for an estimated $2–5 billion in direct health expenses annually, primarily due to prescription medications and clinician visits (Meltzer and Bukstein 2011; Seidman et al. 2015).

Atopic dermatitis is estimated to occur in 20% of children, often with symptoms manifesting in the first year of life and 95% manifesting before the age of 5 years. One in three children will develop an associated food allergy. Other associated atopic disease such as hay fever and asthma are common. A child with severe atopic dermatitis has an estimated 50% risk of developing asthma at some point in life (Thomsen 2015).

The prevalence of food allergies can be harder to estimate correctly due to overlap of food sensitivities and variability in self-reported symptoms. The most common IgE-mediated allergic reactions involve cow's milk, egg, nuts, fish, and shellfish and generally develop in the order in which the child is exposed to the individual foods. Estimated prevalence of true food allergy is 3%–5% of the population, with anaphylaxis to food seen in a limited number estimated at less than 0.01% of the population, although it accounts for the most common cause of anaphylaxis among children and adolescents. Food allergy can wane over life, but sensitivity to tree nuts and peanuts may be life-long (Panel et al. 2010).

Food Allergy and Immunizations

In terms of cross-reactivity with food allergens, it is important to note that influenza vaccine is considered safe in children with egg sensitivity who have tolerated egg without serious reaction, and in children who tolerate cooked egg. Consultation on an individual basis is needed to determine safety in this situation, and facilities delivering vaccines must always be prepared to handle anaphylactic reactions. The measles-mumps-rubella vaccine can be administered to children with egg sensitivity because it does not contain sufficient egg protein to trigger allergic reaction. Some medications are manufactured with egg proteins and care must be taken to screen for history of ana-phylactic reaction. One example is propofol, used in induction of anesthesia (Murphy et al. 2011).

As reported by the CDC, in the U.S. the prevalence of allergies in children varies by race and ethnicity. Hispanic children in the U.S. have been shown to have the lowest prevalence of allergies overall. Non-Hispanic black children have higher prevalence of skin allergies and lower prevalence of respiratory allergies compared to non-Hispanic white children. Food allergy and respiratory allergy increase in children of parents with higher income, but there has been no identified difference in prevalence of skin allergy stratified by socioeconomic level (Jackson, Howie, and Akinbami 2013).

Clinical Manifestations

Different types of allergies manifest in characteristic ways, with reactions ranging from mild to severe. Generally, but not always, first reactions to allergens are mild, worsening with repeated exposure. In the mild situations hives, itching, nasal congestion, rashes, and watery eyes are common symptoms. In some reactions, symptoms such as abdominal cramping or pain, diarrhea, difficulty in swallowing, dizziness, tightness in chest, heart palpitations, swollen eyes, nausea, wheezing, and labored breathing can be observed. Sudden and severe allergic reaction is called anaphylaxis and manifests with airway closure and a dramatic drop in blood pressure requiring immediate emergent care.

Comorbidities

Allergies and asthma are chronic inflammatory illnesses that place children at risk for other allergic conditions. Interference with school, sleep, and daily activities of play and physical exercise are common comorbidities. Avoidance of physical exertion due to overheating and aggravation of itch is also associated with sedentary lifestyle. Mental health concerns such as anxiety, depression, phobias, and other internalizing behaviors have been widely documented as significant comorbidities in children with allergic conditions and can persist into later childhood and into adolescence and adult life. Etiology of this avenue of comorbidity is under active study and likely includes both behavioral and physiologic drivers (Nanda et al. 2016; Jackson, Howie, and Akinbami 2013).

A correlation between childhood asthma and overweight has also been established, although causality remains to be fully determined (Mebrahtu et al. 2015). A large prospective population survey found pediatric allergic disease to be associated with increased prevalence of obesity, hypertension, and hyperlipidemia (Silverberg 2015). Eosinophilic gastroenteritis is a relatively rare condition seen in both children and adults. A history of atopy is common. It has been associated with allergic reaction to food antigens, although its etiology is not yet fully understood (D'Alessandro et al. 2015). Presenting symptoms include a history of dysphagia, non-specific gastrointestinal symptoms, food intolerance, and peripheral eosinophilia (Choi et al. 2015).

Diagnostic Criteria

Detailed description of diagnostic criteria for allergy and asthma is beyond the scope of the chapter. Advances in allergy testing such as the use of molecular diagnostic techniques are beginning to expand options in what has traditionally been a challenging diagnostic process. Accurate diagnosis is important for all allergies, but especially so for food allergies, both to avoid potentially serious exposures and to avoid an overly restrictive diet in children (Caubet and Sampson 2012).

A thorough history and physical are needed to understand symptoms and potential allergic exposures. Family history is important. Vague symptoms can present a diagnostic challenge and may require early elimination diet or avoidance of environmental exposures to narrow the field of suspected triggers. After the identification of a suspected allergen, traditionally three possible types of tests were considered for further diagnosis: skin testing, oral challenge, and serum IgE antibody testing. No one test is the gold standard and a stepwise approach is detailed in widely published international guidelines (Panel et al. 2010).

In the skin test, reaction to the suspected allergen is evaluated by taping it on the skin surface or through intradermal injection. The skin test is helpful related to food allergies, mold, pollen, and animal dander allergy; penicillin allergy; venom allergy or allergic contact dermatitis.

The second type of test is related to food allergy diagnosis and is known as oral challenge testing. A specific food item is removed from the diet for several weeks, then reintroduced and reaction recorded. This requires close supervision.

The third avenue is the blood test through which specific serum IgE antibodies are evaluated (Caubet and Sampson 2012).

Clinician supervised oral challenges are still frequently required due to the low positive predictive value of skin-prick tests and food-specific IgE antibodies (Caubet and Sampson 2012). Any history or suspicion of anaphylactic reaction requires further evaluation and testing under supervision of an experienced pediatric specialist.

Treatment

Conventional Treatment

According to the stage of allergy and its level, there are different types of conventional treatments. Basic approaches include education, optimization of skin care early in life to protect the skin barrier, regular follow-up with a trained specialist, awareness and avoidance of aggravating environments or foods, and routine follow-up with a pediatrician or other clinician to monitor growth and development. The WHO, IOM, and the AAP recommend exclusive breastfeeding until age 6 months to maximize its many benefits (Feldman-Winter 2012); however, current allergy recommendations suggest earlier introduction of solids at 4–6 months to reduce risk of food allergy (Muraro et al. 2014), and the AAP has acknowledged this recommendation in various publications. Individual families should work closely with their child's clinician to determine the best course of individual action based on medical and family history (Greer et al. 2008).

Mild allergy symptoms can be treated through over-the-counter antihistamines such as Benadryl (Albin and Nowak-Wegrzyn 2015). Decongestants, nasal corticosteroids: leukotriene modifiers, cromolyn sodium (controls release of histamine), and nasal atropine (for constriction of blood vessels) are commonly used. For desensitization, immunotherapy treatments are used using high-dose allergen injections to stop the allergic response. This is a long-term treatment, which often takes three to five years but has shown about 80%–90% success rate (Albin and Nowak-Wegrzyn 2015).

Allergen-specific oral immunotherapy has received significant attention in pediatrics and has shown promising results in what was initially perceived as a counterintuitive approach. Some of the early studies in this area were designed to safely desensitize children living with peanut allergy in the hope of reducing serious consequences to accidental exposures. Ongoing studies are evaluating the potential positive benefits in milk and egg allergy (Greenhawt 2015).This is a specialized approach that requires the careful supervision of a trained specialist. Most fatalities in children and adolescents have been associated with unintentional ingestion in food allergy without immediate access to epinephrine. Therefore at risk children and their families should be vigilant in their access to injectable epinephrine at all times (Bock, Munoz-Furlong, and Sampson 2001).

Allergic Rhinitis (Asher et al. 2015)

Overview

Allergic rhinitis is the most commonly occurring allergy, estimated to occur in one out of five to six people. It is characterized by seasonal nasal congestion, runny nose, itchy nose, or sneezing. Common causative factors include pollen, dust mites, animal dander, mold, wood dust, latex, and cat saliva. Annual expenditures related to treatment are estimated in the $2–5 billion range in terms of direct health expenditures. Loss of school and work attendance and productivity are common (Seidman et al. 2015).

Etiology

The immune system mounts an exaggerated response in order to defend the body from the allergen. The process activates immunoglobulin (IgE) antibodies and produces histamine, which triggers the typical symptoms of sneezing and runny nose due to the production of excess mucus. Symptoms can worsen over time as sensitization occurs.

Prevalence

Allergic rhinitis is estimated to affect as many as 40% of the pediatric population, although diagnosis can be challenging if suspicion of acute or chronic infection exists (Turner and Kemp 2012).

Clinical Manifestations

The symptoms of allergic rhinitis become visible immediately after inhalation of allergen; these symptoms include continuous sneezing after waking up in the morning; runny or blocked nose; tickling feeling in throat or a postnasal drip resulting in cough; watery or itchy eyes and itchy nose and throat. It can also include hives, dark circles under eyes, sore throat; pressure under nose and cheeks; and headaches (Turner and Kemp 2012).

Secondary symptoms include a packed nose with sniffing; and difficulty breathing due to congestion. These long-term symptoms may result in sleep disorder; long-lasting cough; difficulty in hearing due to pressure or fluid in ear; and uncomfortable feeling or pain in the face (Turner and Kemp 2012).

Comorbidities

People with rhinitis have a risk of asthma, rhinosinusitis and other upper airway conditions. There is also a direct connection of allergic rhinitis with asthma and sleep disorders due to nasal allergic symptoms (Westman et al. 2012).

Psychological complications of allergic conditions are seen in both children and adults and can include increased prevalence of anxiety, depression, and phobias (Nanda et al. 2016).

Diagnostic Criteria

Clinical symptoms and family medical history are the most common diagnostic tools.

Nasal polyps may be seen due to chronic inflammation and can help confirm diagnosis.

Skin prick test and serum specific IgE testing can be useful in pinpointing triggers, although positive predictive value can be low. Nasal endoscopy may also be needed; and computerized tomography (CT) scan may be used to assess blockage or screen for secondary infection. Routine radiologic screening is not recommended for diagnosis (Westman et al. 2012).

Treatment

Conventional Treatment

Lifestyle approaches include recommendations to avoid known allergens, use of an air filtration system, bed and pillow covers, and environmental exposures. Clinical practice guidelines published by the American Academy of Otolaryngology–Head and Neck Surgery provides an extensive review of treatment approaches for children over 2 years of age through adulthood. Initial steps include intranasal therapy with antihistamines for seasonal symptoms. Combination therapy may be needed, which might include oral antihistamines, intranasal corticosteroids, nasal decongestants or immunotherapy (Seidman et al. 2015).

Integrative Treatment

LIFESTYLE APPROACH

Practical measures include allergen avoidance, an anti-inflammatory whole food diet pattern, regular exercise, adequate hydration, and avoidance of secondary triggers such as tobacco smoke and outdoor air pollution.

COMPLEMENTARY APPROACH

Although many complementary approaches are available, few have been well studied, especially in children (Hon et al. 2015). A typical example is nasal saline irrigation, which is widely used yet has few supporting studies in children. One study of its use by Jeffe et al. has documented good tolerance and compliance with saline irrigation in 61 children ranging in age from less than 5 years to 18 years, despite initial parental skepticism that the child would accept the treatment (Jeffe et al. 2012). Nasal irrigation can be done with a variety of commercially available devices, such as a neti pot (Ragab et al. 2015).

Clinical practice guidelines published by the American Academy of Otolaryngology–Head and Neck Surgery found insufficient supporting literature on a wide variety of herbal therapies, especially Chinese herbal therapies, for allergic rhinitis (Seidman et al. 2015).

There is some supporting literature on positive outcome on the use of oral butterbur (*Petasites hybridus*) in adults with allergic rhinitis, although insufficient supporting evidence exists in children (Sadler et al. 2007).

Although homeopathy use is high in allergic rhinitis globally, and it has obvious parallels to the theory behind the use of immunotherapy in allergy treatment, insufficient studies exist to support standard recommendation. A typical confounder of homeopathy studies is the need for individualization of treatment. Randomized controlled trials are under development to help better determine effectiveness (Banerjee et al. 2014).

The complementary approach with best supporting literature in allergic rhinitis is currently acupuncture, although further studies are needed before routine recommendation is possible (Tille and White 2015).

It is proposed for its immune-modulating effects and ability to resolve blockage of congestion, although its exact mechanism of action is unknown. One randomized pediatric study by Ng et al. showed benefit in the treatment group in a study of 35 children with allergic rhinitis who received acupuncture twice per week for 8 weeks. Acupuncture reduced symptoms scores and number of symptom-free days with no adverse events reported (Ng et al. 2004).

More data on acupuncture is available in adults. A review of acupuncture studies in allergic rhinitis show mixed quality, size and benefit, although several support improvement in quality of life, and in associated pruritus if present with atopic dermatitis (Hauswald and Yarin 2014).

A larger randomized controlled German study of 422 adult patients showed a statistically significant improvement in patient symptoms in a standardized protocol of 12 acupuncture treatments over 8 weeks (Brinkhaus et al. 2013).

A 2015 systematic review and meta-analysis by Feng et al. examined 13 studies involving 2365 adult patients and found an overall positive effect in treatment groups in terms of symptoms and quality of life with no serious adverse events (Feng et al. 2015).

Asthma

Overview

Asthma is a multifactorial illness that involves neuromuscular, inflammatory, and psychological elements that manifest as bronchospasm, airway narrowing and remodeling, and air hunger. Asthma affects people of all ages and has had a sharp increase in prevalence worldwide over the past 30 years, affecting an estimated 300 million people globally, and close to 20 million people in the U.S., 7 million of whom are children (Olin and Wechsler 2014).

Statistics from the 2007 National Health Interview Survey show that asthma is among the top 15 most common medical conditions in which integrative medical therapies are used. Integrative approaches for asthma have been documented in a range of studies in children and adults. A survey of 5435 children with asthma showed that 26.7% had used complementary therapies to treat symptoms in the preceding 12 months, most often in conjunction with conventional therapies (Shen and Oraka 2012). Some of the benefits of the use of integrative therapies in asthma include their potential to improve overall health with lifestyle changes, reduce inflammation and chronic medication exposure, and address psychological stressors associated with living with acute exacerbations and the burden of living with a chronic illness. In part because of its multifactorial nature, asthma lends itself to an integrative approach that can address the multiple components of the disease.

Etiology

Asthma flares can be triggered by a variety of factors, including allergens, environmental pollutants, and internal stressors resulting in bronchoconstriction, mucus plugging, and air hunger. Air quality and presence of very fine particulate matter have been shown to be associated with airway inflammation and remodeling (Guarnieri and Balmes 2014).

Prenatal phthalate and early bisphenol A exposures have also been positively correlated with increased risk of asthma in inner city children (Whyatt et al. 2014).

A review by Robinson and Miller that examines the accumulating research on the effect of both bisphenol A and phthalates on immune modulation and predisposition to allergic and wheezing illnesses finds a growing base of evidence to suggest a link in humans (Robinson and Miller 2015). Genetic factors such as atopy in a parent are important, as are exposure to prenatal smoking (Chhabra et al. 2014), prenatal stressors and diet, and mode of delivery—vaginal versus cesarean (Salam, Zhang, and Begum 2012).

Children with existing allergies have a higher chance of getting asthma; early viral infections of the respiratory tract associated with wheezing are also predictive of a later diagnosis of asthma. Exercise, exposure to air pollution or the environmental factors, outdoor and indoor allergens, tobacco smoke and chemical irritants, and emotional factors such as stress, anger, and fear can all trigger symptoms in susceptible individuals (Salam, Zhang, and Begum 2012).

Prevalence

Asthma is estimated to affect close to one in every eight children in the U.S. and globally (Akinbami, Centers for Disease, and Prevention National Center for Health 2006; Lai et al. 2009).

The disease varies geographically, and by age group, from 0.8% recorded in Tibet to 32.6% in Wellington, New Zealand in 13–14 year olds and 2.4% in Jodhpur, India to 37.6% in Costa Rica in the 6–7 years of age category. Higher income countries overall had higher prevalence of wheeze in children, more so in the older age groups (Lai et al. 2009).

Clinical Manifestations

The word asthma is derived from the Greek *aazein*, to pant or exhale with an open mouth (Banasiak 2016).

Signs and symptoms include: dyspnea; pain or tightness in chest; disturbed sleep patterns; wheezing on exhalation; severe wheezing, or persistent cough with or without wheeze.

Comorbidities

There are many comorbidities of asthma stratified by age with highest rates in adulthood. They include: rhinitis, sinusitis, gastroesophageal reflux disease, bronchitis, obstructive sleep apnea (Banasiak 2016), cardiovascular disease, diabetes, obesity, and psychologic issues such as anxiety and depression. Conditions associated with poor asthma control are psychological dysfunction and paradoxical vocal cord dysfunction (Gershon et al. 2012). Risk of depression and suicidal ideation requires raised awareness and careful screening in children and adolescents (Gerald and Moreno 2016).

Diagnostic Criteria

Asthma is diagnosed on the basis of medical history, physical exams, and signs and symptoms. Lung function tests present a challenge in young children unable to complete forced expirations (Ioan et al. 2015).

Accurate diagnosis in young children can be further complicated by concurrent viral or bacterial respiratory illnesses. Approximately 35%–45% of children diagnosed before the age of 3 years have symptoms after age 6 years (Radhakrishnan et al. 2014). Family asthma history, skin allergies, allergic rhinitis, and prior history of a wheezing illness in infancy increase the likelihood of a positive diagnosis of asthma (Radhakrishnan et al. 2014).

Nocturnal symptoms and sleep disruption are associated with poorer control and decreased quality of life for child and family. Use of biomarkers such as exhaled nitric oxide, serum IgE, and urinary leukotrienes are under active study as useful markers of airway inflammation (Radhakrishnan et al. 2014).

Treatment

Conventional Treatment

The conventional approach towards asthma is based upon two types of treatments and their associated medications: first, quick-relief medications used in urgent and emergency situations; and, second, long-term control medications to prevent exacerbations. Age- and condition-specific guidelines are widely published and updated regularly. One important caveat is to reaffirm diagnosis, inhaler technique, new exposures, and compliance with any current treatment plan before stepping up to a higher intervention. A continuum of care and a clear detailed action plan is an important component of any child's asthma treatment (Reddel et al. 2015).

The quick-relief medications typically include:

- Short-acting beta-2 agonists

- Oral corticosteroid burst
- Inhaled anticholinergics—large airway bronchodilators

The long-term control medications may include:

- Inhaled long-acting beta-agonist
- Inhaled corticosteroids
- Leukotriene modifiers
- Mast cell stabilizers
- Immunomodulator
- Theophylline

Integrative Treatment

LIFESTYLE APPROACH

Lifestyle approaches include avoidance of triggers, including those found in nature, and those that are manmade such as cigarette smoke, chemical perfumes, and environmental substances. Avoidance of windy and dusty outdoor settings may be helpful. Removal of common allergy triggers from the home can also be helpful; for example, removal of carpet and replacement with hard flooring, and use of non-allergic cleaning products (Reddel et al. 2015).

NUTRITION

High Mediterranean diet score in pregnancy has also been associated with a protective effect against persistent wheeze, atopic wheeze, and atopy in children born to mothers adhering to the diet (Chatzi et al. 2008), although a study of 1771 Greek mother–infant pairs failed to find a correlation with maternal Mediterranean diet intake and wheeze in the infant's first 12 months of life. Correlation was made with wheeze and maternal intake of meat and processed meat in this study group (Chatzi et al. 2008).

A Danish cohort of 28,936 mothers showed a significant correlation between high maternal fish intake (2–3 meals/week) and low prevalence of wheeze in offspring at 18 months (p = 0.001), consistent with a Mediterranean diet pattern (Maslova et al. 2013).

The Mediterranean diet pattern has shown benefit in reducing the prevalence of asthma in children in large population studies (Arvaniti et al. 2011; Garcia-Marcos et al. 2013). One cross-sectional study of 1125 Greek children aged 10–12 years old found that each 1-unit increase in Mediterranean diet was associated with a 16% reduction in likelihood of having asthma (Grigoropoulou et al. 2011).

Higher adherence to a Mediterranean diet has also shown a protective effect against wheeze in 287 children aged 9–19 years living in Peru (Rice et al. 2015).

The impact of fiber on inflammatory disease is also a topic of research interest. Animal studies have demonstrated the interface between fiber intake and regulation of the lung's immune system. Studies have shown that dietary fiber can be metabolized by gut microbes into short chain fatty acids that promote the development of regulatory T cells that have a role in reduction of lung inflammation (Huffnagle 2014).

Microbiome and The Lung

Breakthroughs in the study of the microbiome and the respiratory tract have resulted in important strides in understanding of the etiology and course of many diseases, including childhood asthma. These advances will undoubtedly offer new approaches to chronic inflammatory and infectious respiratory conditions. Although many questions remain, studies linking alterations in the microbiome to allergic asthma show a consistent correlation in pediatric studies, and animal studies demonstrate that exposure to antibiotics and dietary changes alter the microbiota and the T-cell–mediated immune system, directly impacting the lung's immune pathways (Dickson et al. 2015).

Probiotics

To date no prospective studies have found beneficial preventive effect of probiotics of various strains, although research remains active in this area (Gorissen et al. 2014).

Exercise

Physical activity can be a two-edged sword for children with exercise-induced asthma, which has been documented in more than one in three children with asthma in some large population studies (Lodrup Carlsen et al. 2006).

Children who participate in endurance and winter sports and swimming have the highest prevalence of exercise-induced asthma. Elite athletes also have higher risk. Avoidance of exercise during extreme cold, heavy pollen loads, and when ill or recovering from respiratory illness is recommended. Repeated exposure to chlorine has shifted thinking about swimming as being a preferred sport for children with asthma, although a 2013 Cochrane Database Systematic Review found benefit in children (Beggs et al. 2013).

Overall fitness has been found to be protective in asthma, and use of short- and long-term beta-agonists as per recent guidelines can help predisposed children exercise safely. Moderate intensity training is an area of active study in animal models and appears to reduce airway smooth muscle hypertrophy, hyperplasia, and remodeling. Studies in humans are demonstrating similar findings (Pakhale et al. 2013), including reduction of allergen-related IgE level (Moreira et al. 2008).

A trial of 36 children randomized to either treadmill or active video game aerobic exercise found improvements in both groups, but significant reduction in exhaled nitric oxide in the video group ($p < 0.005$) after two weekly sessions for an 8-week study period (Del Giacco et al. 2015).

Yoga is an activity that has many potential benefits for the child with asthma due to its focus on controlling the breath and its dual physical and mental relaxation benefits (Rosen et al. 2015).

Despite the encouraging research on physical activity and asthma, children with the disease may be discouraged from participation in physical activity because of social stigma, bullying, or ridicule due to need for medication or inability to keep up with peers (Walker and Reznik 2014).

Obesity is another common and serious barrier to regular physical activity in children (Weinmayr et al. 2014). Every child with asthma or other respiratory conditions will need support and encouragement from adults in their circle to help them incorporate exercise into their asthma treatment successfully.

Complementary Approach

DIETARY SUPPLEMENTS

The use of dietary supplements in both children and adults is common in asthma despite a lack of large high-quality randomized controlled studies supporting their use (Clark et al. 2010; Arnold et al. 2008).

Reasons for their use include a desire to avoid prescription medication, lack of access to other healthcare options, and a desire to maximize overall health. Open discussion and full disclose of use of supplements is very important in all patients, and especially so in those with asthma to avoid possible supplement–drug interactions. One of the more common examples includes a risk of allergic reactions to echinacea and chamomile, both members of the ragweed family Compositae. Exclusive use of supplements may also put patients at risk for delay of appropriate care. There are some supplements that show positive potential as complementary approaches in asthma, including omega-3 fatty acids, vitamin D, and vitamin C.

Omega-3 Fatty Acids   The omega-3 fatty acids have recognized anti-inflammatory and triglyceride-lowering effects and are discussed in detail in Chapter 4, Key Dietary Supplements. They play a role in metabolic disease including reduction of pulmonary inflammation, in part modulated through peroxisome proliferator-activated receptors (PPARs) (Khan et al. 2014).

Reduction of wheeze in offspring has been consistently reported when omega-3 fatty acids are used during pregnancy and lactation, but not when used in children with asthma diagnosis (Muley, Shah, and Muley 2015).

Genetic polymorphisms likely play a role in mixed results in study outcomes, but some studies have shown beneficial effects with minimal adverse effects noted. A systematic review and meta-analysis by Muley et al. of five studies involving 2415 children with asthma showed mixed effects and no specific benefit. Authors cite the need for more randomized controlled trials in children. Synergistic interactions with anticoagulants due to anti-platelet effects have been reported in adult studies (Muley, Shah, and Muley 2015).

Vitamin D   Vitamin D plays an integral role in cell processes and in modulation of the inflammatory cascade. Normal levels are associated with prenatal lung development (Paul et al. 2012). Vitamin D deficiency has been linked to asthma in the pediatric population, correlated with more severe symptoms, more frequent exacerbations, reduction in lung function, and an increased need of prescription medication (Gupta et al. 2012).

A 2015 meta-analysis of eight studies involving 573 children aged 3–18 years reflected a wide variety of study designs and low-quality evidence to support supplementation, but lacked sufficient strength for standard recommendations (Riverin, Maguire, and Li 2015).

Overall maintaining vitamin D in the recommended range of normal in children with asthma is a prudent and low-risk goal. A target range of 30–100 ng/mL is in line with

Endocrine Society guidelines. Vitamin D is discussed in detail in the Chapter 4, Key Dietary Supplements (Holick et al. 2011).

Vitamin C   A Cochrane Database systematic review of five studies involving 214 adults and children found insufficient evidence to support the use of vitamin C for asthma management (Wilkinson et al. 2014).

Butterbur   Butterbur (*Petasites hybridus*), a member of the Asteraceae/Compositae family, has been used for thousands of years for medicinal purposes, including asthma in children. It has an inhibitory effect on leukotriene production among other actions. Some small studies support its use; for example, a prospective randomized open trial in 16 children aged 6–17 years and 64 adults with asthma evaluated butterbur over an 8-week period in addition to their ongoing medications. At 8 weeks, number of attacks had decreased by 48% and duration of attacks decreased by 75%. FEV1 and peak flow had increased by more than 70% and 80% respectively. By week 16 nearly half the patients had decreased their dose of inhaled steroid and short-acting beta agonists (Danesch 2004).

Doses in children range from 50 mg to 150 mg per day divided in to two or three doses. Butterbur extract is standardized to 15% petasins. The raw herb can contain pyrrolizidine alkaloids which are carcinogenic and hepatotoxic.

Morin   Emerging research on morin, a naturally occurring flavonol found in high concentration in herbs in the Moraceae family, has shown it to have both anti-inflammatory and anticancer properties. Animal studies show promising activity against allergic airway inflammation by modulating the complex inflammatory response and reduction of total IgE levels. This and other work on naturally occurring anti-inflammatories will hopefully lead to an expanded range of effective and non-toxic options for asthma (Ma et al. 2016).

Mind–Body Medicine

Mind–body medicine has several important potential benefits in asthma treatment including immune modulation, increased sense of control and self-efficacy, decrease in anxiety and depression, and improved sleep. Some of the most commonly used mind–body therapies in children with asthma include breathing exercises (Shen and Oraka 2012).

Other mind-body therapies useful in asthma include prayer (Luberto et al. 2012), progressive muscle relaxation techniques, which are often combined with guided imagery, and clinical hypnosis, which has a long history of success in children with asthma (Maher-Loughnan et al. 1962; Kohen et al. 1984; McBride, Vlieger, and Anbar 2014).

Mindfulness

Studies on the benefit of an 8-week mindfulness-based stress-reduction course in adults with asthma demonstrate its benefit in improving quality of life and reducing stress, even in the absence of significant change in lung function. Results persisted at 12 months post-intervention follow-up (Pbert et al. 2012).

Yoga

Small studies have shown the benefit of yoga on the quality of life in children with asthma (Galantino, Galbavy, and Quinn 2008).

For example, a randomized study by Tahan et al. in 20 children aged 6–17 years with exercise-induced bronchospasm showed that the treatment group who received two 1-hour yoga sessions weekly for 3 months had a statistically significant improvement in maximum forced expiratory volume following exercise challenge ($p < 0.05$). All exercise positive children became exercise response negative responders after yoga training in this study group (Tahan, Eke Gungor, and Bicici 2014).

Yoga has also been shown to have beneficial effect in overall stress reduction and increase in quality of life for children living with chronic disease and in general has a very low risk profile (Rosen et al. 2015).

While the mind–body therapies are generally very safe and well tolerated, caution must be used in children with a history of any type of abuse or significant trauma. Mind–body therapies should be tailored to the needs and interests of the individual patient, and their use should not delay access to conventional care in acute or chronic situations.

Acupuncture

A systematic review that included seven articles concluded some benefit to the use of traditional acupuncture in children with asthma, although study design variability, differing point placement, session time, duration, and frequency, location inpatient versus outpatient and other variables made conclusions challenging. Serious adverse events were not seen in this group of studies. Authors called for more standardized large-scale studies (Liu and Chien 2015).

Other mind–body therapies such as breathing exercise, music therapy, and biofeedback need larger studies to confirm benefit. Some school-based studies on stress management have shown good acceptance and benefit in children with asthma in pilot studies and further studies are needed (Long et al. 2011).

Conclusion

Allergies and asthma are often interrelated and are, as a group, the most common chronic illnesses in children often accompanied by serious inflammatory-driven comorbidities. Children with these conditions are also at risk for exposure to multiple short- and long-term medications, which although often needed, are accompanied by their own panel of potential side effects. An integrative medicine approach has much to offer in the prevention and treatment of these conditions, beginning in the prenatal period. An emphasis on maternal diet in the form of a Mediterranean diet pattern, avoidance of environmental toxicants, normalization of maternal vitamin D and attention to chronic stressors is important for expectant mothers. Addition of a prenatal probiotic in mothers predisposed to atopy has potential to be protective in their children, especially against the development of atopic dermatitis, considered a first step in the 'atopic march' that can lead to the development of systemic inflammatory conditions such as asthma. Use of all available tools, such as healthy whole food diet, omega-3 fatty acids, moderate vitamin D supplementation, and open-minded exploration of mind–body therapies should be embraced in conjunction with prudent use of conventional therapies to reduce morbidity and medication exposure in children living with these illnesses.

References

Akinbami, L., Control Centers for Disease, and Statistics Prevention National Center for Health. 2006. "The state of childhood asthma, United States, 1980–2005." *Adv Data* 381: 1–24.

Albin, S., and A. Nowak-Wegrzyn. 2015. "Potential treatments for food allergy." *Immunol Allergy Clin North Am* 35(1): 77–100. doi: 10.1016/j.iac.2014.09.011.

Allen, K. J., and J. J. Koplin. 2016. "Prospects for prevention of food allergy." *J Allergy Clin Immunol Pract.* doi: 10.1016/j.jaip.2015.10.010.

Arnold, E., C. E. Clark, T. J. Lasserson, and T. Wu. 2008. "Herbal interventions for chronic asthma in adults and children." *Cochrane Database Syst Rev* 1: CD005989. doi: 10.1002/14651858. CD005989.pub2.

Arvaniti, F., K. N. Priftis, A. Papadimitriou, M. Papadopoulos, E. Roma, M. Kapsokefalou, M. B. Anthracopoulos, and D. B. Panagiotakos. 2011. "Adherence to the Mediterranean type of diet is associated with lower prevalence of asthma symptoms, among 10–12 years old children: the PANACEA study." *Pediatr Allergy Immunol* 22(3): 283–9. doi: 10.1111/j.1399-3038.2010.01113.x.

Asher, B. F., M. D. Seidman, W. D. Reddy, and F. S. Omole. 2015. "Integrative medical approaches to allergic rhinitis." *Curr Opin Otolaryngol Head Neck Surg* 23(3): 221–5. doi: 10.1097/MOO.0000000000000152.

Banasiak, N. C. 2016. "Understanding the relationship between asthma and sleep in the pediatric population." *J Pediatr Health Care.* doi: 10.1016/j.pedhc.2015.11.012.

Banerjee, K., C. Costelloe, R. T. Mathie, and J. Howick. 2014. "Homeopathy for allergic rhinitis: protocol for a systematic review." *Syst Rev* 3: 59. doi: 10.1186/2046-4053-3-59.

Barnes, P. M., B. Bloom, and R. L. Nahin. 2008. "Complementary and alternative medicine use among adults and children: United States, 2007." *Natl Health Stat Report* 12: 1–23.

Beggs, S., Y. C. Foong, H. C. Le, D. Noor, R. Wood-Baker, and J. A. Walters. 2013. "Swimming training for asthma in children and adolescents aged 18 years and under." *Cochrane Database Syst Rev* 4: CD009607. doi: 10.1002/14651858.CD009607.pub2.

Bener, A., M. S. Ehlayel, H. Z. Bener, and Q. Hamid. 2014. "The impact of Vitamin D deficiency on asthma, allergic rhinitis and wheezing in children: an emerging public health problem." *J Family Community Med* 21(3): 154–61. doi: 10.4103/2230-8229.142967.

Bock, S. A., A. Munoz-Furlong, and H. A. Sampson. 2001. "Fatalities due to anaphylactic reactions to foods." *J Allergy Clin Immunol* 107(1): 191–3. doi: 10.1067/mai.2001.112031.

Boyce, J. A., B. Bochner, F. D. Finkelman, and M. E. Rothenberg. 2012. "Advances in mechanisms of asthma, allergy, and immunology in 2011." *J Allergy Clin Immunol* 129(2): 335–41. doi: 10.1016/j.jaci.2011.12.968.

Brinkhaus, B., M. Ortiz, C. M. Witt, S. Roll, K. Linde, F. Pfab, B. Niggemann, J. Hummelsberger, A. Treszl, J. Ring, T. Zuberbier, K. Wegscheider, and S. N. Willich. 2013. "Acupuncture in patients with seasonal allergic rhinitis: a randomized trial." *Ann Intern Med* 158(4): 225–34. doi: 10.7326/0003-4819-158-4-201302190-00002.

Caubet, J. C., and H. A. Sampson. 2012. "Beyond skin testing: state of the art and new horizons in food allergy diagnostic testing." *Immunol Allergy Clin North Am* 32(1): 97–109. doi: 10.1016/j.iac.2011.11.002.

Chatzi, L., M. Torrent, I. Romieu, R. Garcia-Esteban, C. Ferrer, J. Vioque, M. Kogevinas, and J. Sunyer. 2008. "Mediterranean diet in pregnancy is protective for wheeze and atopy in childhood." *Thorax* 63(6): 507–13. doi: 10.1136/thx.2007.081745.

Chhabra, D., S. Sharma, A. T. Kho, R. Gaedigk, C. A. Vyhlidal, J. S. Leeder, J. Morrow, V. J. Carey, S. T. Weiss, K. G. Tantisira, and D. L. DeMeo. 2014. "Fetal lung and placental methylation is associated with in utero nicotine exposure." *Epigenetics* 9(11): 1473–84. doi: 10.4161/15592294.2014.971593.

Choi, J. S., S. J. Choi, K. J. Lee, A. Kim, J. K. Yoo, H. R. Yang, J. S. Moon, J. Y. Chang, J. S. Ko, and G. H. Kang. 2015. "Clinical manifestations and treatment outcomes of eosinophilic gastroenteritis in children." *Pediatr Gastroenterol Hepatol Nutr* 18(4): 253–60. doi: 10.5223/pghn.2015.18.4.253.

Clark, C. E., E. Arnold, T. J. Lasserson, and T. Wu. 2010. "Herbal interventions for chronic asthma in adults and children: a systematic review and meta-analysis." *Prim Care Respir J* 19(4): 307–14. doi: 10.4104/pcrj.2010.00041.

D'Alessandro, A., D. Esposito, M. Pesce, R. Cuomo, G. D. De Palma, and G. Sarnelli. 2015. "Eosinophilic esophagitis: from pathophysiology to treatment." *World J Gastrointest Pathophysiol* 6(4): 150–8. doi: 10.4291/wjgp.v6.i4.150.

Danesch, U. C. 2004. "Petasites hybridus (Butterbur root) extract in the treatment of asthma: an open trial." *Altern Med Rev* 9(1): 54–62.

Del Giacco, S. R., D. Firinu, L. Bjermer, and K. H. Carlsen. 2015. "Exercise and asthma: an overview." *Eur Clin Respir J* 2: 27984. doi: 10.3402/ecrj.v2.27984.

DeVries, A., and D. Vercelli. 2015. "Epigenetics in allergic diseases." *Curr Opin Pediatr* 27(6): 719–23. doi: 10.1097/MOP.0000000000000285.

Dickson, R. P., J. R. Erb-Downward, F. J. Martinez, and G. B. Huffnagle. 2015. "The microbiome and the respiratory tract." *Annu Rev Physiol.* doi: 10.1146/annurev-physiol-021115-105238.

Feldman-Winter, L. 2012. "The AAP updates its policy on breastfeeding and reaches consensus on recommended duration of exclusive breastfeeding." *J Hum Lact* 28(2): 116–7. doi: 10.1177/0890334412442826.

Feng, S., M. Han, Y. Fan, G. Yang, Z. Liao, W. Liao, and H. Li. 2015. "Acupuncture for the treatment of allergic rhinitis: a systematic review and meta-analysis." *Am J Rhinol Allergy* 29(1): 57–62. doi: 10.2500/ajra.2015.29.4116.

Galantino, M. L., R. Galbavy, and L. Quinn. 2008. "Therapeutic effects of yoga for children: a systematic review of the literature." *Pediatr Phys Ther* 20(1): 66–80. doi: 10.1097/PEP.0b013e31815f1208.

Garcia-Marcos, L., J. A. Castro-Rodriguez, G. Weinmayr, D. B. Panagiotakos, K. N. Priftis, and G. Nagel. 2013. "Influence of Mediterranean diet on asthma in children: a systematic review and meta-analysis." *Pediatr Allergy Immunol* 24(4): 330–8. doi: 10.1111/pai.12071.

Gerald, J. K., and F. A. Moreno. 2016. "Asthma and depression: it's complicated." *J Allergy Clin Immunol Pract* 4(1): 74–5. doi: 10.1016/j.jaip.2015.11.020.

Gershon, A. S., J. Guan, C. Wang, J. C. Victor, and T. To. 2012. "Describing and quantifying asthma comorbidity [corrected]: a population study." *PLoS One* 7(5): e34967. doi: 10.1371/journal.pone.0034967.

Gillman, A., and J. A. Douglass. 2012. "Asthma in the elderly." *Asia Pac Allergy* 2(2): 101–8. doi: 10.5415/apallergy.2012.2.2.101.

Gorissen, D. M., N. B. Rutten, C. M. Oostermeijer, L. E. Niers, M. O. Hoekstra, G. T. Rijkers, and C. K. van der Ent. 2014. "Preventive effects of selected probiotic strains on the development of asthma and allergic rhinitis in childhood. The Panda study." *Clin Exp Allergy* 44(11): 1431–3. doi: 10.1111/cea.12413.

Greenhawt, M. 2015. "The learning early about peanut allergy study: the benefits of early peanut introduction, and a new horizon in fighting the food allergy epidemic." *Pediatr Clin North Am* 62(6): 1509–21. doi: 10.1016/j.pcl.2015.07.010.

Greer, F. R., S. H. Sicherer, A. W. Burks, Nutrition American Academy of Pediatrics Committee on, Allergy American Academy of Pediatrics Section on, and Immunology. 2008. "Effects of early nutritional interventions on the development of atopic disease in infants and children: the role of maternal dietary restriction, breastfeeding, timing of introduction of complementary foods, and hydrolyzed formulas." *Pediatrics* 121(1): 183–91. doi: 10.1542/peds.2007-3022.

Grigoropoulou, D., K. N. Priftis, M. Yannakoulia, A. Papadimitriou, M. B. Anthracopoulos, K.

Yfanti, and D. B. Panagiotakos. 2011. "Urban environment adherence to the Mediterranean diet and prevalence of asthma symptoms among 10- to 12-year-old children: The Physical Activity, Nutrition, and Allergies in Children Examined in Athens study." *Allergy Asthma Proc* 32(5): 351–8. doi: 10.2500/aap.2011.32.3463.

Guarnieri, M., and J. R. Balmes. 2014. "Outdoor air pollution and asthma." *Lancet* 383(9928): 1581–92. doi: 10.1016/S0140-6736(14)60617-6.

Gupta, A., A. Bush, C. Hawrylowicz, and S. Saglani. 2012. "Vitamin D and asthma in children." *Paediatr Respir Rev* 13(4): 236–43; quiz 243. doi: 10.1016/j.prrv.2011.07.003.

Hauswald, B., and Y. M. Yarin. 2014. "Acupuncture in allergic rhinitis: a mini-review." *Allergo J Int* 23(4): 115–19. doi: 10.1007/s40629-014-0015-3.

Holick, M. F., N. C. Binkley, H. A. Bischoff-Ferrari, C. M. Gordon, D. A. Hanley, R. P. Heaney, M. H. Murad, C. M. Weaver, and Society Endocrine. 2011. "Evaluation, treatment, and prevention of vitamin D deficiency: an Endocrine Society clinical practice guideline." *J Clin Endocrinol Metab* 96(7): 1911–30. doi: 10.1210/jc.2011-0385.

Hon, K. L., C. K. Fung, A. K. Leung, H. S. Lam, and S. L. Lee. 2015. "Recent Patents of Complementary and Alternative Medicine for Allergic Rhinitis." *Recent Pat Inflamm Allergy Drug Discov* 9(2): 107–19.

Huffnagle, G. B. 2014. "Increase in dietary fiber dampens allergic responses in the lung." *Nat Med* 20(2): 120–1. doi: 10.1038/nm.3472.

Ioan, I., S. Varechova, F. Marchal, and D. A. Plesca. 2015. "A systematic review of lung function testing in asthmatic young children." *Pneumologia* 64(2): 8–12.

Jackson, K. D., L. D. Howie, and L. J. Akinbami. 2013. "Trends in allergic conditions among children: United States, 1997–2011." *NCHS Data Brief* 121: 1–8.

Jeffe J. S., B. Bhushan, and J. W. Schroeder Jr. 2012. "Nasal saline irrigation in children: a study of compliance and tolerance." *Int J Pediatr Otorhinolaryngol* 76: 409–13. doi: 10.1016/j.ijporl.2011.12.022.

Khan, S. A., A. Ali, S. A. Khan, S. A. Zahran, G. Damanhouri, E. Azhar, and I. Qadri. 2014. "Unraveling the complex relationship triad between lipids, obesity, and inflammation." *Mediators Inflamm* 2014: 502749. doi: 10.1155/2014/502749.

Kohen, D. P., K. N. Olness, S. O. Colwell, and A. Heimel. 1984. "The use of relaxation-mental imagery (self-hypnosis) in the management of 505 pediatric behavioral encounters." *J Dev Behav Pediatr* 5(1): 21–5.

Lai, C. K., R. Beasley, J. Crane, S. Foliaki, J. Shah, S. Weiland, Asthma International Study of, and Group Allergies in Childhood Phase Three Study. 2009. "Global variation in the prevalence and severity of asthma symptoms: phase three of the International Study of Asthma and Allergies in Childhood (ISAAC)." *Thorax* 64(6): 476–83. doi: 10.1136/thx.2008.106609.

Liu, C. F., and L. W. Chien. 2015. "Efficacy of acupuncture in children with asthma: a systematic review." *Ital J Pediatr* 41: 48. doi: 10.1186/s13052-015-0155-1.

Lodrup Carlsen, K. C., G. Haland, C. S. Devulapalli, M. Munthe-Kaas, M. Pettersen, B. Granum, M. Lovik, and K. H. Carlsen. 2006. "Asthma in every fifth child in Oslo, Norway: a 10-year follow up of a birth cohort study." *Allergy* 61(4): 454–60. doi: 10.1111/j.1398-9995.2005.00938.x.

Long, K. A., L. J. Ewing, S. Cohen, D. Skoner, D. Gentile, J. Koehrsen, C. Howe, A. L. Thompson, R. K. Rosen, M. Ganley, and A. L. Marsland. 2011. "Preliminary evidence for the feasibility of a stress management intervention for 7- to 12-year-olds with asthma." *J Asthma* 48(2): 162–70. doi: 10.3109/02770903.2011.554941.

Luberto, C. M., M. S. Yi, J. Tsevat, A. C. Leonard, and S. Cotton. 2012. "Complementary and alternative medicine use and psychosocial outcomes among urban adolescents with asthma." *J Asthma* 49(4): 409–15. doi: 10.3109/02770903.2012.672612.

Ma, Y., A. Ge, W. Zhu, Y. N. Liu, N. F. Ji, W. J. Zha, J. X. Zhang, X. N. Zeng, and M. Huang. 2016. "Morin attenuates ovalbumin-induced airway inflammation by modulating oxidative stress-responsive MAPK signaling." *Oxid Med Cell Longev* 2016: 5843672. doi: 10.1155/2016/5843672.

Maher-Loughnan, G. P., A. A. Mason, N. Macdonald, and L. Fry. 1962. "Controlled trial of hypnosis in the symptomatic treatment of asthma." *Br Med J* 2(5301): 371–6.

Maslova, E., M. Strom, E. Oken, H. Campos, C. Lange, D. Gold, and S. F. Olsen. 2013. "Fish intake during pregnancy and the risk of child asthma and allergic rhinitis—longitudinal evidence from the Danish National Birth Cohort." *Br J Nutr* 110(7): 1313–25. doi: 10.1017/S000711451300038X.

McBride, J. J., A. M. Vlieger, and R. D. Anbar. 2014. "Hypnosis in paediatric respiratory medicine." *Paediatr Respir Rev* 15(1): 82–5. doi: 10.1016/j.prrv.2013.09.002.

Mebrahtu, T. F., R. G. Feltbower, D. C. Greenwood, and R. C. Parslow. 2015. "Childhood body mass index and wheezing disorders: a systematic review and meta-analysis." *Pediatr Allergy Immunol* 26(1): 62–72. doi: 10.1111/pai.12321.

Meltzer, E. O., and D. A. Bukstein. 2011. "The economic impact of allergic rhinitis and current guidelines for treatment." *Ann Allergy Asthma Immunol* 106(2 Suppl): S12–16. doi: 10.1016/j.anai.2010.10.014.

Moreira, A., L. Delgado, T. Haahtela, J. Fonseca, P. Moreira, C. Lopes, J. Mota, P. Santos, P. Rytila, and M. G. Castel-Branco. 2008. "Physical training does not increase allergic inflammation in asthmatic children." *Eur Respir J* 32(6): 1570–5. doi: 10.1183/09031936.00171707.

Muley, P., M. Shah, and A. Muley. 2015. "Omega-3 fatty acids supplementation in children to prevent asthma: is it worthy?—a systematic review and meta-analysis." *J Allergy (Cairo)* 2015: 312052. doi: 10.1155/2015/312052.

Muraro, A., S. Halken, S. H. Arshad, K. Beyer, A. E. Dubois, G. Du Toit, P. A. Eigenmann, K. E. Grimshaw, A. Hoest, G. Lack, L. O'Mahony, N. G. Papadopoulos, S. Panesar, S. Prescott, G. Roberts, D. de Silva, C. Venter, V. Verhasselt, A. C. Akdis, A. Sheikh, Eaaci Food Allergy, and Group Anaphylaxis Guidelines. 2014. "EAACI food allergy and anaphylaxis guidelines. Primary prevention of food allergy." *Allergy* 69(5): 590–601. doi: 10.1111/all.12398.

Murphy, A., D. E. Campbell, D. Baines, and S. Mehr. 2011. "Allergic reactions to propofol in egg-allergic children." *Anesth Analg* 113(1): 140–4. doi: 10.1213/ANE.0b013e31821b450f.

Nanda, M. K., G. K. LeMasters, L. Levin, M. E. Rothenberg, A. H. Assa'ad, N. Newman, D. Bernstein, G. Khurana-Hershey, J. E. Lockey, and P. H. Ryan. 2016. "Allergic diseases and internalizing behaviors in early childhood." *Pediatrics* 137(1): 1–10. doi: 10.1542/peds.2015-1922.

Ng, D. K., P. Y. Chow, S. P. Ming, S. H. Hong, S. Lau, D. Tse, W. K. Kwong, M. F. Wong, W. H. Wong, Y. M. Fu, K. L. Kwok, H. Li, and J. C. Ho. 2004. "A double-blind, randomized, placebo-controlled trial of acupuncture for the treatment of childhood persistent allergic rhinitis." *Pediatrics* 114(5): 1242–7. doi: 10.1542/peds.2004-0744.

Olin, J. T., and M. E. Wechsler. 2014. "Asthma: pathogenesis and novel drugs for treatment." *BMJ* 349: g5517. doi: 10.1136/bmj.g5517.

Osawa, R., M. Akiyama, and H. Shimizu. 2011. "Filaggrin gene defects and the risk of developing allergic disorders." *Allergol Int* 60(1): 1–9. doi: 10.2332/allergolint.10-RAI-0270.

Pakhale, S., V. Luks, A. Burkett, and L. Turner. 2013. "Effect of physical training on airway inflammation in bronchial asthma: a systematic review." *BMC Pulm Med* 13: 38. doi: 10.1186/1471-2466-13-38.

Panel, N. IAID-Sponsored Expert, J. A. Boyce, A. Assa'ad, A. W. Burks, S. M. Jones, H. A. Sampson, R. A. Wood, M. Plaut, S. F. Cooper, M. J. Fenton, S. H. Arshad, S. L. Bahna, L. A. Beck, C. Byrd-Bredbenner, C. A. Camargo, Jr., L. Eichenfield, G. T. Furuta, J. M. Hanifin, C. Jones, M. Kraft, B. D. Levy, P. Lieberman, S. Luccioli, K. M. McCall, L. C. Schneider, R. A. Simon, F. E. Simons, S. J. Teach, B. P. Yawn, and J. M. Schwaninger. 2010. "Guidelines for the diagnosis and management of food allergy in the United States: report of the NIAID-sponsored expert panel." *J Allergy Clin Immunol* 126(6 Suppl): S1–58. doi: 10.1016/j.jaci.2010.10.007.

Paul, G., J. M. Brehm, J. F. Alcorn, F. Holguin, S. J. Aujla, and J. C. Celedon. 2012. "Vitamin D and asthma." *Am J Respir Crit Care Med* 185(2): 124–32. doi: 10.1164/rccm.201108-1502CI.

Pawankar, R. 2014. "Allergic diseases and asthma: a global public health concern and a call to action." *World Allergy Organ J* 7(1): 12. doi: 10.1186/1939-4551-7-12.

Pbert, L., J. M. Madison, S. Druker, N. Olendzki, R. Magner, G. Reed, J. Allison, and J. Carmody. 2012. "Effect of mindfulness training on asthma quality of life and lung function: a randomised controlled trial." *Thorax* 67(9): 769–76. doi: 10.1136/thoraxjnl-2011-200253.

Radhakrishnan, D. K., S. D. Dell, A. Guttmann, S. Z. Shariff, K. Liu, and T. To. 2014. "Trends in the age of diagnosis of childhood asthma." *J Allergy Clin Immunol* 134(5): 1057–62 e5. doi: 10.1016/j.jaci.2014.05.012.

Ragab, A., T. Farahat, G. Al-Hendawy, R. Samaka, S. Ragab, and A. El-Ghobashy. 2015. "Nasal saline irrigation with or without systemic antibiotics in treatment of children with acute rhinosinusitis." *Int J Pediatr Otorhinolaryngol* 79(12): 2178–86. doi: 10.1016/j.ijporl.2015.09.045.

Reddel, H. K., E. D. Bateman, A. Becker, L. P. Boulet, A. A. Cruz, J. M. Drazen, T. Haahtela, S. S. Hurd, H. Inoue, J. C. de Jongste, R. F. Lemanske, Jr., M. L. Levy, P. M. O'Byrne, P. Paggiaro, S. E. Pedersen, E. Pizzichini, M. Soto-Quiroz, S. J. Szefler, G. W. Wong, and J. M. FitzGerald. 2015. "A summary of the new GINA strategy: a roadmap to asthma control." *Eur Respir J* 46(3): 622–39. doi: 10.1183/13993003.00853-2015.

Rice, J. L., K. M. Romero, R. M. Galvez Davila, C. T. Meza, A. Bilderback, D. L. Williams, P. N. Breysse, S. Bose, W. Checkley, N. N. Hansel, and Gasp Study Investigators. 2015. "Association between adherence to the Mediterranean diet and asthma in Peruvian children." *Lung* 193(6): 893–9. doi: 10.1007/s00408-015-9792-9.

Riverin, B. D., J. L. Maguire, and P. Li. 2015. "Vitamin D supplementation for childhood asthma: a systematic review and meta-analysis." *PLoS One* 10(8): e0136841. doi: 10.1371/journal.pone.0136841.

Robinson, L., and R. Miller. 2015. "The impact of bisphenol a and phthalates on allergy, asthma, and immune function: a review of latest findings." *Curr Environ Health Rep* 2(4): 379–87. doi: 10.1007/s40572-015-0066-8.

Rosen, L., A. French, G. Sullivan, and Ryt. 2015. "Complementary, holistic, and integrative medicine: yoga." *Pediatr Rev* 36(10): 468–74. doi: 10.1542/pir.36-10-468.

Sadler, C., L. Vanderjagt, S. Vohra, Holistic American Academy of Pediatrics Provisional Section on Complementary, and Medicine Integrative. 2007. "Complementary, holistic, and integrative medicine: butterbur." *Pediatr Rev* 28(6): 235–8.

Salam, M. T., Y. Zhang, and K. Begum. 2012. "Epigenetics and childhood asthma: current evidence and future research directions." *Epigenomics* 4(4): 415–29. doi: 10.2217/epi.12.32.

Schroder, P. C., J. Li, G. W. Wong, and B. Schaub. 2015. "The rural-urban enigma of allergy: what can we learn from studies around the world?" *Pediatr Allergy Immunol* 26(2): 95–102. doi: 10.1111/pai.12341.

Seidman, M. D., R. K. Gurgel, S. Y. Lin, S. R. Schwartz, F. M. Baroody, J. R. Bonner, D. E. Dawson, M. S. Dykewicz, J. M. Hackell, J. K. Han, S. L. Ishman, H. J. Krouse, S. Malekzadeh, J. W. Mims, F. S. Omole, W. D. Reddy, D. V. Wallace, S. A. Walsh, B. E. Warren, M. N. Wilson, L. C. Nnacheta, and Aao-Hnsf Guideline Otolaryngology Development Group. 2015. "Clinical practice guideline: allergic rhinitis." *Otolaryngol Head Neck Surg* 152(1 Suppl): S1–43. doi: 10.1177/0194599814561600.

Shen, J., and E. Oraka. 2012. "Complementary and alternative medicine (CAM) use among children with current asthma." *Prev Med* 54(1): 27–31. doi: 10.1016/j.ypmed.2011.10.007.

Silverberg, J. I. 2015. "Atopic disease and cardiovascular risk factors in US children." *J Allergy Clin Immunol.* doi: 10.1016/j.jaci.2015.09.012.

Spergel, J. M. 2010. "From atopic dermatitis to asthma: the atopic march." *Ann Allergy Asthma Immunol* 105(2): 99–106; quiz 107–9, 117. doi: 10.1016/j.anai.2009.10.002.

Strachan, D. P. 1989. "Hay fever, hygiene, and household size." *BMJ* 299(6710): 1259–60.

Tahan, F., H. Eke Gungor, and E. Bicici. 2014. "Is yoga training beneficial for exercise-induced bronchoconstriction?" *Altern Ther Health Med* 20(2): 18–23.

Thomsen, S. F. 2015. "Epidemiology and natural history of atopic diseases." *Eur Clin Respir J* 2. doi: 10.3402/ecrj.v2.24642.

Thorburn, A. N., L. Macia, and C. R. Mackay. 2014. "Diet, metabolites, and 'western-lifestyle' inflammatory diseases." *Immunity* 40(6): 833–42. doi: 10.1016/j.immuni.2014.05.014.

Tilg, H., and A. R. Moschen. 2015. "Food, immunity, and the microbiome." *Gastroenterology* 148(6): 1107–19. doi: 10.1053/j.gastro.2014.12.036.

Tille, K. S., and K. M. White. 2015. "Acupuncture for seasonal allergic rhinitis: is it ready for prime time?" *Ann Allergy Asthma Immunol* 115(4): 258–9. doi: 10.1016/j.anai.2015.07.007.

Turner, P. J., and A. S. Kemp. 2012. "Allergic rhinitis in children." *J Paediatr Child Health* 48(4): 302–10. doi: 10.1111/j.1440-1754.2010.01779.x.

Von Ehrenstein, O. S., E. Von Mutius, S. Illi, L. Baumann, O. Bohm, and R. von Kries. 2000. "Reduced risk of hay fever and asthma among children of farmers." *Clin Exp Allergy* 30(2): 187–93.

Walker, T. J., and M. Reznik. 2014. "In-school asthma management and physical activity: children's perspectives." *J Asthma* 51(8): 808–13. doi: 10.3109/02770903.2014.920875.

Weinmayr, G., F. Forastiere, G. Buchele, A. Jaensch, D. P. Strachan, G. Nagel, and Isaac Phase Two Study Group. 2014. "Overweight/obesity and respiratory and allergic disease in children: international study of asthma and allergies in childhood (ISAAC) phase two." *PLoS One* 9(12): e113996. doi: 10.1371/journal.pone.0113996.

Westman, M., P. Stjarne, A. Asarnoj, I. Kull, M. van Hage, M. Wickman, and E. Toskala. 2012. "Natural course and comorbidities of allergic and nonallergic rhinitis in children." *J Allergy Clin Immunol* 129(2): 403–8. doi: 10.1016/j.jaci.2011.09.036.

Whyatt, R. M., A. G. Rundle, M. S. Perzanowski, A. C. Just, K. M. Donohue, A. M. Calafat, L. Hoepner, F. P. Perera, and R. L. Miller. 2014. "Prenatal phthalate and early childhood bisphenol A exposures increase asthma risk in inner-city children." *J Allergy Clin Immunol* 134(5): 1195–7 e2. doi: 10.1016/j.jaci.2014.07.027.

Wilkinson, M., A. Hart, S. J. Milan, and K. Sugumar. 2014. "Vitamins C and E for asthma and exercise-induced bronchoconstriction." *Cochrane Database Syst Rev* 6: CD010749. doi: 10.1002/14651858.CD010749.pub2.

Yu, J., K. Ahn, Y. H. Shin, K. W. Kim, D. I. Suh, H. S. Yu, M. J. Kang, K. S. Lee, S. A. Hong, K. Y. Choi, E. Lee, S. I. Yang, J. H. Seo, B. J. Kim, H. B. Kim, S. Y. Lee, S. J. Choi, S. Y. Oh, J. Y. Kwon, K. J. Lee, H. J. Park, P. R. Lee, H. S. Won, S. J. Hong, and Cocoa study group. 2016. "The interaction between prenatal exposure to home renovation and reactive oxygen species genes in cord blood IgE response is modified by maternal atopy." *Allergy Asthma Immunol Res* 8(1): 41–8. doi: 10.4168/aair.2016.8.1.41.

16 Dermatology

Overview

Dermatologic conditions are very common in children and encompass abnormalities of the skin, hair, and nails. The level of mental and physical distress generated by these disorders can be significant, making it important for clinicians to be skilled in their diagnosis and knowledgeable about appropriate timing of referrals. Pediatric dermatology is a specialized field and the intent here is to give an overview of two common conditions, atopic dermatitis and acne, not to attempt an exhaustive review. Addressing the child or adolescent with an integrative approach that considers health in every dimension will help to maximize the patient's potential for healthy skin and may aid in identification and elimination of possible triggers of these common dermatologic conditions, both of which are linked to genetic, environmental, and lifestyle factors.

Children have special characteristics that may predispose them to atopic dermatitis and acne. For example, infant skin is only approximately half as thick as mature adult skin, making it susceptible to damage and predisposing to dehydration and increased absorption of external compounds and toxicants commonly seen in atopic dermatitis. Infants and children also have a proportionally larger surface area of skin compared to adults, making the protective function of the skin even more important. In adolescents, ongoing hormonal influences can precipitate acne. In fact, the skin is a dynamic organ that continues to develop throughout the first years of life both in its internal layers and in the bacterial communities it harbors. The epidermis functions as the front line of protection against pathogenic organisms, external toxicants, and ultraviolet radiation and needs to be healthy for optimal functioning (Telofski et al. 2012).

Atopic Dermatitis

Overview

Atopic dermatitis is a chronic non-infectious inflammatory skin condition and one of the most common skin disorders in infants and children. It is also known as eczema and often has a relapsing course. The word "atopic" from the Greek "different" or "out of place" refers in this instance to an underlying presence of elevated total IgE and frequent sensitization to antigens or triggers in the environment (Gupta 2015). "Dermatitis" refers to inflammation of the skin. The origination of this disease is unknown, but it is linked to disruption of the skin's outer barrier, allowing a range of triggering compounds and potential allergens to invade, subsequently triggering the inflammatory response (Telofski et al. 2012).

Atopic dermatitis is characterized by pruritus, which has a significant impact on the patient's quality of life. It is often present in patients with allergy-driven diseases such as asthma, fever, food sensitivity, and allergic rhinitis. The atopic march theory states that atopic dermatitis creates an environment for progressive atopy by allowing a site for allergic sensitization via the dysfunctional skin barrier. The subsequent T-helper cell imbalance predisposes patients to allergic rhinitis and related airway hyperreactivity (Bantz, Zhu, and Zheng 2014; Gupta 2015; Mortz et al. 2015).

A protective effect against atopy has been seen in children raised in rural settings who are exposed to a wide variety of allergens early in life (Chu et al. 2014).

Etiology

The etiology of atopic dermatitis can be attributed to a combination of genetic predisposition and environmental triggers. Aggravating factors include young age, airborne and food allergens, exposure to harsh soaps or detergents, stress, and other individualized irritants. Breastfeeding appears to have a small protective effect in high risk infants (Blattner and Murase 2014).

If formula feeding is implemented, use of partially hydrolyzed 100% whey-based formulas in infants at risk for atopy has shown to be helpful and cost effective (Spieldenner et al. 2011; von Berg et al. 2008).

Mutation in filaggrin proteins, structural components of the epidermis, are a strong genetic risk factor for atopic dermatitis, especially in children with early onset, more severe, and chronic disease (Dimitriades et al. 2014). The inflammatory response in the skin is complex and involves a disrupted skin barrier, antigen presenting cells, such as Langerhans cells in the epidermal layer with high affinity to IgE receptors which bind the antigen, and subsequent interface with T-helper cells TH2 and TH1 that, in imbalance, trigger cutaneous inflammation (Bieber 2008).

Food allergies have been significantly associated with atopy and atopic dermatitis in children and have been linked to precipitating flares of atopic dermatitis in approximately 30% of affected children who have moderate to severe disease. The offending food acts as a potent inflammatory trigger in the gastrointestinal tract, driving disease symptoms. Gut barrier dysfunction allowing absorption of allergenic food proteins is an identified mechanism in animal studies (Bergmann et al. 2013).

Prevalence varies by age and triggers while individualized offending foods fall into recognizable patterns including: cow's milk, eggs, peanut, wheat, soy, nuts, and fish which have been shown to be responsible for more than 90% of flares. Cow's milk, eggs, soy, and peanut are the most common allergens in young children. Some foods can sensitize through environmental exposure to skin contact; peanut is one well-recognized example (Fox et al. 2009; Bergmann et al. 2013).

In fact, in an approach that inverts earlier thinking, the question of early introduction of peanut and its potential protective role in prevention of peanut allergy is under active study, an approach first proposed by Du Toit et al (Du Toit et al. 2016). Expert panels are evaluating the many questions that remain about the timing of introduction of potentially allergenic foods to infants (Sicherer 2015).

Some of the difficulty in diagnosis of food allergen triggers is the variable pattern of clinical reaction. Some reactions are immediate (within 2 hours) and manifest with visible changes in the skin including urticarial and pruritus, or trigger gastrointestinal, respiratory, or full anaphylactic symptoms. Delayed reactions (6–48 hours after oral exposure) may manifest as flares of cutaneous symptoms. A combination type of reaction involving acute and delayed symptoms has been seen in an estimated 40% of children with a history of positive oral food challenge (Werfel et al. 2007).

Suspicion of food allergy should be supported by a careful history, laboratory evaluation, elimination diet, and possible food challenge. Skin care should be maximized in all children suspected of food allergy. Skin prick tests and or specific IgE measurement in serum can be helpful in some children, although due to the frequency of multiple positive IgE tests in children with atopic dermatitis that lack clinical relevancy these must be interpreted with caution. Skin prick tests have an excellent negative predictive value, but low positive predictive value. Guidelines suggest that a positive skin test be confirmed by elimination diet followed by a carefully monitored food challenge to confirm the diagnosis of food allergy. Similarly, negative serum-specific IgE tests are helpful in ruling out food allergy, but a positive is of low predictive value (Spergel et al. 2015).

New methods such as atopy patch tests are under investigation, but require further study and close supervision by a trained pediatric allergist. Elimination diet over an observation period of 4–6 weeks may be helpful, although this is hard to control and factors such as placebo effect, or removal of masked triggers, such as aerosolized antigens or other unseen triggers, may be involved. Food diary can be a useful tool in this instance (Bergmann et al. 2013).

Prolonged restriction of diet can place children at risk for caloric or specific nutrient deficiency and should be avoided. An oral food challenge is considered the next definitive step in diagnosis in children who had a positive response to elimination diet, but this carries risks and must be done under careful and experienced medical supervision. Standard protocols exist and should be followed (Sampson et al. 2012).

An estimated one of three children outgrow food sensitivity within 1–3 years of its presentation. Foods associated with shorter duration of allergy include cow's milk, eggs, wheat, and soy. Longer duration of allergy has been associated with peanut, fish, and shellfish. Tree nut allergy persists in the majority of affected individuals (Bergmann et al. 2013).

Prevalence

Atopic dermatitis affects one in four children and typically presents early in childhood.

An estimated 60% of cases present in the first 12 months and 90% are diagnosed by the age of 5 years. Among these children, about 70% outgrow the disease before entering adolescence. The disease persists into adulthood in 10%–30% of children (Garg and Silverberg 2015).

An estimated 70% of children have a positive history of related atopic conditions such as asthma, allergic rhinitis, food allergies, and environmental allergies.

Atopy in one parent more than doubles the odds of having atopic dermatitis. Atopic risk increases by three to fivefold in a child who has two atopic parents (Wen et al. 2009).

Prevalence of atopic dermatitis has increased twofold to threefold since the 1970s. Reasons for this sharp increase are not fully understood, but may include a significant reduction in exposure to microorganisms in childhood, often presented as the "hygiene hypothesis," a theory that addresses the changing nature of the gut microbiome and its impact on the immune system and link to atopic diseases. Social elements associated with this hypothesis include smaller family size, increased education, higher socioeconomic level, transformations from rural to urban environment, and the excessive use of antibiotics. Research examining the benefit of probiotics in atopic dermatitis, in part based on this theory, is encouraging, although no specific guidelines currently exist.

Research is very active in this area in both maternal–fetal medicine and in pediatrics (Brown, Arrieta, and Finlay 2013; Storro, Avershina, and Rudi 2013; West 2014). Both indoor (Kim et al. 2015) and outdoor air pollutants have been identified as aggravating factors in atopic dermatitis in children. Examples include tobacco smoke, volatile organic compounds, toluene, nitrogen dioxide, fine particulate matter, among others that may cause skin barrier disruption and precipitate dysregulation of the immune system (Ahn 2014).

Clinical Manifestations

The predominant symptom in atopic dermatitis is intense pruritus, which occurs without fever or other constitutional symptoms. Secondary sleep disturbance is common. The stage of the disease usually determines skin findings. Acute disease manifests as serous exudates or intensely itchy papular rash with vesicles on erythematous base. Sub-acute disease consists of lesions characterized by scaling or plaques on erythematous skin. Chronic disease is defined by lichenification in addition to excoriated papules and nodules. Secondary infection is often seen at this stage in the form of yellow crusting or impetigo or the erythema surrounding characteristic cellulitis present in infected lesions (Gupta 2015).

Comorbidities

In addition to dermatologic symptoms including increased risk of bacterial, viral, and fungal skin infections, large population-based studies connect atopic dermatitis to non-allergic conditions including altered sleep patterns, ADHD, depression and anxiety, and some types of cancers (Romanos et al. 2010). Secondary infection with herpes simplex-1 can also cause recurring flares and can be dangerous especially in the very young or if eye involvement occurs.

An association between pediatric obesity and atopic dermatitis and allergic rhinitis has also been determined, especially in infants who were small for gestational age. Research is active in the effects on late gestational programming of T-helper cells in this population and its impact on inflammatory-mediated diseases such as atopic dermatitis and obesity (Lin, Hsieh et al. 2015).

Some studies have identified a link between increased severity of atopic dermatitis in children over 2 years of age with higher body-mass-index (Koutroulis et al. 2015). A further link between atopic dermatitis, inflammation, and increased risk of cardiovascular disease in adult life reinforces the understanding that the external manifestation of atopic dermatitis is only one part of a complex systemic inflammatory disorder (Yamanaka and Mizutani 2015).

Diagnostic Criteria

Atopic dermatitis has no particular diagnostic test therefore diagnosis is primarily dependent upon history and clinical manifestations. The skin is typically dry and rash is generally erythematous and pruritic with poorly defined papules and plaques. Exudative rash is common in the very young, and superinfection due to itching may make diagnosis more challenging. Under 2 years of age, lesions are more typically seen on the face, neck, scalp, and on extensor surfaces of the extremities. These are the areas that have physical contact with either the infant's hands or surface contact during rolling and crawling. After age 2 years a more typical pattern may develop that involves the flexor surfaces of the antecubital and popliteal fossas. Eyelids, neck, and flexor surfaces of the wrists can also be involved.

Clinical patterns pointing to a diagnosis of atopic dermatitis include sparing of the groin, axilla, and diaper area in part because of the higher moisture in these skin areas.

Differential diagnosis includes: contact dermatitis, scabies, seborrheic dermatitis, ichthyoses, tinea corporis, psoriasis, nutritional deficiencies such as zinc, cutaneous T-cell lymphoma, or rash related to autoimmune illness. Atopic dermatitis is most often diagnosed on the basis of family history of the disease and distribution of lesions.

Skin biopsy can be used to confirm diagnosis, but is not always needed (Gupta 2015).

Treatment

Effective treatment involves reduction of inflammation, prevention of bacterial colonization, and minimizing food-driven flares, all of which can help prevent later sensitization to environmental and other allergens. Treatment goes hand in hand with prevention and restoration of the skin barrier. A first line approach is to moisturize liberally with high-quality fragrance- and dye-free products, especially after bathing. Various moisturizing vehicles, or base ingredients, can be used, each with pros and cons. Ointments have been shown to have the greatest moisturizing effects, but have a greasy texture that can be difficult with clothing and bedding. Lotions may be better tolerated, but may require more frequent application. Creams can be a good option, but some may contain preservatives that can cause stinging on distressed skin. Ceramide-containing creams available over the counter have proven beneficial.

The next step in treatment is to reduce external inflammation. Environmental triggers such as house dust mites can be potential triggers therefore dust mite covers for the bed and pillow are often recommended. Wet wraps for the skin have shown benefit. These involve a wet dressing covering well-moisturized skin covered by a dry wrap, especially effective as an overnight treatment. Topical steroids are considered a mainstay of conventional treatment, but must be used with caution on infants and on and around the face. A range of steroid potency exists, and in general the least potent needed to be effective is preferred. Risks and benefits of all treatments must be considered on an individual basis (Gupta 2015).

Topical calcineurin inhibitors, which inhibit T-cell activation, are also used with or without topical corticosteroids. These are FDA approved for over the age of 2 years, although studies exist supporting their safety and efficacy under 2 years of age (Gupta 2015). Phototherapy and systemic immunosuppressants are other treatment options that may be required if topical treatment fails.

Addressing pruritus resulting from histamine release is an important element of treatment, especially because of its association with disruption of sleep and ability to concentrate. Topical antihistamines are not recommended due to the risk of them causing painful stimulation on irritated skin, leaving systemic treatment as the most common alternative to address the intense itching sensation. Sedating antihistamines have been shown to be the most effective in conventional symptom relief, but have obvious unwanted side effects that limit daytime use.

Management of topical bacterial or viral superinfections is important to reduce the upregulation of inflammation caused by colonization. Minimization of systemic antibiotics is preferred whenever possible. *Staphylococcus aureus* is one of most common pathogens seen in colonization in patients with atopic dermatitis and may be addressed with chlorhexidine soap 4% (Gupta 2015), topical intranasal muciprocin ointment, and dilute bleach baths, which have also been shown to have anti-inflammatory properties (Huang et al. 2009).

In general, it is recommended that baths be limited in duration to reduce drying effects. Mild soaps, warm rather than hot water, and ample moisturizers are recommended.

Integrative Treatment

Lifestyle Approach

Simple measures previously mentioned that spare skin irritation such as avoidance of over-bathing, hot water, harsh soaps, and prevention of skin scratching are standard recommendations. Studies evaluating regional variation in prevalence of atopic dermatitis show lower prevalence in areas with higher humidity, higher ultraviolet index, higher mean temperature, reduced precipitation, and fewer days of use of central heating (Silverberg, Hanifin, and Simpson 2013).

Avoidance of environmental toxicants in indoor and outdoor air and in foods are important as they may precipitate inflammatory factors.

PHYSICAL ACTIVITY

Physical activity might be avoided in people with atopic dermatitis in part due to the worsening of pruritus associated with sweating. Due to the systemic inflammatory nature of the disease it is important for patients to deliberately incorporate exercise into a healthy lifestyle approach to management of the disease to prevent the development of later cardiovascular and metabolic problems, especially obesity. A review by Kim and Silverberg found insufficient data for firm conclusions to be drawn about the best type of exercise. Some factors to consider when counseling patients include awareness of air pollutants that can exacerbate flares, avoidance of overheating, possibility of triggering associated atopic conditions such as asthma and allergic rhinitis, lack of sense of self-efficacy, and self-consciousness due to skin lesions (Kim and Silverberg 2015).

MIND–BODY CONNECTION

Attention to the mind–body connection and effective management of stress and the psychological burden of living with a chronic pruritic inflammatory disease are important to acknowledge and address. A variety of therapies including biofeedback, clinical hypnosis, progressive muscle relaxation, and massage have shown positive effect in overall relaxation and stress management (Bae et al. 2012; Sokel, Lansdown, and Kent 1990).

The use of mind–body tools can help patients cultivate a greater sense of control over their illness and aid in improving sleep quality and self-esteem. Mind–body therapies also have good efficacy in reduction of anxiety in children as young as preschool age (McClafferty 2011). Mind–body therapies must be matched to the interests and expectations of the patient, and a great deal of individual variation exists. These are further discussed in the Chapter 6, Mind–Body Therapies. Support groups have also been shown to be of benefit in stress management in patients with dermatological conditions (Shenefelt 2011).

NUTRITION

Large population studies involving children in Spain, Greece, and Mexico examining the connection between Mediterranean diet and asthma and atopy have shown overall benefit in reduction of atopic and respiratory symptoms (Chatzi and Kogevinas 2009).

Fewer studies have looked at the effect of dietary patterns on atopic dermatitis. One large review by Netting et al. included 42 studies and more than 40,000 children. There were no highly statistically significant associations reported, but a maternal diet most consistent with the Mediterranean diet pattern, rich in fruits and vegetables, fish, and foods containing vitamin D, showed consistent association with a lower risk of atopic disease in children. Conversely, higher risk of atopic disease in children was associated with maternal diets containing margarine, nuts, and fast food and vegetable oil (Netting, Middleton, and Makrides 2014).

Another large population-based study in 20,106 Spanish children aged 6–7 years found no correlation between Mediterranean diet score and atopic dermatitis. A positive association between obesity and atopic dermatitis was seen in secondary analysis (Suarez-Varela et al. 2010).

Although interest is high regarding gluten sensitivity, and some studies have shown a higher incidence of celiac disease in children with atopic dermatitis, there is not currently a robust body of evidence to support gluten elimination in children with atopic dermatitis (Ress et al. 2014).

OUTDOOR TIME AND VITAMIN D

Limited exposure to natural sunlight and normalization of serum vitamin D levels are recommended (Leung and Guttman-Yassky 2014).

In a small randomized pilot study, supplementation of vitamin D (1000 IU daily for 4 weeks) resulted in significant improvement in 11 children with mild to moderate atopic dermatitis with winter-related exacerbations (Sidbury et al. 2008). A larger randomized trial in 107 children aged 2–17 years with atopic dermatitis using the same dose, 1000 IU in concentrated liquid drop form over 4 weeks, showed a similar encouraging result ($p < 0.04$ symptom improvement and $p < 0.03$ global assessment). No adverse effects were reported (Camargo et al. 2014).

Vitamin D is discussed in more detail in Chapter 4, Key Dietary Supplements.

Complementary Therapies

Oral Probiotics

Although no specific guidelines exist, accruing evidence supports the use of probiotics in prevention and treatment of atopic dermatitis (Kalliomaki et al. 2001). For example, a randomized controlled trial by Lin et al. in 40 infants with eczema who received

4 weeks of treatment with *Bifidobacterium bifidum* showed a statistically significant correlation between levels of the *B. bifidum* in the infant's stools and reduction in severity of disease (p < 0.05) (Lin, Qiu et al. 2015).

A study of *Lactobacillus salivarius* (LS01) in 43 children showed improvement in disease severity and reduction in itch in all participants in a 4-week trial (Niccoli et al. 2014).

Recommendations from the World Allergy Organization suggest use of probiotics in pregnant women with a history of atopic disease whose children are at risk for atopy; and use in women who breastfeed infants considered at high risk for developing allergy; and use of probiotics in infants at high risk of developing allergy (Fiocchi et al. 2015).

The forward edge of probiotic research involves the use of non-pathogenic bacteria as topical treatments to reduce skin inflammation. Research is active in this area (Volz et al. 2014).

Omega-3 Fatty Acids

Supplementation with omega-3 fatty acids has been studied in pregnant and breast-feeding women to assess potential for a protective effect in infants at risk for atopy. A Cochrane Systematic Database review of eight randomized trials involving 3366 women and 3175 children showed benefit in certain groups, including reduction in IgE-mediated eczema in children 12–36 months; and reduction of IgE-mediated allergy in children 12–36 months of age, but not older than 36 months. Food allergies were similarly lower in children 12 months and younger whose mothers had supplemented with omega-3 fatty acids. No differences in wheezing or allergic rhinitis were seen in this review. Insufficient evidence currently exists to support specific recommendations for omega-3 fatty acid supplementation, although no adverse effects were reported (Gunaratne, Makrides, and Collins 2015).

Glycyrrhetinic Acid

Glycyrrhetinic acid, MAS063DP, marketed as Atopiclair, is approved for sale in the U.S. and European Union as a non-steroidal topical agent for the treatment of atopic dermatitis. Ingredients include glycyrrhetinic acid 2%, derived from licorice root, *Vitis vinifera* (grapevine extract), and telmestine. Glycyrrhetinic acid has both anti-inflammatory and antipruritic properties. *Vitus vinifera* has been shown to have antioxidant and anti-protease properties. A randomized trial of 142 patients aged 6–12 months using the cream three times a day saw statistically significant improvement in symptoms in a 22-day trial compared to controls (p < 0.0001) (Boguniewicz et al. 2008; Patrizi, Raone, and Neri 2009).

Evening Primrose Oil

Oral evening primrose oil and borage oil, both of which have high levels of gamma-linoleic acid (GLA), have been proposed as treatments for eczema in children and adults. Despite their popularity, a large Cochrane Database Systematic review evaluating 27 studies involving 1596 participants failed to find any difference from placebo. Some concerns exist about potential interaction of evening primrose oil with anticoagulants (Bamford et al. 2013).

Other Botanicals and Supplements

Study of other oral supplements including pyridoxine (vitamin B6), zinc, phosphate, selenium, sea buckthorn seed, or hempseed oil were shown to lack benefit in a Cochrane Systematic Database review (Bath-Hextall et al. 2012).

Chinese Herbal Medicine

A review of seven randomized controlled trials comparing Chinese herbal medicine and Western medicine or placebo found too high a degree in study variability and quality to make firm recommendations, although an overall positive effect on symptoms and quality of life in patients was seen in the majority of studies (Tan et al. 2013).

Homeopathy

Homeopathy is commonly used in children with atopic dermatitis (Silverberg, Lee-Wong, and Silverberg 2014), especially in European countries (Becker-Witt et al. 2004). It has been shown to have mixed benefit, although adverse events are rare (Torley et al. 2013). For example, a prospective multicenter comparative observational trial of homeopathy in children with atopic dermatitis was done in 135 German children who were followed for 6 months before primary analysis. Secondary analysis at 36 months included 99 children. No significant difference was seen in conventional versus homeopathic treatment at 36 months, although disease severity in both groups decreased significantly ($p < 0.001$). Adverse events in either group were rare. Costs were found to be more than twice as high in the homeopathic treatment group, related in part to more frequent doctor's visits and associated fees (Roll et al. 2013).

Another longitudinal study of 213 Italian children with atopic diseases treated with homeopathy followed children for an average of 8 years. Atopic dermatitis was originally diagnosed in 76 of 213 children. Of the 40 seen in follow-up at year 8, 70% had complete resolution of atopic dermatitis, leaving authors to conclude a positive effect, although over this course of time many variables must be considered (Rossi et al. 2012). A typical confounder of homeopathy research remains the individualization of treatment.

Oral

Several oils used in food have shown potential in treatment due to their anti-inflammatory and antibacterial effects. One example is coconut oil that has shown good activity against *Staphylococcus aureus* colonization (DebMandal and Mandal 2011).

Topical

Linoleic acid found in high levels in sunflower oil has been shown to improve skin barrier function and reduce inflammation in pediatric patients with atopic dermatitis (Eichenfield, McCollum, and Msika 2009).

Small studies support the topical use of *Hypericum perforatum* (St. John's wort) using extract standardized to 1.5% hyperforin as compared to control over a 4-week study. Colonization with *Staphylococcus aureus* was also significantly decreased (Schempp et al. 2003). Further studies are needed to confirm the benefit and safety of topical St. John's wort, especially in children (Wolfle, Seelinger, and Schempp 2014).

Acupressure and Acupuncture

Acupressure has also been studied for its benefit in atopic dermatitis and has been shown in small studies to decrease pruritus and lichenification in adults (Lee et al. 2012). Acupuncture has a small but growing body of supporting evidence for improvement of pruritus related to atopic dermatitis (Yu et al. 2015; Pfab et al. 2010; Pfab et al. 2012).

Summary

A written action plan has been shown to have significant value for children and their families coping with atopic dermatitis (Shi et al. 2013).

Expansion of the plan to include integrative treatment approaches that maximize lifestyle measures may help the patient and family minimize disease severity and reduce risk of sensitization and inflammation that occur with disease flares. These approaches might include an emphasis on (Goddard and Lio 2015):

- Nutrition quality with emphasis on the anti-inflammatory Mediterranean diet pattern
- Effective stress management and mastery of mind–body therapies
- Regular enjoyable exercise
- Time in nature and normalization of vitamin D level
- Adequate rest
- Addition of an oral probiotic
- Adequate omega-3 fatty acid intake

Acne

Overview

Acne is a common and distressing skin condition that affects an estimated 95% of adolescents in the U.S. (Zouboulis and Bettoli 2015). Severity can range from mild to severe, and even in mildest presentation can cause significant emotional and physical burden to afflicted adolescents and adults (Zaenglein 2015). It is most common in the range of 12–25 years old, but can persist in adult life.

Etiology

Acne is a chronic inflammatory-driven disease with four main components including excess secretion of sebum driven by the hormonal changes of puberty, altered keratinization of the sebaceous duct which can lead to comedone formation, resultant inflammation of the duct, and bacterial colonization and secondary infection of the hair follicles most commonly by *Propionibacterium acnes* (Williams, Dellavalle, and Garner 2012).

Acne mechanica is seen in athletes and can be exacerbated by heat, friction, moisture, and pressure from equipment. Differential diagnosis of acne is relatively varied and includes milia, rosacea, molluscum contagiosum, flat warts, infection, and drug reaction among others. Some diseases to rule out, especially in prepubertal children, include Cushing syndrome, polycystic ovarian syndrome, gonadal tumor, precocious puberty, and congenital adrenal hyperplasia.

Prevalence

Acne is the most commonly occurring skin disease. The average peak prevalence is seen at 17 years. Approximately 20% of adolescents are affected by moderate-to-severe acne, which has a genetic component (Silverberg and Silverberg 2014).

Clinical Manifestations

Lesions can range from non-inflammatory comedones to inflammatory papules, pustules, or cystic nodules. Distribution can include the face, neck, back, chest, and buttocks. Scarring and inflammatory hyper-pigmentation can occur in typical lesions of acne vulgaris. This can be more common in people with darker complexions and may take months to resolve if not properly treated (Botros, Tsai, and Pujalte 2015).

Comorbidities

In addition to risk of permanent scarring, comorbidities include depression, anxiety, and body dysmorphic disorder leading to social isolation, lack of confidence and self-esteem, depression, suicidal ideation and suicide (Silverberg and Silverberg 2014).

Diagnostic Criteria

Acne is diagnosed after identifying lesions, which can range from noninflammatory open or closed comedones to painful inflammatory lesions. Different grading systems exist, for example grades 1–4 from less serious to more involved, or simply the categories of mild, moderate, and severe (Botros, Tsai, and Pujalte 2015).

Treatment

Conventional treatments for acne have been widely reported and range from topical to systemic depending on severity. Proper skin care is a central theme in treatment, and includes avoidance of harsh cleansers and squeezing or picking of lesions. Mental health screening, especially for depression, is a critical part of every evaluation, as is the offering of hope and reassurance that although treatment may take some time, help is available. Goals of treatment include reduction of inflammation, normalization of sebum production and keratinization, reduction of bacteria, and minimization of permanent scarring.

Conventional Treatments

Topical Over the Counter (Gollnick and Zouboulis 2014)

- Benzoyl peroxide—antibacterial properties, concentration 2.5%–10%
- Salicylic acid—used for unblocking pores

Topical Prescription Drugs

- Retinoids (tretinoin, adapalene, tazarotene)—anti-inflammatory properties, vitamin A derivatives used to rebalance follicular keratinization, and improve post lesion hyperpigmentation. Considered first line treatments.
- Topical antibiotics—typically prescribed with topical retinoids.
- Clindamycin, erythromycin, sulfacetamide, and dapsone.
- Azelaic acid with additional natural anti-inflammatory properties.
- Intralesional glucocorticoid therapy—used selectively for nodular acne.

Oral

- **Antibiotics**—generally limited to inflammatory acne and with involvement of face and chest. Used in conjunction with topical retinoids. Used sparingly to avoid development of bacterial resistance. Minocycline, erythromycin, tetracycline and others.
- **Oral contraceptives**—used for women with hyperandrogenism and acne-related menses.
- **Oral retinoids**—normalize keratinization. Used in severe nodular acne. Highly teratogenic, must be used with birth control. Prescribed by authorized physicians only. Have been linked to depression and suicidal ideation.

Other Approaches

- **Light therapy**—mixed blue-red light has been seen to be most effective in destroying bacteria. FDA approved, requires multiple sessions (Hamilton et al. 2009).
- **Cleansers and peels.**
- **Microdermabrasion.**

Integrative Treatment

Integrative treatments are frequently used to treat acne based on concerns about the side effects associated with prescription treatment, cost, and in some patients due to limited access to healthcare (Cao et al. 2015).

Lifestyle Approach

NUTRITION

The strongest evidence in lifestyle modification and acne points to the benefits of a healthy diet. A comprehensive review by Melnik identifies the three categories with strongest associations: hyperglycemic carbohydrates, dairy products, and excess of saturated fats including trans fats and an imbalance of omega-3 to omega-6 fatty acids (Melnik 2015a).

Emerging research supports the hypothesis that increased insulin-like growth factor-1 (IGF-1) correlates with acne. Elevated IGF-1 has been associated with hyperproliferative activity of the sebaceous follicle leading to clinical manifestation of acne. A simplified overview suggests that involvement of the metabolic transcription factor FoxO1, which is negatively regulated by IGF-1, effects gene expression that effects androgen signaling and subsequent proliferation of sebum production associated with clinical disease. FoxO1 is a negative regulator of the kinase mTORC1 which has been shown to have an important role in acne related to diet. It has been widely reported that a high glycemic load diet worsens acne, and modulates the activity of both free IGF-1 and free serum androgens whereas a low glycemic diet results in improvement of acne (Melnik 2015b). Milk aggravates acne by increasing both serum growth hormone and IGF-1 via the hepatic production of IGF-1 driven by amino acids in cow's milk, not by simple transfer of the factors in the milk. The primary amino acid used in synthesis of IGF-1 is tryptophan, a primary component of the whey protein alpha lactoalbumin (Melnik, John, and Schmitz 2013).

Whey-based supplements frequently used by teenage males for body building or for weight gain have also been associated with acne flares (Silverberg 2012).

Saturated fat intake has been associated with acne. Omega-3 fatty acids inhibit mTORC1 activation, which, in simplified terms, reduces acne. The theory is supported by the prevalence of acne in metabolic conditions such as polycystic ovarian disease that are associated with insulin resistance and increased circulating androgens.

In a comprehensive review, Melnick highlights research that supports an optimal anti-acne diet that consists of a Paleolithic-like pattern with emphasis on low-glycemic vegetables and fruit, and fish. Naturally occurring TORC1 inhibitors have been identified as the primary green tea polyphenol epigallocatechin-3-gallate (EGCG), resveratrol, curcumin (Liu et al. 2015), genistein, and silymarin (Melnik 2015a).

Overarching recommendations include prudent control of overall calorie intake, reduction of sugar, low intake of refined carbohydrates, milk, whey and casein protein, saturated fats, and trans-fats (Melnik 2015a).

A review of 563 patients aged 10–24 years by Grossi et al. echoed these findings, demonstrating connections between acne prevalence and severity and high skim milk and other dairy product consumption, high glycemic carbohydrates, high body-mass-index, and a low consumption of fish, fruits, and vegetables (Grossi et al. 2016).

A 2015 Cochrane Systematic Database Review also found some studies supporting benefit of a low glycemic load diet rich in vegetables and fruits, whole grains, and high-quality lean proteins that includes moderate amounts of organic dairy and that limits processed foods and trans fats (Cao et al. 2015).

Physical activity for acne alone has few supporting studies, but has been shown to be of significant benefit in overall lifestyle and metabolic markers in conditions such as polycystic ovarian disease where acne is often an important early diagnostic marker and a distressing component of the constellation of symptoms (Moran et al. 2011).

MIND–BODY THERAPIES

Mind–body therapies can be used in patients with acne to address self-esteem issues, depression, anxiety, and bullying and social isolation (Magin 2013). It can also be used to redirect habitual picking at lesions (Shenefelt 2004).

Mind–body approaches can be tailored to the individual and should consider interests, availability of therapies, and cost. Many mind–body therapies can be used at home including guided imagery, self-hypnosis, biofeedback, and breathing exercises (Chuh, Wong, and Zawar 2006).

Complementary Therapies

Omega-3 Fatty Acids

Studies on fish oil supplementation in acne have shown mixed results, although inclusion of fish in the diet along with fruits and vegetables has been associated with improvement (Khayef et al. 2012).

Zinc

While some studies have suggested a link between low serum zinc levels and acne, insufficient evidence exists to support routine recommendation of a zinc supplement in acne (Rostami Mogaddam et al. 2014).

One study of 235 patients with acne were treated with a combination product containing zinc, nicotinamide, azelaic acid, pyridoxine, copper, and folic acid (NicAzel, Elorac Inc, Vernon Hills, IL) showed statistically significant improvement in 88% at week 8 of treatment when it was added to their treatment regimen (Shalita et al. 2012).

Vitamin D

The link between vitamin D levels and acne is an area of active research. No definitive recommendations exist, but given the complex role of vitamin D in immune functioning it seems prudent to check and normalize levels in patients suffering from acne (Yildizgoren and Togral 2014).

Topical Tea Tree Oil

Tea tree oil from the Australian tea tree (*Melaleuca alternifolia*) has natural anti-inflammatory properties, and antimicrobial activity against *Propionibacterium acnes*.

Tea tree has a long history of use in acne, and should be used in diluted form (5%–15%) due to the possibility of skin irritation. A Cochrane Database Systematic Review found some support for its use in acne, although the quality of the study was considered low (Cao et al. 2015).

The same review found a paucity of supporting evidence for other herbal medicines in acne, and a similar lack of supporting evidence for acupuncture, wet cupping, or purified bee pollen in acne treatment (Cao et al. 2015).

Green Tea and Pomegranate

In vitro studies of green tea extract, pomegranate juice, and pomegranate extract against *Propionibacterium acnes*, *Staphylococcus aureus*, and *Staphylococcus epidermidis* showed promising antibacterial activity (Li et al. 2015), and use of lotions containing 2% by weight of green tea extract rich in the polyphenol epigallocatechin-3-gallate (EGCG) have shown efficacy in clinical trials in patients with acne (Elsaie et al. 2009; Sharquie, Noaimi, and Al-Salih 2008).

Probiotics

Insufficient evidence currently exists for standard recommendation of probiotics in acne patients, although they have a wide margin of safety in the generally healthy patient.

Summary

Acne is a prevalent disorder that, although distressing both mentally and physically, has several encouraging pathways to treatment. In addition to the well-researched conventional approaches and attention to skin care, nutritional strategies can make a significant difference in the course of the disease. Steps such as avoidance of dairy and emphasis on low-glycemic fruits and vegetables, fish, and plant-based anti-inflammatory and antioxidant compounds such as green tea, while limiting sugary and processed foods, have all been shown to improve clinical outcomes and quality of life. Mind–body therapies to address the challenging and serious psychological consequences of acne treatment are an important part of the treatment plan, as is careful screening for depression and suicidal intent at every visit which can develop due to feelings of hopelessness and social stigma. An integrative approach to acne has the potential to increase the adolescent's sense of self-efficacy and provide an expanded pallet of evidence-based treatment options.

References

Ahn, K. 2014. "The role of air pollutants in atopic dermatitis." *J Allergy Clin Immunol* 134(5): 993–9; discussion 1000. doi: 10.1016/j.jaci.2014.09.023.

Bae, B. G., S. H. Oh, C. O. Park, S. Noh, J. Y. Noh, K. R. Kim, and K. H. Lee. 2012. "Progressive muscle relaxation therapy for atopic dermatitis: objective assessment of efficacy." *Acta Derm Venereol* 92(1): 57–61. doi: 10.2340/00015555-1189.

Bamford, J. T., S. Ray, A. Musekiwa, C. van Gool, R. Humphreys, and E. Ernst. 2013. "Oral evening primrose oil and borage oil for eczema." *Cochrane Database Syst Rev* 4: CD004416. doi: 10.1002/14651858.CD004416.pub2.

Bantz, S. K., Z. Zhu, and T. Zheng. 2014. "The atopic march: progression from atopic dermatitis to allergic rhinitis and asthma." *J Clin Cell Immunol* 5(2): 202. doi: 10.4172/2155-9899.1000202.

Bath-Hextall, F. J., C. Jenkinson, R. Humphreys, and H. C. Williams. 2012. "Dietary supplements for established atopic eczema." *Cochrane Database Syst Rev* 2: CD005205. doi: 10.1002/14651858.CD005205.pub3.

Becker-Witt, C., R. Ludtke, T. E. Weisshuhn, and S. N. Willich. 2004. "Diagnoses and treatment in homeopathic medical practice." *Forsch Komplementarmed Klass Naturheilkd* 11(2): 98–103. doi: 10.1159/000078231.

Bergmann, M. M., J. C. Caubet, M. Boguniewicz, and P. A. Eigenmann. 2013. "Evaluation of food allergy in patients with atopic dermatitis." *J Allergy Clin Immunol Pract* 1(1): 22–8. doi: 10.1016/j.jaip.2012.11.005.

Bieber, T. 2008. "Atopic dermatitis." *N Engl J Med* 358(14): 1483–94. doi: 10.1056/NEJMra074081.

Blattner, C. M., and J. E. Murase. 2014. "A practice gap in pediatric dermatology: does breast-feeding prevent the development of infantile atopic dermatitis?" *J Am Acad Dermatol* 71(2): 405–6. doi: 10.1016/j.jaad.2014.01.868.

Boguniewicz, M., J. A. Zeichner, L. F. Eichenfield, A. A. Hebert, M. Jarratt, A. W. Lucky, and A. S. Paller. 2008. "MAS063DP is effective monotherapy for mild to moderate atopic dermatitis in infants and children: a multicenter, randomized, vehicle-controlled study." *J Pediatr* 152(6): 854–9. doi: 10.1016/j.jpeds.2007.11.031.

Botros, P. A., G. Tsai, and G. G. Pujalte. 2015. "Evaluation and management of acne." *Prim Care* 42(4): 465–71. doi: 10.1016/j.pop.2015.07.007.

Brown, E. M., M. C. Arrieta, and B. B. Finlay. 2013. "A fresh look at the hygiene hypothesis: how intestinal microbial exposure drives immune effector responses in atopic disease." *Semin Immunol* 25(5): 378–87. doi: 10.1016/j.smim.2013.09.003.

Camargo, C. A., Jr., D. Ganmaa, R. Sidbury, Kh Erdenedelger, N. Radnaakhand, and B. Khandsuren. 2014. "Randomized trial of vitamin D supplementation for winter-related atopic dermatitis in children." *J Allergy Clin Immunol* 134(4): 831–5 e1. doi: 10.1016/j.jaci.2014.08.002.

Cao, H., G. Yang, Y. Wang, J. P. Liu, C. A. Smith, H. Luo, and Y. Liu. 2015. "Complementary therapies for acne vulgaris." *Cochrane Database Syst Rev* 1: CD009436. doi: 10.1002/14651858. CD009436.pub2.

Chatzi, L., and M. Kogevinas. 2009. "Prenatal and childhood Mediterranean diet and the development of asthma and allergies in children." *Public Health Nutr* 12(9A): 1629–34. doi: 10.1017/S1368980009990474.

Chu, L. M., D. C. Rennie, D. W. Cockcroft, P. Pahwa, J. Dosman, L. Hagel, C. Karunanayake, W. Pickett, and J. A. Lawson. 2014. "Prevalence and determinants of atopy and allergic diseases among school-age children in rural Saskatchewan, Canada." *Ann Allergy Asthma Immunol* 113(4): 430–9. doi: 10.1016/j.anai.2014.07.003.

Chuh, A., W. Wong, and V. Zawar. 2006. "The skin and the mind." *Aust Fam Physician* 35(9): 723–5.

DebMandal, M., and S. Mandal. 2011. "Coconut (Cocos nucifera L.: Arecaceae): in health promotion and disease prevention." *Asian Pac J Trop Med* 4(3): 241–7. doi: 10.1016/S1995-7645(11)60078-3.

Dimitriades, V., P. C. Rodriguez, J. Zabaleta, and A. C. Ochoa. 2014. "Arginase I levels are decreased in the plasma of pediatric patients with atopic dermatitis." *Ann Allergy Asthma Immunol* 113(3): 271–5. doi: 10.1016/j.anai.2014.06.010.

Du Toit, G., Foong, RM., Lack,G. 2016. "Prevention of food allergy-Early dietary interventions." *Allergol Int* 65(4): 370–7. doi: 10.1016/j.alit.2016.08.001. Epub 2016 Sep 9.

Eichenfield, L. F., A. McCollum, and P. Msika. 2009. "The benefits of sunflower oleo-distillate (SOD) in pediatric dermatology." *Pediatr Dermatol* 26(6): 669–75. doi: 10.1111/j.1525-1470.2009.01042.x.

Elsaie, M. L., M. F. Abdelhamid, L. T. Elsaaiee, and H. M. Emam. 2009. "The efficacy of topical 2% green tea lotion in mild-to-moderate acne vulgaris." *J Drugs Dermatol* 8(4): 358–64.

Fiocchi, A., R. Pawankar, C. Cuello-Garcia, K. Ahn, S. Al-Hammadi, A. Agarwal, K. Beyer, W. Burks, G. W. Canonica, M. Ebisawa, S. Gandhi, R. Kamenwa, B. W. Lee, H. Li, S. Prescott, J. J. Riva, L. Rosenwasser, H. Sampson, M. Spigler, L. Terracciano, A. Vereda-Ortiz, S. Waserman, J. J. Yepes-Nunez, J. L. Brozek, and H. J. Schunemann. 2015. "World Allergy Organization-McMaster University Guidelines for Allergic Disease Prevention (GLAD-P): probiotics." *World Allergy Organ J* 8(1): 4. doi: 10.1186/s40413-015-0055-2.

Fox, A. T., P. Sasieni, G. du Toit, H. Syed, and G. Lack. 2009. "Household peanut consumption as a risk factor for the development of peanut allergy." *J Allergy Clin Immunol* 123(2): 417–23. doi: 10.1016/j.jaci.2008.12.014.

Garg, N., and J. I. Silverberg. 2015. "Epidemiology of childhood atopic dermatitis." *Clin Dermatol* 33(3): 281–8. doi: 10.1016/j.clindermatol.2014.12.004.

Goddard, A. L., and P. A. Lio. 2015. "Alternative, complementary, and forgotten remedies for atopic dermatitis." *Evid Based Complement Alternat Med* 2015: 676897. doi: 10.1155/2015/676897.

Gollnick, H. P., and C. C. Zouboulis. 2014. "Not all acne is acne vulgaris." *Dtsch Arztebl Int* 111(17): 301–12. doi: 10.3238/arztebl.2014.0301.

Grossi, E., S. Cazzaniga, S. Crotti, L. Naldi, A. Di Landro, V. Ingordo, F. Cusano, L. Atzori, F. Tripodi Cutri, M. L. Musumeci, E. Pezzarossa, V. Bettoli, M. Caproni, A. Bonci, and Gised Acne Study Group. 2016. "The constellation of dietary factors in adolescent acne: a semantic connectivity map approach." *J Eur Acad Dermatol Venereol* 30(1): 96–100. doi: 10.1111/jdv.12878.

Gunaratne, A. W., M. Makrides, and C. T. Collins. 2015. "Maternal prenatal and/or postnatal n-3 long chain polyunsaturated fatty acids (LCPUFA) supplementation for preventing allergies in early childhood." *Cochrane Database Syst Rev* 7: CD010085. doi: 10.1002/14651858. CD010085.pub2.

Gupta, D. 2015. "Atopic dermatitis: a common pediatric condition and its evolution in adulthood." *Med Clin North Am* 99(6): 1269–85, xii. doi: 10.1016/j.mcna.2015.07.006.

Hamilton, F. L., J. Car, C. Lyons, M. Car, A. Layton, and A. Majeed. 2009. "Laser and other light therapies for the treatment of acne vulgaris: systematic review." *Br J Dermatol* 160(6): 1273–85. doi: 10.1111/j.1365-2133.2009.09047.x.

Huang, J. T., M. Abrams, B. Tlougan, A. Rademaker, and A. S. Paller. 2009. "Treatment of Staphylococcus aureus colonization in atopic dermatitis decreases disease severity." *Pediatrics* 123(5): e808–14. doi: 10.1542/peds.2008-2217.

Kalliomaki, M., S. Salminen, H. Arvilommi, P. Kero, P. Koskinen, and E. Isolauri. 2001. "Probiotics in primary prevention of atopic disease: a randomised placebo-controlled trial." *Lancet* 357(9262): 1076–9. doi: 10.1016/S0140-6736(00)04259-8.

Khayef, G., J. Young, B. Burns-Whitmore, and T. Spalding. 2012. "Effects of fish oil supplementation on inflammatory acne." *Lipids Health Dis* 11: 165. doi: 10.1186/1476-511X-11-165.

Kim, A., and J. I. Silverberg. 2015. "A systematic review of vigorous physical activity in eczema." *Br J Dermatol.* doi: 10.1111/bjd.14179.

Kim, E. H., S. Kim, J. H. Lee, J. Kim, Y. Han, Y. M. Kim, G. B. Kim, K. Jung, H. K. Cheong, and K. Ahn. 2015. "Indoor air pollution aggravates symptoms of atopic dermatitis in children." *PLoS One* 10(3): e0119501. doi: 10.1371/journal.pone.0119501.

Koutroulis, I., L. Magnelli, J. Gaughan, E. Weiner, and P. Kratimenos. 2015. "Atopic dermatitis is more severe in children over the age of two who have an increased body mass index." *Acta Paediatr* 104(7): 713–7. doi: 10.1111/apa.12970.

Lee, K. C., A. Keyes, J. R. Hensley, J. R. Gordon, M. J. Kwasny, D. P. West, and P. A. Lio. 2012. "Effectiveness of acupressure on pruritus and lichenification associated with atopic dermatitis: a pilot trial." *Acupunct Med* 30(1): 8–11. doi: 10.1136/acupmed-2011-010088.

Leung, D. Y., and E. Guttman-Yassky. 2014. "Deciphering the complexities of atopic dermatitis: shifting paradigms in treatment approaches." *J Allergy Clin Immunol* 134(4): 769–79. doi: 10.1016/j.jaci.2014.08.008.

Li, Z., P. H. Summanen, J. Downes, K. Corbett, T. Komoriya, S. M. Henning, J. Kim, and S. M. Finegold. 2015. "Antimicrobial activity of pomegranate and green tea extract on Propionibacterium acnes, Propionibacterium granulosum, Staphylococcus aureus and Staphylococcus epidermidis." *J Drugs Dermatol* 14(6): 574–8.

Lin, M. H., C. J. Hsieh, J. L. Caffrey, Y. S. Lin, I. J. Wang, W. C. Ho, P. C. Chen, T. N. Wu, and R. S. Lin. 2015. "Fetal growth, obesity, and atopic disorders in adolescence: a retrospective birth cohort study." *Paediatr Perinat Epidemiol* 29(5): 472–9. doi: 10.1111/ppe.12215.

Lin, R. J., L. H. Qiu, R. Z. Guan, S. J. Hu, Y. Y. Liu, and G. J. Wang. 2015. "Protective effect of probiotics in the treatment of infantile eczema." *Exp Ther Med* 9(5): 1593–1596. doi: 10.3892/etm.2015.2299.

Liu, J., X. Mo, D. Wu, A. Ou, S. Xue, C. Liu, H. Li, Z. Wen, and D. Chen. 2015. "Efficacy of a

Chinese herbal medicine for the treatment of atopic dermatitis: a randomised controlled study." *Complement Ther Med* 23(5): 644–51. doi: 10.1016/j.ctim.2015.07.006.

Magin, P. 2013. "Appearance-related bullying and skin disorders." *Clin Dermatol* 31(1): 66–71. doi: 10.1016/j.clindermatol.2011.11.009.

McClafferty, H. 2011. "Complementary, holistic, and integrative medicine: mind-body medicine." *Pediatr Rev* 32(5): 201–3. doi: 10.1542/pir.32-5-201.

Melnik, B. C. 2015a. "Linking diet to acne metabolomics, inflammation, and comedogenesis: an update." *Clin Cosmet Investig Dermatol* 8: 371–88. doi: 10.2147/CCID.S69135.

Melnik, B. C. 2015b. "Western diet-induced imbalances of FoxO1 and mTORC1 signaling promote the sebofollicular inflammasomopathy acne vulgaris." *Exp Dermatol.* doi: 10.1111/exd.12898.

Melnik, B. C., S. M. John, and G. Schmitz. 2013. "Milk is not just food but most likely a genetic transfection system activating mTORC1 signaling for postnatal growth." *Nutr J* 12: 103. doi: 10.1186/1475-2891-12-103.

Moran, L. J., S. K. Hutchison, R. J. Norman, and H. J. Teede. 2011. "Lifestyle changes in women with polycystic ovary syndrome." *Cochrane Database Syst Rev* 2: CD007506. doi: 10.1002/14651858.CD007506.pub2.

Mortz, C. G., K. E. Andersen, C. Dellgren, T. Barington, and C. Bindslev-Jensen. 2015. "Atopic dermatitis from adolescence to adulthood in the TOACS cohort: prevalence, persistence and comorbidities." *Allergy* 70(7): 836–45. doi: 10.1111/all.12619.

Netting, M. J., P. F. Middleton, and M. Makrides. 2014. "Does maternal diet during pregnancy and lactation affect outcomes in offspring? A systematic review of food-based approaches." *Nutrition* 30(11–12): 1225–41. doi: 10.1016/j.nut.2014.02.015.

Niccoli, A. A., A. L. Artesi, F. Candio, S. Ceccarelli, R. Cozzali, L. Ferraro, D. Fiumana, M. Mencacci, M. Morlupo, P. Pazzelli, L. Rossi, M. Toscano, and L. Drago. 2014. "Preliminary results on clinical effects of probiotic Lactobacillus salivarius LS01 in children affected by atopic dermatitis." *J Clin Gastroenterol* 48(Suppl 1): S34–6. doi: 10.1097/MCG.0000000000000233.

Patrizi, A., B. Raone, and I. Neri. 2009. "Atopiclair." *Expert Opin Pharmacother* 10(7): 1223–30. doi: 10.1517/14656560902926106.

Pfab, F., J. Huss-Marp, A. Gatti, J. Fuqin, G. I. Athanasiadis, D. Irnich, U. Raap, W. Schober, H. Behrendt, J. Ring, and U. Darsow. 2010. "Influence of acupuncture on type I hypersensitivity itch and the wheal and flare response in adults with atopic eczema—a blinded, randomized, placebo-controlled, crossover trial." *Allergy* 65(7): 903–10. doi: 10.1111/j.1398-9995.2009.02284.x.

Pfab, F., M. T. Kirchner, J. Huss-Marp, T. Schuster, P. C. Schalock, J. Fuqin, G. I. Athanasiadis, H. Behrendt, J. Ring, U. Darsow, and V. Napadow. 2012. "Acupuncture compared with oral antihistamine for type I hypersensitivity itch and skin response in adults with atopic dermatitis: a patient- and examiner-blinded, randomized, placebo-controlled, crossover trial." *Allergy* 67(4): 566–73. doi: 10.1111/j.1398-9995.2012.02789.x.

Ress, K., T. Annus, U. Putnik, K. Luts, R. Uibo, and O. Uibo. 2014. "Celiac disease in children with atopic dermatitis." *Pediatr Dermatol* 31(4): 483–8. doi: 10.1111/pde.12372.

Roll, S., T. Reinhold, D. Pach, B. Brinkhaus, K. Icke, D. Staab, T. Jackel, K. Wegscheider, S. N. Willich, and C. M. Witt. 2013. "Comparative effectiveness of homoeopathic vs. conventional therapy in usual care of atopic eczema in children: long-term medical and economic outcomes." *PLoS One* 8(1): e54973. doi: 10.1371/journal.pone.0054973.

Romanos, M., M. Gerlach, A. Warnke, and J. Schmitt. 2010. "Association of attention-deficit/hyperactivity disorder and atopic eczema modified by sleep disturbance in a large population-based sample." *J Epidemiol Community Health* 64(3): 269–73. doi: 10.1136/jech.2009.093534.

Rossi, E., P. Bartoli, A. Bianchi, and M. Da Fre. 2012. "Homeopathy in paediatric atopic diseases: long-term results in children with atopic dermatitis." *Homeopathy* 101(1): 13–20. doi: 10.1016/j.homp.2011.09.003.

Rostami Mogaddam, M., N. Safavi Ardabili, N. Maleki, and M. Soflaee. 2014. "Correlation between the severity and type of acne lesions with serum zinc levels in patients with acne vulgaris." *Biomed Res Int* 2014: 474108. doi: 10.1155/2014/474108.

Sampson, H. A., R. Gerth van Wijk, C. Bindslev-Jensen, S. Sicherer, S. S. Teuber, A. W. Burks, A. E. Dubois, K. Beyer, P. A. Eigenmann, J. M. Spergel, T. Werfel, and V. M. Chinchilli. 2012. "Standardizing double-blind, placebo-controlled oral food challenges: American Academy of Allergy, Asthma & Immunology-European Academy of Allergy and Clinical Immunology PRACTALL consensus report." *J Allergy Clin Immunol* 130(6): 1260–74. doi: 10.1016/j.jaci.2012.10.017.

Schempp, C. M., T. Windeck, S. Hezel, and J. C. Simon. 2003. "Topical treatment of atopic dermatitis with St. John's wort cream: a randomized, placebo controlled, double blind half-side comparison." *Phytomedicine* 10(Suppl 4): S31–7.

Shalita, A. R., R. Falcon, A. Olansky, P. Iannotta, A. Akhavan, D. Day, A. Janiga, P. Singri, and J. E. Kallal. 2012. "Inflammatory acne management with a novel prescription dietary supplement." *J Drugs Dermatol* 11(12): 1428–33.

Sharquie, K. E., A. A. Noaimi, and M. M. Al-Salih. 2008. "Topical therapy of acne vulgaris using 2% tea lotion in comparison with 5% zinc sulphate solution." *Saudi Med J* 29(12): 1757–61.

Shenefelt, P. D. 2004. "Using hypnosis to facilitate resolution of psychogenic excoriations in acne excoriee." *Am J Clin Hypn* 46(3): 239–45. doi: 10.1080/00029157.2004.10403603.

Shenefelt, P. D. 2011. "Psychodermatological disorders: recognition and treatment." *Int J Dermatol* 50(11): 1309–22. doi: 10.1111/j.1365-4632.2011.05096.x.

Shi, V. Y., S. Nanda, K. Lee, A. W. Armstrong, and P. A. Lio. 2013. "Improving patient education with an eczema action plan: a randomized controlled trial." *JAMA Dermatol* 149(4): 481–3. doi: 10.1001/jamadermatol.2013.2143.

Sicherer, S. H. 2015. "Early peanut consumption is protective against peanut allergy development." *J Pediatr* 167(1): 209. doi: 10.1016/j.jpeds.2015.04.087.

Sidbury, R., A. F. Sullivan, R. I. Thadhani, and C. A. Camargo, Jr. 2008. "Randomized controlled trial of vitamin D supplementation for winter-related atopic dermatitis in Boston: a pilot study." *Br J Dermatol* 159(1): 245–7. doi: 10.1111/j.1365-2133.2008.08601.x.

Silverberg, J. I., J. Hanifin, and E. L. Simpson. 2013. "Climatic factors are associated with childhood eczema prevalence in the United States." *J Invest Dermatol* 133(7): 1752–9. doi: 10.1038/jid.2013.19.

Silverberg, J. I., M. Lee-Wong, and N. B. Silverberg. 2014. "Complementary and alternative medicines and childhood eczema: a US population-based study." *Dermatitis* 25(5): 246–54. doi: 10.1097/DER.0000000000000072.

Silverberg, J. I., and N. B. Silverberg. 2014. "Epidemiology and extracutaneous comorbidities of severe acne in adolescence: a U.S. population-based study." *Br J Dermatol* 170(5): 1136–42. doi: 10.1111/bjd.12912.

Silverberg, N. B. 2012. "Whey protein precipitating moderate to severe acne flares in 5 teenaged athletes." *Cutis* 90(2): 70–2.

Sokel, B., R. Lansdown, and A. Kent. 1990. "The development of a hypnotherapy service for children." *Child Care Health Dev* 16(4): 227–33.

Spergel, J. M., M. Boguniewicz, L. Schneider, J. M. Hanifin, A. S. Paller, and L. F. Eichenfield. 2015. "Food allergy in infants with atopic dermatitis: limitations of food-specific IgE measurements." *Pediatrics* 136(6): e1530–8. doi: 10.1542/peds.2015-1444.

Spieldenner, J., D. Belli, C. Dupont, F. Haschke, M. Iskedjian, S. Nevot Falco, H. Szajewska, and A. von Berg. 2011. "Partially hydrolysed 100% whey-based infant formula and the prevention of atopic dermatitis: comparative pharmacoeconomic analyses." *Ann Nutr Metab* 59(Suppl 1): S44–52. doi: 10.1159/000334232.

Storro, O., E. Avershina, and K. Rudi. 2013. "Diversity of intestinal microbiota in infancy and the risk of allergic disease in childhood." *Curr Opin Allergy Clin Immunol* 13(3): 257–62. doi: 10.1097/ACI.0b013e328360968b.

Suarez-Varela, M. M., L. G. Alvarez, M. D. Kogan, J. C. Ferreira, A. Martinez Gimeno, I.

Aguinaga Ontoso, C. Gonzalez Diaz, A. Arnedo Pena, B. Dominguez Aurrecoechea, R. M. Busquets Monge, A. Blanco Quiros, J. Batlles Garrido, N. Garcia de Andoain, A. L. Varela, A. Garcia Merino, N. Gimeno Clemente, and A. Llopis Gonzalez. 2010. "Diet and prevalence of atopic eczema in 6 to 7-year-old schoolchildren in Spain: ISAAC phase III." *J Investig Allergol Clin Immunol* 20(6): 469–75.

Tan, H. Y., A. L. Zhang, D. Chen, C. C. Xue, and G. B. Lenon. 2013. "Chinese herbal medicine for atopic dermatitis: a systematic review." *J Am Acad Dermatol* 69(2): 295–304. doi: 10.1016/j.jaad.2013.01.019.

Telofski, L. S., A. P. Morello, 3rd, M. C. Mack Correa, and G. N. Stamatas. 2012. "The infant skin barrier: can we preserve, protect, and enhance the barrier?" *Dermatol Res Pract* 2012: 198789. doi: 10.1155/2012/198789.

Torley, D., M. Futamura, H. C. Williams, and K. S. Thomas. 2013. "What's new in atopic eczema? An analysis of systematic reviews published in 2010–11." *Clin Exp Dermatol* 38(5): 449–56. doi: 10.1111/ced.12143.

Volz, T., Y. Skabytska, E. Guenova, K. M. Chen, J. S. Frick, C. J. Kirschning, S. Kaesler, M. Rocken, and T. Biedermann. 2014. "Nonpathogenic bacteria alleviating atopic dermatitis inflammation induce IL-10-producing dendritic cells and regulatory Tr1 cells." *J Invest Dermatol* 134(1): 96–104. doi: 10.1038/jid.2013.291.

von Berg, A., B. Filipiak-Pittroff, U. Kramer, E. Link, C. Bollrath, I. Brockow, S. Koletzko, A. Grubl, J. Heinrich, H. E. Wichmann, C. P. Bauer, D. Reinhardt, D. Berdel, and G. INIplus study group. 2008. "Preventive effect of hydrolyzed infant formulas persists until age 6 years: long-term results from the German Infant Nutritional Intervention Study (GINI)." *J Allergy Clin Immunol* 121(6): 1442–7. doi: 10.1016/j.jaci.2008.04.021.

Wen, H. J., P. C. Chen, T. L. Chiang, S. J. Lin, Y. L. Chuang, and Y. L. Guo. 2009. "Predicting risk for early infantile atopic dermatitis by hereditary and environmental factors." *Br J Dermatol* 161(5): 1166–72. doi: 10.1111/j.1365-2133.2009.09412.x.

Werfel, T., B. Ballmer-Weber, P. A. Eigenmann, B. Niggemann, F. Rance, K. Turjanmaa, and M. Worm. 2007. "Eczematous reactions to food in atopic eczema: position paper of the EAACI and GA2LEN." *Allergy* 62(7): 723–8. doi: 10.1111/j.1398-9995.2007.01429.x.

West, C. E. 2014. "Gut microbiota and allergic disease: new findings." *Curr Opin Clin Nutr Metab Care* 17(3): 261–6. doi: 10.1097/MCO.0000000000000044.

Williams, H. C., R. P. Dellavalle, and S. Garner. 2012. "Acne vulgaris." *Lancet* 379(9813): 361–72. doi: 10.1016/S0140-6736(11)60321-8.

Wolfle, U., G. Seelinger, and C. M. Schempp. 2014. "Topical application of St. John's wort (Hypericum perforatum)." *Planta Med* 80(2–3): 109–20. doi: 10.1055/s-0033-1351019.

Yamanaka, K., and H. Mizutani. 2015. ""Inflammatory skin march": IL-1-mediated skin inflammation, atopic dermatitis, and psoriasis to cardiovascular events." *J Allergy Clin Immunol* 136(3): 823–4. doi: 10.1016/j.jaci.2015.06.009.

Yildizgoren, M. T., and A. K. Togral. 2014. "Preliminary evidence for vitamin D deficiency in nodulocystic acne." *Dermatoendocrinol* 6(1): e983687. doi: 10.4161/derm.29799.

Yu, C., P. Zhang, Z. T. Lv, J. J. Li, H. P. Li, C. H. Wu, F. Gao, X. C. Yuan, J. Zhang, W. He, X. H. Jing, and M. Li. 2015. "Efficacy of acupuncture in itch: a systematic review and meta-analysis of clinical randomized controlled trials." *Evid Based Complement Alternat Med* 2015: 208690. doi: 10.1155/2015/208690.

Zaenglein, A. L. Md. 2015. "Psychosocial issues in acne management: disease burden, treatment adherence, and patient support." *Semin Cutan Med Surg* 34(5S): S92–4. doi: 110.12788/j.sder.2015.0165.

Zouboulis, C. C., and V. Bettoli. 2015. "Management of severe acne." *Br J Dermatol* 172(Suppl 1): S27–36. doi: 10.1111/bjd.13639.

17 Gastroenterology

Overview

Children experience a surprising variety of gastrointestinal conditions, many of which leave clinicians searching for an expanded range of treatment options. Advancements in understanding of the intricate connections between the gut-inflammatory-immune and neuronal systems have highlighted the value of an integrative approach to gastrointestinal disorders. The material reviews some gastrointestinal conditions where integrative approaches have been shown to be useful in children and is not meant as an exhaustive review of the specialty (Day 2013).

Functional Abdominal Pain

Overview

Chronic abdominal pain without a clear etiology is a very common problem in children, estimated to occur in 10%–30% of children, often in those who have experienced significant stressors or traumatic events (Brown, Beattie, and Tighe 2015).

Abdominal pain-related functional gastrointestinal disorders (AP-FGIDS) is the over-arching term used in the Rome criteria, which encompasses functional abdominal pain, functional abdominal pain syndrome, irritable bowel syndrome (IBS), functional dyspepsia, and abdominal migraine. Recurrent abdominal pain (RAP) is a familiar term coined in the 1950s that is sometimes used interchangeably in the literature (Rasquin et al. 2006).

The Rome III criteria require presence of symptoms consisting of at least three episodes of pain severe enough that the child is unable to continue their daily activities 2 months prior to diagnosis, reduced from 3 months in the Rome II criteria (Korterink et al. 2015).

Functional abdominal pain appears to peak at 4–6 years of age, and again at 9–11 years, although it is not limited to these age groups. The most common pain subtype is irritable bowel syndrome (65%), followed by functional abdominal pain (35%), functional dyspepsia (Brown, Beattie, and Tighe 2015), and abdominal migraine (9%–15%) which is generally accompanied by midline, moderate to severe abdominal pain that lasts a discrete amount of time with vasomotor symptoms such as pallor, and often accompanied by nausea and or vomiting (Carson et al. 2011).

Quality of life is significantly impacted in children experiencing functional abdominal pain and accounts for frequent school absences. Healthcare costs for treatment of functional abdominal pain were more than 2500 euros annually in a study of 258 children in the Netherlands, with significant lost time at work also reported by parents (van Barreveld et al. 2015). A study of the cost of work up for 243 children with functional abdominal pain in the U.S. found an average cost per patient of $6000, with minimal yield from multiple tests (Dhroove, Chogle, and Saps 2010).

The low yield from invasive blood tests and imaging is frustrating for parents and clinicians alike and highlights the importance of clearly explaining the interplay of the gut–brain connection and the many factors that can cause the pain syndrome. Some of these factors include: genetic predisposition, school, social, and family stressors, parental and family pain patterns and behaviors, exercise, diet, gut mobility, and learned coping strategies (Weydert, Ball, and Davis 2003).

The concept of hypersensitivity, which should not be construed as a negative characteristic to a child or adolescent, underlies the most current understanding of the pain sensation. Emerging research on the neural networks involved in irritable bowel syndrome have shown altered levels of emotional arousal in neural imaging studies of patients undergoing rectal distension as compared to controls (Liu et al. 2016).

Stressors that are both physical and mental have been shown to influence pain receptors and the production of pain-mediating neurotransmitters and subsequent symptom flares. This provides an important opening for interventions directed at reduction of psychological stress and a reframing of pain perception. If this approach is framed with skill and compassion, and not presented in a negative manner, as a "weakness" or "all in their head," clinical outcomes are significantly improved (Brown, Beattie, and Tighe 2015).

Etiology

In addition to psychological stressors, genetic factors have been shown to play an important part in etiology, with a parent with IBS being a strong predictor of recurrent abdominal pain in offspring. Maternal depression has also been shown to be a factor in prevalence of functional abdominal pain in children. Highly stressful events in a child's life have also been linked to symptoms, including divorce, family conflict, death, school and sport pressure, and test anxiety, high achiever status in school, separation anxiety, and phobias, among others. Abuse of any kind is another possible hidden etiology that must be considered. Children who are highly emotional, or who internalize worries, are also at higher risk. Studies have shown statistically significant correlation with anxiety, depression, and perceived lower quality of life as predictors of abdominal pain. Children who are less adaptive to change or new stressors are also at higher risk. Recent viral gastrointestinal illness and chronic constipation can also be factors (Brown, Beattie, and Tighe 2015).

Occult constipation, defined as "abdominal pain disappearing with laxative treatment and not reappearing within a 6-month follow up period," was seen in nearly 50% of 200 school-aged children with recurrent abdominal pain (Gijsbers et al. 2014).

Prevalence

International pooled prevalence of recurrent abdominal pain was found to average 13.5% in a large population study with a wide geographic range. Highest rates were seen in South America and Asia at approximately 16.5% of school-aged children, with consistently higher prevalence in girls than in boys (Korterink et al. 2015).

Clinical Manifestations

The symptoms of recurrent abdominal pain vary from child to child and include sharp or dull pain, which may cause pallor, diaphoresis, or crying. Pain can be brief or of longer duration, and may be related to eating, but not always. Pain can occur any time of the day or night, and may lead to skipping meals to avoid provoking pain (Brown, Beattie, and Tighe 2015).

Comorbidities

Recurrent abdominal pain itself creates psychological stress and comorbidities in children and adolescents, including depression and anxiety. Obesity is another frequent comorbidity in children with functional abdominal pain, although the relationship is not fully understood (Malaty et al. 2007).

Overall outlook is positive for symptom resolution over time, although a 5-year follow-up study of 104 patients through the emergency department with non-specific abdominal pain showed that 28% had recurring abdominal pain at year 5 and 13% eventually required diagnostic or therapeutic surgery (Banz et al. 2012).

Diagnostic Criteria

Functional abdominal pain is a clinical diagnosis that considers the frequency, timing, and duration of the pain, as well as what leads to its improvement. Diagnosis can be made more challenging due to a child's inability to fully articulate the presence or characteristics of the pain. Abdominal migraine, a challenging diagnosis in children, can contribute to the complexity of a correct diagnosis (Millichap and Yee 2003).

A detailed history is needed to explore all the relevant areas of a child's life that may be contributing to their pain. General screening tests recommended to rule out other conditions include:

- Complete blood count.
- Basic chemistries.
- C-reactive protein.
- Basic liver function tests.
- Total immunoglobulin A and tissue transglutaminase/endomysial antibody status to rule out celiac disease.
- Consider specific IgE for suspected food allergy.
- Fecal calprotectin if symptoms are suggestive of inflammatory bowel disease.
- Consider screening for *Helicobacter* if upper gastrointestinal symptoms are suggestive and for parasites if history is indicative.
- Consider breath hydrogen test for lactose intolerance if symptoms consistent.
- Erythrocyte sedimentation rate has not been well correlated with symptoms.

Imaging studies are generally not indicated, which can be challenging to explain to concerned parents. In reality pursuit of positive lab and imaging studies in the absence of clinical symptoms can lead to frustration and paradoxically increased worry if negative results continue to accumulate. Ideally clinicians can help children and families feel reassured rather than more anxious by finding ways to skillfully explain the idea of hypersensitivity in an age-appropriate way.

Conversely, signs and symptoms that should raise concern and that require further testing and possible imaging and endoscopy include:

- Weight loss
- Blood in stool
- Diarrhea
- Fever
- Persistent vomiting
- Arthritis
- Certain types of rash, mouth ulcers
- Growth retardation
- Delayed pubertal development
- Difficulty in swallowing
- Night time awakening from pain
- Family history of ulcer or any inflammatory bowel disease

Other possible causes of abdominal pain to rule out include: constipation, stomach virus, irritable or inflammatory bowel disease, food poisoning, food allergies, gallstones, hernia, and trauma among others.

Treatment

Conventional Treatment

It is very important to acknowledge the real pain and discomfort the child is experiencing. Although it sounds deceptively simple, reassurance may be the most important treatment element in this condition. Ideally the information that no abnormal lab tests have been identified, and that long-term outcome is very positive, will serve to speed recovery. Learning to redirect or distract from the pain was shown to be an effective approach for parents in a study by Walker et al. (Walker et al. 2006).

Use of a parent-directed cognitive behavioral therapy approach has also shown to be very effective in reducing pain in a study of 200 children in a three-session intervention over 6 months ($p < 0.01$). Emphasis on the goal of reducing psychological stressors and maximizing daily functioning can help the child gain a sense of greater self-efficacy and teach that they do not have to rely on a medication to feel better. More in-depth psychological consult may be needed to address family conflict or hidden stressors. Medication is rarely indicated and has limited supporting evidence. There is currently no supporting evidence for analgesics, antidepressants, or gabapentin for suspected neuropathic pain. Avoidance of non-steroidal anti-inflammatories is recommended as they can irritate the gut. If dyspepsia is present, H2 antagonists may be considered (Brown, Beattie, and Tighe 2015).

Integrative Treatment

LIFESTYLE APPROACH

For mild recurrent abdominal pain, resting, and immediate measures to reduce stress can be helpful, as can emphasizing the importance of regular good-quality sleep. Maximizing diet quality and avoidance of stimulants such as caffeine and irritants such as carbonation are recommended as is eating small meals including fruits, vegetables, rice, and dry toasts, and avoiding fatty products (Young and Kemper 2013).

There is minimal evidence to support a specific diet approach including lactose free, additional fiber, or fermentable, oligosaccharides, disaccharides, monosaccharides, and polyols diet (FODMAP diet). Probiotics have shown some benefit in irritable bowel syndrome, but not as of yet in functional abdominal pain. There is some evidence to support regular exercise and increasing fruits and vegetables as demonstrated in a study of 925 children with recurrent abdominal pain, where an inverse correlation between fruit intake and recurrent abdominal pain was seen (Malaty et al. 2007).

COMPLEMENTARY APPROACH

Overall the strongest evidence for intervention is stress reduction and behavior interventions. The fact that the gut and nervous system originate from the same embryologic tissue helps clarify the value of considering gut-directed mind–body therapies in the treatment of seemingly unrelated emotional and gastrointestinal conditions. A 2014 Cochrane Systematic Database Review of 37 studies involving 2111 children and pain management in which nine studies involved abdominal pain and found that non-pharmaceutical approaches such as cognitive behavioral therapy and clinical hypnosis were effective with adequate statistical significance to recommend (Eccleston et al. 2014).

This opens the opportunity to explore the full range of mind–body therapies in children to find which will be of most benefit to the individual child and which will fit the child's situation most effectively (McClafferty 2011).

Yoga has shown some benefit in adolescents with irritable bowel syndrome, although not specifically in recurrent abdominal pain. Peppermint oil has similarly shown benefit in irritable bowel syndrome but lacks supporting evidence in recurrent abdominal pain.

Irritable Bowel Syndrome

Overview

Irritable bowel syndrome is the most commonly diagnosed gut condition overall, and the most common subset of functional abdominal pain in children. It is diagnosed in an estimated 9% of children with functional abdominal pain worldwide, often defined by a chronic relapsing course (Korterink et al. 2015).

It differs from recurrent abdominal pain in that it includes a pattern of altered bowel habits in the absence of other identified disease to account for the symptoms. Three main types have been determined: IBS with diarrhea (IBS-D), irritable bowel syndrome with constipation (IBS-C), and irritable bowel pattern-mixed (IBS-M) that can change over time (Chey, Kurlander, and Eswaran 2015).

IBS has been shown to take a significant toll on quality of life, and in adults has been shown to account for more than 3 million outpatient visits, nearly 6 million prescriptions annually, with direct and indirect costs shown to surpass $20 billion (Agarwal and Spiegel 2011).

Complementary therapies are often used by patients with IBS, which makes a working familiarity with integrative approaches important for all clinicians caring for children with this condition (Hussain and Quigley 2006).

Etiology

The etiology of IBS is heterogeneous with two main categories commonly recognized, as follows.

Physiologic Contributors

- Altered pain perception
- Altered brain–gut interaction
- Alteration in gut microbiome
- Increased intestinal permeability
- Increased gut mucosal immune activation
- Visceral hypersensitivity

Studies have shown a striking difference in the fecal microbiome of IBS patients as compared to controls, including a lack of microbial diversity, which may be influenced by a range of factors including antibiotics, genetics, nutrition, stressors, infections, and geographic setting (Collins 2014; Shankar, Reo, and Paliy 2015; Kelly et al. 2015).

External Contributors

- Stressors in early life
- Food intolerance
- Antibiotics
- Gut infection (post-infectious irritable bowel syndrome)

Accruing research shows that short-chain carbohydrates that are rapidly ferment-able and osmotically active such as fructose, lactose, fructans, galactans, and sugar alcohols commonly trigger IBS symptoms. Carbohydrates that are poorly absorbed create osmotic effects and contribute to increased fermentation and gas that have been shown to worsen symptoms in those with IBS. These observations led to the development of the FODMAPs elimination diet that has been shown to have significant benefit in some patients with IBS (Chey, Kurlander, and Eswaran 2015; Brown, Beattie, and Tighe 2015).

Prevalence

Depending on the criteria used, the prevalence of IBS ranges from 10% to 20% internationally. In the U.S. it is estimated at approximately 12% in adults and in 9% of children experiencing functional abdominal pain (Marynowski et al. 2015; Lovell and Ford 2012).

Clinical Manifestations

The basic clinical manifestations of IBS include chronic abdominal pain and changes in bowel habits including constipation, diarrhea, or a mixture of the two. Bloating and flatulence and sensitivity to certain foods can be seen (Chey, Kurlander, and Eswaran 2015).

Comorbidities

Comorbidities in IBS can involve a range of body systems in addition to the gastrointestinal system. For example, in addition to dyspepsia and gastroesophageal reflux, IBS has been associated with a variety of somatic pain syndromes such as migraine headache, fibromyalgia, chronic fatigue syndrome, and chronic pelvic pain in adults. Uncoordinated action of the muscles involved in evacuation can be seen in IBS-constipation, leading to chronic incomplete evacuation of stool. Like recurrent abdominal pain, IBS is associated with anxiety and depression which have been shown to be predictive of worse outcome (Riedl et al. 2008).

Diagnostic Criteria

The Rome III criteria for IBS have been widely published and include the presence of abdominal pain and altered bowel habits in the absence of identifiable disease that occurs at least 3 days in the last month associated with two or more of the following:

- Pain improves with defecation.
- Pain onset is associated with change in stool frequency.
- Pain onset is associated with change in stool consistency.

   In general stool consistency, rather than frequency, is used to differentiate the three major subtypes and has been found to most helpful in directing treatment. A stool diary may be helpful in narrowing the diagnosis (Chey, Kurlander, and Eswaran 2015).
   Symptoms of concern that should trigger further individualized workup (lab, imaging, endoscopy, fecal testing), and possible gastrointestinal referral, include (Chey, Kurlander, and Eswaran 2015):

- Severe or progressive symptoms
- Unexplained weight loss, failure to thrive
- Nocturnal diarrhea
- Family history of significant gut disease
- Rectal bleeding
- Unexplained anemia

   Overlap with symptoms of gluten-related disorders such as celiac disease, non-celiac gluten sensitivity, and wheat allergy can make diagnosis more challenging. Even adoption of a gluten-free diet can improve IBS symptoms in those without a formal diagnosis of gluten-related disorder, making a low threshold for screening for celiac disease appropriate (Makharia, Catassi, and Makharia 2015).
   Irritable bowel disease symptoms can have significant overlap with inflammatory

bowel disease, although studies in adults found a very low incidence of IBD diagnosis by endoscopy (less than 1%) in a study of 900 IBS patients and healthy controls, suggesting that routine endoscopy is not indicated (Chey et al. 2010).

Ultimately the extent of the workup indicated in IBS should be determined based on the child's history, physical, and family history.

Treatment

Conventional Treatment

Recommendations from the American College of Gastroenterology Functional Bowel Disorder Task Force report that over-the counter therapies have not been shown to be very effective in IBS treatment, although they are widely used (Ford et al. 2014).

Interestingly, mainstream recommendations from the group include a patient–physician relationship based on excellent communication skills and trust, patient education, and lifestyle and dietary measures as first-line approaches (Chey, Kurlander, and Eswaran 2015).

Medical treatments for IBS-diarrhea predominant that have been studied include antidiarrheals, serotonin 5-HT3 receptor antagonists, and antispasmodics. Medical treatments for IBS-constipation predominant include fiber supplements, laxatives, prosecretory agents, and rifaximin, a poorly absorbed antibiotic. Centrally acting agents have also been used, especially antidepressants for patients with more severe IBS symptoms.

Overall, medical treatments for IBS in both children and adults have shown mixed results and may put children at risk for unwanted side effects (Sandhu and Paul 2014).

Integrative Treatment

Lifestyle Approach

NUTRITION

Nutrition interventions in IBS patients are an area of active study. Many patients with IBS identify intolerance to specific foods, and although food allergy is frequently considered, it has not been proven to be a prevalent factor in the etiology of IBS (El-Salhy and Gundersen 2015).

More recent research raises the question of whether the improvements often seen in patients with IBS who have non-celiac gluten sensitivity is due to the removal of gluten or to the removal of grain when a gluten-free diet is implemented (Nijeboer et al. 2013).

Other nutrition variables that have shown some promise in studies include increasing dietary fiber, and adoption of a low-fermentable oligosaccharides, disaccharides, monosaccharides and polyols diet (Thomas and Quigley 2015).

Foods that are high in FODMAPs include (Stanford Health Care):

- Fructose (found especially in fruits, honey, high fructose corn syrup)
- Lactose (found in dairy)
- Fructans (found in wheat, garlic, onion, inulin and others)
- Galactans (legumes, lentils, soybeans and others)

- Polyols (sweeteners containing mannitol, xylitol, and sorbitol, and fruits containing stone pits such as avocado, cherry, peaches, plums and others)

The role of the gut microbiome and how it is influenced by dietary changes is a topic at the forefront of research in adult and childhood IBS (Thomas and Quigley 2015; Chumpitazi et al. 2015; Rao, Yu, and Fedewa 2015).

A reasonable early nutrition intervention might include individualized elimination diet and a trial of gluten-free and FODMAP-restricted diet. A food diary may prove to be very useful in narrowing food triggers and to ensure that a healthy variety of foods is being consumed on a regular basis.

PHYSICAL ACTIVITY

Evidence is accruing for the benefit of exercise in IBS treatment. A randomized controlled trial in 102 adults with IBS showed benefit in the treatment group who received individualized instruction on exercise from a physiotherapist and encouragement to increase their physical activity over a 12-week study period. Symptoms decreased in the treatment group, and significantly increased over time in the control group (Johannesson et al. 2011).

Follow-up on 39 women in the treatment group from the 12-week study was done for an average of 5.2 years. A significant improvement in IBS symptoms, quality of life, fatigue, anxiety, and depression was seen in 54% of the women who continued even a relatively small increase in physical activity. In addition to the widely recognized mental health benefits of exercise, more efficient transit of stool has been shown in those with IBS-constipation who exercise. Physical activity has also been shown to improve symptoms of bloating (Johannesson et al. 2011).

Complementary Approach

MIND–BODY THERAPIES

Complementary therapies with strongest evidence in children include clinical hypnosis, which has been shown to be effective in multiple randomized controlled studies with sustained results and absence of adverse events (Whorwell 2013).

Hypnotherapy has been shown to be effective in clinical visits and when used at home with recorded sessions directed at reduction of pain, spasms, and overall balancing of the sympathetic and parasympathetic nervous systems, teaching children how to access the relaxation response (Rutten et al. 2013).

Cognitive behavioral therapy has also shown some benefit and is commonly used in children with IBS (Sandhu and Paul 2014).

Yoga has been studied in children 8–18 years old with both recurrent abdominal pain and IBS and found to be useful in reduction of stress and abdominal pain severity and frequency. Overall quality of life was also shown to be significantly improved in the treatment group (Brands, Purperhart, and Deckers-Kocken 2011).

Some of the determinants of successful treatment with the mind–body therapies involve baseline state of activation of the patient's sympathetic nervous system. One study by Jarett et al. evaluated the most useful biomarkers for determining the success of a comprehensive approach to IBS symptoms. The program included in-person and over the phone interactions linked to a workbook of assignments and homework assignments. Topics covered over eight 60-minute sessions covering autogenic relaxation, identifying false beliefs, and recorded audio relaxation sessions. Markers measured included heart rate variability, salivary cortisol, interleukin-10 production, and intestinal permeability testing through 24-hour urinary lactulose/mannitol ratio. Results of the pilot study in 46 adults with IBS and 46 wait-listed controls showed that the nurse-directed program was more effective in reducing IBS symptoms as compared to the control group. In this study salivary cortisol, IL-10, and lactulose/mannitol ratio were not predictive of improvement with the intervention, although heart rate variability was. The intervention was less successful in patients with higher baseline sympathetic tone. This study gives further insight into the connection between stress and IBS and paves the way for further study in this area (Jarrett et al. 2016).

The forward edge of research in IBS is demonstrated by the use of biomarkers such as salivary cortisol, heart rate variability, and inflammatory serum markers to measure the efficacy of self-management interventions such as cognitively based therapy. Early trends show better efficacy of behavioral interventions in those with lower baseline sympathetic activity.

A study of heart rate variability biofeedback in 27 pediatric patients showed encouraging responses in improvement in both functional abdominal pain and IBS patients. Full remission was achieved by 69.2% of IBS patients, with another 30% achieving partial remission. Of the patients with functional abdominal pain, full remission was seen in 63% and partial remission in 36% (Stern, Guiles, and Gevirtz 2014).

PROBIOTICS

While probiotics have been shown to be effective in randomized clinical trials in a variety of conditions, including: diarrhea associated with rotavirus, antibiotics, and *Clostridium difficile*, traveler's diarrhea, and in some cases of constipation, results in IBS studies have been mixed and questions remain regarding their definitive benefit and efficacy (Cruchet et al. 2015).

For example, a systematic review of 56 papers by Mazurak et al. found a high variability in dose, strain, duration, and benefit. Many studies (27/56) used a variety of strains in combination, adding further complexity to the analysis (Mazurak et al. 2015).

In their review, more than 50% of studies found no benefit. Studies with some of the more positive outcomes were associated with bifidobacteria, although variability of study design remained a confounding factor (Mazurak et al. 2015).

On the other hand, a systematic review and meta-analysis of 15 randomized, double-blind clinical trials involving 1793 patients, in a variety of study designs, concluded overall positive effect of probiotics in reduction of pain and in severity of symptoms in patients with IBS (Didari et al. 2015).

Use of probiotics is frequently considered in pediatric IBS treatment, although relatively few specific randomized controlled trials exist to guide clinicians. One controlled double-blinded randomized trial in 52 children using *Lactobacillus* GG at a daily dose of 1×10 (10) cfu/mL bacteria for 4 weeks found significant improvement in pain severity and frequency in a small study group of 29 children (Kianifar et al. 2015).

PEPPERMINT OIL

Enteric-coated peppermint oil has antispasmodic action, primarily through calcium-blocking action. It has been evaluated in more than 15 trials using a typical dose of 180–200 mg enteric-coated capsules and demonstrated promising effect in reduction of pain.

The most common side effects reported include heartburn and perianal burning in some patients, although in many patients a dose of 1–2 capsules per day was well tolerated (Grigoleit and Grigoleit 2005).

VITAMIN D

Many patients with IBS have been shown to be deficient in vitamin D and small studies suggest this may be correlated with a poorer quality of life, but no randomized controlled trials currently exist in IBS patients to assess the effects of vitamin D supplementation on symptom improvement (Tazzyman et al. 2015).

ACUPUNCTURE

The efficacy of acupuncture in IBS treatment has primarily been evaluated in adults and has shown mixed results (Chao and Zhang 2014). The mechanism is thought to be pain relief through stimulation of endogenous opiates and stimulation of inhibitory serotoninergic pathways (Sandhu and Paul 2014).

A 2012 Cochrane Database Systematic Review of 17 randomized controlled trials involving 1806 patients found a lack of robust data and high study variability, although some studies showed positive outcomes and adverse events were very rare (Manheimer et al. 2012).

Homeopathy is another complementary approach that has high consumer interest, but there are few supporting studies and high study design variability. Again, adverse events have not been reported specifically for the use of homeopathy in IBS (Peckham et al. 2013).

Summary

As is evidenced by the variety of treatments that have been studied, there is not one standardized approach, conventional or integrative, in children with IBS. It is a common and frustrating condition for patients, families, and clinicians. Once other conditions have been ruled out, attention to lifestyle, stressors, healthy nutrition, adequate restful sleep, and development of a personalized approach to pain and gut symptom management is indicated. Ample reassurance and acknowledgement of the painful symptoms, even in the absence of positive workup, is needed. Time to explore the social situation at home and at school to rule out undisclosed bullying, undue academic or sport pressure, or abuse of any kind is indicated in every child. Parental measures such as distraction techniques to redirect attention from the pain have been shown to be helpful. A registered dietician may be needed to help find the dietary pattern that will be best tolerated while still meeting the child's nutritional needs. Probiotics are low risk and may provide some benefit. *Lactobacillus* GG is one of the better studied that has shown benefit. VSL#3 is another well studied probiotic option in children. Gut-directed hypnotherapy or guided imagery have shown benefit with a high margin of safety. Physical activity, including yoga, has shown benefit with low risk. In a way, IBS in children is the ideal condition in which to consider an integrative approach (Sandhu and Paul 2014).

Prognosis in IBS is positive overall, although a 5-year follow-up by Hotopf found that 29% of children had symptoms at year 5. Other large controlled studies (of 268,623 children aged 0–16 years) have shown that hospital admission for non-specific abdominal pain was associated with a later four times increase in relative risk for Crohn's disease, and three times relative risk of celiac disease, suggesting that children with higher severity of symptoms be followed carefully over time (Thornton et al. 2015).

Inflammatory Bowel Disease

Overview

Crohn's disease and ulcerative colitis are the main types of inflammatory bowel conditions seen in children and have a variety of overlapping and distinguishing characteristics that have been widely published. The prevalence of pediatric inflammatory bowel disease has increased worldwide with highest acceleration in the youngest age groups. Approximately 30% of cases are now diagnosed in those in the 4–20 years age group, who have also been shown to have more severe onset, and more involved disease course, including increased risk of development of colorectal cancer later in life. Certain ethnic groups such as Ashkenazi Jews are at high risk, and familial and geographic factors have been widely published with prevalence highest in North America and Western Europe, as well as New Zealand. Increase is being seen in other developing countries, and in children who move from developing to industrialized countries. Industrialization brings a host of environmental factors into play such as changes in microbiome, chemical exposures, medications, and other issues that make understanding of a discrete etiology impossible (M'Koma 2013, Lemberg and Day 2015).

Etiology

Understanding of the underlying etiology for inflammatory bowel disease is not complete, but current theories point to a complex interaction of genetic predisposition, alterations in gut microflora, and disruption of the epithelial lining and host defense that result in dysregulation of the immune system in the susceptible individual. In Crohn's disease, inflammation can affect any part of the gastrointestinal tract, from mouth to anus. Patchy skip lesions may be seen on endoscopy, and chronic granulomatous involvement of the ileocolonic area is common. Strictures and fistulas can be seen over the course of the disease. Perioral ulcers, anal skin tags or perinanal abscess are also common. Ulcerative colitis classically presents as a more continuous inflammatory involvement of the colon, with pan-colitis and bloody diarrhea being common. An estimated 10%–20% of children have an indeterminate disease, which may progress to a more clear diagnosis over time. Variability in symptom presentation and severity can make accurate early diagnosis in children quite challenging (Lemberg and Day 2015), especially in children with onset in early childhood (Nambu et al. 2016).

Prevalence

Global prevalence has increased in inflammatory bowel disease over the past decades, especially in Latin America, Asia, and Eastern Europe, although North America and Northern Europe have higher prevalence overall (Ng et al. 2016).

In the U.S., rates of ulcerative colitis range from 37.5 to 238 per 100,000 people, again with geographic variation (da Silva et al. 2014).

Some countries, such as Scotland, have seen a sharp spike in the prevalence of pediatric IBD, with a 30% increase in juvenile onset of Crohn's disease recorded over the past three decades. Ulcerative colitis cases also increased significantly during that overall time frame (Armitage et al. 2001).

Clinical Diagnosis

Classic presentation for Crohn's disease might include weight loss, anemia, abdominal pain, slowed linear growth, or perianal symptoms. Ulcerative colitis can have an acute presentation of severe colitis and bloody diarrhea, which should be treated as a medical emergency and handled by experienced pediatric specialists in a tertiary setting. Other autoimmune features of inflammatory bowel disease can include joint pain, rash, or uveitis. Diagnosis can be especially challenging in the preschool age which can lead to delayed diagnosis, incorrect treatment and increase need for more aggressive and invasive therapy. A link between proinflammatory cytokines and activity of insulin-like growth factor, which modifies the effects of growth hormone, helps to explain the growth delay common in both conditions (Lemberg and Day 2015).

A comprehensive workup is indicated in children presenting with inflammatory bowel disease to confirm diagnosis and to rule out secondary infection. Magnetic resonance enterography (MRE) is the preferred test to assess mucosal involvement and bowel wall changes while minimizing radiation exposure (Lemberg and Day 2015).

Treatment

The immediate goal in treatment is reduction of the acute inflammatory process and induction of remission, followed by maintenance of remission. Treatment is highly individualized, and detailed review of the treatments is beyond the scope and intent of the chapter, but may include the following.

Induction of remission:

- Enteral nutrition (indicated in Crohn's disease as a first-line approach)
- Antibiotics
- Corticosteroids
- Aminosalicylates
- Biologics
- Surgery (if indicated in more severe disease)

Maintenance of remission:

- Aminosalicylates
- Immunomodulators

- Biologics
- Supplemental enteral nutrition

The overarching goal is to minimize toxicity and invasiveness of treatment while achieving clinical remission on a mucosal level as rapidly as possible.

Integrative Treatment

Use of integrative and complementary therapies is high in children with inflammatory bowel disease, although research in this area remains sparse for many therapies (Day 2013).

A 2002 survey of 92 children attending an Australian IBD clinic found that more than one in three children were being administered some form of complementary treatment (Day 2002).

A subsequent survey of 98 children in the same hospital pediatric gastrointestinal clinic a decade later showed an increase to two in every three children using complementary therapies, although these children did not necessarily carry the diagnosis of IBD. Therapies in order of prevalence used included: nutritional supplements, probiotics, herbal remedies, massage, fish oil, and relaxation techniques (Wadhera et al. 2011).

In a follow-up survey of 48 IBD patients in the clinic, three in four were found to be using some type of complementary therapy. On average children were using two to three therapies, with the most common being fish oil and probiotics. Next tier of prevalence was herbal remedies, homeopathy, and vitamins (Day 2002).

Studies of complementary use in children with IBD worldwide report a similar high prevalence, with the range of therapies reflecting cultural variations (Day 2013).

The goals of complementary medicine use in children and adolescents with IBD include a desire to maximize overall health and nutrition and to reduce pain and inflammation. Stress management for acute flares, and to help manage the chronic nature of the disease, is another frequently identified reason.

The prevalence of integrative medicine use in this population highlights the importance of encouraging disclosure of all therapies and remaining open to discussion of all options. Many families do not report use of complementary therapies, which can put the child at risk for drug–supplement and other types of interactions. In response to the high prevalence of complementary use identified in children with chronic conditions, including IBD, seen in outpatient clinics in Canada, Adams et al. developed example questions that may be useful to clinicians who wish to invite open discussion with families. "It would help me to know if other healthcare providers are involved in your child's care," and "What else do you do to support your child's health?" are two useful examples (Adams et al. 2013).

NUTRITION

Optimizing nutrition at every phase of diagnosis and treatment is a critical component in inflammatory bowel disease in children and adolescents to maximize growth and to address common nutrient deficiencies. Some patients require exclusive enteral nutrition for 8–12 weeks, which has been shown to be a factor in inducing remission in some children with Crohn's disease. Other patients are able to take a whole food diet, which optimally would be of high quality, and prioritize a variety of fresh organic foods. There is currently no universally recommended dietary preference, although a prospective study of 366,351 patients showed a positive correlation between "high sugar and soft drinks pattern" and low vegetable intake in terms of increased risk for ulcerative colitis. More research is needed in this important area (Racine et al. 2016).

The range of nutrient deficiencies is highly variable based on individual factors, disease distribution in the gut, socioeconomic status, geographic setting, and age. Attention to ferritin and vitamin D, and B12 levels, are important for optimal growth and development (Wedrychowicz, Zajac, and Tomasik 2016).

The importance of maintaining normal levels of vitamin D should be stressed given the link between vitamin D, immune functioning, and increased prevalence of colon cancer, an area of active research (Meeker and Ferguson 2011).

PROBIOTICS

To date the best studied probiotic in pediatric inflammatory bowel disease is VSL3#, a combination of eight strains: four strains of *Lactobacillus* (*L. paracasei*, *L. plantarum*, *L. acidophilus*, and *L. delbrueckii* subsp. *bulgaricus*), three strains of *Bifidobacterium* (*B. longum*, *B. breve*, and *B. infantis*), and one strain of *Streptococcus salivarius* subsp. *thermophilus*. In one prospective, randomized, double-blind study 29 pediatric patients with new diagnosis of ulcerative colitis received standard care and either VSL#3 in a weight-based dose or placebo. Remission was achieved in 92.8% of patients treated with VSL#3 versus 36.4% of those in the placebo group. Additionally, 21.4% of those in the treatment group relapsed within 1 year as opposed to 73% in the placebo group. At 6 months, 12 months or at time of relapse, the patients in the treatment group had significantly lower evidence of disease severity than those in the placebo group (Miele et al. 2009).

An open label study of 13 pediatric patients with mild-to-moderate ulcerative colitis receiving daily VSL#3 in two divided doses per day for 8 weeks showed remission in 56% of patients and a combined remission-positive response rate of 61%. Rectal biopsy post treatment with VSL#3 reflected a change in the bacterial taxonomy in the gut that was postulated to be associated with VSL#3 treatment (Huynh et al. 2009). And a meta-analysis of 23 randomized controlled trials involving 1763 participants found significantly higher rates of remission in patients treated with VSL#3 over placebo ($p < 0.0001$), and a significant reduction in remission rates when VSL#3 was added in treatment for pouchitis. No significant adverse events were reported. No benefit was seen in patients with Crohn's disease in this analysis. A clear mechanism for probiotics is not yet understood, although VSL#3 has been shown to decrease tumor necrosis factor-alpha, IL-6 and to protect the epithelial barrier through protection of tight junction proteins among other actions (Chibbar and Dieleman 2015; Shen, Zuo, and Mao 2014).

OMEGA-3 FATTY ACIDS

Omega-3 fatty acids are polyunsaturated fats of interest in IBD due to their anti-inflammatory effects, although their benefit, especially in pediatric IBD, remains unclear. A systematic review of omega-3 fatty acids in 19 randomized controlled trials involving more than 600 adult and pediatric patients failed to find compelling evidence for benefit of their use in patients with ulcerative colitis or Crohn's disease (Cabre, Manosa, and Gassull 2012).

Overall risk profile is low, and they have other beneficial properties, such as lowering triglycerides in adults with elevated levels. Care should be taken if patients are at risk for bleeding disorders due to their antiplatelet effects.

CURCUMIN

Curcumin is a principal natural curcuminoid and active ingredient found in the rhizomes of the plant *Curcuma longa* (turmeric). It is a member of the ginger family (Zingiberaceae). Curcumin has a long history of use in India and in the Ayurvedic tradition as a potent anti-inflammatory. It has been shown in many studies to inhibit tumor necrosis factor, IL-12, and IL-2, all highly proinflammatory cytokines. Curcumin has been studied in a variety of autoimmune conditions such as rheumatoid arthritis and IBD in adults and has shown benefit. A prospective forced-dose titration study examining the tolerability of curcumin in pediatric patients with IBD showed good tolerability and minimal adverse effect (gassiness in two patients) of a dose of 2 grams per day for 3 weeks.

Three of 11 patients in the study had improvement in their overall disease symptom score, suggesting potential for use as a complementary therapy in pediatric patients with IBD (Suskind et al. 2013).

Some of the other botanicals that have been reviewed for use in IBD include oral *Aloe vera* gel, *Boswellia serrata* or Indian frankincense, *Andrographis paniculata* (Acanthaceae) or Indian echinacea, and *Artemisia absinthium* (Compositae) known as wormwood.

Some small studies exist to support each of their use in either adult ulcerative colitis (curcumin, aloe vera, *Boswellia*, *Andrographis paniculata*) or Crohn's disease (wormwood), but insufficient evidence exist to support their routine recommendation in pediatrics (Algieri et al. 2015).

EMERGING RESEARCH

Mouse studies in induced colitis show that lupeol (a pentacyclic triterpene and naturally occurring anti-inflammatory found in a variety of fruits and vegetables such as white cabbage, pepper, cucumber, tomato, olive, fig, mango, strawberry, red grapes, and in American ginseng), was able to switch macrophages from a pro-inflammatory M1 to an anti-inflammatory M2 phenotype with resultant amelioration of the colitis (Zhu et al. 2016).

ACUPUNCTURE

Acupuncture has been shown to be effective in improving IBD symptoms in some adult studies but a lack of data in pediatric IBD patients prohibits definitive recommendation.

Acupuncture has been shown to be well tolerated in children and is used in a variety of academic settings for treatment of pain, nausea, and vomiting (Langhorst et al. 2015; Shiu-Lin 2015).

MIND–BODY THERAPIES

Perceived stress has been identified as a predictive factor in flare of adult ulcerative colitis in a prospective study of 75 patients followed for an average of a year (Langhorst et al. 2013). Perceived stress and avoidance coping behavior were similarly associated with relapse in 101 adult patients with Crohn's disease in medical remission in a prospective study of patients followed over 12 months (Bitton et al. 2008).

Perceived stress, and psychosocial factors at school and home, play a significant role in quality of life in children and adolescents with IBD, making acquisition of coping and self-regulatory skills very important. An accruing number of studies show the benefit of the mind–body therapies in children and adolescents with IBD. For example, a survey study of 67 adolescents with IBD showed that the majority used some type of relaxation therapy at least weekly to help in symptom management, including prayer (62%), relaxation (40%), and imagery (21%), and younger patients expressed interest in learning meditation and yoga (Cotton et al. 2010).

A prospective randomized controlled trial of 39 adult outpatients with IBD showed a statistically significant reduction in pain and anxiety and improvement in stress levels and quality of life after three in-person training sessions and use of an audio disk for home use (Mizrahi et al. 2012).

Somatic symptoms and coping skills were found to be improved after a 1-day teaching pilot program that included relaxation training and cognitively based disease-related coping skills in 13 adolescent girls and their parent or caretaker (McCormick et al. 2010).

Clinical gut-directed hypnotherapy has also been shown to have positive effect in patients with IBD, although more studies are needed to substantiate positive effect in children. Targets are pain, immune modulation, and overall relaxation (Moser 2014).

Overall, exercise is beneficial for optimal bone health and plays an important role in mental health and wellbeing. Although randomized controlled trials are limited in this area in children, finding an exercise that is tolerable and enjoyable can help children and adolescents cultivate a sense of self-efficacy while maintaining overall fitness for optimum health throughout the life cycle. A trial of yoga in 25 adolescents with IBS was found to be beneficial, although similar studies are lacking in children with IBD (Kuttner et al. 2006; Peters, Muir, and Gibson 2015).

Attention to caretaker stress is also indicated in families of children living with chronic illness. A small study on the benefit of an 8-week program on reducing caretaker burnout shows positive effect in reduction of burnout in families with children living with type-1 diabetes and IBD (Lindstrom et al. 2015).

Summary

Children living with inflammatory bowel disease face a challenging course in adjusting to a systemic inflammatory illness with significant psychosocial implications. Harnessing the full range of therapies to support a healthy lifestyle, optimal diet, and use of evidence-based complementary therapies such as VSL#3 in ulcerative colitis, and mind–body therapies to address stress, pain, procedural anxiety, and immune modulation can help smooth the way and provide a greater sense of control and self-efficacy. The high prevalence of complementary medicine use in this population suggests that every clinician working in this area be knowledgeable about the range of evidence-based options available.

Functional Constipation

Overview

Functional constipation is commonly seen in children worldwide with an estimated prevalence range of approximately 0% to 30%. It can be due to delayed transit time in the colon, or to dysfunction of pelvic floor muscles. It is characterized by painful bowel movements, hard stools, and fecal incontinence, which can take a significant toll on a child's quality of life. Many factors can come into play, including: exercise, nutrition, cow's milk allergy, stressors, gut microbiome, socioeconomic status, and fluid intake among other things. Some studies have demonstrated an association between overweight and obesity and functional constipation, but this has not been consistently seen (Koppen, Velasco-Benitez et al. 2016).

Regular access to safe, clean bathrooms, especially at school, seems intuitive, but lack of privacy, bullying, unhygienic conditions, and feeling unsafe in school toilets has been associated with stool withholding and both urinary and abdominal pain and complications in both lower elementary and high school students (Norling et al. 2015).

Clinical Manifestations

In addition to the physical discomfort and difficulty passing hard or very large stools, children can complain of reduced appetite and have increased flatulence. Certain conditions such as autism are associated with a high prevalence of gastrointestinal disorders, including constipation, which may be associated with altered gut microbiota (Wang et al. 2014).

Passage of a large, hard stool can be frightening for a young child and cause further withholding behavior. One in three children have been shown to continue to experience problems into puberty (Tabbers and Benninga 2015).

Comorbidities

Urinary tract infection secondary to vesicoureteral reflux has been associated with chronic constipation (Shaikh et al. 2016). Constipation can cause psychological comorbidities such as anxiety, stress, and depression as well as frustration and social stigma with episodes of fecal incontinence.

Diagnostic Criteria

Presence of signs and symptoms require a thorough evaluation of the patient, including careful history and physical examination. Organic diseases and their symptoms should be ruled out, including IBS-constipation, which may be challenging.

Treatment

Conventional Treatment

Acute care may require manual disimpaction. Next steps include modification of the dietary plan and increasing fluids and physical activity. An oral laxative such as polyethylene glycol (Miralax) is commonly used in children (Koppen et al. 2015).

Integrative Treatment

Lifestyle Approach

Proactive measures in diet modification and increased physical activity can help in preventing constipation and developing regular bowel movements. Increasing natural fiber in meals, including whole grains, fruits, and vegetables, adding breakfast cereals with extra fiber and fruits such as prunes which are natural laxatives, and increasing water intake are simple first steps that can help a child avoid the need for an artificial laxative. Whole fruit juices in moderation can also have a laxative effect (Bae 2014).

Recommended total fiber intake in children older than 1 year can be estimated at approximately 0.5 g/kg. Fiber in a child's diet has many benefits including increasing stool bulk and speeding transit time; natural fermentation of fiber produces short chain fatty acids that can also accelerate stool transit time, and these short chain fatty acids also have a beneficial effect on the gut microbiome; and fiber draws water into the gut.

Complementary Approach

Probiotics

A variety of studies suggest promise in the potential for the use of probiotics, although insufficient evidence exists to make a firm recommendation. Risk of adverse effect is low in an otherwise healthy child. *Lactobacillus* GG and VSL#3 are some of the probiotics that have been studied in constipation (Koppen, Di Lorenzo et al. 2016).

Biofeedback involving pelvic floor muscle retraining has shown positive benefit and is under further study with randomized controlled studies in children (van Engelenburg-van Lonkhuyzen et al. 2013). Other complementary approaches, such as acupuncture, have been studied but lack sufficient supporting data, especially in children (Wang and Yin 2015).

Gastroesophageal Reflux Disease (GERD) and Functional Dyspepsia

Overview

Mechanical gastroesophageal reflux is seen commonly in infants who often have decreased tone in the lower gastroesophageal sphincter. This differs from (Lightdale et al. 2013) gastroesophageal reflux disease (GERD) and functional dyspepsia which are seen in an estimated 5%–10% of children (Carbone, Holvoet, and Tack 2015).

Gastroesophageal reflux disease describes the symptoms that can occur when stomach contents pass into the esophagus, but it also causes symptoms of discomfort such as heartburn, epigastric pain, feeding difficulties, dysphagia, and what are known as aerodigestive disorders such as asthma, aspiration, or chronic cough. The two main categories of this condition are GERD, and functional dyspepsia. GERD is characterized by erosive esophagitis or gastritis on endoscopy, whereas functional dyspepsia is described in the Rome III criteria as: persistent upper abdominal pain or discomfort that is not exclusively relieved by defecation or associated with changes in the stool; and as pain unexplained by organic disease. No sign of endoscopic change is seen in functional dyspepsia. Pain must be present at least once per week for at least 2 months prior to diagnosis. There is discussion regarding subdividing the group functional dyspepsia into two subgroups: meal-related dyspepsia or post-prandial distress syndrome, and meal-unrelated dyspepsia or epigastric pain syndrome. Because of the high over-lap in the groups, there is a question about the clinical usefulness of this distinction (Carbone, Holvoet, and Tack 2015).

Etiology

The etiology of gastroesophageal reflux is considered multifactorial. It is not erosive in every case. A familial component has been identified in up to 20% of patients (Katle, Hatlebakk, and Steinsvag 2013). Children with predisposing conditions, such as neu-rologic impairment or congenital disorders of the GI system, are at higher risk. Reflux can be caused by a loose lower esophageal sphincter, or by increased pressure in the GI system due to obesity, chronic constipation, or mechanical blockage from strictures, hiatal hernia, or rarely solid tumors. Some children suffer from dysmotility issues. In preterm infants other factors can include cardiac anomalies, diaphragmatic hernia, infection, necrotizing enterocolitis, a range of congenital anomalies, especially gastro-intestinal and respiratory such as bronchopulmonary dysplasia, as well as complex vascular anomalies (Katle, Hatlebakk, and Steinsvag 2013).

Diet, medications, acidic beverages, and alcohol have all been studied and may be contributors in some individuals (Katle, Hatlebakk, and Steinsvag 2013).

Prevalence

Prevalence of GERD in United States is estimated at 10%–20% in the overall population.

An estimated 7% of school-aged children and up to 8% of adolescents are affected (Hyams et al. 1996).

Gastroesophageal reflux was seen in 10.3% of 567 preterm infants in one retrospec-tive neonatal ICU study, which was associated with on average an additional 30 days' stay in the NICU and on average more than $70,000 in additional cost (Jadcherla et al. 2013).

Clinical Manifestations

There are many symptoms associated with GERD, in which heartburn and acid regur-gitation are among the most common. Diagnosis can be challenging in infants and children and may manifest as regurgitation, vomiting, irritability, food refusal, weight loss, arching of the back during feedings, coughing or choking during feeds, recurrent wheeze or other respiratory symptoms. All can point to GERD and should raise suspi-cions (Badillo and Francis 2014).

Adolescents more closely mimic adult symptoms, for example heartburn, sour stom-ach, chest pain, nocturnal symptoms, chronic cough, wheezing, and chronic sinusitis may be due to GERD and require appropriate workup. Symptoms can be worse after meals, and with reclined position. Chronic GERD has been shown to have a significant negative effect on quality of life in children and adults (Lightdale et al. 2013).

Comorbidities

There are several types of comorbidities present in GERD patients. Heartburn is the main symptom and reported by the majority of its population. Asthma-related comorbidities and rhinitis may also be aggravated. Dental erosion can occur, as can recurrent otitis media. Constipation can be a comorbidity of the primary disease and of pharmaceutical treatment, and can worsen reflux (Badillo and Francis 2014). In adults particularly, severe erosive esophagitis, Barrett esophagus, and esophageal adenocarcinoma can be seen (Lightdale et al. 2013).

Diagnostic Criteria

Diagnosis can be made by consideration of clinical presentation and history, and be confirmed by upper endoscopy and esophageal pH monitoring. A trial of medication is sometimes used presumptively before full workup is done. Barium esophagram is no longer the test of choice in primary diagnosis of GERD (Badillo and Francis 2014).

Multiple intraluminal impedance is on the forward edge of technology to clarify diagnosis and is designed to differentiate and measure acidic versus non-acidic fluids, solids, and air in the esophagus as well as speed, volume, and length of esophageal boluses (Lightdale et al. 2013).

Treatment

Conventional Treatment

Probably one of the most important steps is for clinicians to reassure parents that many children have uncomplicated gastroesophageal reflux without erosive disease that generally resolves without intervention. Normal weight gain is a primary indicator of good overall health in children and serves as an important positive finding. Conversely, weight loss in a child with gastroesophageal reflux is a red flag that should prompt further workup.

In children, lifestyle changes are emphasized as the first line of treatment. Medication may be needed, and surgery is considered as a last option unless a child is failing to thrive. Simple measures such as controlling the speed of feeding and elevating the head are first steps. Milk protein allergy should be excluded. The traditional thickening of formula with rice cereal has been shown to help in some studies, although the added calories must be watched to avoid overfeeding. Thickening of feeds should not be done in preterm infants. In older children and adolescents, weight loss, avoidance of smoking, alcohol, spicy foods, and caffeine may be helpful (Lightdale et al. 2013).

Several small studies in children have shown the benefit of chewing sugar-free gum after meals to reduce reflux (Moazzez, Bartlett, and Anggiansah 2005).

Traditionally two main classes of medications have been used: acid suppressants, and prokinetic agents. The prokinetics, such as metoclopramide and cisapride, have fallen out of favor due to their high incidence of side effects. Cisapride was removed from the market in the U.S. in 2000 due to an association with fatal arrhythmias, long QT syndrome and sudden death. Metoclopramide, a widely used prokinetic, received a black box warning in 2009. As a group the prokinetics are not recommended for treatment of GERD in infants or children (Lightdale et al. 2013).

Acid suppressants are considered the mainstay of treatment, and may be used as a trial to help clarify diagnosis. This can be very effective in healing erosive changes in the esophagus, but may not make a difference in patients with non-erosive symptoms. The main groups of acid suppressors include: antacids, histamine-2 receptor blockers, and proton pump inhibitors (PPIs). Of the three groups, the antacids have the least sup-porting evidence and have been linked with aluminum toxicity. Chronic use of antacid therapy is not recommended in children (Lightdale et al. 2013).

Histamine-2 receptor blockers such as cimetidine are widely used in children as first-line treatment. They work by partially blocking the histamine-2 receptors on acid-producing parietal cells in the stomach mucosa. Although they have been shown to be effective, their effect wanes after approximately 6 weeks. Of note, cimetidine has also been linked to liver disease and gynecomastia (Lightdale et al. 2013).

Proton pump inhibitors have moved up in popularity, in part because they have been shown to have better sustained efficacy in acid reduction. The U.S. FDA has approved several of these drugs for use in pediatrics such as: omeprazole, lansoprazole, and esomeprazole for children 12 months and older. Despite this endorsement, many concerns exist due to a high prevalence of serious adverse events, including lower respi-ratory tract infections (Vandenplas et al. 2009).

Despite safety concerns and lack of established efficacy, PPI use remains high in infants and children. A retrospective chart analysis of 2469 infants who were pre-scribed PPIs in a large healthcare network showed that prescriptions rose by a factor of 4 in the early 2000s. Nearly one in every two of the claims (49%) occurred by age 4 months; 85% of the infants were on the medication by age 9 months. Two of every three infants had already been tried on an H2 blocker. Longer duration of use was associated with increased number of comorbidities. Reasons for use of the prescription included crying and spitting up, yet PPI performed no better than placebo in its effect (Barron et al. 2007).

Interestingly, a study in *Pediatrics* examining parental perception of the disease label "GERD" had a significant effect on the parents' interest in a prescription medication to treat the illness, even when guidelines suggested that medication was not effective (Scherer et al. 2013).

Overuse of the proton pump inhibitors in infants has generated significant concern in the medical community, not only because benefit has not been clearly shown in infants, but also because of the wide range of side effects seen in older children and adults including headache, diarrhea, constipation, and nausea. Other concerns include the risk of malabsorption of iron, magnesium, calcium, and vitamin B12. Rebound hyper-secretion of acid is another physiologic effect seen when the drug is stopped in some people. In addition, because gastric acid plays a role in immune function, suppression of gastric acid may play a role in increased rates of community-acquired pneumonia, fungal infections, and necrotizing enterocolitis in preterm infants (Lightdale et al. 2013).

In severe cases, or when medication fails, surgery is done; however, this too has risks and has not been shown to prevent symptom recurrence (Lightdale et al. 2013).

Integrative Treatment

Lifestyle Approach

There are many simple lifestyle approaches that can improve GERD, such as: elevating the head of the bed 6–8 inches, remaining upright after eating, weight reduction in over-weight children and adolescents, and avoidance of trigger foods (typically spicy, acidic, or fatty foods, caffeine, alcohol). Elimination diets can be considered, but screening for celiac disease should be done prior to removal of all gluten. Avoidance of constipation is important and can be addressed with adequate fluids, physical activity, and fiber in the diet in a majority of children (Badillo and Francis 2014).

Complementary Approach

The gut–brain connection is the subject of intense research, which puts the mind–body tools forward as an important tool in the non-pharmacologic treatment of patients suffering from GERD or functional dyspepsia. The buffet of options in mind–body therapies encourages children and adolescents to try various types to see which holds most potential. Examples include breathing exercises, progressive muscle relaxation, guided imagery, clinical hypnosis, yoga, and biofeedback. More studies are needed in children, but small studies on hypnosis show encouraging results in reduction of pain in related conditions including irritable bowel syndrome and functional abdominal pain as discussed earlier (Rutten et al. 2013).

Mind–body therapies can be helpful in addressing the stressors that can precipitate or accompany GERD and functional dyspepsia. Children with functional dyspepsia have been shown to have a higher incidence of psychosocial issues such as anxiety and depression, or somatic complaints and a lower quality of life in adolescence and into early adulthood (Rippel et al. 2012).

Mental health referral may be indicated in more severe situations, in which case mind–body therapies may be used as adjunctive treatment.

Several dietary supplements have been evaluated in small studies in the treatment of GERD and functional dyspepsia. Although none have strong enough data to recommend routinely, familiarity with their benefits and risks is important for the clinician treating a child or adolescent with gastroesophageal reflux.

IBEROGAST

Iberogast (manufactured by STW-5-Medical Futures Inc. Richmond Hill, Ontario, Canada), on the commercial market for more than five decades, is a compound product consisting of nine herbal extracts. In adults it has been found to be effective in small studies for functional dyspepsia and irritable bowel syndrome. Components include a proprietary blend of chamomile flower, lemon balm leaf, bitter candy tuft, caraway fruit, licorice root, angelica root, milk thistle fruit, peppermint leaf, and greater celadine herb. Adverse events have not been reported. To date, no randomized controlled trials exist in children (Ottillinger et al. 2013).

LICORICE

The deglycyrrhizinated form of licorice (DGL) is rich in flavonoids and has historically been used in the treatment of ulcers, functional dyspepsia, and GERD. It has been shown in small randomized controlled studies in adults to be more effective than placebo, although studies are lacking in children. In part its mechanism of action is thought to be inhibition of prostaglandin and other inflammatory cytokines (Raveendra et al. 2012).

GINGER

Ginger, specifically the rhizome of *Zingiber officinale*, has a similar long history in the treatment of gastrointestinal conditions. It has been shown to improve gastric emptying and gastroduodenal motility in human studies, primarily through the actions of ginerols and shogaols, which have been shown to stimulate gut motility. Ginger is widely used in the treatment of nausea in pregnancy, post-operative nausea and vomiting (Giacosa et al. 2015), and chemotherapy-induced nausea (Marx, Ried et al. 2015) with a good safety profile. The recommended dose ranges from 1 to 1.5 grams per day of dried herb. Doses in excess of 5 grams per day have been associated with symptoms including diarrhea, heartburn, and stomach pain. Dried root powder has a significantly lower potency than ginger rhizome extract. Potential contraindications to ginger include cross reactions with anti-clotting medications due to its anti-platelet effect, although studies are contradictory. It should not be taken perioperatively for the same potential reasons (Marx, McKavanagh et al. 2015).

Studies are lacking in children, although its safety profile in nausea and vomiting in early pregnancy is reassuring (Oates-Whitehead 2004). Many forms are available that may be more appealing to children, including chewables, hard candies, and teas, although dosing is less exact.

MELATONIN

Accruing research has shown melatonin to have an important protective role on the gut mucosa, where it is produced by the gut's enterochromaffin cells at levels higher than those produced by the pineal gland. Its role is to regulate gut motility, decrease inflammation and modulate visceral sensation, although many questions remain about its role (Siah, Wong, and Ho 2014). Small studies in adults have shown a positive relationship between melatonin and GERD as compared to placebo (Kandil et al. 2010).

Other research on dietary supplements and botanicals is beginning to unravel the complex interactions of anti-inflammatory and antioxidant compounds found in traditional herbal medicines such as Rhei Rhizoma (rhubarb) and their potential in the treatment of reflux esophagitis which appears promising in animal studies (Kwon et al. 2016).

Eosinophilic Esophagitis

Overview

Eosinophilic esophagitis is a chronic inflammatory condition characterized by eosinophilic infiltration and disruption of normal esophageal activity. Although atopic disease is commonly seen as a comorbidity, and IgE sensitization to foods allergens has been associated as an initial trigger, emerging research finds the pathogenesis of the condition unrelated to IgE-mediated food allergy and many questions remain to be answered about its impact or interaction with gut microbiota, diet, and best treatment approaches (Simon et al. 2016).

Prevalence

It is relatively common, estimated to occur in 1 in 2000 people in the general population.

Eosinophilic esophagitis in children is characterized by nonspecific gastrointestinal symptoms such as feeding problems, vomiting and abdominal pain.

Clinical Manifestations

In adolescents the pattern of symptoms more closely resembles adult symptoms of dysphagia and food impaction. Heartburn is a common symptom that does not respond to typical medical approaches. It is thought to be an inflammatory food allergy driven condition that manifests with physical changes in the esophagus including edema and strictures and is often accompanied by other allergic conditions.

Comorbidities

Peripheral eosinophilia is seen in up to half of patients and total serum IgE is commonly elevated (Miehlke 2015). Atopic disease is common.

Diagnostic Criteria

Many questions remain about the specifics of diagnosis (Martin et al. 2015).

Treatment

Treatment is variable but some patients respond well to food elimination diets, or elemental diets if indicated. An empiric six-food elimination diet has been found to significantly reduce eosinophilia in children (Kagalwalla et al. 2011) and adults. Removal of cereal, milk, eggs, fish/seafood, legumes/peanuts, and soy for 6 weeks followed by reintroduction of all single foods identified a single food allergen in 35% of 67 adults, two foods triggers in 31%, and three or more food triggers were seen in 33%. In both studies, cow's milk was the most common trigger (Lucendo et al. 2013).

Celiac Disease/Gluten Sensitivity

Overview

Celiac disease is a chronic inflammatory condition that combines food intolerance with an autoimmune inflammatory element. It is seen in children and adults and is triggered by gluten in predisposed individuals. It has been widely reported and researched, and manifests with a range of clinical expressions, including failure to thrive, malabsorption and abdominal pain in children (Lebwohl, Ludvigsson, and Green 2015).

Common sources of dietary gluten include (Lebwohl, Ludvigsson, and Green 2015):

- Wheat
- Rye
- Barley (malt)

Hidden sources include:

- Oats (if harvested with wheat, may be gluten free if harvested separately from wheat)
- Sauces such as soy sauce or others
- Prescription and over-the-counter drug, and dietary supplement, fillers
- Cross-contamination from shared foods or cooking pots or utensils
- Processed meats

Etiology

The condition is triggered by the storage proteins from the endosperm of wheat (gliadins) and barley (hordeins) and rye (secalins) in susceptible individuals. The disease centers on the mucosa of the proximal small intestine manifested by villous atrophy and inflammatory changes, which heals when the triggering gluten is removed from the diet (Lebwohl, Ludvigsson, and Green 2015).

Prevalence

Prevalence in the U.S. is estimated at approximately 1%–3%, with a recognized familial component of up to 5%–30% recorded in some studies. It has been widely reported in the United Kingdom, Sweden, Germany, Netherlands, Ireland, Finland, and Italy among other countries and is increasing worldwide—although prevalence is lowest in populations where gluten intake is either at the highest or lowest extremes. Higher prevalence has been reported in individuals with other autoimmune illnesses, for example type-1 diabetes and autoimmune thyroid disorders. An estimated 95% of patients with celiac disease carry the HLA-DQ2 alleles associated with susceptibility to autoimmune disorders. Individuals with Down's syndrome, Turner syndrome, and Williams syndrome are also at increased risk (Meijer, Shamir, and Mearin 2015).

Clinical Manifestations

Celiac disease can present with a wide range of symptoms due to its systemic autoimmune etiology. In children, abdominal pain and failure to thrive are common presentations. Diarrhea is less commonly seen, and if present, it presents in younger children. In adults, anemia, osteoporosis, dermatitis herpetiformis, abdominal pain, infertility, aphthous ulcers (Lebwohl, Ludvigsson, and Green 2015), and neurologic or psychiatric problems such as ataxia and cerebellar degeneration, seizures, anxiety, migraine, neuropathy, and multiple sclerosis among others (Jackson et al. 2012).

Large population studies have not determined an association between autism and biopsy-proven celiac disease, although positive serology for IgA and IgG was seen (Ludvigsson et al. 2013).

Comorbidities

The most common association has been seen with autoimmune diseases such as type-1 diabetes mellitus and autoimmune thyroid disorders. A variety of cancers, especially lymphoma, can be seen. Liver disorders, primary sclerosing cholangitis and primary biliary cirrhosis are associations. Celiac patients may also suffer from neurological and psychiatric conditions, though no specific disorder has been found established. Reproductive problems have been reported in women (Lebwohl, Ludvigsson, and Green 2015).

Diagnostic Criteria

Diagnosis is primarily through blood tests: a high level of anti-endomysium (EMA) and anti-tissue transglutaminase (tTGA) antibodies (IgA and IgG), and deamidated gliadin peptide antibodies. Confirmation is done with duodenal biopsy as the gold standard. Discussion is active in the literature regarding guidelines for a non-biopsy diagnosis in some subsets of patients, particularly in pediatrics where in some groups serology reaches more than 95% specificity (Mills and Murray 2016).

Non-celiac gluten sensitivity is another clinical condition that can cause diagnostic confusion. Gastrointestinal symptoms are noted after ingestion of gluten in the absence of characteristic changes in the mucosa. Theories include sensitivity to other grain proteins separate from gluten, but a definitive etiology has not been determined. Randomized trials are lacking in children. Further clouding diagnosis are reports of headache, joint pains, fatigue, anemia or behavioral changes. Food allergy is more common, but other autoimmune conditions are not associated. One of the challenges in children with apparent sensitivity to gluten in the absence of a clear diagnosis is inappropriate narrowing of the diet, which can lead to unintended nutrient deficiencies (Meijer, Shamir, and Mearin 2015).

Treatment

Conventional Treatment

The conventional approach includes a lifelong gluten-free dietary plan to allow time to heal the villi and improve absorption of food. It is highly advisable not to stop gluten-free food completely before definitive diagnosis to avoid masking clinical findings.

Integrative Treatment

LIFESTYLE APPROACH

The lifestyle approach revolves around food measures. All the gluten-based food products are strictly avoided after diagnosis; similarly grains and starches should also be gluten free in order to produce a balanced diet. Fresh meat, fish, poultry which are not breaded, coated or marinated, fruits, dairy products, potatoes, rice, and vegetables should be used in the diet. All the processed food, pasta, baked items should be avoided completely to avoid inadvertent exposure. Care must be taken to avoid micronutrient deficiencies, and to avoid processed gluten-free foods that are high in empty calories. Input from a registered dietician can be helpful, especially in growing children (Theethira and Dennis 2015).

COMPLEMENTARY APPROACH

Few complementary treatments have been well studied in celiac disease, although use of dietary supplements was seen in approximately one in four in a survey of 423 patients with biopsy-proven celiac disease. The most frequently used in this group was probiotics (Nazareth et al. 2015).

Some evidence is accruing to support the use of probiotics in children with celiac disease. In one double-blinded, placebo-controlled trial of 49 patients, treatment with *Bifidobacterium breve* was shown to reduce production of TNF-alpha, a highly proinflammatory cytokine (Klemenak et al. 2015).

Research is active in interplay of the microbiota and diet in the evolution and treatment of celiac disease (Cenit et al. 2015).

References

Adams, D., S. Dagenais, T. Clifford, L. Baydala, W. J. King, M. Hervas-Malo, D. Moher, and S. Vohra. 2013. "Complementary and alternative medicine use by pediatric specialty outpatients." *Pediatrics* 131(2): 225–32. doi: 10.1542/peds.2012-1220.

Agarwal, N., and B. M. Spiegel. 2011. "The effect of irritable bowel syndrome on health-related quality of life and health care expenditures." *Gastroenterol Clin North Am* 40(1): 11–9. doi: 10.1016/j.gtc.2010.12.013.

Algieri, F., A. Rodriguez-Nogales, M. E. Rodriguez-Cabezas, S. Risco, M. A. Ocete, and J. Galvez. 2015. "Botanical drugs as an emerging strategy in inflammatory bowel disease: a review." *Mediators Inflamm* 2015: 179616. doi: 10.1155/2015/179616.

Armitage, E., H. E. Drummond, D. C. Wilson, and S. Ghosh. 2001. "Increasing incidence of both juvenile-onset Crohn's disease and ulcerative colitis in Scotland." *Eur J Gastroenterol Hepatol* 13(12): 1439–47.

Badillo, R., and D. Francis. 2014. "Diagnosis and treatment of gastroesophageal reflux disease." *World J Gastrointest Pharmacol Ther* 5(3): 105–12. doi: 10.4292/wjgpt.v5.i3.105.

Bae, S. H. 2014. "Diets for constipation." *Pediatr Gastroenterol Hepatol Nutr* 17(4): 203–8. doi: 10.5223/pghn.2014.17.4.203.

Banz, V. M., O. Sperisen, M. de Moya, H. Zimmermann, D. Candinas, S. G. Mougiakakou, and A. K. Exadaktylos. 2012. "A 5-year follow up of patients discharged with nonspecific abdominal pain: out of sight, out of mind?" *Intern Med J* 42(4): 395–401. doi: 10.1111/j.1445-5994.2010.02288.x.

Barron, J. J., H. Tan, J. Spalding, A. W. Bakst, and J. Singer. 2007. "Proton pump inhibitor utilization patterns in infants." *J Pediatr Gastroenterol Nutr* 45(4): 421–7. doi: 10.1097/MPG.0b013e31812e0149.

Bitton, A., P. L. Dobkin, M. D. Edwardes, M. J. Sewitch, J. B. Meddings, S. Rawal, A. Cohen, S. Vermeire, L. Dufresne, D. Franchimont, and G. E. Wild. 2008. "Predicting relapse in Crohn's disease: a biopsychosocial model." *Gut* 57(10): 1386–92. doi: 10.1136/gut.2007.134817.

Brands, M. M., H. Purperhart, and J. M. Deckers-Kocken. 2011. "A pilot study of yoga treatment in children with functional abdominal pain and irritable bowel syndrome." *Complement Ther Med* 19(3): 109–14. doi: 10.1016/j.ctim.2011.05.004.

Brown, L. K., R. M. Beattie, and M. P. Tighe. 2015. "Practical management of functional abdominal pain in children." *Arch Dis Child.* doi: 10.1136/archdischild-2014-306426.

Cabre, E., M. Manosa, and M. A. Gassull. 2012. "Omega-3 fatty acids and inflammatory bowel diseases: a systematic review." *Br J Nutr* 107(Suppl 2): S240–52. doi: 10.1017/S0007114512001626.

Carbone, F., L. Holvoet, and J. Tack. 2015. "Rome III functional dyspepsia subdivision in PDS and EPS: recognizing postprandial symptoms reduces overlap." *Neurogastroenterol Motil* 27(8): 1069–74. doi: 10.1111/nmo.12585.

Carson, L., D. Lewis, M. Tsou, E. McGuire, B. Surran, C. Miller, and T. A. Vu. 2011. "Abdominal migraine: an under-diagnosed cause of recurrent abdominal pain in children." *Headache* 51(5): 707–12. doi: 10.1111/j.1526–4610.2011.01855.x.

Cenit, M. C., M. Olivares, P. Codoner-Franch, and Y. Sanz. 2015. "Intestinal microbiota and celiac disease: cause, consequence or co-evolution?" *Nutrients* 7(8): 6900–23. doi: 10.3390/nu7085314.

Chao, G. Q., and S. Zhang. 2014. "Effectiveness of acupuncture to treat irritable bowel syndrome: a meta-analysis." *World J Gastroenterol* 20(7): 1871–7. doi: 10.3748/wjg.v20.i7.1871.

Chey, W. D., J. Kurlander, and S. Eswaran. 2015. "Irritable bowel syndrome: a clinical review." *JAMA* 313(9): 949–58. doi: 10.1001/jama.2015.0954.

Chey, W. D., B. Nojkov, J. H. Rubenstein, R. R. Dobhan, J. K. Greenson, and B. D. Cash. 2010. "The yield of colonoscopy in patients with non-constipated irritable bowel syndrome: results from a prospective, controlled US trial." *Am J Gastroenterol* 105(4): 859–65. doi: 10.1038/ajg.2010.55.

Chibbar, R., and L. A. Dieleman. 2015. "Probiotics in the management of ulcerative colitis." *J Clin Gastroenterol* 49(Suppl 1): S50–5. doi: 10.1097/MCG.0000000000000368.

Chumpitazi, B. P., J. L. Cope, E. B. Hollister, C. M. Tsai, A. R. McMeans, R. A. Luna, J. Versalovic, and R. J. Shulman. 2015. "Randomised clinical trial: gut microbiome biomarkers are associated with clinical response to a low FODMAP diet in children with the irritable bowel syndrome." *Aliment Pharmacol Ther* 42(4): 418–27. doi: 10.1111/apt.13286.

Collins, S. M. 2014. "A role for the gut microbiota in IBS." *Nat Rev Gastroenterol Hepatol* 11(8): 497–505. doi: 10.1038/nrgastro.2014.40.

Cotton, S., Y. Humenay Roberts, J. Tsevat, M. T. Britto, P. Succop, M. E. McGrady, and M. S. Yi. 2010. "Mind-body complementary alternative medicine use and quality of life in adolescents with inflammatory bowel disease." *Inflamm Bowel Dis* 16(3): 501–6. doi: 10.1002/ibd.21045.

Cruchet, S., R. Furnes, A. Maruy, E. Hebel, J. Palacios, F. Medina, N. Ramirez, M. Orsi, L. Rondon, V. Sdepanian, L. Xochihua, M. Ybarra, and R. A. Zablah. 2015. "The use of probiotics in pediatric gastroenterology: a review of the literature and recommendations by Latin-American experts." *Paediatr Drugs* 17(3): 199–216. doi: 10.1007/s40272-015-0124-6.

da Silva, B. C., A. C. Lyra, R. Rocha, and G. O. Santana. 2014. "Epidemiology, demographic characteristics and prognostic predictors of ulcerative colitis." *World J Gastroenterol* 20(28): 9458–67. doi: 10.3748/wjg.v20.i28.9458.

Day, A. S. 2002. "Use of complementary and alternative therapies and probiotic agents by children attending gastroenterology outpatient clinics." *J Paediatr Child Health* 38(4): 343–6.

Day, A. S. 2013. "A review of the use of complementary and alternative medicines by children with inflammatory bowel disease." *Front Pediatr* 1: 9. doi: 10.3389/fped.2013.00009.

Dhroove, G., A. Chogle, and M. Saps. 2010. "A million-dollar work-up for abdominal pain: is it worth it?" *J Pediatr Gastroenterol Nutr* 51(5): 579–83. doi: 10.1097/MPG.0b013e3181de0639.

Didari, T., S. Mozaffari, S. Nikfar, and M. Abdollahi. 2015. "Effectiveness of probiotics in irritable bowel syndrome: updated systematic review with meta-analysis." *World J Gastroenterol* 21(10): 3072–84. doi: 10.3748/wjg.v21.i10.3072.

Eccleston, C., T. M. Palermo, A. C. Williams, A. Lewandowski Holley, S. Morley, E. Fisher, and E. Law. 2014. "Psychological therapies for the management of chronic and recurrent pain in children and adolescents." *Cochrane Database Syst Rev* 5: CD003968. doi: 10.1002/14651858.CD003968.pub4.

El-Salhy, M., and D. Gundersen. 2015. "Diet in irritable bowel syndrome." *Nutr J* 14: 36. doi: 10.1186/s12937-015-0022-3.

Ford, A. C., P. Moayyedi, B. E. Lacy, A. J. Lembo, Y. A. Saito, L. R. Schiller, E. E. Soffer, B. M. Spiegel, E. M. Quigley, and Disorders Task Force on the Management of Functional Bowel. 2014. "American College of Gastroenterology monograph on the management of irritable bowel syndrome and chronic idiopathic constipation." *Am J Gastroenterol* 109(Suppl 1): S2–26; quiz S27. doi: 10.1038/ajg.2014.187.

Giacosa, A., P. Morazzoni, E. Bombardelli, A. Riva, G. Bianchi Porro, and M. Rondanelli.

2015. "Can nausea and vomiting be treated with ginger extract?" *Eur Rev Med Pharmacol Sci* 19(7): 1291–6.

Gijsbers, C. F., C. M. Kneepkens, Y. Vergouwe, and H. A. Buller. 2014. "Occult constipation: faecal retention as a cause of recurrent abdominal pain in children." *Eur J Pediatr* 173(6): 781–5. doi: 10.1007/s00431-013-2257-3.

Grigoleit, H. G., and P. Grigoleit. 2005. "Peppermint oil in irritable bowel syndrome." *Phytomedicine* 12(8): 601–6. doi: 10.1016/j.phymed.2004.10.005.

Hotopf, M., S. Carr, R. Mayou, M. Wadsworth, W. Wessely. 1998. "Why do children have chronic abdominal pain, and what happens to them when they grow up? Population based cohort study." *Br Med J* 316: 1196–200.

Hussain, Z., and E. M. Quigley. 2006. "Systematic review: complementary and alternative medicine in the irritable bowel syndrome." *Aliment Pharmacol Ther* 23(4): 465–71. doi: 10.1111/j.1365-2036.2006.02776.x.

Huynh, H. Q., J. deBruyn, L. Guan, H. Diaz, M. Li, S. Girgis, J. Turner, R. Fedorak, and K. Madsen. 2009. "Probiotic preparation VSL#3 induces remission in children with mild to moderate acute ulcerative colitis: a pilot study." *Inflamm Bowel Dis* 15(5): 760–8. doi: 10.1002/ibd.20816.

Hyams, J. S., G. Burke, P. M. Davis, B. Rzepski, and P. A. Andrulonis. 1996. "Abdominal pain and irritable bowel syndrome in adolescents: a community-based study." *J Pediatr* 129(2): 220–6.

Jackson, J. R., W. W. Eaton, N. G. Cascella, A. Fasano, and D. L. Kelly. 2012. "Neurologic and psychiatric manifestations of celiac disease and gluten sensitivity." *Psychiatr Q* 83(1): 91–102. doi: 10.1007/s11126-011-9186-y.

Jadcherla, S. R., J. L. Slaughter, M. R. Stenger, M. Klebanoff, K. Kelleher, and W. Gardner. 2013. "Practice variance, prevalence, and economic burden of premature infants diagnosed with GERD." *Hosp Pediatr* 3(4): 335–41. doi: 10.1542/hpeds.2013-0036.

Jarrett, M. E., K. C. Cain, P. G. Barney, R. L. Burr, B. D. Naliboff, R. Shulman, J. Zia, and M. M. Heitkemper. 2016. "Balance of autonomic nervous system predicts who benefits from a self-management intervention program for irritable bowel syndrome." *J Neurogastroenterol Motil* 22(1): 102–11. doi: 10.5056/jnm15067.

Johannesson, E., M. Simren, H. Strid, A. Bajor, and R. Sadik. 2011. "Physical activity improves symptoms in irritable bowel syndrome: a randomized controlled trial." *Am J Gastroenterol* 106(5): 915–22. doi: 10.1038/ajg.2010.480.

Kagalwalla, A. F., A. Shah, B. U. Li, T. A. Sentongo, S. Ritz, M. Manuel-Rubio, K. Jacques, D. Wang, H. Melin-Aldana, and S. P. Nelson. 2011. "Identification of specific foods responsible for inflammation in children with eosinophilic esophagitis successfully treated with empiric elimination diet." *J Pediatr Gastroenterol Nutr* 53(2): 145–9. doi: 10.1097/MPG.0b013e31821cf503.

Kandil, T. S., A. A. Mousa, A. A. El-Gendy, and A. M. Abbas. 2010. "The potential therapeutic effect of melatonin in gastro-esophageal reflux disease." *BMC Gastroenterol* 10: 7. doi: 10.1186/1471-230X-10-7.

Katle, E. J., J. G. Hatlebakk, and S. Steinsvag. 2013. "Gastroesophageal reflux and rhinosinusitis." *Curr Allergy Asthma Rep* 13(2): 218–23. doi: 10.1007/s11882-013-0340-5.

Kelly, J. R., P. J. Kennedy, J. F. Cryan, T. G. Dinan, G. Clarke, and N. P. Hyland. 2015. "Breaking down the barriers: the gut microbiome, intestinal permeability and stress-related psychiatric disorders." *Front Cell Neurosci* 9: 392. doi: 10.3389/fncel.2015.00392.

Kianifar, H., S. A. Jafari, M. Kiani, H. Ahanchian, S. V. Ghasemi, Z. Grover, L. Z. Mahmoodi, R. Bagherian, and M. Khalesi. 2015. "Probiotic for irritable bowel syndrome in pediatric patients: a randomized controlled clinical trial." *Electron Physician* 7(5): 1255–60. doi: 10.14661/1255.

Klemenak, M., J. Dolinsek, T. Langerholc, D. Di Gioia, and D. Micetic-Turk. 2015. "Administration of Bifidobacterium breve decreases the production of TNF-alpha in children with celiac disease." *Dig Dis Sci* 60(11): 3386–92. doi: 10.1007/s10620-015-3769-7.

Koppen, I. J., C. Di Lorenzo, M. Saps, P. G. Dinning, D. Yacob, M. A. Levitt, and M. A. Benninga.

2016. "Childhood constipation: finally something is moving!" *Expert Rev Gastroenterol Hepatol* 10(1): 141–55. doi: 10.1586/17474124.2016.1098533.

Koppen, I. J., L. A. Lammers, M. A. Benninga, and M. M. Tabbers. 2015. "Management of functional constipation in children: therapy in practice." *Paediatr Drugs* 17(5): 349–60. doi: 10.1007/s40272-015-0142-4.

Koppen, I. J., C. A. Velasco-Benitez, M. A. Benninga, C. Di Lorenzo, and M. Saps. 2016. "Is There an association between functional constipation and excessive bodyweight in children?" *J Pediatr*. doi: 10.1016/j.jpeds.2015.12.033.

Korterink, J. J., K. Diederen, M. A. Benninga, and M. M. Tabbers. 2015. "Epidemiology of pediatric functional abdominal pain disorders: a meta-analysis." *PLoS One* 10(5): e0126982. doi: 10.1371/journal.pone.0126982.

Kuttner, L., C. T. Chambers, J. Hardial, D. M. Israel, K. Jacobson, and K. Evans. 2006. "A randomized trial of yoga for adolescents with irritable bowel syndrome." *Pain Res Manag* 11(4): 217–23.

Kwon, O. J., B. K. Choo, J. Y. Lee, M. Y. Kim, S. H. Shin, B. I. Seo, Y. B. Seo, M. H. Rhee, M. R. Shin, G. N. Kim, C. H. Park, and S. S. Roh. 2016. "Protective effect of Rhei Rhizoma on reflux esophagitis in rats via Nrf2-mediated inhibition of NF-kappaB signaling pathway." *BMC Complement Altern Med* 16(1): 7. doi: 10.1186/s12906-015-0974-z.

Langhorst, J., A. Hofstetter, F. Wolfe, and W. Hauser. 2013. "Short-term stress, but not mucosal healing nor depression was predictive for the risk of relapse in patients with ulcerative colitis: a prospective 12-month follow-up study." *Inflamm Bowel Dis* 19(11): 2380–6. doi: 10.1097/MIB.0b013e3182a192ba.

Langhorst, J., H. Wulfert, R. Lauche, P. Klose, H. Cramer, G. J. Dobos, and J. Korzenik. 2015. "Systematic review of complementary and alternative medicine treatments in inflammatory bowel diseases." *J Crohns Colitis* 9(1): 86–106. doi: 10.1093/ecco-jcc/jju007.

Lebwohl, B., J. F. Ludvigsson, and P. H. Green. 2015. "Celiac disease and non-celiac gluten sensitivity." *BMJ* 351:h4347. doi: 10.1136/bmj.h4347.

Lemberg, D. A., and A. S. Day. 2015. "Crohn disease and ulcerative colitis in children: an update for 2014." *J Paediatr Child Health* 51(3): 266–70. doi: 10.1111/jpc.12685.

Lightdale, J. R., D. A. Gremse, Hepatology Section on Gastroenterology, and Nutrition. 2013. "Gastroesophageal reflux: management guidance for the pediatrician." *Pediatrics* 131(5): e1684–95. doi: 10.1542/peds.2013-0421.

Lindstrom, C., J. Aman, A. Anderzen-Carlsson, and A. Lindahl Norberg. 2015. "Group intervention for burnout in parents of chronically ill children: a small-scale study." *Scand J Caring Sci*. doi: 10.1111/scs.12287.

Liu, X., A. Silverman, M. Kern, B. D. Ward, S. J. Li, R. Shaker, and M. R. Sood. 2016. "Excessive coupling of the salience network with intrinsic neurocognitive brain networks during rectal distension in adolescents with irritable bowel syndrome: a preliminary report." *Neurogastroenterol Motil* 28(1): 43–53. doi: 10.1111/nmo.12695.

Lovell, R. M., and A. C. Ford. 2012. "Global prevalence of and risk factors for irritable bowel syndrome: a meta-analysis." *Clin Gastroenterol Hepatol* 10(7): 712–721 e4. doi: 10.1016/j.cgh.2012.02.029.

Lucendo, A. J., A. Arias, J. Gonzalez-Cervera, J. L. Yague-Compadre, D. Guagnozzi, T. Angueira, S. Jimenez-Contreras, S. Gonzalez-Castillo, B. Rodriguez-Dominguez, L. C. De Rezende, and J. M. Tenias. 2013. "Empiric 6-food elimination diet induced and maintained prolonged remission in patients with adult eosinophilic esophagitis: a prospective study on the food cause of the disease." *J Allergy Clin Immunol* 131(3): 797–804. doi: 10.1016/j.jaci.2012.12.664.

Ludvigsson, J. F., A. Reichenberg, C. M. Hultman, and J. A. Murray. 2013. "A nationwide study of the association between celiac disease and the risk of autistic spectrum disorders." *JAMA Psychiatry* 70(11): 1224–30. doi: 10.1001/jamapsychiatry.2013.2048.

M'Koma, A. E. 2013. "Inflammatory bowel disease: an expanding global health problem." *Clin Med Insights Gastroenterol* 6: 33–47. doi: 10.4137/CGast.S12731.

Makharia, A., C. Catassi, and G. K. Makharia. 2015. "The overlap between irritable bowel syndrome and non-celiac gluten sensitivity: a clinical dilemma." *Nutrients* 7(12): 10417–26. doi: 10.3390/nu7125541.

Malaty, H. M., S. Abudayyeh, K. Fraley, D. Y. Graham, M. A. Gilger, and D. R. Hollier. 2007. "Recurrent abdominal pain in school children: effect of obesity and diet." *Acta Paediatr* 96(4): 572–6. doi: 10.1111/j.1651-2227.2007.00230.x.

Manheimer, E., K. Cheng, L. S. Wieland, L. S. Min, X. Shen, B. M. Berman, and L. Lao. 2012. "Acupuncture for treatment of irritable bowel syndrome." *Cochrane Database Syst Rev* 5: CD005111. doi: 10.1002/14651858.CD005111.pub3.

Martin, L. J., J. P. Franciosi, M. H. Collins, J. P. Abonia, J. J. Lee, K. A. Hommel, J. W. Varni, J. T. Grotjan, M. Eby, H. He, K. Marsolo, P. E. Putnam, J. M. Garza, A. Kaul, T. Wen, and M. E. Rothenberg. 2015. "Pediatric Eosinophilic Esophagitis Symptom Scores (PEESS v2.0) identify histologic and molecular correlates of the key clinical features of disease." *J Allergy Clin Immunol* 135(6): 1519–28 e8. doi: 10.1016/j.jaci.2015.03.004.

Marx, W., D. McKavanagh, A. L. McCarthy, R. Bird, K. Ried, A. Chan, and L. Isenring. 2015. "The effect of ginger (Zingiber officinale) on platelet aggregation: a systematic literature review." *PLoS One* 10(10): e0141119. doi: 10.1371/journal.pone.0141119.

Marx, W., K. Ried, A. L. McCarthy, L. Vitetta, A. Sali, D. McKavanagh, and E. Isenring. 2015. "Ginger—mechanism of action in chemotherapy-induced nausea and vomiting: a review." *Crit Rev Food Sci Nutr*. doi: 10.1080/10408398.2013.865590.

Marynowski, M., A. Likonska, H. Zatorski, and J. Fichna. 2015. "Role of environmental pollution in irritable bowel syndrome." *World J Gastroenterol* 21(40): 11371–8. doi: 10.3748/wjg.v21.i40.11371.

Mazurak, N., E. Broelz, M. Storr, and P. Enck. 2015. "Probiotic therapy of the irritable bowel syndrome: why is the evidence still poor and what can be done about it?" *J Neurogastroenterol Motil* 21(4): 471–85. doi: 10.5056/jnm15071.

McClafferty, H. 2011. "Complementary, holistic, and integrative medicine: mind-body medicine." *Pediatr Rev* 32(5): 201–3. doi: 10.1542/pir.32-5-201.

McCormick, M., B. Reed-Knight, J. D. Lewis, B. D. Gold, and R. L. Blount. 2010. "Coping skills for reducing pain and somatic symptoms in adolescents with IBD." *Inflamm Bowel Dis* 16(12): 2148–57. doi: 10.1002/ibd.21302.

Meeker, J. D., and K. K. Ferguson. 2011. "Relationship between urinary phthalate and bisphenol A concentrations and serum thyroid measures in U.S. adults and adolescents from the National Health and Nutrition Examination Survey (NHANES) 2007–2008." *Environ Health Perspect* 119(10): 1396–402. doi: 10.1289/ehp.1103582.

Meijer, C. R., R. Shamir, and M. L. Mearin. 2015. "Coeliac disease and noncoeliac gluten sensitivity." *J Pediatr Gastroenterol Nutr* 60(4): 429–32. doi: 10.1097/MPG.0000000000000708.

Miehlke, S. 2015. "Clinical features of eosinophilic esophagitis in children and adults." *Best Pract Res Clin Gastroenterol* 29(5): 739–48. doi: 10.1016/j.bpg.2015.09.005.

Miele, E., F. Pascarella, E. Giannetti, L. Quaglietta, R. N. Baldassano, and A. Staiano. 2009. "Effect of a probiotic preparation (VSL#3) on induction and maintenance of remission in children with ulcerative colitis." *Am J Gastroenterol* 104(2): 437–43. doi: 10.1038/ajg.2008.118.

Millichap, J. G., and M. M. Yee. 2003. "The diet factor in pediatric and adolescent migraine." *Pediatr Neurol* 28(1): 9–15.

Mills, J. R., and J. A. Murray. 2016. "Contemporary celiac disease diagnosis: is a biopsy avoidable?" *Curr Opin Gastroenterol* 32(2): 80–5. doi: 10.1097/MOG.0000000000000245.

Mizrahi, M. C., R. Reicher-Atir, S. Levy, S. Haramati, D. Wengrower, E. Israeli, and E. Goldin. 2012. "Effects of guided imagery with relaxation training on anxiety and quality of life among patients with inflammatory bowel disease." *Psychol Health* 27(12): 1463–79. doi: 10.1080/08870446.2012.691169.

Moazzez, R., D. Bartlett, and A. Anggiansah. 2005. "The effect of chewing sugar-free gum on gastro-esophageal reflux." *J Dent Res* 84(11): 1062–5.

Moser, G. 2014. "The role of hypnotherapy for the treatment of inflammatory bowel diseases." *Expert Rev Gastroenterol Hepatol* 8(6): 601–6. doi: 10.1586/17474124.2014.917955.

Nambu, R., S. I. Hagiwara, M. Kubota, and S. Kagimoto. 2016. "Difference between early onset and late onset pediatric ulcerative colitis." *Pediatr Int*. doi: 10.1111/ped.12935.

Nazareth, S., B. Lebwohl, C. A. Tennyson, S. Simpson, H. Greenlee, and P. H. Green. 2015. "Dietary supplement use in patients with celiac disease in the United States." *J Clin Gastroenterol* 49(7): 577–81. doi: 10.1097/MCG.0000000000000218.

Ng, S. C., Z. Zeng, O. Niewiadomski, W. Tang, S. Bell, M. A. Kamm, P. Hu, H. J. de Silva, M. A. Niriella, W. S. Udara, D. Ong, K. L. Ling, C. J. Ooi, I. Hilmi, K. Lee Goh, Q. Ouyang, Y. F. Wang, K. Wu, X. Wang, P. Pisespongsa, S. Manatsathit, S. Aniwan, J. Limsrivilai, J. Gunawan, M. Simadibrata, M. Abdullah, S. W. Tsang, F. H. Lo, A. J. Hui, C. M. Chow, H. H. Yu, M. F. Li, K. K. Ng, J. Y. Ching, V. Chan, J. C. Wu, F. K. Chan, M. Chen, J. J. Sung, Crohn's Asia-Pacific, and Group Colitis Epidemiology Study. 2016. "Early course of inflammatory bowel disease in a population-based inception cohort study from 8 countries in Asia and Australia." *Gastroenterology* 150(1): 86–95 e3. doi: 10.1053/j.gastro.2015.09.005.

Nijeboer, P., H. J. Bontkes, C. J. Mulder, and G. Bouma. 2013. "Non-celiac gluten sensitivity. Is it in the gluten or the grain?" *J Gastrointestin Liver Dis* 22(4): 435–40.

Norling, M., K. Stenzelius, N. Ekman, and A. Wennick. 2015. "High school students' experiences in school toilets or restrooms." *J Sch Nurs*. doi: 10.1177/1059840515611476.

Oates-Whitehead, R. 2004. "Nausea and vomiting in early pregnancy." *Clin Evid* 11: 1840–52.

Ottillinger, B., M. Storr, P. Malfertheiner, and H. D. Allescher. 2013. "STW 5 (Iberogast(R)): a safe and effective standard in the treatment of functional gastrointestinal disorders." *Wien Med Wochenschr* 163(3–4): 65–72. doi: 10.1007/s10354-012-0169-x.

Peckham, E. J., E. A. Nelson, J. Greenhalgh, K. Cooper, E. R. Roberts, and A. Agrawal. 2013. "Homeopathy for treatment of irritable bowel syndrome." *Cochrane Database Syst Rev* 11: CD009710. doi: 10.1002/14651858.CD009710.pub2.

Peters, S. L., J. G. Muir, and P. R. Gibson. 2015. "Review article: gut-directed hypnotherapy in the management of irritable bowel syndrome and inflammatory bowel disease." *Aliment Pharmacol Ther* 41(11): 1104–15. doi: 10.1111/apt.13202.

Racine, A., F. Carbonnel, S. S. Chan, A. R. Hart, H. B. Bueno-de-Mesquita, B. Oldenburg, F. D. van Schaik, A. Tjonneland, A. Olsen, C. C. Dahm, T. Key, R. Luben, K. T. Khaw, E. Riboli, O. Grip, S. Lindgren, G. Hallmans, P. Karling, F. Clavel-Chapelon, M. M. Bergman, H. Boeing, R. Kaaks, V. A. Katzke, D. Palli, G. Masala, P. Jantchou, and M. C. Boutron-Ruault. 2016. "Dietary patterns and risk of inflammatory bowel disease in Europe: results from the EPIC Study." *Inflamm Bowel Dis* 22(2): 345–54. doi: 10.1097/MIB.0000000000000638.

Rao, S. S., S. Yu, and A. Fedewa. 2015. "Systematic review: dietary fibre and FODMAP-restricted diet in the management of constipation and irritable bowel syndrome." *Aliment Pharmacol Ther* 41(12): 1256–70. doi: 10.1111/apt.13167.

Rasquin, A., C. Di Lorenzo, D. Forbes, E. Guiraldes, J. S. Hyams, A. Staiano, and L. S. Walker. 2006. "Childhood functional gastrointestinal disorders: child/adolescent." *Gastroenterology* 130(5): 1527–37. doi: 10.1053/j.gastro.2005.08.063.

Raveendra, K. R., Jayachandra, V. Srinivasa, K. R. Sushma, J. J. Allan, K. S. Goudar, H. N. Shivaprasad, K. Venkateshwarlu, P. Geetharani, G. Sushma, and A. Agarwal. 2012. "An extract of Glycyrrhiza glabra (GutGard) alleviates symptoms of functional dyspepsia: a randomized, double-blind, placebo-controlled study." *Evid Based Complement Alternat Med* 2012: 216970. doi: 10.1155/2012/216970.

Riedl, A., M. Schmidtmann, A. Stengel, M. Goebel, A. S. Wisser, B. F. Klapp, and H. Monnikes. 2008. "Somatic comorbidities of irritable bowel syndrome: a systematic analysis." *J Psychosom Res* 64(6): 573–82. doi: 10.1016/j.jpsychores.2008.02.021.

Rippel, S. W., S. Acra, H. Correa, M. Vaezi, C. Di Lorenzo, and L. S. Walker. 2012. "Pediatric patients with dyspepsia have chronic symptoms, anxiety, and lower quality of life as adolescents and adults." *Gastroenterology* 142(4): 754–61. doi: 10.1053/j.gastro.2011.12.043.

Rutten, J. M., J. B. Reitsma, A. M. Vlieger, and M. A. Benninga. 2013. "Gut-directed hypnotherapy for functional abdominal pain or irritable bowel syndrome in children: a systematic review." *Arch Dis Child* 98(4): 252–7. doi: 10.1136/archdischild-2012-302906.

Sandhu, B. K., and S. P. Paul. 2014. "Irritable bowel syndrome in children: pathogenesis, diagnosis and evidence-based treatment." *World J Gastroenterol* 20(20): 6013–23. doi: 10.3748/wjg.v20.i20.6013.

Scherer, L. D., B. J. Zikmund-Fisher, A. Fagerlin, and B. A. Tarini. 2013. "Influence of 'GERD' label on parents' decision to medicate infants." *Pediatrics* 131(5): 839–45. doi: 10.1542/peds.2012-3070.

Shaikh, N., A. Hoberman, R. Keren, N. Gotman, S. G. Docimo, R. Mathews, S. Bhatnagar, A. Ivanova, T. K. Mattoo, M. Moxey-Mims, M. A. Carpenter, H. G. Pohl, and S. Greenfield. 2016. "Recurrent urinary tract infections in children with bladder and bowel dysfunction." *Pediatrics* 137(1): 1–7. doi: 10.1542/peds.2015-2982.

Shankar, V., N. V. Reo, and O. Paliy. 2015. "Simultaneous fecal microbial and metabolite profiling enables accurate classification of pediatric irritable bowel syndrome." *Microbiome* 3(1): 73. doi: 10.1186/s40168-015-0139-9.

Shen, J., Z. X. Zuo, and A. P. Mao. 2014. "Effect of probiotics on inducing remission and maintaining therapy in ulcerative colitis, Crohn's disease, and pouchitis: meta-analysis of randomized controlled trials." *Inflamm Bowel Dis* 20(1): 21–35. doi: 10.1097/01.MIB.0000437495.30052.be.

Shiu-Lin, Tsai. 2015. "Acupuncture for pediatrics: a new frontier emerges" *Medical Acupuncture* 27(6): 406–8. doi: 10.1089.

Siah, K. T., R. K. Wong, and K. Y. Ho. 2014. "Melatonin for the treatment of irritable bowel syndrome." *World J Gastroenterol* 20(10): 2492–8. doi: 10.3748/wjg.v20.i10.2492.

Simon, D., A. Cianferoni, J. M. Spergel, S. Aceves, M. Holbreich, C. Venter, M. E. Rothenberg, I. Terreehorst, A. Muraro, A. J. Lucendo, A. Schoepfer, A. Straumann, and H. U. Simon. 2016. "Eosinophilic esophagitis is characterized by a non-IgE-mediated food hypersensitivity." *Allergy*. doi: 10.1111/all.12846.

Stanford Health Care, Digestive Health Center Nutrition Services. "The Low FODMAP Diet (FODMAP=Fermentable Oligo-Di-Monosaccharides and Polyols." https://stanfordhealthcare.org/content/dam/SHC/for-patients-component/programs-services/clinical-nutrition-services/docs/pdf-lowfodmapdiet.pdf.

Stern, M. J., R. A. Guiles, and R. Gevirtz. 2014. "HRV biofeedback for pediatric irritable bowel syndrome and functional abdominal pain: a clinical replication series." *Appl Psychophysiol Biofeedback* 39(3–4): 287–91. doi: 10.1007/s10484-014-9261-x.

Suskind, D. L., G. Wahbeh, T. Burpee, M. Cohen, D. Christie, and W. Weber. 2013. "Tolerability of curcumin in pediatric inflammatory bowel disease: a forced-dose titration study." *J Pediatr Gastroenterol Nutr* 56(3): 277–9. doi: 10.1097/MPG.0b013e318276977d.

Tabbers, M. M., and M. A. Benninga. 2015. "Constipation in children: fibre and probiotics." *BMJ Clin Evid* 2015.

Tazzyman, S., N. Richards, A. R. Trueman, A. L. Evans, V. A. Grant, I. Garaiova, S. F. Plummer, E. A. Williams, and B. M. Corfe. 2015. "Vitamin D associates with improved quality of life in participants with irritable bowel syndrome: outcomes from a pilot trial." *BMJ Open Gastroenterol* 2(1): e000052. doi: 10.1136/bmjgast-2015-000052.

Theethira, T. G., and M. Dennis. 2015. "Celiac disease and the gluten-free diet: consequences and recommendations for improvement." *Dig Dis* 33(2): 175–82. doi: 10.1159/000369504.

Thomas, A., and E. M. Quigley. 2015. "Diet and irritable bowel syndrome." *Curr Opin Gastroenterol* 31(2): 166–71. doi: 10.1097/MOG.0000000000000158.

Thornton, G. C., M. J. Goldacre, R. Goldacre, and L. J. Howarth. 2015. "Diagnostic outcomes following childhood non-specific abdominal pain: a record-linkage study." *Arch Dis Child*. doi: 10.1136/archdischild-2015-308198.

van Barreveld, M., J. Rutten, A. Vlieger, C. Frankenhuis, E. George, M. Groeneweg, O. Norbruis,

A. Ten W. Tjon, H. van Wering, M. Merkus, M. Benninga, and M. Dijkgraaf. 2015. "Cost-effectiveness and cost-utility of home-based hypnotherapy using compact disc versus individual hypnotherapy by a therapist for pediatric irritable bowel syndrome and functional abdominal pain (syndrome)." *Value Health* 18(7): A628. doi: 10.1016/j.jval.2015.09.2214.

van Engelenburg-van Lonkhuyzen, M. L., E. M. Bols, M. A. Benninga, W. A. Verwijs, N. M. Bluijssen, and R. A. de Bie. 2013. "The effect of pelvic physiotherapy on reduction of functional constipation in children: design of a multicentre randomised controlled trial." *BMC Pediatr* 13: 112. doi: 10.1186/1471-2431-13-112.

Vandenplas, Y., C. D. Rudolph, C. Di Lorenzo, E. Hassall, G. Liptak, L. Mazur, J. Sondheimer, A. Staiano, M. Thomson, G. Veereman-Wauters, T. G. Wenzl, Hepatology North American Society for Pediatric Gastroenterology, Nutrition, Hepatology European Society for Pediatric Gastroenterology, and Nutrition. 2009. "Pediatric gastroesophageal reflux clinical practice guidelines: joint recommendations of the North American Society for Pediatric Gastroenterology, Hepatology, and Nutrition (NASPGHAN) and the European Society for Pediatric Gastroenterology, Hepatology, and Nutrition (ESPGHAN)." *J Pediatr Gastroenterol Nutr* 49(4): 498–547. doi: 10.1097/MPG.0b013e3181b7f563.

Wadhera, V., D. A. Lemberg, S. T. Leach, and A. S. Day. 2011. "Complementary and alternative medicine in children attending gastroenterology clinics: usage patterns and reasons for use." *J Paediatr Child Health* 47(12): 904–10. doi: 10.1111/j.1440-1754.2011.02100.x.

Walker, L. S., S. E. Williams, C. A. Smith, J. Garber, D. A. Van Slyke, and T. A. Lipani. 2006. "Parent attention versus distraction: impact on symptom complaints by children with and without chronic functional abdominal pain." *Pain* 122(1–2): 43–52. doi: 10.1016/j.pain.2005.12.020.

Wang, L., M. A. Conlon, C. T. Christophersen, M. J. Sorich, and M. T. Angley. 2014. "Gastrointestinal microbiota and metabolite biomarkers in children with autism spectrum disorders." *Biomark Med* 8(3): 331–44. doi: 10.2217/bmm.14.12.

Wang, X., and J. Yin. 2015. "Complementary and alternative therapies for chronic constipation." *Evid Based Complement Alternat Med* 2015: 396396. doi: 10.1155/2015/396396.

Wedrychowicz, A., A. Zajac, and P. Tomasik. 2016. "Advances in nutritional therapy in inflammatory bowel diseases: review." *World J Gastroenterol* 22(3): 1045–66. doi: 10.3748/wjg.v22.i3.1045.

Weydert, J. A., T. M. Ball, and M. F. Davis. 2003. "Systematic review of treatments for recurrent abdominal pain." *Pediatrics* 111(1): e1–11.

Whorwell, P. J. 2013. "Hypnotherapy: first line treatment for children with irritable bowel syndrome?" *Arch Dis Child* 98(4): 243–4. doi: 10.1136/archdischild-2012-303178.

Young, L., and K. J. Kemper. 2013. "Integrative care for pediatric patients with pain." *J Altern Complement Med* 19(7): 627–32. doi: 10.1089/acm.2012.0368.

Zhu, Y., X. Li, J. Chen, T. Chen, Z. Shi, M. Lei, Y. Zhang, P. Bai, Y. Li, and X. Fei. 2016. "The pentacyclic triterpene Lupeol switches M1 macrophages to M2 and ameliorates experimental inflammatory bowel disease." *Int Immunopharmacol* 30: 74–84. doi: 10.1016/j.intimp.2015.11.031.

18 Infectious Disease: Upper Respiratory Infections and Otitis Media

Upper Respiratory Infections

Overview

Acute upper respiratory infections (URI), or the common cold, are among the most common infections seen in the world and among the top reason for visits to the doctor. They are also among the leading causes of morbidity and mortality in children (Bezerra et al. 2011).

URIs are generally due to infection with rhinovirus or adenovirus and can occur year round in all age groups. Symptoms can range from mild to severe and may involve various parts of the respiratory tract, resulting tonsillitis, pharyngitis, laryngitis, sinusitis, otitis media, or pneumonia (Chonmaitree et al. 2008).

An estimated 3.5 million deaths are attributable to URI-associated pneumonia globally every year, especially in areas of high poverty, low medical resources, and high rates of serious illnesses such as HIV-AIDS (Murray and Lopez 1997).

Influenza and respiratory syncytial virus are also important pathogens in children that can cause more serious illness. URI is highly contagious from contact with infected respiratory droplets, and can spread especially rapidly in close quarters. Viral–bacterial etiology is also common, and can involve common strains such as *Streptococcus pneumoniae* responsible for a range of secondary infections (Bosch et al. 2013).

Etiology

It has been estimated that almost one in three healthy and asymptomatic children carry several respiratory viruses at any given time. The epithelial layer of the respiratory mucosa is considered the first defensive line against infections. Breach of the mucosa can allow rapid viral replication. Infection triggers rapid upregulation of the inflammatory response to combat the infection. The healthy airway actually hosts a local microbiome that is part of the surveillance mechanism to protect against infection along with cilia to prevent pathogenic virus or bacteria from invading and causing disease. When these defenses have been conquered pathogens are usually very efficient in their reproductive cycle (Bosch et al. 2013).

Prevalence

Upper respiratory tract infection is one of the most common diseases observed around the world. Adults average a common cold two to four times per year, children an estimated six to eight times annually. URI accounts for billions of dollars in healthcare expenditures globally (Murray and Lopez 1997).

Influenza and respiratory syncytial virus also account for significant morbidity and mortality in infants, children, and adolescents and have been widely covered in the medical literature.

Clinical Manifestation

Commonly observed signs and symptoms in an average respiratory illness include coughing, sore throat, runny nose, nasal congestion, low-grade fever, sneezing and feeling of increased pressure in the face. The early symptoms start off with a simple congestion in the nasal sinuses and pathways or an uncomfortable tickle in the airways. The next stage is a runny nose, termed as rhinorrhea. The cough develops with time and irritates the entire tracheal region, causing a significant disturbance in children. The cough itself causes more inflammation and discomfort in the throat. Body fatigue and fever are common occurrences. Infant and children may be fussy and have difficulty eating and drinking. Other symptoms that can occur include a scratchy throat, which becomes inflamed, making swallowing painful. Loss of smell can also occur, as can conjunctivitis. Some people also experience vomiting, diarrhea, and dehydration.

In children, the symptoms of URI are often observed in the lower part of the respiratory tract. Usually laryngotracheitis is noticed in this age group, which features a series of symptoms such as dry cough, hoarseness, loss of voice, barking or deep cough, gagging, and thick mucus secretion. Upper respiratory tract infection symptoms are usually seen to last for a period of 3 to 14 days (Bosch et al. 2013).

Comorbidities

- Sinusitis
- Otitis media: by age 3 years an estimated 80% of children have had at least one episode of otitis media and 40% have had six or more episodes by age 7 years
- Pharyngitis
- Bronchitis
- Pneumonia
- Bronchospasm
- Dehydration
- Conjunctivitis
- Epiglottitis with bacterial secondary infection in unimmunized children
- Mastoiditis

Diagnostic Criteria

Common cold is typically a clinical diagnosis in children. Nasal swabs and polymerase chain reaction assays can help to identify other pathogens such as influenza or respiratory syncytial virus. Comorbidities such as pneumonia may require x-ray to confirm.

Pharyngitis, ear infections, and most other comorbidities can be confirmed clinically. Deeper infections such as mastoiditis may require CT or MRI imaging.

Treatment

No specific cure is available. The goal of treatment is to decrease symptoms and support the patient while allowing the disease to pass at its own pace. Maintenance of hydration throughout the illness is especially important in infants and children.

Conventional Treatment

Although concerned parents often push for treatment, antibiotics are not effective for the common cold, and many of the over-the-counter and prescription medications to manage symptoms cause serious side effects in the pediatric population. Due to the high number of serious adverse events, their use has been advised against in children under age 2 years by the U.S. FDA since 2007, with a formalized statement published in 2008 against their use, including warning labels on over-the-counter products. Since then, reports of adverse events have continued to accrue. Advisories have now expanded to include recommending against their use in children under the age of 6 years (Mazer-Amirshahi et al. 2014).

A 2012 Annual Report of American Association of Poison Control Centers includes over-the-counter cough-cold medicines in the top three substances associated with death in children younger than 5 years (Mowry et al. 2013).

Some of the common classes of conventional over-the-counter drugs available include the following.

ANTIHISTAMINES

Shown in a 2015 Cochrane Database Systematic Review to have no demonstrated efficacy in URI in adults or children including no measurable effect on nasal obstruction or rhinorrhea. Side effects can include: drowsiness, paradoxical agitation, and dystonic reaction (De Sutter, Saraswat, and van Driel 2015).

DECONGESTANTS

By default phenylephrine has become the primary decongestant in children's over-the-counter cough and cold medicines despite a widely published lack of effectiveness or supporting safety studies. It was approved by the FDA in 1976 after previous related man-made decongestants fell out of favor: pseudoephedrine because of its role in methamphetamine manufacture, phenylpropanolamine because of its association with stroke. Side effects can include irregular heart rhythms, agitation, irritability, headaches, and dystonic reactions, among other symptoms (Hatton et al. 2007).

MUCOLYTICS

One of the most common substances available to manage mucus in pediatric over-the-counter products is guaifenesin, sourced from the bark of the guaiac tree. It was approved by the FDA for over-the-counter use in 1952; however, large randomized controlled trials have not supported its efficacy. Side effects can include: either drowsiness or agitation, severe respiratory suppression, nausea, and vomiting (Hoffer-Schaefer et al. 2014).

COUGH SUPPRESSANTS

Dextromethorphan was approved by the FDA in 1958 and is a common ingredient in children's over-the-counter medicines as a cough suppressant. It is a man-made chemical with similarities to opioids, but is non-addictive. American Academy of Pediatrics policy statements have raised concerns about dextromethorphan for decades because ultimately cough suppression is undesirable and often dangerous in children, especially in young children, who rely on their powerful gag reflex to protect their airway. Side effects include: irritability, agitation, and hallucinations (Academy of Pediatrics Committee on Drugs 1997).

Like codeine, dextromethorphan works centrally and in high doses acts as a dissociative anesthetic, making it a popular drug of abuse (Finkelstein et al. 2015).

Many of the pediatric over-the-counter cough-cold medications have added acetaminophen or non-steroidal anti-inflammatories to address fever and pain. This makes the risk of double dosing these drugs in the presence of fever or pain a real possibility, especially if multiple caretakers are involved. Overdose of both has been associated with serious side effects in young children (Wood et al. 2010).

Use of over-the-counter medication can also delay medical care in infants or young children with potentially serious respiratory syncytial virus or influenza. Any infant with a fever, who appears to have labored breathing, who is unable to maintain hydration, or who is inconsolable, must be evaluated for serious illness in an appropriate care facility as quickly as possible.

Integrative Treatment

One of the most challenging issues in the clinical encounter can be educating parents that supportive care is a more prudent approach than medication for URI in children. Basic steps such as rest, ample fluids, plenty of sleep, and warm supportive care are important and carry far less risk than conventional treatments. Nursing infants should continue to breastfeed throughout a URI if at all possible (Fashner, Ericson, and Werner 2012).

PREVENTIVE MEASURES

Standard preventive measures should be encouraged, such as influenza vaccines in eligible children, good hand washing, and rest at the first signs of illness to promote more rapid healing.

ZINC

A 2011 Cochrane Database Systematic Review of 13 studies involving 1360 individuals found that the use of oral zinc sulfate has been associated with a decrease in severity and duration of cold symptoms in some studies if taken within the first 24 hours of illness. In children it was found to reduce the number of school absences and number of prescriptions received when it was taken over a longer time span averaging at least 5 months. Metallic taste and texture palatability were two downsides (Singh and Das 2011).

PROBIOTICS

Variable evidence exists to support the use of probiotics as a preventive measure against acute upper respiratory infections. A Cochrane Database Systematic Review of 12 randomized controlled trials involving 3720 children and adults found that probiotics were better than placebo, but lacked sufficient evidence to make formal recommendation for their use in URI prevention. Studies included a wide variety of strains, dosing, and duration of treatment (Quick 2015).

A 2009 randomized controlled trial in *Pediatrics* in 326 children aged 3–5 years given either *Lactobacillus acidophilus* alone or in combination with *Bifidobacterium animalis* twice daily for 6 months versus placebo showed that children in the treatment groups had significant reductions in fevers, cough, rhinorrhea, prescription use, and number of days absent. The combination strain was slightly more significant than the single strain ($p < 0.001$ versus $p = 0.002$ respectively) (Leyer et al. 2009).

VITAMIN C

A 2007 Cochrane Database Systematic Review found consistent benefit in URI prevention in 13% of children who took 1 gram of vitamin C daily versus control groups. No difference was seen in treatment of URI however (Douglas et al. 2007).

Treatments with Supporting Evidence

In URI treatment, familiarity with interventions that have supporting evidence in pediatrics is helpful. These include the following.

DECONGESTANTS

- Nasal irrigation
- Humidity
- Menthol vapor rub (keep out of reach of children and avoid use in infants)

MUCOLYTICS

Warm liquids given in small amounts by syringe or spoon can help to thin mucus. Typical dose recommended by the American Academy of Pediatrics is one to three teaspoons three to four times per day in infants over 3 months of age.

COUGH SUPPRESSION

Evidence continues to accrue to support the use of dark honey (Buckwheat honey) for cough in children over 1 year of age. Honey has been shown to be as or more effective than over-the-counter cough suppressants, with a significant safety margin. Of note, however, is that honey must be avoided in children under age 1 year due to the real risk of botulism. If spores are ingested in contaminated honey, they may colonize in the young child's gut and produce botulinum toxin, which has potent neurotoxic effects (Oduwole et al. 2014).

Doses of honey vary by age (Fashner, Ericson, and Werner 2012). See Table 18.1.

Table 18.1 Doses of Honey by Age

Age Range	Dosage
2–5 years	2.5 mL
6–11 years	5 mL
12–18 years	10 mL

PELARGONIUM SIDOIDES (UMCKA COLDCARE)

A 2008 Cochrane Database Systematic Review found that *Pelargonium sidoides*, a homeopathic preparation derived from the medicinal plant, may have some efficacy in improving symptoms of URI in children, although mechanism is not well understood (Timmer et al. 2008).

School-aged children who have a reliable gag reflex can add a hard lozenge to suck on to sooth the throat and reduce cough.

Popular measures that are commonly used but that have been shown to lack efficacy in children to prevent or treat URI include most echinacea products, over-the-counter medications, and steroids.

ELDERBERRY FOR INFLUENZA

In cases of proven influenza, black elderberry (*Sambucus nigra*) has been shown to have inhibitory effects on both influenza virus and against *Streptococcus pyogenes* and group C and G *Streptococci*, and gram-negative *Branhamella catarrhalis*. Liquid elderberry extract exists for children, although no standard dosage recommendations have been published. Adverse events have not been reported (Krawitz et al. 2011).

Otitis Media and Otalgia

Overview

Otitis media is a common comorbidity in pediatric URI and may be due to viral or bacterial infection, or a combination of the two (Nokso-Koivisto, Marom, and Chonmaitree 2015).

It has been estimated that the majority of children (~80%) experience at least one episode of otitis media by preschool age, with peak incidence occurring between 6–15 months. An estimated 10%–15% of cases become chronic. Due to concerns about antibiotic overuse, including: development of resistant organisms, lack of efficacy in addressing pain or preventing tympanic rupture, and high rate of spontaneous remission, many pediatric organizations, including the American Academy of Pediatrics, have adopted watchful waiting periods of 2–3 days, followed by re-examination prior to recommending or starting antibiotic treatment. Adverse effects from antibiotic treatment in children with otitis are common; of every 14 children treated, it has been shown that one will suffer an adverse event such as gastrointestinal upset, rash, or allergic reaction. It is currently recommended that antibiotics be reserved for children under age 2 years with bilateral infection, or with unilateral infection and tympanic membrane perforation. Management in other groups should focus on pain management, with ear recheck in 2–3 days (Venekamp et al. 2015).

Integrative Medicine Treatment

Although many therapies have been explored for treatment and symptom relief of otitis media in children, one of the few therapies with a small body of supporting research is homeopathy (Marom et al. 2016).

Challenges in interpreting the study results include variable remedies, use of combination remedies, and variable dosing and duration of treatment (Marom et al. 2016).

A small number of randomized controlled trials have shown promise. The first compared homeopathic ear drops versus placebo in 75 children and showed a statistically significant decrease in pain at 24 hours and 64 hours after treatment (Jacobs, Springer, and Crothers 2001).

The second was a study in 81 Indian children randomized to receive antipyretics and analgesics versus homeopathic drops. No child in the homeopathic group in this study required antibiotics, compared to the majority in the conventional treatment group (Sinha et al. 2012).

And in a prospective study of 230 children by Frei, the children treated with homeopathic drops had pain resolution that was 2.4 times more rapid than that of the conventional group and no adverse events were noted (Frei and Thurneysen 2001).

References

Academy of Pediatrics Committee on Drugs. 1997. "Use of codeine-and dextromethorphan-containing cough remedies in children." *Pediatrics* 99(6): 918–20.

Bezerra, P. G., M. C. Britto, J. B. Correia, C. Duarte Mdo, A. M. Fonceca, K. Rose, M. J. Hopkins, L. E. Cuevas, and P. S. McNamara. 2011. "Viral and atypical bacterial detection in acute respiratory infection in children under five years." *PLoS One* 6(4): e18928. doi: 10.1371/journal.pone.0018928.

Bosch, A. A., G. Biesbroek, K. Trzcinski, E. A. Sanders, and D. Bogaert. 2013. "Viral and bacterial interactions in the upper respiratory tract." *PLoS Pathog* 9(1): e1003057. doi: 10.1371/journal.ppat.1003057.

Chonmaitree, T., K. Revai, J. J. Grady, A. Clos, J. A. Patel, S. Nair, J. Fan, and K. J. Henrickson. 2008. "Viral upper respiratory tract infection and otitis media complication in young children." *Clin Infect Dis* 46(6): 815–23. doi: 10.1086/528685.

De Sutter, A. I., A. Saraswat, and M. L. van Driel. 2015. "Antihistamines for the common cold." *Cochrane Database Syst Rev* 11: CD009345. doi: 10.1002/14651858.CD009345.pub2.

Douglas, R. M., H. Hemila, E. Chalker, and B. Treacy. 2007. "Vitamin C for preventing and treating the common cold." *Cochrane Database Syst Rev* 3: CD000980. doi: 10.1002/14651858. CD000980.pub3.

Fashner, J., K. Ericson, and S. Werner. 2012. "Treatment of the common cold in children and adults." *Am Fam Physician* 86(2): 153–9.

Finkelstein, Y., G. Goel, J. R. Hutson, J. Armstrong, C. R. Baum, P. Wax, J. Brent, and Consortium Toxicology Investigators. 2015. "Drug misuse in adolescents presenting to the emergency department." *Pediatr Emerg Care.* doi: 10.1097/PEC.0000000000000571.

Frei, H., and A. Thurneysen. 2001. "Homeopathy in acute otitis media in children: treatment effect or spontaneous resolution?" *Br Homeopath J* 90(4): 180–2.

Hatton, R. C., A. G. Winterstein, R. P. McKelvey, J. Shuster, and L. Hendeles. 2007. "Efficacy and safety of oral phenylephrine: systematic review and meta-analysis." *Ann Pharmacother* 41(3): 381–90. doi: 10.1345/aph.1H679.

Hoffer-Schaefer, A., H. J. Rozycki, M. A. Yopp, and B. K. Rubin. 2014. "Guaifenesin has no effect on sputum volume or sputum properties in adolescents and adults with acute respiratory tract infections." *Respir Care* 59(5): 631–6. doi: 10.4187/respcare.02640.

Jacobs, J., D. A. Springer, and D. Crothers. 2001. "Homeopathic treatment of acute otitis media in children: a preliminary randomized placebo-controlled trial." *Pediatr Infect Dis J* 20(2): 177–83.

Krawitz, C., M. A. Mraheil, M. Stein, C. Imirzalioglu, E. Domann, S. Pleschka, and T. Hain. 2011. "Inhibitory activity of a standardized elderberry liquid extract against clinically-relevant human respiratory bacterial pathogens and influenza A and B viruses." *BMC Complement Altern Med* 11: 16. doi: 10.1186/1472-6882-11-16.

Leyer, G. J., S. Li, M. E. Mubasher, C. Reifer, and A. C. Ouwehand. 2009. "Probiotic effects on cold and influenza-like symptom incidence and duration in children." *Pediatrics* 124(2): e172–9. doi: 10.1542/peds.2008-2666.

Marom, T., P. Marchisio, S. O. Tamir, S. Torretta, H. Gavriel, and S. Esposito. 2016. "Complementary and alternative medicine treatment options for otitis media: a systematic review." *Medicine (Baltimore)* 95(6): e2695. doi: 10.1097/MD.0000000000002695.

Mazer-Amirshahi, M., I. Rasooly, G. Brooks, J. Pines, L. May, and J. van den Anker. 2014. "The impact of pediatric labeling changes on prescribing patterns of cough and cold medications." *J Pediatr* 165(5): 1024–8 e1. doi: 10.1016/j.jpeds.2014.07.047.

Mowry, J. B., D. A. Spyker, L. R. Cantilena, Jr., J. E. Bailey, and M. Ford. 2013. "2012 Annual Report of the American Association of Poison Control Centers' National Poison Data System (NPDS): 30th Annual Report." *Clin Toxicol (Phila)* 51(10): 949–1229. doi: 10.3109/15563650.2013.863906.

Murray, C. J., and A. D. Lopez. 1997. "Global mortality, disability, and the contribution of risk factors: Global Burden of Disease Study." *Lancet* 349(9063): 1436–42. doi: 10.1016/S0140-6736(96)07495-8.

Nokso-Koivisto, J., T. Marom, and T. Chonmaitree. 2015. "Importance of viruses in acute otitis media." *Curr Opin Pediatr* 27(1): 110–15. doi: 10.1097/MOP.0000000000000184.

Oduwole, O., M. M. Meremikwu, A. Oyo-Ita, and E. E. Udoh. 2014. "Honey for acute cough in children." *Cochrane Database Syst Rev* 12: CD007094. doi: 10.1002/14651858.CD007094.pub4.

Quick, M. 2015. "Cochrane Commentary: probiotics for prevention of acute upper respiratory infection." *Explore (NY)* 11(5): 418–20. doi: 10.1016/j.explore.2015.07.012.

Singh, M., and R. R. Das. 2011. "Zinc for the common cold." *Cochrane Database Syst Rev* 2: CD001364. doi: 10.1002/14651858.CD001364.pub3.

Sinha, M. N., V. A. Siddiqui, C. Nayak, V. Singh, R. Dixit, D. Dewan, and A. Mishra. 2012. "Randomized controlled pilot study to compare homeopathy and conventional therapy in acute otitis media." *Homeopathy* 101(1): 5–12. doi: 10.1016/j.homp.2011.08.003.

Timmer, A., J. Gunther, G. Rucker, E. Motschall, G. Antes, and W. V. Kern. 2008. "Pelargonium sidoides extract for acute respiratory tract infections." *Cochrane Database Syst Rev* 3: CD006323. doi: 10.1002/14651858.CD006323.pub2.

Venekamp, R. P., S. L. Sanders, P. P. Glasziou, C. B. Del Mar, and M. M. Rovers. 2015. "Antibiotics for acute otitis media in children." *Cochrane Database Syst Rev* 6: CD000219. doi: 10.1002/14651858.CD000219.pub4.

Wood, D. M., E. English, S. Butt, H. Ovaska, F. Garnham, and P. I. Dargan. 2010. "Patient knowledge of the paracetamol content of over-the-counter (OTC) analgesics, cough/cold remedies and prescription medications." *Emerg Med J* 27(11): 829–33. doi: 10.1136/emj.2009.085027.

19 Mental Health: Toxic Stress, Peer Victimization (Bullying), Anxiety, Depression

It seems counterintuitive that children would encounter stress, victimization, anxiety, depression, and other mental health conditions in their formative years when ideally they would be surrounded by a stable and collaborative network of nurturing family, teachers, and community members. Any experienced pediatric clinician understands the gritty reality behind this image for all too many children. In fact, the prevalence of abuse, victimization, and mental health disease in children is sobering, and has been shown in an accruing body of research to take a severe mental and physical toll on the child's developing mind and body. Clinicians who are tuned into this topic can serve as critical advocates for children and can learn to offer a range of options to assist them, and to help children learn to assist themselves, even in the absence of an ideal home or school scenario. This chapter covers toxic stress, bullying, anxiety, and depression, only a small sample of the wide range of mental health conditions that affect the pediatric population. Although the field is in its early stages, integrative therapies are under active study to offer expanded treatment approaches to children and their families struggling with mental health and wellbeing (Edwards et al. 2013).

Toxic Stress

Overview

Self-limited stress is a protective mechanism, in simple terms characterized by the familiar "fight or flight response," which prepares the individual for immediate action by catalyzing instant physiologic response on a neurologic and cellular level. The biology of stress has been well characterized by Cannon, Seyle, and other pioneers in this field of study and will not be reviewed in detail here (Szabo, Tache, and Somogyi 2012).

Ideally, the body reacts to a specific stressor with appropriate and incremental emotional and physiologic responses and quickly regains homeostasis when the stress passes. In fact, not all stress is bad for children. Positive stress might help shape coping skills and is characterized as a short-term stressor in which a child is well supported by individuals and their community such that the obstacle is mastered and the child buffered from the extremes of the stress reaction. This type of stress can build resilience, grit, self-confidence, and sense of self-efficacy. Examples might include a science fair presentation, changing schools, or starting a new sport (Thompson 2014).

Tolerable stress has a longer duration, and more potential for harm. It may require the ongoing support of parents, caretakers, school, or community resources to be sure the child weathers the stressor successfully. Examples here might include family disruption through a divorce or remarriage, death of a family member or close friend, environmental event such as a flood or tornado, or other serious yet time-limited stressor. This category tests both the child's and caretaker's capacity for coping and may involve accessing community or professional support as needed (Thompson 2014).

Toxic stress moves beyond the self-limited to a level of chronic pressure impossible for the child to mitigate alone. Conditions for this scenario often exist even before birth, negatively influencing the developing fetus (Johnson et al. 2013).

Toxic stress leaves the child vulnerable to adverse physiologic consequences. Examples include the range of high-level socioeconomic stressors such as poverty, lack of safe housing, food insecurity, family dysfunction, harsh or emotionally distant parents, lack of access to basic healthcare, and the range of potential opportunities for physical, sexual, and emotional abuse and exploitation. It is important to remember that the potential for toxic stress is not limited to underserved populations. Children at every socioeconomic level are vulnerable. Parallels exist with research in the child maltreatment literature, also seen at every socioeconomic level. Toxic stress might be thought of as the invisible damage inflicted by a range of difficult situations outside of the child's control (Shonkoff et al. 2012).

Prenatal Toxic Stress

The reality is that the fetus and newborn infant must adapt to both the environmental and behavioral elements of their surroundings in order to survive. Repeated studies have shown that exposure to prenatal stress results in children who may be more highly reactive to threats and challenges and with corresponding changes in brain architecture and intricate influences on the developing immune and inflammatory systems (Thompson 2014).

Seminal work by Shonkoff et al. published in *Pediatrics* in 2012, presented a new framework for understanding the consequence of the experience of unremitting stress experienced by children due to the range of adverse experiences. Their development of a paradigm-shifting framework examining the relationships between Ecology (the social and physical environment), Biology (physiological adaptations and disruptions), and Health and Development (learning, behavior, and physical and mental wellbeing) has provided a new direction of study and research that links the physiologic events associated with chronic stress to physical and mental disease later in life (Shonkoff et al. 2012).

They have organized their work around research demonstrating that ongoing dysregulation of the neuro-endocrine-immune axis has a cascading effect on the body's finely tuned regulatory systems which eventually must succumb to chronic pressure with resultant inability to compensate. Crossing this threshold predisposes the body to elevated cortisol activation, chronic upregulation of the inflammatory cascade, disruption of the development of normal brain architecture, and ultimately end organ dysfunction involving serious effects on both mental and physical health. Toxic stress can affect both adults and children. In this chapter the focus will be placed on children and their caretakers. A working definition of childhood toxic stress is exposure to severe, prolonged, or repetitive adversity that is not met with appropriate support or nurturance by the child's caregiver, resulting in an abnormal and ongoing stress response (Garner et al. 2012).

Researchers are actively pursuing further understanding of the physiologic and epigenetic links behind these theories, which is well documented in the work through the Center on the Developing Child at Harvard University (Harvard University).

Early findings have shown that the effects of toxic stress influence the acquisition of both cognitive and social skills. Behavior is shaped in the sense of learning adaptive and maladaptive responses to stressors faced later in life. Negative conditions can set up the child for a widening gap of health and socioeconomic disparities, with the potential to take an enormous toll on both the individual and population health. Leaders organizing around this initiative call for a new framework of policy, leadership, and education that attends to the three overlapping domains of ecology, biology, and development to address new policies and approaches that impact on the individual, family, community, and national level to prevent and reverse harm that begins in the earliest stages of infancy and early childhood (Garner et al. 2012).

Because pediatricians and other clinicians caring for children are uniquely positioned at the intersection of child and family health and community impact, they have an important opportunity to identify, and intervene at multiple levels to help reverse the effects of, poverty, discrimination, and childhood maltreatment that can potentially benefit children's health over a lifetime. This highlights the need to introduce a new skill set for addressing toxic stress into the pediatric medical home setting (Garner et al. 2012).

Etiology

It has been determined that high-level stressors and early-life adversities faced by children without the buffering presence of an engaged caretaker can result in dysregulation of the hypothalamic-pituitary-adrenal (HPA) axis. The HPA axis is part of an intricate feedback loop system that involves both the inflammatory and immune systems, details of which have been widely described elsewhere in the medical literature (Webster, Tonelli, and Sternberg 2002).

Glucocorticoid plays a central role in the stress biology feedback loop. In excess it suppresses normal immune function, and in insufficient amounts it allows unchecked cascade of the inflammatory response with resulting release of multiple proinflammatory cytokines that impact all body tissues and organs, including the brain and nervous system (Johnson et al. 2013).

Immune system development occurs prenatally and continues throughout childhood. It has been established that significant immune system calibration occurs in these early critical time windows, and that maternal stress, anxiety, and depression have important effects on the child's immune system development. This patterning lays the groundwork for patterns of disease susceptibility and resilience that speak to the intricate connections between mother and developing fetus and offer insight into opportunities to lay a foundation of health (Entringer, Buss, and Wadhwa 2015).

Brain and nervous system development occur in the same critical time windows as the immune system, and continue to develop throughout childhood and adolescence into adult life. The idea that even minor negative influences in fetal development or early childhood life are magnified substantially over time form the basis of the urgent initiatives for change (Buss et al. 2012).

Brain development is highly influenced by the same hormonal and immune systems involved in the stress response. Imaging studies have shown that mothers who suffered from significant anxiety at specific points of the second trimester had children with patterns of reduction in brain grey matter that correlated with decreased executive functioning later in childhood (Buss et al. 2010; Buss et al. 2011).

Encouraging Progress

The highly plastic brain of an infant and preschooler is especially responsive to stimuli, which means that the early intervention has good potential for positive outcome. Later interventions have still been shown to be of great value, but early interventions are better. Epigenetic influences make generalization impossible, as evidenced by variability in outcome studies in children raised in institutional settings such as orphanages (Fries, Shirtcliff, and Pollak 2008).

For example, the immune systems of children who are raised in a nurturing environment have been shown to have better resistance to new infections and better able to keep dormant infections quiescent (Johnson et al. 2013). Some children appear to be more naturally tolerant to stress than others, but this is not a fixed outcome. Resilience can be learned.

Studies have also shown that an adolescent mother's direct experience of violence, and subsequent level of depressive symptoms, has an effect on her preschooler's behavior, even when the child has not directly witnessed violence. Labeled *maternal distress*, this was found to be highly predictive of behavioral problems in young offspring (Mitchell et al. 2011).

Study is also active on the effects of maternal stress on the upregulation of cytokines in infant cord blood and their implications for future health (Sternthal et al. 2009).

Other studies show that children exposed to early stressors have upregulation of the inflammatory response predictive of adult inflammatory related disease (Danese et al. 2007; Hennessy, Deak, and Schiml-Webb 2010).

Optimal timing, "dose," and type of interventions are the basis of active study and many questions remain about specific etiologies and individual variations (Entringer, Buss, and Wadhwa 2015).

Prevalence

Although exact numbers are hard to quantify, it has been estimated that up to 50%–96% of urban youth have directly witnessed violence in their communities (Gorman-Smith, Henry, and Tolan 2004).

According to statistics from the Department of Health and Human Services, in 2009 alone the estimated child victimization rate in the U.S. was approximately 10 per 1000 children, with an estimated 80% of these children being maltreated by a parent. An estimated 50%–78% of adult depression, suicide attempts, and substance abuse have been attributed to adverse childhood experiences, and the prevalence of the continuation of intergenerational cycles of maltreatment have been well documented (Valentino et al. 2012).

Globally, an estimated 8%–31% of girls and an estimated 3%–17% of boys experience sexual abuse as reported in a systematic review and meta-analysis by Barth and colleagues (Barth et al. 2013).

In a survey study of 6787 Swiss teenagers, prevalence of sexual abuse and harassment was 40.2% in girls and 17.2% of boys, most frequently via the Internet, an important source of bullying and chronic stress in children and adolescents (Mohler-Kuo et al. 2014).

Ongoing studies of toxic stress will help to better delineate and quantify other types of stressors in the different age groups.

Clinical Manifestations

Behavioral markers of stress in children can be challenging to identify, especially in younger children. Some of the following examples from the AAP Task Force on the Family give an overview of children's stress behavior by age (Schor and American Academy of Pediatrics Task Force on the 2003).

Infants (Simpson et al. 2016)

- Regression and detachment
- Gaze aversion
- Flat affect
- Increased crying
- Irritability
- Sleep disruption
- Decrease in appetite
- Increased startle response

Children Under One Year (Schor and American Academy of Pediatrics Task Force on the 2003)

In addition to the above signs, may also show exaggerated separation anxiety.

Toddlers and Preschoolers

- Increase in irritability and negativity
- Temper tantrums
- Physicality such as pushing
- Sleep disruption
- Night terrors
- Behavioral and skill regression
- Clinging
- Loss of appetite
- Regression in toilet training
- Somatic complaints such as stomachache and headache

School-Aged Children

- Sleep disruption
- Regressive behaviors and separation anxiety
- Somatic complaints (abdominal pain, headache)
- Fatigue
- School resistance

- Bed-wetting
- Acting out and increased negativity

Adolescents

- Increased irritability
- Anger, verbal outbursts
- Fatigue, change in sleep patterns (increased sleep or insomnia), nightmares
- Lightheadedness, dizziness
- Somatic complaints (migraine, abdominal pain, nausea, chest pain)
- Change in appetite
- School avoidance
- Social withdrawal
- Depression
- Conversion reactions
- Increased risk-taking behaviors such as drug use or sexual activity; suicidal thoughts or attempts

Other behavioral symptoms might include hypervigilance, difficulty concentrating, difficulty with emotional regulation, and difficulty with memory, all of which impact school performance. In social settings, difficulty connecting with peers in a constructive and enjoyable manner can be hard due to a higher level of emotional reactivity and lack of appropriate self-regulation skills. Signs and symptoms of special concern include deficits in communication, restricted or repetitive behaviors, and inappropriate sexual behaviors. Passive acceptance and emotional shutdown also fall into the high-risk category. This may be reflected physiologically by depression of normal diurnal cortisol variation, essentially an under-reaction to stress which has been demonstrated in children living in homes marked by domestic violence and in children in foster care, which has many metabolic and immune system implications (Dozier et al. 2006; Bernard et al. 2010).

The full picture of toxic stress in childhood may not manifest until later in life through development of unhealthy lifestyles including substance abuse, inferior nutrition and lack of regular physical activity, lack of success in school and gainful employment, and poor mental and physical health such as cancer, diabetes, gastrointestinal disorders, metabolic syndrome, and cardiovascular disease, or autoimmune illnesses (Danese et al. 2009; Thompson 2014).

Comorbidities

Large longitudinal studies have correlated the number of adverse childhood events and subsequent risk of health issues which manifest in a graded pattern with a 20% increase in coronary heart disease for each additional type of childhood adversity experienced (Felitti et al. 1998).

Large population-based studies in adolescents using data from the National Longitudinal Study on Adolescent Health showed correlation between adverse childhood events and cell-mediated immune function in adulthood, with highest correlation in those reporting abuse in earlier childhood (Slopen et al. 2013; Miller, Chen, and Parker 2011).

Childhood adversity is an identified risk factor for clinical depression and increased risk of worse mental health outcomes, including increased risk for suicidal ideation and attempts (Tunnard et al. 2014).

Children suffering from toxic stress may be at higher risk for serious infectious illnesses. Toxic stress in the family can also prevent the individual from seeking or receiving help due to decreased caretaker self-efficacy. The family may also suffer dissociation from the society and its norms. In these cases, self-neglect and suicidal tendencies can be seen. An increase in the number of diseases such as cancer, tuberculosis, bronchitis, digestive ailments and tumors has also been seen in toxic stress patients highlighting the importance of early intervention (Thompson 2014).

Diagnostic Criteria

Diagnosis of a child suffering from toxic stress is a complex task and is not defined by a single physical or laboratory test. Clinical diagnosis often falls to the pediatrician or family practitioner, and may require the input of a specialist in pediatric mental health. It may be very difficult to identify a vulnerable child, especially at very young ages, or if the family is not forthcoming, if language barriers exist, or if the child is non-verbal or has only sporadic access to healthcare. Clinicians should be aware of risk factors common to their communities and have a high index of suspicion if a family appears to be in need of social or mental health services. One of the most useful methods may be to assess the level of chronic stress in the child's caretaker, as this has been determined to be an important predictive factor, and reduction of caretaker stress has been correlated with improvement of physiologic markers of chronic stress in children (Thompson 2014).

Widely published AAP policy statements and clinical reports outline steps and resources for involvement of family services. Family-specific red flags that should prompt careful screening include maternal depression, exposure to domestic or community violence, food insecurity, substance abuse in the home, or a lack of robust social connections, non-biologically related male living in the home, young parents, evidence of low parental self-esteem, or unemployment (Flaherty et al. 2010).

Obtaining information in a skillful and mindful way is critical to piecing together the full story of the child's life and may require involvement of an inter-professional team of healthcare providers, school nurses, and teachers. Early suspicion, diagnosis, and organized intervention will ideally facilitate earlier treatment.

Treatment

Heightened awareness is the first step in effective treatment of toxic stress. Although admittedly challenging, interventions must be instituted on societal, community, and individual levels to help provide competent and caring adult buffers to protect children from the full force of adverse experiences. The importance of the parent or caretaker–child interaction cannot be overemphasized. In an assessment of multisystem biological risk, parental or caretaker warmth and affection was found to be highly protective in children. Core areas of attention include stable nurturing relationships, safe and supportive physical environment, and sound and appropriate nutrition from the prenatal period forward (Carroll et al. 2013).

This may involve school and community programs, early childhood intervention programs, social support workers, and collaboration between all levels of legal and foster care. Ideally interventions would include an infusion of support for families in distress, increased access to trained mental health workers, and growth of trauma-directed cognitive therapies along the lines of national programs such as Zero to Three (National Center for Infants) and the American Academy of Pediatrics Bright Futures supported by the maternal and Child Health Bureau, Health Resources and Services Administration (American Academy of Pediatrics).

Conventional Treatment

Assuming no obvious treatable illness has been identified on history and physical, a 2012 policy statement by the AAP provides a roadmap for pediatricians to improve care in this area, and includes steps to incentivize fair reimbursement for clinician time and screening, and recommendations on how to identify and coordinate individual, school, and community resources to help mitigate the early-life origins of adult disease. Careful screening at each well visit, and review of anticipatory guidance tuned in to the clinical signs and symptoms associated with stress, are of high importance (Shonkoff et al. 2012).

Efforts are underway to emphasize the medical home as a seat for screening and recognition of children at risk for toxic stress, including prenatal recognition, family support, parenting techniques, and ensuring maximal social and community support.

Individual variation through incompletely understood epigenetic factors and a child's prior experiences understandably make the process more complex.

The Importance of Resilience

One of the primary goals in treatment for toxic stress is the cultivation of resilience, defined by Merriam-Webster as "the capability of a strained body to recover its size and shape after deformation caused especially by compressive stress, and an ability to recover from or adjust easily to misfortune or change" (Webster).

Some of the earliest work in this area has been done in children in the foster care system, where programs to develop warm and consistent connections and a more robust social support system for foster parents resulted in normalization of the HPA reactivity of the preschooler's stress response. Children who have a history of exposure to high-level chronic stressors need the opportunity to reset their biological stress response with repeated opportunities to experience situations of reduced threat, experience of consistency and adult support, and the opportunity to master self-regulatory skills. They also need warm and supportive feedback that encourages them to incrementally gain a sense of self-efficacy. This often takes the introduction of an adult outside of the family unit, whether it be a grandparent, teacher, social worker, or other trusted professional or community member (Thompson 2014).

Strengthening of resilience can be done at many levels, including home, school, and in the community setting; for example, through sports programs and in emerging mindfulness and yoga programs tailored to children. At school the teacher can play an especially important role in helping the child cultivate resilience outside of a potentially toxic home setting. A trained mental health practitioner who has gained the child's trust may be able to provide structured training and input on whether any bridging medications to address anxiety or depression may be needed. Goals of resilience training include increasing confidence, self-efficacy, empathic skills, greater social connectivity and problem-solving skills, and a positive self-concept, among other factors that change over time depending on the child's age, stage of development, and personality (Miller-Lewis et al. 2013; Rutter 2013).

Integrative Treatment

In an integrative approach, once the child's safety at home and at school have been established, first steps are to maximize preventive measures and address core lifestyle elements such as a healthy physical environment, nutrition, sleep, and social support. This approach also involves evaluation of the child's situation for things that may be removed or reduced; for example, excessive screen time, a noisy chaotic environment, exposure to light at night, delayed sleep onset, excessive intake of sugar-sweetened beverages, and lack of safe time outdoors for free play.

Introduction to self-regulation skills is an early priority which can be accomplished in children as young as preschool age using simple mind–body therapies, discussed in more detail below. The overarching goal is for each child and caretaker to learn to access their physiologic "relaxation response," first described by Benson in the 1970s. This is accomplished through stimulation of the parasympathetic nervous system and describes a state of lowered sympathetic activation, which counteracts the classic stress response. Physiologically it consists of slowed heart rate, lowered blood pressure, increased heart rate variability, and slowed respiratory rate (Benson, Beary, and Carol 1974).

A detailed overview of the foundations of health—nutrition, sleep, environmental health, physical activity, and common dietary supplements—are provided in Section II, Foundations of Health. The family may need financial, social, and/or community support to meet even the child's basic needs, a role often coordinated through the pediatrician.

Mind–Body Skills

The relaxation response is accessed through four basic behaviors that can be applied in a multitude of ways to best meet the individual's age and developmental stage. Overall they consist of repetition of a sound or phrase, inward focus to minimize distraction, relaxed position, and quiet surroundings (Benson, Beary, and Carol 1974).

Young children who have been exposed to both acute and chronic stress can be encouraged to learn simple breath counting, belly breathing, progressive muscle relaxation exercises (with or without accompanying music or guided imagery), simple yoga poses, and basic mindfulness skills by a trained clinician or associate. All these gentle and non-pharmacologic therapies can be tailored to meet a variety of ages, developmental stages, and venues. For example, preschool children through adolescents have been shown to have success with clinical hypnosis to help them access the relaxed state. Any child who has experienced physical or sexual abuse should be screened prior to the use of mind–body therapies to prevent trigger of a PTSD-type setback (Olness 1996).

Work on introducing mindfulness to urban adolescents who face significant stressors has shown beneficial effect when delivered through public school systems in low-income neighborhoods. One of the few randomized trials of mindfulness done in children is a 2016 study by Sibinga et al., involving 300 adolescents with a mean age of 12 years, in a 12-week mindfulness program taught by experienced mindfulness-based stress reduction instructors. The study found a significant reduction in depressive symptoms, self-hostility, somatization, negative mood, negative coping, and posttraumatic symptoms (Sibinga et al. 2016).

Small studies are beginning to accrue examining the benefit of weekly yoga in school-aged children who had experienced interpersonal trauma. In one study by Beltran of 10 boys aged 8–12 years old, a series of 12 weekly yoga sessions at an urban-based healthcare center resulted in significant improvements in interpersonal functioning (Beltran et al. 2016).

A meta-review on the use of yoga by Macy et al. highlights the need for larger well-designed research studies, but at the same time identifies encouraging preliminary data for this low-risk intervention (Macy et al. 2015).

The introduction of mind–body therapies to address caretaker, child, and adolescent stressors is one way to help individuals at risk acquire gentle, portable, non-pharmacologic tools to increase self-efficacy and coping skills.

Peer Victimization (Bullying)

Overview

Commonly known as bullying, peer victimization is the targeted intimidation or humiliation of a selected individual based on an imbalance of power that sets it apart from simple aggression. Bullying can take the form of physical or verbal aggression (direct), but may be more insidious such as social isolation, rumor spreading, and cyber aggression including text, video, email, and other social media (indirect) that target the victim's reputation and social status while allowing the perpetrator to remain anonymous. Typically bullying is a pattern that often occurs at least weekly and persists for months, but may also be as harmful and effective in isolated incidents. Characteristics of children who practice indirect bullying have been identified as high social status, sophisticated social skills, and a calculating lack of empathy, with an ability to orchestrate group dynamics to their advantage. Bullying is prevalent in middle school and high school, a time of extensive social and physical reordering in childhood, making it a highly strategic behavior. An inflated view of self has been commonly reported in bullies in academic and sporting endeavors, and it has been reported that bullies often receive positive social feedback from bystanders eager to avoid becoming targets themselves.

The bystander role is also complex, and has been categorized as having three subcomponents: co-victim, isolate, and confederate which carry their own set of stressors including risk of posttraumatic stress, and internalizing behaviors (Rivers 2012).

Bullying can be a source of significant chronic stress and may manifest with physical and mental symptoms. Often tolerated as a "rite of passage," bullying has been identified as a serious societal problem due to its long-lasting detrimental effects. Peer victimization is commonly observed in schools and in academic institutions and can cut across age groups from preschool to senior populations. Predictive risk factors for victimization include obesity, a low sense of social rank, sensitive nature, insecure, anxious, submissive, early or late pubertal development, overprotective parents, low self-esteem, lack of confidence in social settings, and a history of being previously bullied. Other targeted groups include: lesbian, gay, bisexual, transgender, short stature, underweight, special needs, learning disabilities, visible skin conditions such as eczema, burns, acne, and children who have any deviation from the physical norm or other healthcare needs, such as use of an inhaler for asthma during gym class or similar situations (Andersen et al. 2015).

Essentially any "lack of fit" with the group makes the child a potential target. Children who react emotionally to bullies initially provide a response that bullies find rewarding, and may inadvertently set themselves up for further harassment. This is one of the many factors that reinforce the argument to equip children and adolescents with advanced coping skills that build resilience and allow them to more effectively adapt to challenging circumstances (Andersen et al. 2015).

Research shows that individuals involved in all three bullying roles (bully, bystander, victim) are subject to detrimental health effects over time. Bullying often goes unreported for a variety of reasons including fear of retaliation, shame, ongoing intimidation or escalation after reporting, feelings of helplessness and isolation, or follow through of actual physical or sexual assault (Andersen et al. 2015).

Longitudinal outcome studies in adults with a history of involvement in the cycle of bullying consistently show correlation with chronic physical and mental health conditions such as depression, anxiety, substance abuse, and increased risk of self-harm (Lereya et al. 2015).

Etiology

The causes of peer harassment are variable and depend on the situation and mindset of the individuals involved. A pattern of bullies being the bully-victim either at home or school has been identified in some children. Teachers who are dismissive of bullying complaints, or who are themselves bullies, perpetuate a culture lacking adult oversight.

Bullying is related to social status in the group, including popularity, preference of the group, school performance, and socioeconomic standing. It is possible that growing up in a lower socioeconomic setting predisposes to higher stress, less stable family structure, and more illness which in itself may compromise teaching of robust adaptive coping skills that are protective against risk of being bullied. Parental neglect and over-authoritarian parenting have both been found to be predictive of bullying. A correlation has been established between being bullied at school and risk of being bullied as an adult in the workplace, especially in obese individuals (Andersen et al. 2015).

Prevalence

A pair of large population surveys of 218,000 adolescents in 66 countries demonstrate wide geographic variation, but on average more than one in three adolescents aged 11–15 years reported at least one bullying event in the preceding 2 months (Andersen et al. 2015).

Large studies in Western populations indicate that approximately 4%–9% of children bully, approximately 25% are bullied, and there are some subsets of children who are bully-victims depending on social circumstances (Juvonen and Graham 2014).

An important 2015 review of cyberbullying by Hamm et al. in *JAMA Pediatrics* examined 36 studies in 34 publications primarily in U.S. children and found a median prevalence of approximately one in four children reporting being cyberbullied. Reasons for bullying others in this study were listed as: a lack of confidence in themselves, a desire to feel better about themselves, a desire for control, entertainment, and retaliation among others (Hamm et al. 2015).

In schools, almost 54% of the handicapped children may suffer victimization at the hands of their peers, with school climate and tolerance for bullying being an important determining factor (Wang et al. 2014).

Clinical Manifestation

It is important to remember that the detrimental mental and physical effects involved in bullying are experienced by all involved in the triad: victim, bully, and bystander (Rivers 2012).

Peer victimization is often considered to be primarily a psychological issue and has been shown to inflict shame, humiliation, embarrassment, loneliness, social isolation, general and social anxiety, diminished self-esteem, depression, and suicidal ideation, cutting behavior, and completed suicide. However, bullying also significantly impacts physical health. In its most obvious form, physical impact may be seen from the injuries inflicted during the process of the abuse when many bullies find it empowering to hit the bullied individual (Andersen et al. 2015).

Stress-related illness due to bullying has been related to dysregulation of the hypothalamic-pituitary axis as referenced in the toxic stress discussion above. Neuroimaging studies have correlated the area of the brain that processes pain (in the cingulate cortex) with the area that lights up on functional MRI in an experimental model of social exclusion. Activity in the same area was also associated with increased depressive symptoms in children in the study 1 year later, which has raised the question about the connection between bully victims and somatic complaints (Andersen et al. 2015).

Comorbidities

The frequency, occurrence, and stage of comorbidities experienced vary from person to person, as does the level of adversity or outright brutality executed in the bullying process. Depression is a common comorbidity and is seen in all ages of bullied children, adolescents, and adults. This depression can be linked physiologically as a root cause of other malignant diseases like hypertension, diabetes, heart diseases, and endocrine problems. Social isolation and lack of friends can perpetuate the victim role. Development of self-blame and suicidal tendencies are another serious comorbidity. School attendance, performance, and grades also commonly suffer. Avoidance, worrying, and self-blame have all been associated with poorer outcomes for children who have been bullied (Fisher et al. 2012; Geoffroy et al. 2016; Juvonen and Graham 2014).

Diagnostic Criteria

The diagnosis of bullying can be challenging if not disclosed to a trusted parent, caretaker, clinicians, coach, school nurse or other supportive adult (Narayanan and Betts 2014).

Many children suffer in fear and in silence to avoid the risk of retaliation or further humiliation. An adult recipient of a child's disclosure of bullying must also be careful not to frame and blame the child as "victim" or as a weak individual. Some of the most heartbreaking cases can be the children who are bullied for physical or mental disability. This becomes a societal issue that must be addressed at every level of family, school, and government to extinguish (Vaz et al. 2015).

Once the issue has been disclosed, the clinician can react to help the child. Bullying is recognized in the International Statistical Classification of Diseases and Related Health Problems 10th Revision (ICD-10), which has a bullying diagnosis, "victim of bullying," found within ICD-10-CM Z65.8 "Other specified problems related to psychosocial circumstances." Comorbidities such as anxiety and depression can be coded separately accordingly.

Although gaining attention in the medical community in some areas, for example, North America, Europe, and Australia, bullying is not yet recognized as a serious social, educational, and environmental hazard in many other areas of the world. Hopefully this will change over time as research continues to accrue (Stevens et al. 2015).

Treatment

In addition to addressing the individual's symptoms, especially anxiety and depression, discussed in more detail below, a developing theme in the literature is "school belongingness," an approach that emphasizes inclusion, adopts a whole-school anti-bullying approach, increases the number of positive interactions among both teacher–student and student–student, and addresses physical differences among students as positive attributes of strength and character, and deliberately develops expectations for social acceptance, problem-solving skills, and coping strategies (Vaz et al. 2015).

Although some programs have shown short-term success, long-term benefits have yet to be documented and research remains very active in this area (Cantone et al. 2015).

School-wide interventions to alter school climate around bullying include:

- Increased awareness
- Heightened monitoring
- Systematic and consistent responses to bullying, and clear consequences for staff and students
- Full staff engagement and training

Some Examples of School Programs (Juvonen and Graham 2014)

- *KiVa (kiusaamista vastaan)*: From the Finnish "against bullying," designed to develop empathy in bystanders and encourage them to intervene.
- *WITS (Walk away, Ignore, Talk it out, Seek help)*: A Canadian based program for early elementary students.
- *Steps to Respect*: An American program directed toward relational aggression such as gossip and shunning that involves observation of playground behavior to address bullying behavior.

Targeted interventions can be directed towards specific individuals in the bullying triad. Programs have been evaluated that address antisocial behavior in early childhood and provide longitudinal intervention and academic tutoring. One example is Fast Track, where target areas include social information processing, social problem solving, emotional understanding, self-control and communication skills. Involvement of parents in the training is another important element (Juvonen and Graham 2014).

Fewer organized programs have been developed or studied on the interpretation of the victims' plight to lessen their feeling of self-blame or humiliation. This is an area where reframing through mind–body therapies may have significant potential to shift the perception of "I am a loser," or "This wouldn't happen if I was cooler" to gain the perspective of "I was in the wrong place at the wrong time," or "This person bullying me has issues that have nothing to do with me," "This is not my fault."

It has been well established that the treatment of bullying can be highly challenging.

One theory involves "coherence," a sense of perception of control and agency—the ability of the child to comprehend, grasp the underlying meaning, and have a sense of access to adequate resources for coping with the immediate situation. A strong sense of coherence has been shown to have protective effects against bullying. Having even one friend has been shown to have an important protective effect in both bullying episodes and in the extent of distress experienced if bullied. Any adult who has been bullied can appreciate the difficulty of gaining perspective in a complex social situation for a young child, middle school child, or developing adolescent (Juvonen and Graham 2014).

Conventional Treatment

Awareness, parental suspicion, discussion, and disclosure in a non-judgmental environment are all essential to encouraging a victimized child, or a traumatized bystander, to begin to take control of a situation that may feel impossible. Parents may then engage the help of the child's clinician, who becomes an important ally in addressing the situation. Some parents find it difficult to reach out due to embarrassment that their child has been perceived as "weak," which can unfortunately stall appropriate intervention for the child, and some clinicians are not well prepared to offer assistance. Teachers, principals, and at times law enforcement must be engaged. School nurses, counselors, or mental health professionals may be crucial members of the inter-professional team. In many cases engagement from supportive adults is needed to help children caught in this toxic cycle (Rudolph et al. 2014).

Integrative Treatment

Although not specifically integrative, elements of the KiVa program that emphasize bystander dynamics, such as encouraging disapproval of bullying, standing up for and expressing empathy for victims, help to diminish the positive social motivation often experienced by bullies by shifting the peer group dynamic away from reinforcing behavior that can be driven by fear of becoming a victim. This involves increasing the empathic skills of students, which has been shown to be effective in reducing bullying, in direct counterpoint to bystanders laughing or otherwise reinforcing the social capital of the bully, which has been shown to perpetuate the behavior in the overall classroom.

Teacher reaction to bullying has also been shown to be pivotal to its perpetuation or extinction in the classroom (Saarento, Boulton, and Salmivalli 2015).

Another initiative gathering momentum is the implementation of school-wide training programs that include student and teaching training as well as introduction to a mindfulness-based social and emotional skills curriculum, which has shown positive uptake in English secondary schools (Bonell et al. 2015).

Summary

Bullying is pervasive and highly detrimental with potential to cause harmful long-term mental and physical effects. At a minimum, clinicians must be aware of this dynamic and prepared to assist children and their families with positive and effective steps. Two of the most important steps are to protect the child from ongoing harm, and to empower the child and family to stop the destructive cycle.

Anxiety

Overview

Anxiety is very common and is experienced by the vast majority of people at some point in life as a normal human emotion. In contrast, an anxiety disorder manifests as an amplified and distorted feeling of anxiety that can occur at irregular periods of time, in the form of feelings of hypervigilance, fear, threat, anguish, and distress. Anxiety disorders are often comorbid with other mental health conditions, such as depression or irritability. Anxiety disorders in children and adolescents should be regarded as serious and treated accordingly. Anxiety disorder can be subtle in children and may go unnoticed by parents or unreported by the child, which is concerning because anxiety is negatively associated with multiple physiologic effects in both children and adults. Some of the common sub-categories in children include separation anxiety, social anxiety, phobias, and panic attacks. Untreated anxiety disorders in children and adolescents often persist into adult life (Polanczyk et al. 2015; Cornacchio et al. 2016).

Understanding the pathophysiology of anxiety is important, because it has been shown to affect not only decision making and mood, but also critical elements of structural brain plasticity such as neuronal replacement, dendritic remodeling, and synapse turnover that particularly affect the hippocampus, amygdala, and prefrontal cortex—all associated with fear as well as cognition (McEwen et al. 2012).

Etiology

Anxiety disorders affecting day-to-day activity have a multifactorial etiology and are associated with a variety of conditions, including those associated with toxic stress, discussed in detail above. Heritability is high at an estimated 20%–65%, paralleling that of major depressive disorder. Study is very active examining the molecular basis of anxiety disorders, and their association with epigenetic marks, including families involved in wars and natural catastrophes (Sakolsky, McCracken, and Nurmi 2012).

These unremitting stress conditions cause dysregulation of the hypothalamic-pituitary axis and upregulation of the inflammatory response that can lead to chronic disease (McEwen et al. 2012).

Anxiety can manifest as a result of a wide range of social and situational conditions, including bullying (Rose and Tynes 2015), abuse (Fonzo et al. 2015), poverty (Heberle and Carter 2015; Flouri, Midouhas, and Joshi 2014), food insecurity (Knowles et al. 2016), and parental divorce (Merikangas et al. 2010).

Neurodevelopmental diseases such as autism (Rodgers et al. 2016), and ADHD, are also known drivers of anxiety (Lahey et al. 2016).

Prevalence

Worldwide pooled prevalence of all pediatric mental health disorders is estimated at

13.4% based on data from 87,742 subjects in a broad meta-analysis by Polanczyk and colleagues. In this sample, any anxiety disorder was estimated at 6.5%. All types of anxiety disorders were more prevalent in females (Polanczyk et al. 2015).

U.S. estimates are higher, with a prevalence of 31% recorded in adolescents in the National Comorbidity Survey-Adolescent Supplement, a survey of 10,123 adolescents aged 13–18 years. Median age of anxiety onset was 6 years in this group (Merikangas et al. 2010).

Clinical Manifestations (Siegel and Dickstein 2012)

Anxiety can manifest along a spectrum from normal anticipation to extreme agitation, and escalate to fear, dread, hypervigilance, and panic that prevent the sufferer from experiencing the normal joys and rhythms of life. In school-aged children this might include performance anxiety, school phobia, or fear of speaking up in class.

An acute onset of anxiety can occur without any warning signs and leaves the person in a twist of fear, accelerated excitement, or feelings of distress and terror. Another type of anxiety can lead to an intensely phobic personality, which becomes afraid of everyday tasks and routines. An acute anxiety attack can be accompanied by physiologic changes such as a spike in blood pressure, increased heart rate and respiratory rate—mimicking the typical fight or flight response. Nausea, vertigo, breathlessness, "suffocation false alarm," and a feeling of threat from surrounding people can occur and feel very real (Preter and Klein 2014).

Comorbidities

Anxiety disorders have a range of comorbidities, including self-isolation, depression, substance abuse, phobias, migraine headache, eating disorders and in serious cases self-harming behavior, suicidal ideation, and completed suicide—especially in those with a history of childhood trauma (Carlier et al. 2016).

Diagnostic Criteria

Anxiety disorder is defined in the updated DSM-V and can often be confused with low-level depression or may be interpreted as an attempt by the child or adolescent to garner attention. It is only when the disease worsens that caregivers may actually realize the presence of a disorder. Formal diagnosis is done by a psychologist or psychiatrist (Siegel and Dickstein 2012) who can be of significant help to the child and family if a relationship of trust can be built and sustained.

Diseases that can be associated with anxiety disorders and may cloud diagnosis include vitamin B12 deficiency, cardiac arrhythmia, pheochromocytoma, hyperthyroidism, and some variations of pediatric autoimmune neuropsychiatric disorders associated with streptococcal infections (PANDAS), among others.

Treatment

The treatment process involved in anxiety disorder is individualized and often requires several components including individual and family behavioral therapy and possibly medication. Exacerbating conditions must be ruled out, including over-the-counter prescriptions, and dietary supplements; for example, SAMe which can cause anxiety, other prescription medications, caffeine consumption, asthma medications, thyroid medication, corticosteroids, ADHD psychostimulants, energy drinks, or stimulant drugs of abuse such as cocaine, methamphetamine, or alcohol.

Conventional Treatment

Conventional treatment is determined by disease severity, patient history, age, and comorbid conditions. Extreme care must be taken in children started on selective serotonin reuptake inhibitors (SSRIs) and serotonin norepinephrine reuptake inhibitor (SNRIs), where a certain percentage can develop suicidal ideation and complete suicide, especially in the early stages of drug treatment. This finding generated a black box warning for the drugs as a class in children aged 13–17 years in 2004. The warning was subsequently expanded to cover all antidepressants, and the age range expanded to include those 18–24 years in 2007. These drugs are commonly used in the treatment of both anxiety and depression in children and adolescents. Updates on the FDA black box warnings can be accessed at (Bushnell et al. 2015): http://www.fda.gov/Drugs/DrugSafety/PostmarketDrugSafetyInformationforPatientsandProviders/ucm111085.htm

Side effects of the SSRIs and SNRIs include:

- Headache and nausea
- Drowsiness
- Agitation
- Reduced sex drive
- Weight gain

Serotonin syndrome is a potentially serious side effect that can be precipitated by combining SSRI with medications that increase serotonergic activity in the central nervous system, such as a monoamine oxidase inhibitor (MAO inhibitor). Other drugs include triptans, lithium fentanyl, and other antidepressants. Herbs such as St. John's wort, ginseng, and supplements such as SAMe and 5-HTP may also precipitate the syndrome. Symptoms include agitation, confusion, hallucinations, spike in blood pressure, and other systemic symptoms including dangerously elevated core temperature.

Cognitive behavioral therapy (James et al. 2015) and other types of behavioral counseling are often used in the conventional approach to anxiety (Bushnell et al. 2015).

Integrative Treatment

Integrative treatment approaches to anxiety can be used alone or in conjunction with conventional therapies. Lifestyle approaches form the foundation, and should include an assessment of nutrition, including screening for regular intake of high-quality foods and elimination of stimulants such as caffeine in sodas, coffee, tea, or energy drinks. Review of diet should emphasize a healthy whole food approach, with an emphasis on organic foods as feasible.

SLEEP

Sleep disorders including insomnia, separation anxiety, and nightmares are common in children with anxiety disorders, which should prompt the clinician's inquiry about sleep hygiene at each visit along with screening for stimulants and excessive screen time. Studies have shown that cognitive behavioral therapy and in certain children sertraline have been helpful. However, non-pharmacologic approaches should also be considered in the form of a child-directed bedtime ritual, relaxation, and self-regulation therapies such as breath work and progressive muscle relaxation, guided imagery, music therapy, aromatherapy, and other complementary approaches that may not yet have robust research support, but are also safe with few adverse events reported. Approaches to sleep are discussed in more detail in Chapter 7, Sleep (Caporino et al. 2015).

An integrative interview would ideally make time for a full discussion of the child's typical home and school day, which can be a useful approach to identifying recurring areas of concern; for example, peer pressure, family friction, test anxiety, or sports performance issues. Regular enjoyable exercise is an important element lifestyle element, although large studies are lacking. Interestingly, a study by Gadomski and colleagues showed that pet ownership was associated with lower prevalence of anxiety in a study of 643 children, median age 6.7 years of age (p = 0.002) (Gadomski et al. 2015).

EXERCISE

Relatively few studies exist examining the specific effects of exercise in children's mental health. A review by Biddle and colleagues found wide variability in study quality and design, and few studies on anxiety alone. Conclusions included an overall improvement in short-term self-esteem, and some improvement in academic performance and cognitive performance in some small studies. Overall more data is needed before definitive conclusions can be made, although the downside of age-appropriate, adequately supervised physical activity seems low and overall benefits positive (Biddle and Asare 2011).

One promising intervention for anxiety appears to be yoga. A systematic review by Weaver of 16 studies found an overall positive effect, although again study size and design were identified as limiting factors (Weaver and Darragh 2015).

A second systematic review by Rosen and colleagues of 15 controlled yoga studies and four systematic reviews also showed positive benefit in a variety of small studies, especially for emotional and behavioral regulation of a variety of conditions, including anxiety, but study size and variability again limited generalized recommendation. Adverse events were not reported (Rosen et al. 2015).

Work is ongoing to identify how yoga can best be inserted into treatment plans for traumatized and anxious children and adolescents, but again overall risk appears to be very low (Macy et al. 2015).

For example, yoga has been successfully embedded into psychotherapy groups in a small study of 10 urban boys aged 8–12 years over 12 once-a-week sessions and was found to benefit interpersonal strength and family involvement scores (Beltran 2016) (p = 0.004).

Another area showing positive benefit in chronically stressed urban youth is work by Sibinga and colleagues using mindfulness in school-based programs through introduction of mindfulness-based stress reduction programs, which have shown improvement in coping, self-hostility, rumination, depression and negative affect (Sibinga et al. 2016).

Compassion-based cognitive therapy based on self-compassion has been shown to be beneficial in a study of 132 adolescents. The approach included six components described by authors as: self-kindness, common humanity, mindfulness, self-judgment, isolation, and over-identification. Earlier studies in college students have shown that higher scores on self-compassion are associated with less negative emotions and a more accepting attitude towards personal failures consistent with higher resilience (Muris et al. 2016).

Clinical hypnosis is another mind–body therapy that has shown efficacy and excellent safety profile in pediatric anxiety (Adinolfi and Gava 2013; McClafferty 2011).

DIETARY SUPPLEMENTS AND BOTANICALS

Relatively few trials have been done on dietary supplements to treat anxiety in children.

Inositol   Inositol, which is part of the B-vitamin complex, with an important role in nerve transmission and cell membrane structure, has generated interest, although to date insufficient evidence exists to support its use in children (Mukai et al. 2014).

Chamomile   Chamomile (*Matricaria recutita*) has a record of safe documented use over thousands of years for its calming effect in health conditions such as sleeplessness, stomach upset, colic, and anxiety. It can be used in teas, tinctures, and capsules. The dried flower contains flavonoids and terpenoids thought to be responsible for its soothing properties. Its mechanism of action in anxiety is not completely understood, although research is active in examining its effects on GABA, dopamine, and serotonin neurotransmission. Chamomile is approved by the German Commission E for anxiety and restlessness. Cooled teas are often used in children to sooth restlessness sand colic. An excellent overview of chamomile and its medicinal uses can be found in a review by Srivastava and colleagues (Singh et al. 2011). There is a low risk of allergic reaction with chamomile, especially in people sensitive to ragweed or chrysanthemums or other members of the Compositae family.

Lemon Balm   Lemon balm (*Melissa officinalis*) alone or in combination with fennel has been shown in small studies to help with anxiety in children. It has been used to relieve stress and anxiety throughout history, and has a strong safety record. It is often used in children as a cooled tea and may also be taken as a capsule. A small study in children younger than 12 years of age found that the combination of valerian and lemon balm reduced restlessness and improved sleep (Muller and Klement 2006).

Although not specifically directed towards anxiety, a more recent prospective study involving 169 school-aged children with a history of restlessness, difficulty concentrating, and impulsive behavior showed benefit with a standardized daily dose of 640 mg valerian and 320 mg lemon balm extracts taken over a 7-week study period (Gromball et al. 2014).

Other herbals and dietary supplements have small supporting studies in adults for anxiety; for example, valerian, rhodiola, passion flower, and L-theanine. However, supporting evidence is insufficient at this time to routinely recommend for children.

ACUPUNCTURE

Small studies support the use of acupuncture in anxiety, although a review by Errington-Evans points to high variability in protocols, duration of treatments, and outcome measures. More studies are needed in children and adolescents before generalized recommendation can be made, although serious adverse events were not reported (Errington-Evans 2012).

THERAPEUTIC MASSAGE

Therapeutic massage has been safely used in adolescents, children, infants, and preterm infants for relaxation and to relieve stress, although randomized controlled studies are limited. When performed by a trained practitioner, or by an appropriately trained parent, massage can be a safe complementary therapy for children in inpatient or outpatient settings (Valji et al. 2013; Field 2014).

MUSIC THERAPY

Music therapy is becoming more widely used in the hospital setting; for example, in preprocedural anxiety in children where it has been shown to be helpful. It has also been used in palliative care and oncology settings. While larger studies are needed, risk is low (van der Heijden et al. 2015).

Other low-risk therapies that lack robust supporting data but might be considered if an experienced practitioner is available, and no contraindications exist, include therapeutic touch, healing touch, reiki, and aromatherapy.

Summary

Every child or adolescent with anxiety needs a thorough evaluation to determine cause, and requires effective intervention to prevent development of a chronic condition which can lead to unwanted mental and physical morbidities. An integrative approach that considers nutrition, appropriate dietary supplements, and that emphasizes healthy lifestyle and development of a strong sense of self-efficacy and resilience can help the child gain a sense of mastery over their symptoms and move through life's challenges more confidently and successfully. This requires supportive adults that may by necessity include those outside of their immediate family. The clinician can play a key role in advocating for the child to receive all appropriate treatment options.

Depression

Overview

The World Health Organization reports depression as the leading cause of disability and estimates that by 2020 it will rank second overall for causes of disability globally, cutting across categories of age, gender, race, and communities.

Although major depression is less common in childhood, risk increases with age and raises substantially in adolescence to between 8.4% and 15%. In children depression has been shown to negatively impact family, school, and physical functioning and can go unidentified due to internalizing behaviors. Risk of suicidal ideation and completed suicide are disturbingly high in children with depression, and a range of serious comorbidities, outlined below, raise the stakes for effective treatment. Classic work by Kovacs has reported that depression in childhood is associated with a 70% risk of relapse within 5 years, indicating that long-term surveillance is also important (Kovacs et al. 1984).

Unfortunately, many of the people globally suffering from depression may receive no medical attention for the condition, despite the fact that it is treatable, and in many cases curable. An integrative approach with an emphasis on prevention and healthy lifestyle measures has much to offer in the form of expanded, non-pharmacologic treatment options.

Etiology

The etiology of depression appears to be multifactorial, with genetic, environmental, lifestyle, and likely epigenetic components involved. Dysregulation of the hypothalamic-pituitary-adrenal axis is implicated, with subsequent impact on inflammatory and immune processes, opening the door to its many associated comorbidities in addition to its direct effect on neurotransmitters and neuroplasticity in the brain (Lopresti, Hood, and Drummond 2013; Cattaneo et al. 2015).

Various high-level stressors can trigger depression, such as a death or other significant loss, abuse, or exposure to violence. Children living with chronic illness often suffer depression as a comorbidity; for example, those with cystic fibrosis (Kopp et al. 2016), cancer (Lowe et al. 2015), asthma (Ahmadiafshar et al. 2016), and gastrointestinal diseases such as inflammatory bowel disease (van Tilburg et al. 2015).

Excessive technology use including smartphones and television (Bickham, Hswen, and Rich 2015) and compulsive online gaming have also been implicated in depression in children and adolescents (Han et al. 2016).

Microbiome

The connection between the gut microbiome, the inflammatory system, and mood disorders is an area of high research interest. Etiologic connections and therapeutic options are under study, and this will be an exciting area to follow for potential new approaches (Mangiola et al. 2016).

Prevalence

Worldwide pooled prevalence of all mental health disorders is estimated at 13.4% in children and adolescents based on data from 87,742 subjects. In this sample, any depressive disorder was estimated at 2.6% (Polanczyk et al. 2015).

In the U.S., statistics show a prevalence of mood disorders at 14.3% in the National Comorbidity Survey-Adolescent Supplement, a survey of 10,123 adolescents aged 13–18 years. The average of onset of major depression and dysthymia was 11–14 years in this group, with prevalence increasing steadily throughout adolescence.

Statistics from the National Institute of Mental Health indicate that nearly 20% of adolescents will suffer depression at some time, and on any given day approximately 2% of school-aged children and slightly more than 8% of adolescents will meet the criteria for major depression. In 2007, suicide was the leading cause of death in those aged 15–24 years (Forman-Hoffman et al. 2016).

Clinical Manifestations

People who suffer from depression experience dysphoria and have a sense of depleted energy and vitality. Adolescents may manifest depression by sickness behavior, school avoidance, excessive worry, or a feeling of being more moody than usual. Negativity, hopelessness, and guilt are also common, as are irritability, a critical and cynical nature, and the inability to concentrate. Adolescents with depression have a predilection for substance abuse and may have very disrupted sleep cycles with a tendency toward insomnia. Physically, energy levels are low and they tend to become weak, exhausted, and depleted even after doing small tasks. Somatic complaints are common. Suicidal ideation and completed suicide are risks (Forman-Hoffman et al. 2016).

Comorbidities

Depression causes a number of comorbidities which can become serious over time.

Some of the primary systems targeted include the cardiovascular system with hypertension and cardiovascular disease, weight gain, metabolic syndrome, diabetes, and obesity (Muhlig et al. 2016).

The interplay between depression and obesity is not fully understood, but is an area of active study. Adolescent girls who are depressed carry an increased risk of adult obesity, more so than depressed boys (Mihalopoulos and Spigarelli 2015).

Increased prevalence of chronic pain and sleep disorders, particularly decreased slow wave sleep, are frequently observed in adults with depression (Tesler et al. 2016).

Changes in sleep architecture in pediatric patients with depression have also been identified and remain an area of active study. Immune competency can be affected, predisposing to a variety of infectious illnesses.

Diagnostics Criteria

The signs and symptoms of depression can be subtle in their initial presentation in children and are outlined in the DSM-V. The faster the patient comes to treatment, generally the easier they are to treat. One of the challenges with depression is that signs and symptoms of depression overlap with those of other diseases, such as nutrient deficiency or a developing chronic illness, hence the patient should be worked up by a general physician to ascertain the diagnosis before (or concurrently with) mental health assessment. Family history is important as depression has an established hereditary link.

Treatment

Conventional Treatment

Classically, conventional therapy includes talk therapy, often in the form of cognitive behavioral therapy, and may involve antidepressants. Efficacy rates of the medications suggests only minimal to moderate effect. These medications also carry risk of serious side effects in the form of FDA black box warnings regarding suicidal thoughts, aggression, and risk of completed suicide (Sharma et al. 2016).

Medication also fails to address overall wellbeing, self-esteem, or quality of life measures and may encourage the child to view the pill as the cure, undermining their sense of self-efficacy (Spielmans and Gerwig 2014).

Integrative Treatment

Research on an integrative approach to depression in children and adolescents is still evolving, although some studies targeting lifestyle measures show encouraging promise. One of the challenging issues in those with depression is that summoning the energy to take even the smallest step in self-care can seem overwhelming. In children this can be made more complicated by comorbidity within the family dynamic and compounded by mental illness or poverty. Although not common as of yet, the idea of an integrative medical home would ideally serve as a hub to support development of a strong foundation of lifestyle practices from the earliest ages and help identify families in need of additional support. Lifestyle measures with the most robust supporting evidence in depression to date include exercise, nutrition, and sleep.

NUTRITION

Research is accruing on the benefit of a Mediterranean-type diet in depression in children that parallels that seen in adults where several meta-analyses have now shown an inverse and, in some studies, dose dependent correlation between Mediterranean diet pattern and depression (Psaltopoulou et al. 2013; Rahe, Unrath, and Berger 2014).

A systematic review of 12 pediatric articles (n = 82,779 children aged 4.5–18 years) by O'Neil and colleagues found a significant relationship between unhealthy diet patterns (Western diet, high intake of processed foods, sugary beverages) and mental health. Possible etiologies include lack of essential micronutrients, especially folate, magnesium, and zinc—each associated with depression in deficiency states.

The link with systemic inflammation, unhealthy diet and depression is also under active study in children. Confounders noted by authors included socioeconomic status which was not reported in all studies and variables in physical activity. Prospective longitudinal and intervention studies are needed to further pursue this important association (O'Neil et al. 2014).

An important point in considering nutrition in depression is the correlation with obesity, touched on above, to be sure the child and family have adequate information on meal balancing and portion control to avoid the development of overweight or obesity.

DIETARY SUPPLEMENTS

Omega-3 Fatty Acids   The inherent anti-inflammatory properties of the omega-3 fatty acids are believed to be in part responsible for their beneficial effects as demonstrated in some studies. Omega-3 fatty acids are also involved in neurotransmission and promotion of neuroplasticity, as well as in cell membrane integrity. Animal models have also shown that omega-3 fatty acids in models of depression have effects on serotonin and dopamine production and may have a role in influencing cortisol regulation (O'Neil et al. 2014).

Meta-analyses in adults have shown that higher ratios of EPA compared to DHA are associated with better outcomes in depression, although both EPA and DHA have shown benefit in various studies in adults.

In children, higher intake of omega-3 fatty acids in foods has shown mixed results in several studies, and to date randomized controlled trials of omega-3 fatty acid supplements are still needed. Low red blood cell omega-3 fatty acid levels have been repeatedly correlated with depressed mood. In particular, an association with low red cell DHA and SSRI resistant major depressive disorder in adolescents has been reported in a small study by McNamara. Improvement in depressive symptoms was seen with repletion in both low-dose and higher-dose omega-3 fatty acid treatment groups. Full remission of residual depressive symptoms was seen in the high-dose group (n = 7) (p < 0.0001) who received 16.2 grams per day of EPA 10.8 g + DHA 5.4 g over the 10-week study. A positive trend (p = 0.06) was seen in the low-dose treatment group (n = 10) 2.4 g/day of EPA 1.6 g + DHA 0.8 g. Fish oil supplement was shown to correct the red cell omega-3 fatty acid deficits. No serious adverse effects were seen (McNamara et al. 2014).

Further work in this area in pediatrics will hopefully provide further promising outcomes. Until more is known, encouraging mixed EPA/DHA omega-3 fatty acid intake either naturally in fish (one serving two to three times per week) or in supplement form (minimum ~1–2 grams per day in school-aged children) is a low risk and potentially high yield step in children with depression, in conjunction with a full evaluation and close clinical monitoring if on a conventional antidepressant.

S-Adenosyl Methionine (SAMe)   S-adenosyl methionine has been evaluated as a supplement in adult depression with some positive effects. It serves as a methyl donor for a variety of physiologic functions, including the methylation of neurotransmitters, but overall studies are lacking in children and adolescents. Because of its encouraging effects in adult depression, further studies in pediatrics are indicated. SAMe can precipitate anxiety and should not be used in those suspected of bipolar illness or with comorbid anxiety. SAMe might predispose to serotonin syndrome in an individual on an SSRI. Adult dose usually begins at 200 mg twice a day and gradually increases to a maximum of 1600 mg in three divided doses.

Adolescents have safely used doses of 400–1200 mg/day (O'Neil et al. 2014).

Vitamin D   Several studies have shown an association with insufficient vitamin D and depressive symptoms in children, but small study size and variable quality make definitive conclusions about routine supplementation for depression in children premature. Larger, randomized trials are needed to address questions about dosing, duration, and best candidates for supplementation. In general, ensuring a vitamin D level as measured by serum 25 OH D in the "sufficient" range (30–100 ng/mL) per U.S. Endocrine Society recommendations is a safe addition to the treatment plan (Hogberg et al. 2012).

B Vitamins   Well-controlled studies in adult depression evaluating the effects of B vitamins, including B9 (folate), B12, and B6, have shown benefit. The B vitamins play a role in neurotransmitter synthesis and many other key metabolic and mitochondrial functions. To date there is insufficient data on their use as supplements in children or adolescents with depression.

Overall given the paucity of research in the use of individual supplements to address pediatric depression, healthy whole food diets and use of a high-quality multivitamin to fill potential nutrition gaps appears to be an important approach. Further work will likely shed more light on how and when individual supplements might be of benefit and on their safety and long-term effects.

Vitamin C   A small study of vitamin C (1000 mg) has shown promise in pediatric depression as an adjunctive treatment to fluoxetine as compared to placebo. However, further studies are lacking to support broad recommendation (Amr et al. 2013).

Zinc   Zinc has shown some promise in adult depression but to date studies in children are also lacking.

BOTANICALS

St. John's wort (*Hypericum perforatum*) has shown some efficacy in the treatment of adult depression. It has been shown to be superior to placebo in some studies in major depression. Three open labeled trials have confirmed it to have equivalent efficacy to the SSRIs with fewer side effects in mild to moderate depression (Lopresti 2015).

Overall, in these adult studies, conclusions are limited by study quality and variable study design. St. John's wort can induce cytochrome P450 and subsequently may reduce the bioavailability of some drugs such as oral contraceptives and some immunosuppressants. It should not be taken with monoamine oxidase or serotonin reuptake inhibitors due to risk of serotonin syndrome (Qaseem et al. 2016).

At present there is a paucity of research on the use of St. John's wort in pediatric depression.

EXERCISE

A 2013 Cochrane Database Systematic Review of exercise in depression evaluated 37 trials involving 2326 adults and concluded that exercise was moderately more effective than a control intervention (Cooney et al. 2013).

A second review of 16 studies involving the use of exercise in 1191 children with depression or anxiety found a similar small overall positive effect, compounded by variable study design and quality. Overall, however, given the risks associated with antidepressants in children and young adults, maximizing all lifestyle elements, including exercise seems advisable. Yoga has shown some promise in children with depression in both school and community-based programs (Larun et al. 2006).

Another important element tied to exercise is time in nature with exposure to natural light. Although research is limited in children, some adult studies have demonstrated benefit in reduction of depressive symptoms.

Light therapy has also been used in the hospital setting to address depression. A pilot study of bright light therapy in hospitalized cystic fibrosis patients with mild or moderate depression using 10,000lx for 30 minutes daily for 7 consecutive days resulted in a significant decrease in depressive symptoms for all patients ($p < 0.0001$). No adverse effects were noted (Kopp et al. 2016).

Sleep disturbance is a common comorbidity in depression, and should be addressed in a comprehensive manner in children suffering with the condition. Evolving research on changes in slow wave sleep and its relationship with pediatric and adolescent depression precludes simplistic recommendations, but attention to basic sleep hygiene such as reduction of light at night, limiting stimulants such as caffeine, and child-directed bedtime routines are low-risk interventions that may be beneficial (Piotrowicz, Edlin, and McCartney 1985).

An important relationship has been established between sleep and cortical plasticity, which is a major process in adolescent brain development (Hobson and Pace-Schott 2002).

MIND–BODY THERAPIES

As seen in the developing literature on toxic stress and anxiety in school-aged children, use of mind–body therapies, particularly mindfulness, is the focus of active study in children and adolescents who have suffered trauma and ongoing high-level stressors. Mindfulness and other programs are being introduced into schools and communities to help children acquire an expanded skill set in self-regulatory skills (Sibinga et al. 2016).

Mastery of other mind–body skills ranging from simple breath work and progressive muscle relaxation to more complex use of clinical hypnosis or guided imagery sessions have potential to benefit children and adolescents with depression and encourage reduction of comorbid anxiety and enhancement of self-regulation skills. To date large studies are lacking in this area. Mind–body therapies are highly individualized and should be carefully selected in children and adolescents with depression to avoid precipitating re-experiencing of a prior trauma.

Another emerging thread of research is prevention of depression in high-risk youth by the introduction of long-term cognitive behavioral training in adolescents whose parents have a history of depression. In one study of 316 adolescents, eight weekly 90-minute sessions, and a follow-up of 6-monthly "continuation sessions," resulted in lower incidence of depression and a lower incidence of new depressive episodes in the first 9 months of the program. In this long-term study, benefits continued to be seen 6 years later (Brent et al. 2015).

Other techniques such as healing touch, therapeutic touch, and massage therapy may have a calming effect on the patient, but lack robust supporting evidence.

Summary

Depression is a common and serious condition in children that becomes more prevalent in adolescence and can persist throughout adult life. Identification of high-risk youth is critical, and early work in preventive behavioral interventions appears very encouraging. Prescription medications may be effective in some children, but are associated with a concerning risk of suicidal ideation and completed suicide and must therefore be used with due caution and close monitoring. Integrative approaches with the most robust support to date include healthy nutrition, exercise, and maximizing restorative sleep.

References

Adinolfi, B., and N. Gava. 2013. "Controlled outcome studies of child clinical hypnosis." *Acta Biomed* 84(2): 94–7.

Ahmadiafshar, A., A. Ghoreishi, S. Afkhami Ardakani, P. Khoshnevisasl, S. Faghihzadeh, and P. Nickmehr. 2016. "The high prevalence of depression among adolescents with asthma in Iran." *Psychosom Med* 78(1): 113–14. doi: 10.1097/PSY.0000000000000286.

American Academy of Pediatrics. "Bright Futures." https://brightfutures.aap.org/Pages/default. aspx.

Amr, M., A. El-Mogy, T. Shams, K. Vieira, and S. E. Lakhan. 2013. "Efficacy of vitamin C as an adjunct to fluoxetine therapy in pediatric major depressive disorder: a randomized, double-blind, placebo-controlled pilot study." *Nutr J* 12: 31. doi: 10.1186/1475-2891-12-31.

Andersen, L. P., M. Labriola, J. H. Andersen, T. Lund, and C. D. Hansen. 2015. "Bullied at school, bullied at work: a prospective study." *BMC Psychol* 3: 35. doi: 10.1186/s40359-015-0092-1.

Barth, J., L. Bermetz, E. Heim, S. Trelle, and T. Tonia. 2013. "The current prevalence of child sexual abuse worldwide: a systematic review and meta-analysis." *Int J Public Health* 58(3): 469–83. doi: 10.1007/s00038-012-0426-1.

Beltran, M., A. N. Brown-Elhillali, A. R. Held, P. C. Ryce, M. E. Ofonedu, D. W. Hoover, K. M. Ensor, and H. M. Belcher. 2016. "Yoga-based psychotherapy groups for boys exposed to trauma in urban settings." *Altern Ther Health Med* 22(1): 39–46.

Benson, H., J. F. Beary, and M. P. Carol. 1974. "The relaxation response." *Psychiatry* 37(1): 37–46.

Bernard, K., Z. Butzin-Dozier, J. Rittenhouse, and M. Dozier. 2010. "Cortisol production patterns in young children living with birth parents vs children placed in foster care following involvement of Child Protective Services." *Arch Pediatr Adolesc Med* 164(5): 438–43. doi: 10.1001/archpediatrics.2010.54.

Bickham, D. S., Y. Hswen, and M. Rich. 2015. "Media use and depression: exposure, household rules, and symptoms among young adolescents in the USA." *Int J Public Health* 60(2): 147–55. doi: 10.1007/s00038-014-0647-6.

Biddle, S. J., and M. Asare. 2011. "Physical activity and mental health in children and adolescents: a review of reviews." *Br J Sports Med* 45(11): 886–95. doi: 10.1136/bjsports-2011-090185.

Bonell, C., A. Fletcher, N. Fitzgerald-Yau, D. Hale, E. Allen, D. Elbourne, R. Jones, L. Bond, M. Wiggins, A. Miners, R. Legood, S. Scott, D. Christie, and R. Viner. 2015. "Initiating change locally in bullying and aggression through the school environment (INCLUSIVE): a pilot randomised controlled trial." *Health Technol Assess* 19(53): 1–109, vii–viii. doi: 10.3310/hta19530.

Brent, D. A., S. M. Brunwasser, S. D. Hollon, V. R. Weersing, G. N. Clarke, J. F. Dickerson, W. R. Beardslee, T. R. Gladstone, G. Porta, F. L. Lynch, S. Iyengar, and J. Garber. 2015. "Effect of a cognitive-behavioral prevention program on depression 6 years after implementation among at-risk adolescents: a randomized clinical trial." *JAMA Psychiatry* 72(11): 1110–18. doi: 10.1001/jamapsychiatry.2015.1559.

Bushnell, G. A., T. Sturmer, S. A. Swanson, D. White, D. Azrael, V. Pate, and M. Miller. 2015. "Dosing of selective serotonin reuptake inhibitors among children and adults before and after the FDA black-box warning." *Psychiatr Serv*. doi: 10.1176/appi.ps.201500088.

Buss, C., E. P. Davis, C. J. Hobel, and C. A. Sandman. 2011. "Maternal pregnancy-specific anxiety is associated with child executive function at 6–9 years age." *Stress* 14(6): 665–76. doi: 10.3109/10253890.2011.623250.

Buss, C., E. P. Davis, L. T. Muftuler, K. Head, and C. A. Sandman. 2010. "High pregnancy anxiety during mid-gestation is associated with decreased gray matter density in 6–9-year-old children." *Psychoneuroendocrinology* 35(1): 141–53. doi: 10.1016/j.psyneuen.2009.07.010.

Buss, C., S. Entringer, J. M. Swanson, and P. D. Wadhwa. 2012. "The role of stress in brain development: the gestational environment's long-term effects on the brain." *Cerebrum* 2012: 4.

Cantone, E., A. P. Piras, M. Vellante, A. Preti, S. Danielsdottir, E. D'Aloja, S. Lesinskiene, M. C.

Angermeyer, M. G. Carta, and D. Bhugra. 2015. "Interventions on bullying and cyberbullying in schools: a systematic review." *Clin Pract Epidemiol Ment Health* 11(Suppl 1 M4): 58–76. doi: 10.2174/1745017901511010058.

Caporino, N. E., K. L. Read, N. Shiffrin, C. Settipani, P. C. Kendall, S. N. Compton, J. Sherrill, J. Piacentini, J. Walkup, G. Ginsburg, C. Keeton, B. Birmaher, D. Sakolsky, E. Gosch, and A. M. Albano. 2015. "Sleep-related problems and the effects of anxiety treatment in children and adolescents." *J Clin Child Adolesc Psychol*: 1–11. doi: 10.1080/15374416.2015.1063429.

Carlier, I. V., J. G. Hovens, M. F. Streevelaar, Y. R. van Rood, and T. van Veen. 2016. "Characteristics of suicidal outpatients with mood, anxiety and somatoform disorders: the role of childhood abuse and neglect." *Int J Soc Psychiatry*. doi: 10.1177/0020764016629701.

Carroll, J. E., T. L. Gruenewald, S. E. Taylor, D. Janicki-Deverts, K. A. Matthews, and T. E. Seeman. 2013. "Childhood abuse, parental warmth, and adult multisystem biological risk in the Coronary Artery Risk Development in Young Adults study." *Proc Natl Acad Sci U S A* 110(42): 17149–53. doi: 10.1073/pnas.1315458110.

Cattaneo, A., F. Macchi, G. Plazzotta, B. Veronica, L. Bocchio-Chiavetto, M. A. Riva, and C. M. Pariante. 2015. "Inflammation and neuronal plasticity: a link between childhood trauma and depression pathogenesis." *Front Cell Neurosci* 9: 40. doi: 10.3389/fncel.2015.00040.

Cooney, G. M., K. Dwan, C. A. Greig, D. A. Lawlor, J. Rimer, F. R. Waugh, M. McMurdo, and G. E. Mead. 2013. "Exercise for depression." *Cochrane Database Syst Rev* 9: CD004366. doi: 10.1002/14651858.CD004366.pub6.

Cornacchio, D., K. I. Crum, S. Coxe, D. B. Pincus, and J. S. Comer. 2016. "Irritability and severity of anxious symptomatology among youth with anxiety disorders." *J Am Acad Child Adolesc Psychiatry* 55(1): 54–61. doi: 10.1016/j.jaac.2015.10.007.

Danese, A., T. E. Moffitt, H. Harrington, B. J. Milne, G. Polanczyk, C. M. Pariante, R. Poulton, and A. Caspi. 2009. "Adverse childhood experiences and adult risk factors for age-related disease: depression, inflammation, and clustering of metabolic risk markers." *Arch Pediatr Adolesc Med* 163(12): 1135–43. doi: 10.1001/archpediatrics.2009.214.

Danese, A., C. M. Pariante, A. Caspi, A. Taylor, and R. Poulton. 2007. "Childhood maltreatment predicts adult inflammation in a life-course study." *Proc Natl Acad Sci U S A* 104(4): 1319–24. doi: 10.1073/pnas.0610362104.

Dozier, M., M. Manni, M. K. Gordon, E. Peloso, M. R. Gunnar, K. C. Stovall-McClough, D. Eldreth, and S. Levine. 2006. "Foster children's diurnal production of cortisol: an exploratory study." *Child Maltreat* 11(2): 189–97. doi: 10.1177/1077559505285779.

Edwards, E., D. Mischoulon, M. Rapaport, B. Stussman, and W. Weber. 2013. "Building an evidence base in complementary and integrative healthcare for child and adolescent psychiatry." *Child Adolesc Psychiatr Clin N Am* 22(3): 509–29, vii. doi: 10.1016/j.chc.2013.03.007.

Entringer, S., C. Buss, and P. D. Wadhwa. 2015. "Prenatal stress, development, health and disease risk: a psychobiological perspective-2015 Curt Richter Award Paper." *Psychoneuroendocrinology* 62: 366–75. doi: 10.1016/j.psyneuen.2015.08.019.

Errington-Evans, N. 2012. "Acupuncture for anxiety." *CNS Neurosci Ther* 18(4): 277–84. doi: 10.1111/j.1755-5949.2011.00254.x.

Felitti, V. J., R. F. Anda, D. Nordenberg, D. F. Williamson, A. M. Spitz, V. Edwards, M. P. Koss, and J. S. Marks. 1998. "Relationship of childhood abuse and household dysfunction to many of the leading causes of death in adults. The Adverse Childhood Experiences (ACE) Study." *Am J Prev Med* 14(4): 245–58.

Field, T. 2014. "Massage therapy research review." *Complement Ther Clin Pract* 20(4): 224–9. doi: 10.1016/j.ctcp.2014.07.002.

Fisher, H. L., T. E. Moffitt, R. M. Houts, D. W. Belsky, L. Arseneault, and A. Caspi. 2012. "Bullying victimisation and risk of self harm in early adolescence: longitudinal cohort study." *BMJ* 344: e2683. doi: 10.1136/bmj.e2683.

Flaherty, E. G., J. Stirling, Jr., Abuse American Academy of Pediatrics. Committee on Child, and Neglect. 2010. "Clinical report: the pediatrician's role in child maltreatment prevention." *Pediatrics* 126(4): 833–41.

Flouri, E., E. Midouhas, and H. Joshi. 2014. "Family poverty and trajectories of children's emotional and behavioural problems: the moderating roles of self-regulation and verbal cognitive ability." *J Abnorm Child Psychol* 42(6): 1043–56. doi: 10.1007/s10802-013-9848-3.

Fonzo, G. A., H. J. Ramsawh, T. M. Flagan, A. N. Simmons, S. G. Sullivan, C. B. Allard, M. P. Paulus, and M. B. Stein. 2015. "Early life stress and the anxious brain: evidence for a neural mechanism linking childhood emotional maltreatment to anxiety in adulthood." *Psychol Med*: 1–18. doi: 10.1017/S0033291715002603.

Forman-Hoffman, V., E. McClure, J. McKeeman, C. T. Wood, J. C. Middleton, A. C. Skinner, E. M. Perrin, and M. Viswanathan. 2016. "Screening for major depressive disorder in children and adolescents: a systematic review for the U.S. Preventive Services Task Force." *Ann Intern Med*. doi: 10.7326/M15-2259.

Fries, A. B., E. A. Shirtcliff, and S. D. Pollak. 2008. "Neuroendocrine dysregulation following early social deprivation in children." *Dev Psychobiol* 50(6): 588–99. doi: 10.1002/dev.20319.

Gadomski, A. M., M. B. Scribani, N. Krupa, P. Jenkins, Z. Nagykaldi, and A. L. Olson. 2015. "Pet dogs and children's health: opportunities for chronic disease prevention?" *Prev Chronic Dis* 12: E205. doi: 10.5888/pcd12.150204.

Garner, A. S., J. P. Shonkoff, Child Committee on Psychosocial Aspects of, Health Family, Adoption Committee on Early Childhood, Care Dependent, Developmental Section on, and Pediatrics Behavioral. 2012. "Early childhood adversity, toxic stress, and the role of the pediatrician: translating developmental science into lifelong health." *Pediatrics* 129(1): e224–31. doi: 10.1542/peds.2011-2662.

Geoffroy, M. C., M. Boivin, L. Arseneault, G. Turecki, F. Vitaro, M. Brendgen, J. Renaud, J. R. Seguin, R. E. Tremblay, and S. M. Cote. 2016. "Associations between peer victimization and suicidal ideation and suicide attempt during adolescence: results from a prospective population-based birth cohort." *J Am Acad Child Adolesc Psychiatry* 55(2): 99–105. doi: 10.1016/j. jaac.2015.11.010.

Gorman-Smith, D., D. B. Henry, and P. H. Tolan. 2004. "Exposure to community violence and violence perpetration: the protective effects of family functioning." *J Clin Child Adolesc Psychol* 33(3): 439–49. doi: 10.1207/s15374424jccp3303_2.

Gromball, J., F. Beschorner, C. Wantzen, U. Paulsen, and M. Burkart. 2014. "Hyperactivity, concentration difficulties and impulsiveness improve during seven weeks' treatment with valerian root and lemon balm extracts in primary school children." *Phytomedicine* 21(8–9): 1098–103. doi: 10.1016/j.phymed.2014.04.004.

Hamm, M. P., A. S. Newton, A. Chisholm, J. Shulhan, A. Milne, P. Sundar, H. Ennis, S. D. Scott, and L. Hartling. 2015. "Prevalence and effect of cyberbullying on children and young people: a scoping review of social media studies." *JAMA Pediatr* 169(8): 770–7. doi: 10.1001/ jamapediatrics.2015.0944.

Han, D. H., S. M. Kim, S. Bae, P. F. Renshaw, and J. S. Anderson. 2016. "A failure of suppression within the default mode network in depressed adolescents with compulsive internet game play." *J Affect Disord* 194: 57–64. doi: 10.1016/j.jad.2016.01.013.

Harvard University. "Center on the Developing Child." http://www.developingchild.harvard.edu

Heberle, A. E., and A. S. Carter. 2015. "Cognitive aspects of young children's experience of economic disadvantage." *Psychol Bull* 141(4): 723–46. doi: 10.1037/bul0000010.

Hennessy, M. B., T. Deak, and P. A. Schiml-Webb. 2010. "Early attachment-figure separation and increased risk for later depression: potential mediation by proinflammatory processes." *Neurosci Biobehav Rev* 34(6): 782–90. doi: 10.1016/j.neubiorev.2009.03.012.

Hobson, J. A., and E. F. Pace-Schott. 2002. "The cognitive neuroscience of sleep: neuronal systems, consciousness and learning." *Nat Rev Neurosci* 3(9): 679–93. doi: 10.1038/nrn915.

Hogberg, G., S. A. Gustafsson, T. Hallstrom, T. Gustafsson, B. Klawitter, and M. Petersson. 2012. "Depressed adolescents in a case-series were low in vitamin D and depression was ameliorated by vitamin D supplementation." *Acta Paediatr* 101(7): 779–83. doi: 10.1111/j.1651-2227.2012.02655.x.

James, A. C., G. James, F. A. Cowdrey, A. Soler, and A. Choke. 2015. "Cognitive behavioural therapy for anxiety disorders in children and adolescents." *Cochrane Database Syst Rev* 2: CD004690. doi: 10.1002/14651858.CD004690.pub4.

Johnson, S. B., A. W. Riley, D. A. Granger, and J. Riis. 2013. "The science of early life toxic stress for pediatric practice and advocacy." *Pediatrics* 131(2): 319–27. doi: 10.1542/peds.2012-0469.

Juvonen, J., and S. Graham. 2014. "Bullying in schools: the power of bullies and the plight of victims." *Annu Rev Psychol* 65: 159–85. doi: 10.1146/annurev-psych-010213-115030.

Knowles, M., J. Rabinowich, S. Ettinger de Cuba, D. B. Cutts, and M. Chilton. 2016. "'Do you wanna breathe or eat?': parent perspectives on child health consequences of food insecurity, trade-offs, and toxic stress." *Matern Child Health J* 20(1): 25–32. doi: 10.1007/s10995-015-1797-8.

Kopp, B. T., D. Hayes, Jr., P. Ghera, A. Patel, S. Kirkby, R. A. Kowatch, and M. Splaingard. 2016. "Pilot trial of light therapy for depression in hospitalized patients with cystic fibrosis." *J Affect Disord* 189: 164–8. doi: 10.1016/j.jad.2015.08.056.

Kovacs, M., T. L. Feinberg, M. A. Crouse-Novak, S. L. Paulauskas, and R. Finkelstein. 1984. "Depressive disorders in childhood. I. A longitudinal prospective study of characteristics and recovery." *Arch Gen Psychiatry* 41(3): 229–37.

Lahey, B. B., S. S. Lee, M. H. Sibley, B. Applegate, B. S. Molina, and W. E. Pelham. 2016. "Predictors of adolescent outcomes among 4–6-year-old children with attention-deficit/hyperactivity disorder." *J Abnorm Psychol* 125(2): 168–81. doi: 10.1037/abn0000086.

Larun, L., L. V. Nordheim, E. Ekeland, K. B. Hagen, and F. Heian. 2006. "Exercise in prevention and treatment of anxiety and depression among children and young people." *Cochrane Database Syst Rev* 3: CD004691. doi: 10.1002/14651858.CD004691.pub2.

Lereya, S. T., W. E. Copeland, E. J. Costello, and D. Wolke. 2015. "Adult mental health consequences of peer bullying and maltreatment in childhood: two cohorts in two countries." *Lancet Psychiatry* 2(6): 524–31. doi: 10.1016/S2215-0366(15)00165-0.

Lopresti, A. L. 2015. "A review of nutrient treatments for paediatric depression." *J Affect Disord* 181: 24–32. doi: 10.1016/j.jad.2015.04.014.

Lopresti, A. L., S. D. Hood, and P. D. Drummond. 2013. "A review of lifestyle factors that contribute to important pathways associated with major depression: diet, sleep and exercise." *J Affect Disord* 148(1): 12–27. doi: 10.1016/j.jad.2013.01.014.

Lowe, K., C. Escoffery, A. C. Mertens, and C. J. Berg. 2015. "Distinct health behavior and psychosocial profiles of young adult survivors of childhood cancers: a mixed methods study." *J Cancer Surviv*. doi: 10.1007/s11764-015-0508-1.

Macy, R. J., E. Jones, L. M. Graham, and L. Roach. 2015. "Yoga for trauma and related mental health problems: a meta-review with clinical and service recommendations." *Trauma Violence Abuse*. doi: 10.1177/1524838015620834.

Mangiola, F., G. Ianiro, F. Franceschi, S. Fagiuoli, G. Gasbarrini, and A. Gasbarrini. 2016. "Gut microbiota in autism and mood disorders." *World J Gastroenterol* 22(1): 361–8. doi: 10.3748/wjg.v22.i1.361.

McClafferty, H. 2011. "Complementary, holistic, and integrative medicine: mind-body medicine." *Pediatr Rev* 32(5): 201–3. doi: 10.1542/pir.32-5-201.

McEwen, B. S., L. Eiland, R. G. Hunter, and M. M. Miller. 2012. "Stress and anxiety: structural plasticity and epigenetic regulation as a consequence of stress." *Neuropharmacology* 62(1): 3–12. doi: 10.1016/j.neuropharm.2011.07.014.

McNamara, R. K., J. Strimpfel, R. Jandacek, T. Rider, P. Tso, J. A. Welge, J. R. Strawn, and M. P. Delbello. 2014. "Detection and treatment of long-chain omega-3 fatty acid deficiency in adolescents with SSRI-resistant major depressive disorder." *PharmaNutrition* 2(2): 38–46. doi: 10.1016/j.phanu.2014.02.002.

Merikangas, K. R., J. P. He, M. Burstein, S. A. Swanson, S. Avenevoli, L. Cui, C. Benjet, K.

Georgiades, and J. Swendsen. 2010. "Lifetime prevalence of mental disorders in U.S. adolescents: results from the National Comorbidity Survey Replication—Adolescent Supplement (NCS-A)." *J Am Acad Child Adolesc Psychiatry* 49(10): 980–9. doi: 10.1016/j.jaac.2010.05.017.

Mihalopoulos, N. L., and M. G. Spigarelli. 2015. "Comanagement of pediatric depression and obesity: a clear need for evidence." *Clin Ther* 37(9): 1933–7. doi: 10.1016/j.clinthera.2015.08.009.

Miller, G. E., E. Chen, and K. J. Parker. 2011. "Psychological stress in childhood and susceptibility to the chronic diseases of aging: moving toward a model of behavioral and biological mechanisms." *Psychol Bull* 137(6): 959–97. doi: 10.1037/a0024768.

Miller-Lewis, L. R., A. K. Searle, M. G. Sawyer, P. A. Baghurst, and D. Hedley. 2013. "Resource factors for mental health resilience in early childhood: an analysis with multiple methodologies." *Child Adolesc Psychiatry Ment Health* 7(1): 6. doi: 10.1186/1753-2000-7-6.

Mitchell, S. J., A. Lewin, A. Rasmussen, I. B. Horn, and J. G. Joseph. 2011. "Maternal distress explains the relationship of young African American mothers' violence exposure with their preschoolers' behavior." *J Interpers Violence* 26(3): 580–603. doi: 10.1177/0886260510363423.

Mohler-Kuo, M., M. A. Landolt, T. Maier, U. Meidert, V. Schonbucher, and U. Schnyder. 2014. "Child sexual abuse revisited: a population-based cross-sectional study among Swiss adolescents." *J Adolesc Health* 54(3): 304–11 e1. doi: 10.1016/j.jadohealth.2013.08.020.

Muhlig, Y., J. Antel, M. Focker, and J. Hebebrand. 2016. "Are bidirectional associations of obesity and depression already apparent in childhood and adolescence as based on high-quality studies? A systematic review." *Obes Rev* 17(3): 235–49. doi: 10.1111/obr.12357.

Mukai, T., T. Kishi, Y. Matsuda, and N. Iwata. 2014. "A meta-analysis of inositol for depression and anxiety disorders." *Hum Psychopharmacol* 29(1): 55–63. doi: 10.1002/hup.2369.

Muller, S. F., and S. Klement. 2006. "A combination of valerian and lemon balm is effective in the treatment of restlessness and dyssomnia in children." *Phytomedicine* 13(6): 383–7. doi: 10.1016/j.phymed.2006.01.013.

Muris, P., C. Meesters, A. Pierik, and B. de Kock. 2016. "Good for the self: self-compassion and other self-related constructs in relation to symptoms of anxiety and depression in non-clinical youths." *J Child Fam Stud* 25: 607–17. doi: 10.1007/s10826-015-0235-2.

Narayanan, A., and L. R. Betts. 2014. "Bullying behaviors and victimization experiences among adolescent students: the role of resilience." *J Genet Psychol* 175(1–2): 134–46. doi: 10.1080/00221325.2013.834290.

National Center for Infants, Toddlers, and Families. "Zero to Three." http://www.zerotothree.org

O'Neil, A., S. E. Quirk, S. Housden, S. L. Brennan, L. J. Williams, J. A. Pasco, M. Berk, and F. N. Jacka. 2014. "Relationship between diet and mental health in children and adolescents: a systematic review." *Am J Public Health* 104(10): e31–42. doi: 10.2105/AJPH.2014.302110.

Olness, K. 1996. "Hypnosis and biofeedback with children and adolescents; clinical, research, and educational aspects. Introduction." *J Dev Behav Pediatr* 17(5): 299.

Piotrowicz, B. I., S. E. Edlin, and A. C. McCartney. 1985. "A sensitive chromogenic Limulus amoebocyte lysate micro-assay for detection of endotoxin in human plasma and in water." *Zentralbl Bakteriol Mikrobiol Hyg A* 260(1): 108–12.

Polanczyk, G. V., G. A. Salum, L. S. Sugaya, A. Caye, and L. A. Rohde. 2015. "Annual research review: a meta-analysis of the worldwide prevalence of mental disorders in children and adolescents." *J Child Psychol Psychiatry* 56(3): 345–65. doi: 10.1111/jcpp.12381.

Preter, M., and D. F. Klein. 2014. "Lifelong opioidergic vulnerability through early life separation: a recent extension of the false suffocation alarm theory of panic disorder." *Neurosci Biobehav Rev* 46 Pt 3: 345–51. doi: 10.1016/j.neubiorev.2014.03.025.

Psaltopoulou, T., T. N. Sergentanis, D. B. Panagiotakos, I. N. Sergentanis, R. Kosti, and N. Scarmeas. 2013. "Mediterranean diet, stroke, cognitive impairment, and depression: a meta-analysis." *Ann Neurol* 74(4): 580–91. doi: 10.1002/ana.23944.

Qaseem, A., M. J. Barry, D. Kansagara, and Physicians Clinical Guidelines Committee of the American College of. 2016. "Nonpharmacologic versus pharmacologic treatment of adult patients with major depressive disorder: a clinical practice guideline from the American College of Physicians." *Ann Intern Med*. doi: 10.7326/M15-2570.

Rahe, C., M. Unrath, and K. Berger. 2014. "Dietary patterns and the risk of depression in adults: a systematic review of observational studies." *Eur J Nutr* 53(4): 997–1013. doi: 10.1007/s00394-014-0652-9.

Rivers, I. 2012. "Morbidity among bystanders of bullying behavior at school: concepts, concerns, and clinical/research issues." *Int J Adolesc Med Health* 24(1): 11–16. doi: 10.1515/ijamh.2012.003.

Rodgers, J., S. Wigham, H. McConachie, M. Freeston, E. Honey, and J. R. Parr. 2016. "Development of the anxiety scale for children with autism spectrum disorder (ASC-ASD)." *Autism Res*. doi: 10.1002/aur.1603.

Rose, C. A., and B. M. Tynes. 2015. "Longitudinal associations between cybervictimization and mental health among U.S. adolescents." *J Adolesc Health* 57(3): 305–12. doi: 10.1016/j.jadohealth.2015.05.002.

Rosen, L., A. French, G. Sullivan, and Ryt. 2015. "Complementary, holistic, and integrative medicine: yoga." *Pediatr Rev* 36(10): 468–74. doi: 10.1542/pir.36-10-468.

Rudolph, K. D., J. E. Lansford, A. M. Agoston, N. Sugimura, D. Schwartz, K. A. Dodge, G. S. Pettit, and J. E. Bates. 2014. "Peer victimization and social alienation: predicting deviant peer affiliation in middle school." *Child Dev* 85(1): 124–39. doi: 10.1111/cdev.12112.

Rutter, M. 2013. "Annual Research Review: resilience—clinical implications." *J Child Psychol Psychiatry* 54(4): 474–87. doi: 10.1111/j.1469-7610.2012.02615.x.

Saarento, S., A. J. Boulton, and C. Salmivalli. 2015. "Reducing bullying and victimization: student- and classroom-level mechanisms of change." *J Abnorm Child Psychol* 43(1): 61–76. doi: 10.1007/s10802-013-9841-x.

Sakolsky, D. J., J. T. McCracken, and E. L. Nurmi. 2012. "Genetics of pediatric anxiety disorders." *Child Adolesc Psychiatr Clin N Am* 21(3): 479–500. doi: 10.1016/j.chc.2012.05.010.

Schor, E. L., and Family American Academy of Pediatrics Task Force on the. 2003. "Family pediatrics: report of the Task Force on the Family." *Pediatrics* 111(6 Pt 2): 1541–71.

Sharma, T., L. S. Guski, N. Freund, and P. C. Gotzsche. 2016. "Suicidality and aggression during antidepressant treatment: systematic review and meta-analyses based on clinical study reports." *BMJ* 352: i65. doi: 10.1136/bmj.i65.

Shonkoff, J. P., A. S. Garner, Child Committee on Psychosocial Aspects of, Health Family, Adoption Committee on Early Childhood, Care Dependent, Developmental Section on, and Pediatrics Behavioral. 2012. "The lifelong effects of early childhood adversity and toxic stress." *Pediatrics* 129(1): e232–46. doi: 10.1542/peds.2011-2663.

Sibinga, E. M., L. Webb, S. R. Ghazarian, and J. M. Ellen. 2016. "School-based mindfulness instruction: an RCT." *Pediatrics* 137(1): 1–8. doi: 10.1542/peds.2015-2532.

Siegel, R. S., and D. P. Dickstein. 2012. "Anxiety in adolescents: update on its diagnosis and treatment for primary care providers." *Adolesc Health Med Ther* 3: 1–16. doi: 10.2147/AHMT.S7597.

Simpson, T. E., E. Condon, R. M. Price, B. K. Finch, L. S. Sadler, and M. R. Ordway. 2016. "Demystifying infant mental health: what the primary care provider needs to know." *J Pediatr Health Care* 30(1): 38–48. doi: 10.1016/j.pedhc.2015.09.011.

Singh, O., Z. Khanam, N. Misra, and M. K. Srivastava. 2011. "Chamomile (Matricaria chamomilla L.): an overview." *Pharmacogn Rev* 5(9): 82–95. doi: 10.4103/0973-7847.79103.

Slopen, N., K. A. McLaughlin, E. C. Dunn, and K. C. Koenen. 2013. "Childhood adversity and cell-mediated immunity in young adulthood: does type and timing matter?" *Brain Behav Immun* 28: 63–71. doi: 10.1016/j.bbi.2012.10.018.

Spielmans, G. I., and K. Gerwig. 2014. "The efficacy of antidepressants on overall well-being and self-reported depression symptom severity in youth: a meta-analysis." *Psychother Psychosom* 83(3): 158–64. doi: 10.1159/000356191.

Sternthal, M. J., M. B. Enlow, S. Cohen, M. J. Canner, J. Staudenmayer, K. Tsang, and R. J.

Wright. 2009. "Maternal interpersonal trauma and cord blood IgE levels in an inner-city cohort: a life-course perspective." *J Allergy Clin Immunol* 124(5): 954–60. doi: 10.1016/j.jaci.2009.07.030.

Stevens, G. W., S. D. Walsh, T. Huijts, M. Maes, K. R. Madsen, F. Cavallo, and M. Molcho. 2015. "An internationally comparative study of immigration and adolescent emotional and behavioral problems: effects of generation and gender." *J Adolesc Health* 57(6): 587–94. doi: 10.1016/j.jadohealth.2015.07.001.

Szabo, S., Y. Tache, and A. Somogyi. 2012. "The legacy of Hans Selye and the origins of stress research: a retrospective 75 years after his landmark brief 'letter' to the editor# of nature." *Stress* 15(5): 472–8. doi: 10.3109/10253890.2012.710919.

Tesler, N., M. Gerstenberg, M. Franscini, O. G. Jenni, S. Walitza, and R. Huber. 2016. "Increased frontal sleep slow wave activity in adolescents with major depression." *Neuroimage Clin* 10: 250–6. doi: 10.1016/j.nicl.2015.10.014.

Thompson, R. A. 2014. "Stress and child development." *Future Child* 24(1): 41–59.

Tunnard, C., L. J. Rane, S. C. Wooderson, K. Markopoulou, L. Poon, A. Fekadu, M. Juruena, and A. J. Cleare. 2014. "The impact of childhood adversity on suicidality and clinical course in treatment-resistant depression." *J Affect Disord* 152–154: 122–30. doi: 10.1016/j.jad.2013.06.037.

Valentino, K., A. K. Nuttall, M. Comas, J. G. Borkowski, and C. E. Akai. 2012. "Intergenerational continuity of child abuse among adolescent mothers: authoritarian parenting, community violence, and race." *Child Maltreat* 17(2): 172–81. doi: 10.1177/1077559511434945.

Valji, R., D. Adams, S. Dagenais, T. Clifford, L. Baydala, W. J. King, and S. Vohra. 2013. "Complementary and alternative medicine: a survey of its use in pediatric oncology." *Evid Based Complement Alternat Med* 2013: 527163. doi: 10.1155/2013/527163.

van der Heijden, M. J., S. Oliai Araghi, M. van Dijk, J. Jeekel, and M. G. Hunink. 2015. "The effects of perioperative music interventions in pediatric surgery: a systematic review and meta-analysis of randomized controlled trials." *PLoS One* 10(8): e0133608. doi: 10.1371/journal.pone.0133608.

van Tilburg, M. A., R. L. Claar, J. M. Romano, S. L. Langer, L. S. Walker, W. E. Whitehead, B. Abdullah, D. L. Christie, and R. L. Levy. 2015. "Role of coping with symptoms in depression and disability: comparison between inflammatory bowel disease and abdominal pain." *J Pediatr Gastroenterol Nutr* 61(4): 431–6. doi: 10.1097/MPG.0000000000000841.

Vaz, S., M. Falkmer, M. Ciccarelli, A. Passmore, R. Parsons, T. Tan, and T. Falkmer. 2015. "The personal and contextual contributors to school belongingness among primary school students." *PLoS One* 10(4): e0123353. doi: 10.1371/journal.pone.0123353.

Wang, W., T. Vaillancourt, H. L. Brittain, P. McDougall, A. Krygsman, D. Smith, C. E. Cunningham, J. D. Haltigan, and S. Hymel. 2014. "School climate, peer victimization, and academic achievement: results from a multi-informant study." *Sch Psychol Q* 29(3): 360–77. doi: 10.1037/spq0000084.

Weaver, L. L., and A. R. Darragh. 2015. "Systematic review of yoga interventions for anxiety reduction among children and adolescents." *Am J Occup Ther* 69(6): 6906180070p1–9. doi: 10.5014/ajot.2015.020115.

Webster, J. I., L. Tonelli, and E. M. Sternberg. 2002. "Neuroendocrine regulation of immunity." *Annu Rev Immunol* 20: 125–63. doi: 10.1146/annurev.immunol.20.082401.104914.

Webster, Merriam. http://www.merriam-webster.com/dictionary/resilience.

20 Neurodevelopmental Disorders: ADHD and Autism

Attention-Deficit/Hyperactivity Disorder (ADHD)

Overview

Attention-deficit/hyperactivity disorder (ADHD) is considered one the most common neurodevelopmental disorders in children and was one of the first psychiatric diagnoses to be labeled and treated in children. Use of stimulant medication in children was introduced in 1937. ADHD persists into adulthood in an estimated 50% of individuals (Goldman et al. 1998).

National Health Interview Survey data shows the prevalence at 11% of children aged 4–17 years in the United States, an increase of 42% over the time span 2003–2011. This accounts for an estimated increase of approximately 2 million children living with the diagnosis over a relatively short time span. An estimated 69% of these children were reported to be taking medication for the condition in 2011 (Visser et al. 2014).

The disorder is characterized by chronic, pervasive, and impairing inattention, impulsivity, emotional lability, and hyperactivity that occurs consistently in more than one setting; for example, both at school and at home. ADHD can have a significant negative impact on a child's life. Integrative options are important in ADHD for several reasons, among them the fact that even with combined medical and psychiatric treatment, more than 30% of children remain symptomatic (Swanson et al. 2001).

Etiology

The etiology of ADHD has not been clearly delineated, although a variety of factors have been found to be associated, such as: a genetic predisposition, epigenetic factors, prenatal exposures to alcohol, tobacco, lead, pesticides, bisphenol A, and chronic maternal stress (Thapar et al. 2013).

Environmental exposures to certain pyrethroid pesticides have also been associated with ADHD diagnosis, in males more than females. These are the class of pesticides most commonly used currently in residential and public health control of vector-borne disease, also widely used in agricultural spraying. Animal studies have shown correlation between these pesticides and hyperactive behavior (Wagner-Schuman et al. 2015).

Human data reflects this association. Data from the 2001–2002 National Health and Nutrition Examination Survey including 687 children aged 8–15 years old showed a dose response relationship between urinary pesticide metabolite excretion and hyperactive-impulsive symptoms in a ratio of 50% worsening of symptoms for every 10-fold increase in urinary metabolite level (Wagner-Schuman et al. 2015).

Other possible etiologies for ADHD proposed include dietary factors, although studies have shown that only approximately 8% of children with ADHD have true food sensitivity (Millichap and Yee 2012). Sugar had been long been suspected as a primary causative factor, but no link has been identified in more recent studies (Nigg et al. 2012).

Several micronutrient deficiencies have been studied as possible etiologic factors, including: zinc, magnesium, and ferritin. Although none have been identified as direct causative factors, they may have some role in treatment in certain subsets of children and are discussed in more detail below (Nigg et al. 2012).

Ultimately a definitive etiology remains unclear and is likely to be a multifactorial combination of genetic predisposition, environment, and social factors.

Prevalence

ADHD is estimated to affect approximately 11% of children in the U.S., a significant increase over the past decade (Visser et al. 2014).

Global prevalence of ADHD was estimated to be approximately 5.5% from statistics sourced for the 2013 Global Burden of Disease Study, but deficits in available data, especially in sub-Saharan Africa, highlight many data gaps. Of the 187 countries surveyed, 124 had no data available on any mental health disorder (Erskine et al. 2016).

Clinical Manifestations

ADHD-affected children can be overtly active, highly sensitive, distractible, and impulsive. Younger children may be disruptive, engage in very active play, and aggravate teachers and classmates if not redirected. Forgetfulness is common, and can lead to confusion and anxiety, especially in the school setting when assignments and homework may become scattered and they may present as chronically late and disorganized (Visser et al. 2014; Gray et al. 2015).

Interrupting conversations and difficulty in social situations are common. They are also seen to be bored of one thing, appear inquisitive and restless, and quick to drop one activity for another. They are often socially awkward, and may become socially isolated for this reason. On the other hand, symptoms of ADHD can be associated with high creativity, energy, and drive. A range of lay resources are available to help children, adolescents, and adults living with ADHD connect socially and find academic settings and careers where their unique strengths can be used to greatest advantage.

Comorbidities

A number of mental and physical comorbidities have been associated with ADHD. One important connection is a link with obesity. ADHD has frequently been associated with irritability, depression, anxiety, and sleep disorders—especially short sleep duration insomnia associated with delayed onset of melatonin release, all of which compound obesity risk. In patients not on medication, ADHD has been related to binge eating and impulsiveness, meal skipping due to poor planning, short sleep duration and subsequent craving of carbohydrate-rich foods, and may be related to addictive behaviors, in particular through dysregulation of dopamine (Tanofsky-Kraff and Yanovski 2004).

Starting a stimulant prescription has been related to a 2–3 kg drop in weight, which appears to be self-limited in the absence of additional changes to diet and lifestyle habits in those who are overweight or obese. Assistance with meal planning and life-style change has been associated with healthy weight loss in some studies (Kooij 2016).

A large systematic review and meta-analysis by Cortese et al. in more than 48,000 adults and children showed an increased risk for obesity over time in those with ADHD. Those who were treated for ADHD with stimulant medication reduced their obesity risk back to that of the general population, clarifying two important points: untreated ADHD symptoms can drive obesity, and the combined treatment of ADHD and obesity appear to be more effective than treatment of obesity alone—meaning that overweight and obese individuals must be carefully screened for ADHD, and if present, early treatment of ADHD should be considered in conjunction with comprehensive approach to obesity lifestyle treatment if lifestyle measures alone are unsuccessful (Cortese et al. 2016).

Preliminary data in children analyzed from ongoing research by Nigg and colleagues examining pediatric data only in 43 studies in children and adolescents found a significantly smaller association with ADHD and obesity, although adolescent girls with depression and conduct disorder remained at higher risk (Nigg et al. 2016).

Overall, although research is still accruing, current information points to a need for increased awareness and early reinforcement of healthy lifestyle measures in children both at risk for and diagnosed with ADHD (Kooij 2016).

An estimated 50%–70% of children with ADHD have an externalizing disorder (oppositional defiant disorder, conduct disorder) and an estimated 64% present with an internalizing disorder (depression, anxiety, separation anxiety, social phobia, obsessive-compulsive disorder). Externalizing behaviors have been associated with higher levels of peer relationships, and internalizing behaviors were associated with poorer family quality of life (Armstrong et al. 2015).

Armstrong and colleagues found that children with co-existing externalizing and internalizing behaviors had an especially difficult time, related to higher reporting of peer-related problems, difficulties with daily functioning, and an overall worse quality of life measure, independent of severity of ADHD symptoms (Armstrong et al. 2015).

Comorbid anxiety in children has been associated with high levels of maternal anxiety, overprotectiveness, and a lack of positive parenting skills, reinforcing the importance of assessment of the overall family dynamic in treatment (Pfiffner and McBurnett 2006).

Clinically impairing irritability has been reported in 25%–45% of children with ADHD (Fernandez de la Cruz et al. 2015). Bullying behavior, and bully victimization, are also prevalent in children with ADHD (Verlinden et al. 2015).

ADHD is associated with increased risk of suicidal ideation and completed suicide, seen in 12% of a study of 287 adolescents in a study of Taiwanese adolescents by Chou and colleagues (Chou et al. 2016).

Traumatic injuries, increased risk of physical and sexual abuse, and eating disorder are also important comorbidities that may trigger diagnosis (Pon et al. 2015).

Diagnostic Criteria

ADHD can be difficult to diagnose clinically and often takes input from a variety of sources such as teachers, parents, and tutors. One of the challenges is that children go through many behavioral, psychological, and physical changes in the course of normal development, and may naturally become impatient or encounter frustration at not being able to master a developmentally inappropriate task. These behaviors may mimic ADHD, but the differentiating factor is that they are not sustained (Visser et al. 2014).

For this reason, a detailed history is needed to establish normal developmental milestones, and to rule out precipitating factors such as physical, sexual, or emotional abuse, or school bullying. Mental health assessment is usually indicated, and referral is common, ideally to a mental health professional specializing in this pediatric ADHD. To confirm an ADHD diagnosis, symptoms must persist for at least 6 months and reach a level of severity that interrupts daily activity in more than one setting. Diagnosis often involves collaboration between parent, teacher, and pediatrician (Armstrong et al. 2015).

Competing diagnosis must be ruled out, which may involve screening for low ferritin, zinc, and red blood cell magnesium which have each been associated with worsening of ADHD symptoms in certain subsets of children (Villagomez 2014).

Although pesticide exposure has been associated with ADHD symptoms, it has not been categorized as a diagnostic factor and routine screening is not currently recommended. It is conceivable that this may change in the future as compelling research continues to accrue correlating urinary pesticide metabolite levels to ADHD (Wagner-Schuman et al. 2015; Richardson et al. 2015).

To date ADHD remains a clinical diagnosis often made with input from teachers and parents, but emerging technologies are beginning to allow expansion of the diagnostic capabilities in many neuropsychiatric disorders, including ADHD. Multimodal neuroimaging, a combination of magnetic resonance imaging (MRI), positron emission tomography (PET), electroencephalography (EEG), and magnetoencephalography (MEG), allows measurement of changes on a scale that was previously impossible. Early research shows changes in functional brain metabolism and neural activity (functional MRI, PET, and EEG/MEG) and brain anatomy and neural fiber tracts (structural MRI and diffusion MRI). Other conditions under study include epilepsy, stroke, obsessive-compulsive disorder, autism, bipolar disorder and others. Some of the abnormalities that may be seen in children with ADHD include decreased total brain volume and changes in predictable brain regions. Emerging data suggests evidence of disruption of interconnected structural networks in the white matter of the developing brain (Liu et al. 2015).

Treatments

Treatment is highly individualized and may include a variety of approaches with the overarching goal of minimizing dysfunction and improving overall quality of life at home and at school (Fernandez de la Cruz et al. 2015).

It is a sobering fact that 30% of children will remain symptomatic even despite well-established conventional treatment (Visser et al. 2014).

Conventional Treatment

Conventional treatment often includes the use of prescription medication. The primary categories of medications used are psychostimulants that, somewhat paradoxically, refer to drugs that help bring stability and calmness in the patient. Commonly used stimulants include amphetamine and methylphenidate, but they are not without side effects, including: abuse, dependence, tolerability, growth delay, insomnia, restless sleep, hallucinations, indigestion, overeating, weight loss and loss of appetite (Childress 2016).

If the side effects remain persistent, consultation may result in a medication change, which is relatively frequent among children with ADHD. Non-stimulant options include atomoxetine, FDA approved for use in children in 2002, which now accounts for an estimated 6% of prescriptions for pediatric ADHD. Studies have shown improvement in quality of life and reduction in some comorbidities; however, clinical improvements are not necessarily sustained. Studies to date have not reported growth delay or interference with sexual development (Childress 2016).

Despite some reports of success, many children with ADHD continue to have significant impairment on a day-to-day basis, even on mono- or poly-pharmaceutical treatment (Baweja et al. 2016).

Conventional treatment typically also involves counseling, and may include behavioral classes to help the child become more socially adept. Parenting programs are also used in a comprehensive model of treatment (Fernandez de la Cruz et al. 2015).

It should be kept in mind that there is no one specific treatment-cure for ADHD. The use of pharmaceutical medications may help reduce the symptoms and comorbidities of ADHD, smooth social interactions, and steer children toward improved school performance. Medications, while not always needed, may also serve as a bridge as lifestyle changes and integrative treatments are implemented.

Integrative Treatment

An integrative approach can be used alone or as a complement to conventional treatment to help bring more peace, control, organization, and confidence into a child's life. The approach of practicing healthy lifestyle in a healthy environment resonates especially well in the treatment of ADHD where so many opportunities exist to make a significant difference in a child and family's quality of life.

NUTRITION

In general families should strive to provide a diet made with as many high-quality whole foods as possible. Ideally foods with artificial colors and flavors would be eliminated, and fresh foods would be sourced from local organic grocers. In reality of course this is rarely the case, but parents can be taught to become more savvy food label readers and learn to avoid foods high in pesticides and those with an ingredient list filled with unrecognizable chemicals (Nigg and Holton 2014).

A review of the literature by Nigg and colleagues concludes that dietary interventions for ADHD have a less than 50–50 chance for succeeding. They may also be very challenging for the family to undertake, although they may still very useful in some children (Nigg and Holton 2014).

For example, the Impact of Nutrition on Children with ADHD (INCA) study, a randomized controlled trial in two stages, open-label with masked measurements followed by a double-blind crossover in 100 children aged 4–8 years in the Netherlands and Belgium, saw a significant improvement in the initial treatment group after 5 weeks ($p<0.0001$), and a significant relapse rate in the second challenge phase ($p<0.0001$). In the challenge phase, 63% of the children had relapse of symptoms, regardless of whether their IgG blood levels were high or low to the specific foods eaten. Authors reinforced the lack of efficacy of the IgG testing, and stated that a strictly supervised elimination diet may serve as a valuable aid in diagnosing food-driven ADHD symptoms (Pelsser et al. 2011).

If true food allergy is suspected, formal evaluation with an allergist is indicated for controlled challenge to avoid possible serious reactions.

In summary, a general shift to a healthier diet should be encouraged for all children with ADHD. Food additives should be eliminated as a trial (Millichap and Yee 2012), especially artificial colors, as it appears that approximately 8% of children with ADHD have reproducible sensitivity to artificial colors and preservatives. Despite popular belief to the contrary, sugar intake, per se, has not been shown to be specifically correlated with ADHD symptoms (Millichap and Yee 2012).

The correlation between obesity and ADHD discussed above is an important reason to monitor nutrition in a balanced and non-punitive manner. This may require collaboration with a registered dietician who can help ensure adequate intake of calories, and of critical micronutrients, especially of iron, magnesium, and zinc.

DIETARY SUPPLEMENTS

Several dietary supplements under active study in ADHD including ferritin, zinc, magnesium, vitamin D, and omega-3 fatty acids. While none have enough evidence to recommend as a sole treatment strategy in all children with ADHD, each has shown promise in certain subsets of patients. A detailed review can be found in a 2014 review by Villagomez and Ramtekkar (Villagomez 2014).

Ferritin Briefly, ferritin is integral to the synthesis of a variety of both dopamine and catecholamines. Ferritin is a reliable biomarker for peripheral iron stores, and low levels have been associated in some studies with ADHD. One of the few randomized controlled placebo trials in children with ADHD was a study of 23 children with ADHD identified as having low ferritin (< 30 ng/mL). Replacement with 80 mg elemental iron resulted in measurable improvement in the study group (Konofal et al. 2008).

Review of the literature confirms mixed results in other studies and a need for larger trials, but it is a reasonable and low-risk step to screen for and correct low ferritin in children and adolescents with ADHD (Cortese et al. 2012).

Zinc The interplay between zinc and ADHD is not fully understood, although zinc is intricately involved as a cofactor in hundreds of enzymes and plays an important role in immune, neurologic, and inflammatory processes. It is also a necessary component of vitamin B6 synthesis, a critical step in the manufacture of serotonin and melatonin, and is necessary in the regulation of dopamine transport used by many of the prescription psychostimulants used in ADHD treatment. Measurements of plasma or serum zinc levels are not considered a reliable reflection of body stores and are not done routinely in children, therefore clinical suspicion is important. In research studies hair analysis is used to reflect long-term zinc status, and urine and red cell zinc to quantify more recent intake (Villagomez 2014).

Small studies have indicated some promise in treatment with zinc supplementation; for example, a randomized study by Arnold and colleagues in children aged 6–14 with ADHD showed that although clinical outcomes were not significantly improved, the treatment group who received 30 mg zinc glycinate in two divided doses was associated with a 37% reduction in dose of psychostimulant medication. The same did not hold true with the study arm receiving 15 mg daily, or in the control group (Arnold et al. 2011).

Zinc deficiency is a widely recognized nutritional issue in developing countries. Another consideration is the possibility of reduced dietary zinc intake in children in developed countries on stimulant medication who often experience appetite suppression. Monitoring by an experienced registered dietician should be done in children who are losing weight or in any child with early signs of failure to thrive. No adverse events were seen.

Magnesium Magnesium has been identified as a deficiency in some children with ADHD, although the mechanism of action is unclear and insufficient data exists to support standard recommendation. Measurement of magnesium was most commonly done by red blood cell magnesium in available studies to reflect intracellular levels as plasma or serum magnesium does not accurately reflect body stores. A dose response curve was identified where doses over 200 mg/day were associated with adverse effects (or 10 mg/kg/day up to a maximum of 200 mg). No double blind randomized controlled clinical trials have been done to date. A trial of appropriately dosed magnesium may be considered in those suspected of magnesium deficiency, or in response to established insufficient level of red blood cell magnesium; however, no standardized treatment guidelines exist for duration of treatment. Attention to adequate magnesium intake in a healthy balanced diet rich in magnesium-rich whole grains, nuts, legumes, leafy greens, and seafood can complement ADHD treatment (Arnold, Hurt, and Lofthouse 2013).

Vitamin D In general, because of its important role in a range of immune and neurologic functions, vitamin D should be normalized in all children being evaluated for a possible ADHD diagnosis. Some studies correlate low levels with increased ADHD symptoms, although randomized controlled studies are lacking (Goksugur et al. 2014).

Omega-3 Fatty Acids Historically research outcomes have been mixed on the benefit of omega-3 fatty acids in ADHD; however, recent work suggests a potential positive benefit. For example, in a double-blind randomized controlled trial involving 79 boys with ADHD (40 in treatment group) receiving 650 mg of eicosapentaenoic acid (EPA)/docosahexaenoic acid (DHA) versus placebo in enriched margarine over the course of a 16-week intervention, treatment group showed a significant decrease in ADHD symptoms as measured by improvement in inattention. Results suggested that the omega-3 fatty acids were beneficial in reducing the dose of stimulant medication needed. Of interest, omega-3 fatty acids have also been found to improve task performance in typically developing children (Bos et al. 2015).

Bacopa monnieri (CDRI 08) CDRI 08 is an extract of *Bacopa monnieri* from the family Scrophulariaceae, used for thousands of years in the Ayurvedic tradition for its memory, antiepileptic, anti-inflammatory, and mild sedating effects. Active components are believed to be bacosides A and B, which appear to have anxiolytic effects (Russo and Borrelli 2005).

CDRI 08 is an extract of not less than 55% bacosides, which has been tested in animal models and in adult humans with positive results on memory, mood, and cognition. No randomized controlled studies exist to date in children, but studies are planned such as a 14-week randomized trial in 120 males with ADHD by Russo which will measure hyperactivity and inattention and a range of behavioral and psychologic measures (Kean et al. 2015).

PHYSICAL ACTIVITY

Physical activity, especially combined with time outdoors in nature, has increasingly been identified as important in children's health, even giving rise to the "park prescription" movement developing nationally in line with the Healthy Parks Healthy People initiative of the U.S. National Park Service and the White House's Every Kid in a Park program. In addition to helping with overall physical fitness, improving test scores, and buffering stress, reduced behavioral symptoms related to ADHD have been recorded in a number of studies (Seltenrich 2015).

Effects are thought to be due to the restorative mental effect, identified as a rest and restoration of focus and concentration, and the positive social benefits of the shared experience. Enhanced immune function has also been recorded (Seltenrich 2015).

Three of the most active programs in the U.S. include the City of San Francisco, which has fully adopted the Park Prescriptions model into the Department of Public Health, and a program associated with Unity Health Care in Washington D.C., where the park system and green spaces have been entered into a database that can be linked to the patient's electronic medical record, to date reaching more than 100,000 patients. A third program is Prescription Trails in New Mexico, in existence since 2008 (Seltenrich 2015).

YOGA

Small studies of children and adolescents have shown promise in reduction of ADHD symptoms when delivered in group sessions, often in complement to standard medication. Larger well-controlled trials are needed, but positive effects have been recorded. For example, a study of nine children aged 5–16 years being treated in-patient for ADHD received daily yoga sessions for an average of eight sessions and showed good skill acquisition and improvement at initial follow-up, although none maintained the practice once home at 2 and 3-month follow-up (Hariprasad et al. 2013).

In another study by Jensen, 14 Australian boys aged 8–13 years participated in a randomized crossover trial and received a total of 20 1-hour per week yoga sessions. Parent ratings on a range of behavioral scales for attention, impulsivity, and behavior in the treatment group were significantly improved as compared to controls in this study (Jensen and Kenny 2004).

MINDFULNESS

Interest in mindfulness training for children with ADHD is growing and, like yoga, small studies have shown promise. A feasibility study by Zylowska in 24 adults and 8 adolescents used a simple workbook to introduce basic background and provided initiation into meditation in 5-minute increments. This was supplemented with home-guided meditation on CD, and showed good acceptance by 78% and a 30% overall reduction of ADHD symptoms (Zylowska et al. 2008).

In another 8-week mindfulness training study, 10 adolescents with ADHD, and their parents (n = 19), received instruction in parallel groups. Both adolescents and parents saw improvements in attention over the 8-week course. Adolescents showed a decrease in behavioral problems and an improvement in mindfulness score. Mothers showed improvement in over-reactive parenting, although fathers showed an overall increase in this measure. Improvement was progressive over the course of the trial, but not sustained at 16-week follow-up (van de Weijer-Bergsma et al. 2012).

A review by Modesto-Lowe and colleagues highlights the benefits of mindfulness training in ADHD as improvements in self-regulation, task completion, and impulse control, including conflict monitoring and prioritizing incoming stimuli to determine what action to take next (Modesto-Lowe et al. 2015).

Overall risk is very low, and mindfulness training shows promise in children and adolescents with ADHD.

NEUROFEEDBACK

Neurofeedback training, which leverages the brain's plasticity, is the subject of intense study as a treatment intervention for children, adolescents, and adults with ADHD (Albrecht et al. 2015).

Its intention is to train a child or adolescent to regulate a single measure of the brain's electrical activity as measured by electroencephalogram in a real-time biofeedback model using auditory and visual feedback. In early studies the goal has been to learn to suppress theta waves and increase beta wave activity. New measurement tools and approaches are under study (Micoulaud-Franchi et al. 2014).

Overall, benefits have been shown, especially for inattention and impulsivity, with improvements recorded up to 2 years post intervention in some studies. A school-based study by Steiner and colleagues of 104 children 7–11 years old with ADHD provided 40 sessions (three per week) over a 6-month period and resulted in significant improvement in the treatment group. Positive findings were seen in attention, executive functioning, and impulsivity. Children in the treatment group were able to maintain, rather than increase, medication dosages in contrast to the control who had overall significant increases in medication dosages over the study period (Steiner et al. 2014).

Discussion is active now around which interventions are most effective and on the importance of presenting neurofeedback as a learned skill that can be mastered over recurring sessions, rather than as a game or entertainment (Arns, Heinrich, and Strehl 2014).

Some of the downsides of neurofeedback are cost, number of sessions needed, which depends on the individual but is typically 20–40 on average, and variable insurance reimbursement.

Other integrative therapies that have less robust research support include the following.

SLEEP HYGIENE

Behavioral sleep disorders are common in children with ADHD and may be aggravated by stimulant medication (Mulraney et al. 2016).

Some basic steps in addition to those outlined in Chapter 7, Sleep, include minimizing light at night, encouragement of a child-directed, relaxing bedtime ritual that might include guided imagery, aromatherapy, journaling, gentle yoga or other options. Other steps include limiting screen time throughout the day and especially in the evening, and use of a blue light blocker on computers and smart phones.

ENVIRONMENTAL HEALTH HYGIENE

Practical steps can be taken to reduce exposures in all children and this may be especially important in children with ADHD. In addition to the measures outlined in Chapter 8, Environmental Health, those such as limiting exposures to endocrine-disrupting chemicals including pesticides and plasticizers can be an important first step in children suspected of ADHD. Concrete measures such as purchasing organic produce when possible and limiting intake of foods and beverages packaged or prepared in plastic are logical first steps (McClafferty 2016).

Specific attention should be given to avoidance of organophosphate and pyrethroid pesticide exposure; for example, from agriculture spray drift, excess pesticide use around the home, or use of harsh cleaning chemicals in the home. Parents should also be aware of possible pesticides that they may be tracking in from work on clothes, shoes, or equipment.

Other complementary approaches with insufficient data in ADHD yet good safety profiles for encouraging relaxation include aromatherapy, breath work, progressive muscle relaxation, bioenergetic therapies such as therapeutic touch, and therapeutic massage, discussed in earlier chapters. Insufficient data currently exists on the use of acupuncture in pediatric ADHD (Yang et al. 2015).

Attention to caretaker stress and self-care, and encouraging mastery of effective parenting strategies that are neither too lenient nor too harsh, are also a cornerstone of ADHD treatment.

Autism

Overview

The autism spectrum disorder (ASD) describes a set of related neurodevelopmental conditions that consist of persistent deficits in social interaction and communication, repetitive and rigid behavior patterns, and extreme reactivity to sensory input that causes significant impairment in day-to-day functioning, and that lacks a better alternative diagnosis. Symptoms commonly manifest between the age of 1–3 years and can be subtle and easily overlooked in the early stages given the inherent variability in child development. Delayed speech is one of the reasons many children come to diagnosis (Smith, Reichow, and Volkmar 2015).

Autism is a condition that is now estimated to affect 1 in every 68 children in the U.S., with males slightly more than four times as likely to be diagnosed. Prevalence has spiked dramatically, yet a full understanding of the condition's etiology remains elusive (Klein and Kemper 2016).

The level of clinical expression is highly variable from one child to another. Some children have significant disability, while others have a keen intellect and unique gifts and strengths (Treffert and Rebedew 2015).

Although the life of an autistic child can be very challenging in the U.S., internationally the lack of services and understanding of the disease can result in autistic children and their families left to manage both the primary disease and associated comorbidities without adequate diagnostic tools, interventions, or access to ongoing care, which is predictive of poorer outcomes (Lagunju, Bella-Awusah, and Omigbodun 2014; Al Shirian and Al Dera 2015).

Because of the variability and severity of symptoms, lack of easy treatment, and impact on the caretaker and the whole family, families of children with autism spectrum disorders often incorporate one or more complementary therapies into their child's treatment plan. Studies show that these range from therapies with sufficient supporting evidence to recommend, to those that are not well supported by current evidence, or even contraindicated (Levy and Hyman 2015).

Etiology

Many theories exist on the etiology of autism, but none have been proven. A growing consensus points to a multifactorial etiology of genetics and prenatal environmental exposures, which have been reviewed in detail elsewhere in the medical literature. Alterations in immune and inflammatory functions and in neural synaptogenesis are other mechanisms under active study (Edmonson, Ziats, and Rennert 2016; Hens, Peeters, and Dierickx 2016; Lyall, Schmidt, and Hertz-Picciotto 2014).

More recent large studies of sibling pairs have determined a correlation between cesarean section delivery and autism, with an increased risk of 20% in those born by cesarean section. Theories for this correlation include change in microbiota, anesthesia exposure, and altered stress response, although a clear etiology has not been identified (Curran et al. 2015).

Prevalence

Autism is found in all the regions of the world with an average global prevalence according to the World Health Organization of 1 in every 160 people, although detailed geographical variation is not well documented in many areas (Elsabbagh et al. 2012; Al Shirian and Al Dera 2015).

Prevalence in the United States has continued to increase sharply and is currently estimated at 1 in 68 children, with males four and a half times more likely to have the diagnosis. The steady rise in prevalence is attributed to a variety of factors, including changes in diagnostic criteria and screening measures which may skew the numbers to a certain extent but do not fully explain the significant increase (Klein and Kemper 2016).

Clinical Manifestations

Clinical manifestations of autism are expressed across a range of behaviors and may include deficits in social verbal interaction, social reciprocity and facial recognition; repetitive behaviors; and narrowed interests. Delayed speech in early childhood can be seen. Some children with autism cannot tolerate social gatherings and if forced may become agitated or even violent. Other children with autism have savant characteristics, which can manifest in a variety of extraordinary skills and talents (Treffert and Rebedew 2015).

Comorbidities

Autism has been associated with a high prevalence of psychiatric comorbidity, such as attention-deficit/hyperactivity disorder (ADHD) or simply attention deficit disorder (ADD), other externalizing behaviors associated with physical aggression and self-injury, psychotic disorders, seizures, and anxiety. Skin allergy, food allergy, and a variety of gastrointestinal symptoms may be present (Klein and Kemper 2016).

Targeted bullying is highly prevalent in children with autism and should be considered as a comorbidity given the well-documented detrimental mental and physical effects of peer victimization (Maiano et al. 2015).

Diagnostic Criteria

In addition to the clinical manifestations of deficits in social interaction reciprocity, impaired abilities in communication, repetitive behaviors, and narrowed interests, multimodal neuroimaging studies have identified changes in the volumes of both gray and white matter in affected children and have demonstrated both structural and functional abnormalities in the brain. Although multimodal neural imaging is currently used primarily in research, eventually it may become a powerful early diagnostic tool in infants and children as the field matures (Liu et al. 2015).

Treatment

Treatment of autism remains an area of intense research activity, with no single intervention identified as most effective. To date the areas with most potential hinge on early diagnosis in the first 2 years of life, early speech training, and structured behavioral training, especially with consistent parental involvement and training (Bradshaw et al. 2015).

Conventional Treatment

An overall approach to healthy lifestyle may not seem feasible in a child with severe symptoms, but covering the basics of preventive health is important for all children to the highest extent possible. Relatively few randomized controlled trials of lifestyle intervention currently exist, but the clinician could confidently recommend regular enjoyable exercise as tolerated, supervised time outdoors in nature, upgrade of nutrition quality of tolerated foods (including addition of organic foods if possible), limiting light at night and excessive screen time, and attention to sleep hygiene. The FDA has approved risperidone and aripiprazole for the treatment of severe disruptive behavioral symptoms, although side effects are a concern—including metabolic changes such as dyslipidemia, and weight gain, and neurologic symptoms of tremor and sedation. Typical anti-seizure medications may also be used in children suffering from epilepsy. Some children require special diets to avoid triggering food sensitivity, which requires a highly individualized approach (Klein and Kemper 2016).

Integrative Treatment

Integrative treatment of autism might be considered in a four-category framework to help reduce confusion. A model by Klein and Kemper simplifies the options based on assessment of safety and efficacy using a "recommended," "monitored," "tolerate," and "avoid" model that is highly practical (Klein and Kemper 2016). To meet the bar for the recommended category, a minimum of two randomized controlled trials were needed. Currently recommended interventions include attention to healthy lifestyle (exercise, outdoor time, stress management, environmental health hygiene to reduce unwanted exposures to toxicants, and the use of melatonin to address sleep latency and maintenance). Another recommended intervention is music therapy, which is a low-risk therapy that has encouraging supporting research in improving social skills and emotional reciprocity, as well as promise in improving the parent–child interaction in small studies (Ghasemtabar et al. 2015). Neurofeedback is another approach that has shown promise in small studies, although price, access, and number of sessions needed may be significant obstacles for some families (Klein and Kemper 2016).

"Monitored" therapies in the Klein-Kemper model include a restricted diet such as the gluten-free-casein-free diet. Although popular, limited supporting evidence is available, and children are at risk for undernutrition in the form of micro and macronutrients, possible calorie restriction, and peer victimization due to the restricted foods eaten. A gluten-free-casein-free diet would ideally be used only in those with proven sensitivity and be monitored closely for appropriate nutrition and caloric content.

"Tolerated" therapies include those that appear to be safe, yet lack adequate supporting evidence. This may be the largest category of therapies, as families want to take any measure to improve the health of their child. Some of the most common options in this category include the dietary supplements (omega-3 fatty acids, vitamins B6 or B12, folate, vitamin C, vitamin D), sensory integration therapy, animal-assisted therapy, yoga, massage, acupuncture, and therapies that address the spiritual or bioenergetic aspects of the child's condition and might include prayer, therapeutic touch, reiki, and homeopathy. Insufficient evidence currently exists for any of these therapies in autism, but they appear low risk if used by a trained practitioner who has experience working with children with disabilities. Clinicians should encourage families to keep them apprised of all therapies being used. None of the dietary supplements mentioned have sufficient supporting data to meet the "recommended" category, and any "mega-dose" approach to dietary supplements should be actively discouraged. Ideally children would receive a healthy balance of nutrients in the diet, although if this is not the case, dietary consult and repletion of vitamins and other supplements such as omega-3 fatty acids should be done in a thoughtful and systematic way in conjunction with the child's primary care provider.

Vitamin D should be normalized in all children and is discussed in detail in Chapter 4 (Klein and Kemper 2016).

Also in the "tolerated" category are therapeutic approaches such as sensory integration (Section On Complementary and Integrative Medicine et al. 2012), occupational therapy, animal-assisted therapy using dogs and horses (Borgi et al. 2016; Siewertsen, French, and Teramoto 2015), and yoga (Bremer, Crozier, and Lloyd 2016).

In each of these some small studies show potential benefit. Therapeutic massage has also been shown to be helpful in some small studies, but may not be tolerated by some children with autism who dislike being touched. Acupuncture has been shown to have some potential, but study quality has been highly variable, leaving insufficient data to conclude consistent benefit (Klein and Kemper 2016).

Insufficient evidence exists to support the use of chiropractic in autism, and special attention must be paid to the pediatric training of any type of manual medicine practice in children, especially if non-verbal.

In the Klein-Kemper model, therapies that are contraindicated include hyperbaric oxygen, chelation to remove heavy metals, and secretin to address gastrointestinal symptoms, all due to a lack of sufficient supporting evidence and risk of unwanted side effects (Klein and Kemper 2016).

Possibly one of the most important approaches for the child with autism is to address the chronic stress of the caretaker which can be significant and may impair immune response and upregulate the inflammatory system, leading to a range of comorbidities seen in toxic stress (De Andres-Garcia, Moya-Albiol, and Gonzalez-Bono 2012).

Use of all appropriate therapies for adults involved in caring for autistic children is recommended, including parents, other caretakers, and clinicians. This might include healthy whole foods, adequate time off or respite, adequate sleep, regular physical activity, robust social connections, and use of the range of mind–body tools to cultivate resilience, self-control, sense of meaning and purpose, and a sense of equilibrium in a highly challenging situation. Clinicians working with families of autistic children face unique challenges and high potential stressors dealing with the complex needs, chronic care, and lack of available financial and social support for these families. Appropriate self-care modeling by clinicians and consistent encouragement to take time for their own self-renewal has the potential to benefit these special caretakers.

References

Al Shirian, S., and H. Al Dera. 2015. "Descriptive characteristics of children with autism at Autism Treatment Center, KSA." *Physiol Behav* 151: 604–8. doi: 10.1016/j.physbeh.2015.09.001.

Albrecht, B., H. Uebel-von Sandersleben, H. Gevensleben, and A. Rothenberger. 2015. "Pathophysiology of ADHD and associated problems-starting points for NF interventions?" *Front Hum Neurosci* 9: 359. doi: 10.3389/fnhum.2015.00359.

Armstrong, D., K. Lycett, H. Hiscock, E. Care, and E. Sciberras. 2015. "Longitudinal associations between internalizing and externalizing comorbidities and functional outcomes for children with ADHD." *Child Psychiatry Hum Dev* 46(5): 736–48. doi: 10.1007/s10578-014-0515-x.

Arnold, L. E., R. A. Disilvestro, D. Bozzolo, H. Bozzolo, L. Crowl, S. Fernandez, Y. Ramadan, S. Thompson, X. Mo, M. Abdel-Rasoul, and E. Joseph. 2011. "Zinc for attention-deficit/hyperactivity disorder: placebo-controlled double-blind pilot trial alone and combined with amphetamine." *J Child Adolesc Psychopharmacol* 21(1): 1–19. doi: 10.1089/cap.2010.0073.

Arnold, L. E., E. Hurt, and N. Lofthouse. 2013. "Attention-deficit/hyperactivity disorder: dietary and nutritional treatments." *Child Adolesc Psychiatr Clin N Am* 22(3): 381–402, v. doi: 10.1016/j.chc.2013.03.001.

Arns, M., H. Heinrich, and U. Strehl. 2014. "Evaluation of neurofeedback in ADHD: the long and winding road." *Biol Psychol* 95: 108–15. doi: 10.1016/j.biopsycho.2013.11.013.

Baweja, R., P. J. Belin, H. H. Humphrey, L. Babocsai, M. E. Pariseau, D. A. Waschbusch, M. T. Hoffman, O. O. Akinnusi, J. L. Haak, W. E. Pelham, and J. G. Waxmonsky. 2016. "The effectiveness and tolerability of central nervous system stimulants in school-age children with attention-deficit/hyperactivity disorder and disruptive mood dysregulation disorder across home and school." *J Child Adolesc Psychopharmacol.* doi: 10.1089/cap.2015.0053.

Borgi, M., D. Loliva, S. Cerino, F. Chiarotti, A. Venerosi, M. Bramini, E. Nonnis, M. Marcelli, C. Vinti, C. De Santis, F. Bisacco, M. Fagerlie, M. Frascarelli, and F. Cirulli. 2016. "Effectiveness of a standardized equine-assisted therapy program for children with autism spectrum disorder." *J Autism Dev Disord* 46(1): 1–9. doi: 10.1007/s10803-015-2530-6.

Bos, D. J., B. Oranje, E. S. Veerhoek, R. M. Van Diepen, J. M. Weusten, H. Demmelmair, B. Koletzko, M. G. de Sain-van der Velden, A. Eilander, M. Hoeksma, and S. Durston. 2015. "Reduced symptoms of inattention after dietary omega-3 fatty acid supplementation in boys with and without attention deficit/hyperactivity disorder." *Neuropsychopharmacology* 40(10): 2298–306. doi: 10.1038/npp.2015.73.

Bradshaw, J., A. M. Steiner, G. Gengoux, and L. K. Koegel. 2015. "Feasibility and effectiveness of very early intervention for infants at-risk for autism spectrum disorder: a systematic review." *J Autism Dev Disord* 45(3): 778–94. doi: 10.1007/s10803-014-2235-2.

Bremer, E., M. Crozier, and M. Lloyd. 2016. "A systematic review of the behavioural outcomes following exercise interventions for children and youth with autism spectrum disorder." *Autism*. doi: 10.1177/1362361315616002.

Childress, A. C. 2016. "A critical appraisal of atomoxetine in the management of ADHD." *Ther Clin Risk Manag* 12: 27–39. doi: 10.2147/TCRM.S59270.

Chou, W. J., T. L. Liu, H. F. Hu, and C. F. Yen. 2016. "Suicidality and its relationships with individual, family, peer, and psychopathology factors among adolescents with attention-deficit/hyperactivity disorder." *Res Dev Disabil* 53–54: 86–94. doi: 10.1016/j.ridd.2016.02.001.

Cortese, S., M. Angriman, M. Lecendreux, and E. Konofal. 2012. "Iron and attention deficit/hyperactivity disorder: What is the empirical evidence so far? A systematic review of the literature." *Expert Rev Neurother* 12(10): 1227–40. doi: 10.1586/ern.12.116.

Cortese, S., C. R. Moreira-Maia, D. St Fleur, C. Morcillo-Penalver, L. A. Rohde, and S. V. Faraone. 2016. "Association between ADHD and obesity: a systematic review and meta-analysis." *Am J Psychiatry* 173(1): 34–43. doi: 10.1176/appi.ajp.2015.15020266.

Curran, E. A., C. Dalman, P. M. Kearney, L. C. Kenny, J. F. Cryan, T. G. Dinan, and A. S. Khashan. 2015. "Association between obstetric mode of delivery and autism spectrum disorder: a population-based sibling design study." *JAMA Psychiatry* 72(9): 935–42. doi: 10.1001/jamapsychiatry.2015.0846.

De Andres-Garcia, S., L. Moya-Albiol, and E. Gonzalez-Bono. 2012. "Salivary cortisol and immunoglobulin A: responses to stress as predictors of health complaints reported by caregivers of offspring with autistic spectrum disorder." *Horm Behav* 62(4): 464–74. doi: 10.1016/j.yhbeh.2012.08.003.

Edmonson, C. A., M. N. Ziats, and O. M. Rennert. 2016. "A non-inflammatory role for microglia in autism spectrum disorders." *Front Neurol* 7: 9. doi: 10.3389/fneur.2016.00009.

Elsabbagh, M., G. Divan, Y. J. Koh, Y. S. Kim, S. Kauchali, C. Marcin, C. Montiel-Nava, V. Patel, C. S. Paula, C. Wang, M. T. Yasamy, and E. Fombonne. 2012. "Global prevalence of autism and other pervasive developmental disorders." *Autism Res* 5(3): 160–79. doi: 10.1002/aur.239.

Erskine, H. E., A. J. Baxter, G. Patton, T. E. Moffitt, V. Patel, H. A. Whiteford, and J. G. Scott. 2016. "The global coverage of prevalence data for mental disorders in children and adolescents." *Epidemiol Psychiatr Sci*: 1–8. doi: 10.1017/S2045796015001158.

Fernandez de la Cruz, L., E. Simonoff, J. J. McGough, J. M. Halperin, L. E. Arnold, and A. Stringaris. 2015. "Treatment of children with attention-deficit/hyperactivity disorder (ADHD) and irritability: results from the multimodal treatment study of children with ADHD (MTA)." *J Am Acad Child Adolesc Psychiatry* 54(1): 62–70 e3. doi: 10.1016/j.jaac.2014.10.006.

Ghasemtabar, S. N., M. Hosseini, I. Fayyaz, S. Arab, H. Naghashian, and Z. Poudineh. 2015. "Music therapy: An effective approach in improving social skills of children with autism." *Adv Biomed Res* 4: 157. doi: 10.4103/2277-9175.161584.

Goksugur, S. B., A. E. Tufan, M. Semiz, C. Gunes, M. Bekdas, M. Tosun, and F. Demircioglu. 2014. "Vitamin D status in children with attention-deficit-hyperactivity disorder." *Pediatr Int* 56(4): 515–19. doi: 10.1111/ped.12286.

Goldman, L. S., M. Genel, R. J. Bezman, and P. J. Slanetz. 1998. "Diagnosis and treatment of attention-deficit/hyperactivity disorder in children and adolescents. Council on Scientific Affairs, American Medical Association." *JAMA* 279(14): 1100–17.

Gray, S. A., P. Fettes, S. Woltering, K. Mawjee, and R. Tannock. 2015. "Symptom manifestation and impairments in college students with ADHD." *J Learn Disabil*. doi: 10.1177/0022219415576523.

Hariprasad, V. R., R. Arasappa, S. Varambally, S. Srinath, and B. N. Gangadhar. 2013. "Feasibility and efficacy of yoga as an add-on intervention in attention deficit-hyperactivity disorder: an exploratory study." *Indian J Psychiatry* 55(Suppl 3): S379–84. doi: 10.4103/0019-5545.116317.

Hens, K., H. Peeters, and K. Dierickx. 2016. "The ethics of complexity. Genetics and autism, a literature review." *Am J Med Genet B Neuropsychiatr Genet*. doi: 10.1002/ajmg.b.32432.

Jensen, P. S., and D. T. Kenny. 2004. "The effects of yoga on the attention and behavior of boys with attention-deficit/hyperactivity disorder (ADHD)." *J Atten Disord* 7(4): 205–16.

Kean, J. D., J. Kaufman, J. Lomas, A. Goh, D. White, D. Simpson, A. Scholey, H. Singh, J. Sarris, A. Zangara, and C. Stough. 2015. "A randomized controlled trial investigating the effects of a special extract of Bacopa monnieri (CDRI 08) on hyperactivity and inattention in male children and adolescents: BACHI Study Protocol (ANZCTRN12612000827831)." *Nutrients* 7(12): 9931–45. doi: 10.3390/nu7125507.

Klein, N., and K. J. Kemper. 2016. "Integrative approaches to caring for children with autism." *Curr Probl Pediatr Adolesc Health Care*. doi: 10.1016/j.cppeds.2015.12.004.

Konofal, E., M. Lecendreux, J. Deron, M. Marchand, S. Cortese, M. Zaim, M. C. Mouren, and I. Arnulf. 2008. "Effects of iron supplementation on attention deficit hyperactivity disorder in children." *Pediatr Neurol* 38(1): 20–6. doi: 10.1016/j.pediatrneurol.2007.08.014.

Kooij, J. J. 2016. "ADHD and Obesity." *Am J Psychiatry* 173 (1): 1–2. doi: 10.1176/appi. ajp.2015.15101315.

Lagunju, I. A., T. T. Bella-Awusah, and O. O. Omigbodun. 2014. "Autistic disorder in Nigeria: profile and challenges to management." *Epilepsy Behav* 39: 126–9. doi: 10.1016/j. yebeh.2014.08.020.

Levy, S. E., and S. L. Hyman. 2015. "Complementary and alternative medicine treatments for children with autism spectrum disorders." *Child Adolesc Psychiatr Clin N Am* 24(1): 117–43. doi: 10.1016/j.chc.2014.09.004.

Liu, S., W. Cai, S. Liu, F. Zhang, M. Fulham, D. Feng, S. Pujol, and R. Kikinis. 2015. "Multimodal neuroimaging computing: a review of the applications in neuropsychiatric disorders." *Brain Inform* 2: 167–80. doi: 10.1007/s40708-015-0019-x.

Lyall, K., R. J. Schmidt, and I. Hertz-Picciotto. 2014. "Maternal lifestyle and environmental risk factors for autism spectrum disorders." *Int J Epidemiol* 43(2): 443–64. doi: 10.1093/ije/dyt282.

Maiano, C., C. L. Normand, M. C. Salvas, G. Moullec, and A. Aime. 2015. "Prevalence of school bullying among youth with autism spectrum disorders: a systematic review and meta-analysis." *Autism Res*. doi: 10.1002/aur.1568.

McClafferty, H. 2016. "Environmental health: childrens health, a clinician's dilemma." *Curr Probl Pediatr Adolesc Health Care*. doi: 10.1016/j.cppeds.2015.12.003.

Micoulaud-Franchi, J. A., P. A. Geoffroy, G. Fond, R. Lopez, S. Bioulac, and P. Philip. 2014. "EEG neurofeedback treatments in children with ADHD: an updated meta-analysis of randomized controlled trials." *Front Hum Neurosci* 8: 906. doi: 10.3389/fnhum.2014.00906.

Millichap, J. G., and M. M. Yee. 2012. "The diet factor in attention-deficit/hyperactivity disorder." *Pediatrics* 129(2): 330–7. doi: 10.1542/peds.2011-2199.

Modesto-Lowe, V., P. Farahmand, M. Chaplin, and L. Sarro. 2015. "Does mindfulness meditation improve attention in attention deficit hyperactivity disorder?" *World J Psychiatry* 5(4): 397–403. doi: 10.5498/wjp.v5.i4.397.

Mulraney, M., R. Giallo, K. Lycett, F. Mensah, and E. Sciberras. 2016. "The bidirectional relationship between sleep problems and internalizing and externalizing problems in children with ADHD: a prospective cohort study." *Sleep Med* 17: 45–51. doi: 10.1016/j.sleep.2015.09.019.

Nigg, J. T., and K. Holton. 2014. "Restriction and elimination diets in ADHD treatment." *Child Adolesc Psychiatr Clin N Am* 23(4): 937–53. doi: 10.1016/j.chc.2014.05.010.

Nigg, J. T., J. M. Johnstone, E. D. Musser, H. G. Long, M. T. Willoughby, and J. Shannon. 2016. "Attention-deficit/hyperactivity disorder (ADHD) and being overweight/obesity: new data and meta-analysis." *Clin Psychol Rev* 43: 67–79. doi: 10.1016/j.cpr.2015.11.005.

Nigg, J. T., K. Lewis, T. Edinger, and M. Falk. 2012. "Meta-analysis of attention-deficit/hyperactivity disorder or attention-deficit/hyperactivity disorder symptoms, restriction diet, and synthetic food color additives." *J Am Acad Child Adolesc Psychiatry* 51(1): 86–97 e8. doi: 10.1016/j.jaac.2011.10.015.

Pelsser, L. M., K. Frankena, J. Toorman, H. F. Savelkoul, A. E. Dubois, R. R. Pereira, T. A.

Haagen, N. N. Rommelse, and J. K. Buitelaar. 2011. "Effects of a restricted elimination diet on the behaviour of children with attention-deficit hyperactivity disorder (INCA study): a randomised controlled trial." *Lancet* 377(9764): 494–503. doi: 10.1016/S0140-6736(10)62227-1.

Pfiffner, L. J., and K. McBurnett. 2006. "Family correlates of comorbid anxiety disorders in children with attention deficit/hyperactivity disorder." *J Abnorm Child Psychol* 34(5): 725–35. doi: 10.1007/s10802-006-9060-9.

Pon, N., B. Asan, S. Anandan, and A. Toledo. 2015. "Special considerations in pediatric psychiatric populations." *Emerg Med Clin North Am* 33(4): 811–24. doi: 10.1016/j.emc.2015.07.008.

Richardson, J. R., M. M. Taylor, S. L. Shalat, T. S. Guillot, 3rd, W. M. Caudle, M. M. Hossain, T. A. Mathews, S. R. Jones, D. A. Cory-Slechta, and G. W. Miller. 2015. "Developmental pesticide exposure reproduces features of attention deficit hyperactivity disorder." *FASEB J* 29(5): 1960–72. doi: 10.1096/fj.14-260901.

Russo, A., and F. Borrelli. 2005. "Bacopa monniera, a reputed nootropic plant: an overview." *Phytomedicine* 12(4): 305–17. doi: 10.1016/j.phymed.2003.12.008.

Section on Complementary and Integrative Medicine, Council on Children with Disabilities, American Academy of Pediatrics, M. Zimmer, and L. Desch. 2012. "Sensory integration therapies for children with developmental and behavioral disorders." *Pediatrics* 129(6): 1186–9. doi: 10.1542/peds.2012-0876.

Seltenrich, N. 2015. "Just what the doctor ordered: using parks to improve children's health." *Environ Health Perspect* 123(10): A254–9. doi: 10.1289/ehp.123-A254.

Siewertsen, C. M., E. D. French, and M. Teramoto. 2015. "Autism spectrum disorder and pet therapy." *Adv Mind Body Med* 29 (2): 22–5.

Smith, I. C., B. Reichow, and F. R. Volkmar. 2015. "The effects of DSM-5 Criteria on number of individuals diagnosed with autism spectrum disorder: a systematic review." *J Autism Dev Disord* 45(8): 2541–52. doi: 10.1007/s10803-015-2423-8.

Steiner, N. J., E. C. Frenette, K. M. Rene, R. T. Brennan, and E. C. Perrin. 2014. "In-school neurofeedback training for ADHD: sustained improvements from a randomized control trial." *Pediatrics* 133(3): 483–92. doi: 10.1542/peds.2013-2059.

Swanson, J. M., H. C. Kraemer, S. P. Hinshaw, L. E. Arnold, C. K. Conners, H. B. Abikoff, W. Clevenger, M. Davies, G. R. Elliott, L. L. Greenhill, L. Hechtman, B. Hoza, P. S. Jensen, J. S. March, J. H. Newcorn, E. B. Owens, W. E. Pelham, E. Schiller, J. B. Severe, S. Simpson, B. Vitiello, K. Wells, T. Wigal, and M. Wu. 2001. "Clinical relevance of the primary findings of the MTA: success rates based on severity of ADHD and ODD symptoms at the end of treatment." *J Am Acad Child Adolesc Psychiatry* 40(2): 168–79. doi: 10.1097/00004583-20010 2000-00011.

Tanofsky-Kraff, M., and S. Z. Yanovski. 2004. "Eating disorder or disordered eating? Non-normative eating patterns in obese individuals." *Obes Res* 12(9): 1361–6. doi: 10.1038/oby.2004.171.

Thapar, A., M. Cooper, O. Eyre, and K. Langley. 2013. "What have we learnt about the causes of ADHD?" *J Child Psychol Psychiatry* 54(1): 3–16. doi: 10.1111/j.1469-7610.2012.02611.x.

Treffert, D. A., and D. L. Rebedew. 2015. "The Savant Syndrome Registry: a preliminary report." *WMJ* 114(4): 158–62.

van de Weijer-Bergsma, E., A. R. Formsma, E. I. de Bruin, and S. M. Bogels. 2012. "The effectiveness of mindfulness training on behavioral problems and attentional functioning in adolescents with ADHD." *J Child Fam Stud* 21(5): 775–87. doi: 10.1007/s10826-011-9531-7.

Verlinden, M., P. W. Jansen, R. Veenstra, V. W. Jaddoe, A. Hofman, F. C. Verhulst, P. Shaw, and H. Tiemeier. 2015. "Preschool attention-deficit/hyperactivity and oppositional defiant problems as antecedents of school bullying." *J Am Acad Child Adolesc Psychiatry* 54(7): 571–9. doi: 10.1016/j.jaac.2015.05.002.

Villagomez, A.; Ramtekkar. 2014. "Iron, magnesium, vitamin D, and zinc deficiencies in children presenting with symptoms of attention-deficit/hyperactivity disorder." *Children* 1: 261–79.

Visser, S. N., M. L. Danielson, R. H. Bitsko, J. R. Holbrook, M. D. Kogan, R. M. Ghandour, R.

Perou, and S. J. Blumberg. 2014. "Trends in the parent-report of health care provider-diagnosed and medicated attention-deficit/hyperactivity disorder: United States, 2003–2011." *J Am Acad Child Adolesc Psychiatry* 53(1): 34–46 e2. doi: 10.1016/j.jaac.2013.09.001.

Wagner-Schuman, M., J. R. Richardson, P. Auinger, J. M. Braun, B. P. Lanphear, J. N. Epstein, K. Yolton, and T. E. Froehlich. 2015. "Association of pyrethroid pesticide exposure with attention-deficit/hyperactivity disorder in a nationally representative sample of U.S. children." *Environ Health* 14: 44. doi: 10.1186/s12940-015-0030-y.

Yang, C., Z. Hao, L. L. Zhang, and Q. Guo. 2015. "Efficacy and safety of acupuncture in children: an overview of systematic reviews." *Pediatr Res* 78(2): 112–19. doi: 10.1038/pr.2015.91.

Zylowska, L., D. L. Ackerman, M. H. Yang, J. L. Futrell, N. L. Horton, T. S. Hale, C. Pataki, and S. L. Smalley. 2008. "Mindfulness meditation training in adults and adolescents with ADHD: a feasibility study." *J Atten Disord* 11(6): 737–46. doi: 10.1177/1087054707308502.

21 Obesity and Metabolic Disease

Obesity

Overview

The prevalence of childhood obesity in developed countries increased by a staggering 47.1% globally between 1980 and 2013 yet a definitive etiology for the epidemic remains elusive. Taken in perspective, development of the obesity epidemic has been fast, significant, and highly resistant to preventive measures, with no countries reporting significant downward trends in prevalence in the past 30 years. Obesity tracks through adolescence into adulthood, a point of significant concern because data from large pooled studies have conclusively shown that BMI greater than $23\,kg/m^2$ in adults is associated with progressive increase in risk of cardiovascular disease, cancer, diabetes, chronic renal disease, and osteoarthritis (Ng et al. 2014).

Commercial and environmental initiatives that devalue pediatric health, intersecting with a complex matrix of genetic and epigenetic factors, have created a perfect storm, resulting in one in three children in North America either overweight or obese, a ratio mirrored globally in developed and developing countries (Ng et al. 2014).

The small number of reported successful interventions has contributed to a growing consensus among leading pediatric organizations that a deliberate and urgent shift towards primary prevention is needed (Daniels, Hassink, and Committee On 2015).

This requires pediatricians to become skilled educators, trained to recognize early signs of overweight in infants and children and be prepared to offer effective intervention if a child is heading off track. To this end, rather than provide a detailed overview of less common causes of obesity; for example, Prader-Willi syndrome, Cushing's syndrome, or the pharmacologic or surgical treatment of obesity in children, the following material will focus on information that can help pediatricians be more successful in primary obesity prevention.

Etiology

Obesity is a highly complex inflammatory-driven disorder (Martinez-Fernandez et al. 2015) that is characterized by non-proportionate increase in the fat content of the body mass. Unhealthy lifestyle combining excess consumption of high caloric food and insufficient physical activity is considered the main driver. Parental overweight has been shown to be the most significant risk factor for pediatric obesity in some studies (Agras and Mascola 2005), due to a mix of genetic, epigenetic, environmental, social, and lifestyle influences, including early modeling of food, beverage, and physical activity behaviors. Lifestyle issues can affect children at each end of the socioeconomic spectrum for different reasons based on access to healthy food, safe outlets for physical activity, and a diverse range of cultural factors (Ogden et al. 2014; Brown et al. 2015).

An emerging area of interest is the impact of the intrauterine environment and early post-natal exposures on the developmental origins of obesity. Some predictive factors include being either small or large for gestational age, maternal smoking, and maternal obesity at time of conception (Gilmore, Klempel-Donchenko, and Redman 2015; Gurnani, Birken, and Hamilton 2015). Prenatal exposures to systemic antibiotics (Mor et al. 2015), and some types of persistent organic pollutants have been associated with increased body-mass-index in early childhood in large population studies (Mor et al. 2015). These and other intrauterine exposures are areas of active study (Penfold and Ozanne 2015). Systematic review of 15 studies involving 163,796 adults has shown correlation of overweight and obesity with history of cesarean delivery (Darmasseelane et al. 2014), raising questions about the association between altered gut microbiome and the potential influence of the circumstances unique to a cesarean section birth (Goedert et al. 2014). Alteration in the microbiome in toddlers born to obese mothers also raises questions about the possibility of transmission of obesogenic maternal microbes driving pediatric obesity (Galley et al. 2014). This range of research questions highlight the incredible complexity of the human microbiome, and introduces exciting frontiers that may lead to important insights into obesity prevention.

Early growth trajectory and feeding methods (breast versus bottle and timing of introduction of solid foods) are also under study, although data is somewhat mixed at present (Vehapoglu et al. 2014). For example, some studies show that high birth weight and a rapid trajectory of growth have been shown to correlate with obesity, although confounding variables make definitive interpretation difficult. Early introduction of solid foods, at less than 3 or 5 months depending on the study, has also been correlated with obesity risk in some studies (Pearce and Langley-Evans 2013; McPherson and Lindsay 2012).

Food insecurity is another important factor associated with obesity in children. Data from the National Health and Nutrition Examination Study (NHANES) measuring adolescents 12–18 years from 1999 to 2006 showed a significant correlation with overweight in moderate and low food secure children. Children in marginally food secure households were 1.3 times more likely to be obese, with nearly 1 in 4 children in all groups (marginal, low, very low food secure) reported to have central obesity, a figure 1.4 to 1.5 times higher than children in the high food security group. Risk factors for metabolic syndrome were identified in 3.1% of the low food security children (Holben and Taylor 2015).

A longitudinal study of 28,353 children aged 2–5 years in the Massachusetts Special Supplemental Nutrition Program for Women, Infants, and Children showed that persistent food insecurity was associated with 22% greater odds of childhood obesity compared to children in food secure homes (p<0.05). Approximately 17.1% of the children were obese at their 5-year-old health visit. Mothers experiencing higher food insecurity had greater odds of a child with obesity. The etiology of the paradoxical link between food scarcity, food insecurity, and obesity are not fully understood. Due to the high prevalence of pediatric obesity in these scenarios it is very important for pediatricians to be aware that children, and their mothers, living with ongoing food insecurity issues in very difficult socioeconomic conditions may still be overweight or obese and at high risk for the complications associated with the metabolic syndrome (Metallinos-Katsaras, Must, and Gorman 2012).

Exposure to direct advertising and marketing of energy-dense, nutrient-poor foods and beverages to children is another important contributor to pediatric obesity. For example, despite industry wide promises to curb direct advertising to children in the Children's Food and Beverage Advertising Initiative (CFBAI), an estimated U.S.$1.8 billion was spent in direct non-nutritive food marketing to children in 2009 alone through a variety of avenues including television, product endorsement, and Internet media marketing (Powell, Harris, and Fox 2013).

Intake of unhealthy foods and beverages has been widely correlated with exposure to embedded commercial food marketing within children's television shows (Kelly et al. 2015; Jenkin et al. 2014; Cornwell, McAlister, and Polmear-Swendris 2014).

Child-directed marketing cues, for example cartoon characters on packaging, have even been shown to significantly influence taste preference in controlled studies in preschool-aged children (Enax et al. 2015). AAP policy recommendations have consistently called for reduction of the presence of non-nutritive foods in all areas of school food distribution (school meals, vending machines, school stores, informal fundraisers, parties, and rewards) (Council on School Health and Committee on Nutrition 2015).

Federal, state, and local changes in policy and regulations have also been designed to upgrade food and beverage quality delivered to children in the school setting, where an estimated 35%–40% of children's daily energy intake occurs during the school day (Cullen et al. 2015). For example, parents and caretakers may unwittingly perpetuate the problem by turning to processed convenience foods or frequent eating out to compensate for busy days and long work hours. These types of meal options are often high in fat and sugar, served in disproportionate portion sizes, and frequently incentivized by including children's toys and other marketing materials. Families with a pattern of high fast food intake have been shown to complete their overall food intake with a less healthy Western diet, a finding shown to be independently associated with obesity and overweight in large population surveys of children and adults (Poti, Duffey, and Popkin 2014).

Food addiction can also be a factor in children and has been correlated with depression and in both preadolescent and adolescents' groups (Laurent and Sibold 2015; Meule, Hermann, and Kubler 2015). Overweight or obesity related to food addiction, binge eating, and other types of stress-related eating should raise a flag of concern for the possibility of emotional, sexual, or physical abuse and deserves careful investigation by the pediatrician (Mason et al. 2015).

Several of the environmental toxicants classified as endocrine-disrupting chemicals have been shown to be obesogens and metabolic disruptors, raising another issue of concern. One of the most ubiquitous, and best-studied toxicants is bisphenol A (BPA) used in polycarbonate plastic and resin manufacturing. Both in vivo and in vitro studies have shown BPA's disruptive effect on regulation of genes involved in fat metabolism and insulin homeostasis (Menale et al. 2015). BPA has also been shown to increase the expression of pro-inflammatory cytokines and act to stimulate adipogenesis in cell studies using omental biopsies in children (Wang et al. 2013).

Other environmental toxicants associated with obesity are discussed in Chapter 8, Environmental Health.

Antibiotic exposure before 6 months of age, or repeatedly in infants younger than 1 year, has also been associated with a trend towards obesity in healthy children (Azad et al. 2014). For example, in a large population-based cohort of 12,062 healthy children in Finland, antibiotic exposure in infancy was associated with increase in both height and weight by age 24 months. Macrolide antibiotics were found to have the greatest effect in this study. Effects were more pronounced in boys who had received more overall exposures to antibiotics (Saari et al. 2015).

Intense research interest exists around the connection between antibiotic exposures, obesity, and alterations in gut microbiome. Work in animal models has shown how antibiotics affect gene expression involved in the conversion of carbohydrates to short chain fatty acids, increasing energy harvest, among other metabolic changes (Cho et al. 2012; Turnbaugh et al. 2006).

The wide range of contributing etiologies of the pediatric obesity epidemic reflect the complex nature of the disease, and at the same time provide windows into promising areas of intervention. Awareness of the areas under active study can help the clinician plan strategies for primary prevention.

Summary of etiologic factors of childhood obesity:

- Parental overweight
- Unhealthy lifestyle
- Prenatal environment
- Antibiotics
- Cesarean delivery
- Microbiome
- Decision to breast or bottle feed, timing of solid food introduction
- Food insecurity
- Exposure to food marketing and advertising
- Food addiction
- Abuse, chronic stressors
- Federal, state, local governmental nutrition policies
- Environmental exposures

Diagnostic Criteria

Obesity Under Age 24 Months

In general, the World Health Organization (WHO) growth standards are recommended for monitoring growth in children younger than 2 years. The CDC growth charts are based solely on U.S. populations at various points over the past 30–40 years, whereas the WHO charts use healthy breastfed infants from a range of countries as the benchmark for normal growth. In the WHO growth charts the 97.7th percentile is recommended as the cutoff for obesity compared to the 95th percentile in the CDC charts. Although differences in the charts are relatively small, gaining weight more rapidly on the WHO charts, for example jumping percentiles, may reflect early signs of overweight in the infant and should be monitored closely (Grummer-Strawn et al. 2010; Ogden et al. 2014).

Obesity Aged 2–19 Years

Body-mass-index is at or above 95th percentile of gender specific CDC BMI-for-age growth charts. Overweight in this age group is defined as BMI-for-age greater than or equal to 85th–95th percentiles.

Class 2 obesity (more severe obesity) is defined as BMI greater than 120% of the 95th percentile for age or gender, or a BMI of 35 or greater, whichever is lower.

Class 3 obesity is defined as a BMI of greater than 140% of the 95th percentile for age or sex, or a BMI greater or equal to 40, whichever is lower. Both class 2 and 3 obesity are considered high risk and are associated with early mortality (Berrington de Gonzalez et al. 2010).

Prevalence

There has been no significant reduction in the prevalence of obesity in children, although in some age groups the rate of increase has slowed. In 2011–2012 approximately one in three North American children (31.8%) were either overweight or obese. Nearly 10% of infants and toddlers are overweight or obese; more than 8% of 2–5 year olds were obese; 17.7% of 6–11 year olds; and 20.5% of 12–19 year olds were obese. In addition, 5.9% of children fell into the class 2 category for obesity, and 2.1% fit criteria for class 3 obesity. All classes of obesity have increased prevalence in U.S. children over the past 14 years (Skinner and Skelton 2014; Ogden et al. 2014), with low-income children almost twice as likely to be obese as their middle and upper-income peers (Anderson and Whitaker 2009).

Large global population surveys show that on average in 2013, 23.8% of boys and 22.6% of girls in developed countries were overweight or obese. Children and adolescents in certain ethnic groups are particular targets of overweight and obesity and associated risk of metabolic syndrome and type-2 diabetes. Some of the most rapid increases in obesity have been seen in children in Mexico (41.8%), Brazil (22.1%), India (22.0%), and Argentina (19.3%). Countries on a rapid upward trajectory for childhood obesity prevalence include Brazil (from 4.1 % to 13.9% between 1974 and 1997), China (6.4% to 7.7% between 1991 and 1997), and India (4.9% to 6.6% in the span of 2003–2006)(Gupta et al. 2013).

Adult prevalence of adults with body-mass-index greater than 25 kg/m^2 has also increased significantly in developed countries to 36.9% in men and 38% in women (Ogden et al. 2014; Ng et al. 2014; Brown et al. 2015).

Clinical Manifestations

Recognition of obesity may be challenging for parents because of difficulty differentiating between their child's body growth and excessive increase in body fat. This is especially so in young children, where parents often view rapid growth as a sign of a healthy child (Lupi et al. 2014).

It has been shown that many parents of overweight children fail to identify their child as overweight, especially in the age range of 2–6 years, and confusion is common regarding meaning and importance of BMI measurement (Rietmeijer-Mentink et al. 2013; Francescatto et al. 2014).

A need to purchase clothes in sizes meant for older children, or the child growing out of their current clothes very quickly, may serve as early indicators of concern for parents regarding children's weight. Parents can be reluctant to label their child as overweight, and may benefit from direct discussion with their child's pediatrician about methods to identify overweight and clear action steps to address the issue, including specific nutrition counseling or involvement of a registered dietician (Lupi et al. 2014).

Overweight and obese children may themselves begin to notice a decline in their ability to keep up with peers. Running may become very difficult and even walking may cause exertion. This may precipitate bullying or ridicule, which can cause subsequent avoidance of physical activity, further deteriorating the situation (Latzer and Stein 2013).

Comorbidities

Overweight and obese children can experience serious comorbidities involving physiologic, structural, or emotional issues (Bass and Eneli 2015). Physiologic complications are primarily cardiovascular in origin and have been identified in more than one in three overweight children in some large population surveys (I'Allemand et al. 2008). For example, it is estimated that obese children in the U.S. have an approximately three-fold risk of hypertension than children of normal weight. Family history of hypertension is an important predictor in children (Sorof and Daniels 2002). A sample of 3383 adolescents aged 12–19 years in an NHANES survey showed a prevalence of 14% prehypertension, 22% for borderline dyslipidemia, 6% for more serious dyslipidemia, and 15% for prediabetes and diabetes during the survey period 1999–2008, with a consistent increase in prevalence with each increase in weight category. At least one cardiovascular risk factor was seen in 43% of the children studied. Overweight children in the study had a 49% chance of having a cardiovascular risk factor, while obese children had a prevalence of 61% (May, Kuklina, and Yoon 2012).

Screening Guidelines

Universal screening for dyslipidemia is recommended for children 9–11 years, and again between 17 and 19 years, by the National Heart, Lung, and Blood Institute through the Expert Panel on Integrated Guidelines for Cardiovascular Health and Risk Reduction in Children and Adolescents (Tables 21.1 and 21.2). Childhood dyslipidemia has been closely associated with atherosclerotic changes in overweight and obese children, established by both imaging and autopsy studies, and are highly predictive of dyslipidemia and atherosclerotic changes in adulthood (May, Kuklina, and Yoon 2012). If level of HDL cholesterol is elevated, lifestyle measures are the first target of treatment. If these are unsuccessful, medication has been recommended for children as young as 10 years of age. This policy change highlights the prevalence of the problem and the urgent need for effective lifestyle approaches in children (Expert Panel on Integrated Guidelines for Cardiovascular et al. 2011).

LIPIDS AND LIPOPROTEIN LEVELS

Importantly, elevated cardiovascular risk factors in children have been shown to be reversible by healthy lifestyle measures. In 1809 children followed for 27 years in a Finnish study, healthy lifestyle was correlated with beneficial lipid ratios, healthy BMI, and reduced progression of atherosclerotic changes (Juonala, Viikari, and Raitakari 2013).

Table 21.1 Acceptable, Borderline-High, and High Plasma Lipid, Lipoprotein, and Apolipoprotein Concentrations for Children and Adolescents

Category	Low, mg/dL [a]	Acceptable, mg/dL	Borderline-High, mg/dL	High, mg/dL[a]
TC	–	<170	170–199	≥200
LDL cholesterol	–	<110	110–129	≥130
Non-HDL cholesterol	–	<120	120–144	≥145
Apolipoprotein B		<90	90–109	≥110
Triglycerides				
0–9 years	–	<70	75–99	≥100
10–19 years	–	<90	90–129	≥130
HDL cholesterol	<40	>45	40–45	–
Apolipoprotein A-1	<115	>120	115–120	–

Note: Values for plasma lipid and lipoprotein levels are from the NCEP Expert Panel on Cholesterol Levels in Children. Non-HDL cholesterol values from the Bogalusa Heart Study are equivalent to the NCEP Pediatric Panel cut points for LDL cholesterol. Values for plasma apolipoprotein B and apolipoprotein A-1 are from the National Health and Nutrition Examination Survey III. Note that values shown are in mg/dL; to convert to SI units, divide the results for TC, LDL cholesterol, HDL cholesterol, and non-HDL cholesterol by 38.6; for triglycerides, divide by 88.6.

[a] Low cut points for HDL cholesterol and apolipoprotein A-1 represent approximately the 10th percentile. The cut points for high and borderline-high represent approximately the 95th and 75th percentiles, respectively.

Table 21.2 Recommended Cut Points for Lipid and Lipoprotein Levels in Young Adults

Category	Low, mg/dL[a]	Borderline-Low, mg/dL	Acceptable, mg/dL	Borderline-High, mg/dL	High, mg/dL [a]
TC	–	–	<170	170–100	≥200
LDL cholesterol	–	–	<120	120–159	≥160
Non-HDL Cholesterol	–	–	<150	150–189	≥190
Triglycerides	–	–	<115	115–189	≥190
HDL cholesterol	<40	40–44	>45	–	–

Source: Expert Panel on Integrated Guidelines for Cardiovascular Health and Risk Reduction in Children and Adolescents, National Heart, Lung, and Blood and Institute. 2011. "Expert panel on integrated guidelines for cardiovascular health and risk reduction in children and adolescents: summary report." *Pediatrics* 128(Suppl 5): S213–56. doi: 10.1542/peds.2009-2107C.

Note: Values provided are from the Lipid Research Clinics Prevalence Study. The cut points for TC, LDL cholesterol, and non HDL cholesterol and non HDL cholesterol represent the 95th percentile for 20 to 24-year-old subjects and are not identical with the cut points used in the most recent NHLBI adult guidelines, Adult Treatment Panel III ("Third Report of the Expert Panel on Detection, Evaluation, and Treatment of High Blood Cholesterol in Adults"), which are derived from combined data on adults of all ages. The age specific cut points given here are provided for pediatric care providers to use in managing this young adult age group. For TC, LDL cholesterol, and non HDL cholesterol, borderline high values are between the 75th and 94th percentiles, whereas acceptable value are at the <75th percentile. The high triglyceride cut point represents approximately the 90th percentile; borderline high values are between the 75th and 89th percentiles, and acceptable values are at the <75th percentile. The low HDL cholesterol cut point represents approximately the 25th percentile; borderline low values are between the 26th and 50th percentiles, and acceptable values are at the >50th percentile.

Type-2 Diabetes

Prevalence of type-2 diabetes has increased by an estimated 30.5% in youth between 2001 and 2009, and now accounts for 20%–50% of new onset diabetes cases in children, with disproportionate impact on racial and ethnic minority groups including American Indians, African American, Hispanic, and Asian/Pacific Islanders. Prevalence in all groups in 2009 is estimated at 0.46 per 1000 (Dabelea et al. 2014).

A high correlation with obesity exists, although the etiology of type-2 diabetes is not completely understood in children. Type-2 diabetes is discussed in more detail later in the chapter.

Polycystic Ovarian Syndrome (PCOS)

PCOS is another illness related to obesity and insulin resistance in female adolescents. PCOS occurs in ≥8% of young women 18 to 25 years of age, with prevalence varying depending on the definition used. Adolescents with polycystic ovarian syndrome are often overweight or obese and demonstrate insulin resistance, type-2 diabetes, or the full metabolic syndrome (Moran et al. 2011).

Lifestyle modification, targeted weight management, and adequate physical activity are important components of management. Weight loss has been positively correlated with improvement in insulin resistance and with improvement in menstrual irregularity in PCOS (Marzouk and Sayed Ahmed 2015).

Slipped Capital Femoral Epiphysis and Tibia Vara

Structural comorbidities such as slipped capital femoral epiphysis, have been shown to be associated with both high weight load and metabolic or endocrine abnormalities. Delayed sexual maturation and metabolic factors, such as insulin-like growth hormone and leptin, are thought to play a role (Witbreuk et al. 2013). Blount disease (tibia vara) is another structural abnormality seen in obese children which manifests as bowing of the lower extremity. Both slipped capital femoral epiphysis and tibia vara have also been associated with hypertension in obese youth, although the association is not yet fully understood (Taussig et al. 2015). Excess fat can also compress a range of organs impacting functioning, and can impair respiratory effort, resulting in reduced lung function (Cibella et al. 2015).

Non-Alcoholic Fatty Liver Disease (NALFD)

NALFD is the most common type of chronic liver disease in children, primarily seen in pediatric obesity, where prevalence may reach as high as 70%–80%. Hispanic children have shown the highest prevalence in several studies (Mencin and Lavine 2011). The definitive etiology of NALFD is unknown, but is thought to be multi-factorial, involving elements such as genetic susceptibility, epigenetic overlay, lifestyle measures such as lack of physical activity, and excess energy intake. Increased fatty acid delivery to the liver results in elevated hepatic triglyceride accumulation, increased lipogenesis, and interruption of normal fatty acid metabolism in hepatocytes. Accumulation of hepatic fat interferes with insulin receptors, increasing insulin resistance (Samuel et al. 2004). The disease is characterized by fat accumulation in the liver (steatosis), and considered the hepatic manifestation of metabolic syndrome, often associated with insulin resistance, elevated cholesterol and triglycerides, elevated serum glucose, and hypertension. Recent studies show that inflammation, alteration of gut microbiota, and increased gut permeability all play a role in the complex pathology of NALFD. Children at risk should be screened with serum liver transaminases and liver ultrasound (Frasinariu et al. 2013). In advanced stages NALFD progresses to nonalcoholic steatohepatitis (NASH), which is characterized by fibrosis that may progress to cirrhosis and end-stage-liver disease. Liver biopsy is the diagnostic standard, although other methods are under study; for example, the pediatric NALFD fibrosis index (PNFI) based on age, waist circumference, and triglyceride levels. This has been shown to be a potentially useful tool, but less reliable than liver biopsy (Nobili et al. 2009). There is no approved pharmacological treatment for NALFD in children, who are also at increased risk of cardiovascular disease. Lifestyle approaches with careful monitoring and multispecialty and inter-professional support including gastroenterology, cardiology, dieticians, and endocrinologists are recommonded to address the multifactorial elements of treatment (Aggarwal et al. 2014; Berardis and Sokal 2014). First-line treatment targets safe weight loss using a balanced diet usually under the close guidance of a registered dietician. Improvement in insulin resistance has been shown to be the factor most closely associated with improvement in NAFLD pathology (Reinehr et al. 2009). Probiotics have been evaluated in NALFD and have been shown to reduce liver inflammation and improve the epithelial function of the gut barrier. Both VSL #3 and *Lactobacillus* GG have shown benefit in children in small studies (Ferolla et al. 2015). Omega-3 fatty acids have also been shown to have a beneficial effect in reduction of inflammation and in reduction of insulin resistance in adult studies. A small randomized, double blind controlled trial of 250 mg, versus 500 mg of omega-3-docosahexaenoic acid (DHA) improved liver steatosis and insulin sensitivity. Both doses were effective in this study. Lowering of triglycerides was seen at 24 months follow-up. Studies in children are needed before definitive recommendations can be made, but risk of adverse effects is low (Nobili et al. 2013). Despite some progress on these dietary supplements, the mainstay of treatment for NASH remains lifestyle measures targeting weight loss and using a healthy whole food diet (Nobili et al. 2015).

Obstructive Sleep Apnea Syndrome (OSAS)

OSAS consists of periods of prolonged partial upper airway obstruction associated with decreased oxygenation, wakening, and repeated sleep fragmentation. Estimated prevalence is approximately 6% of children. Obesity is an independent risk factor for OSAS in children and has been partly explained by alteration in leptin and ghrelin balance and subsequent appetite stimulation. Daytime sleepiness is also associated with decreased physical activity (Spruyt et al. 2010).

Severity of symptoms may vary based on fat distribution in the upper body and neck. First-line treatment incudes adenotonsillectomy, although post-operative complications, including need for intubation, are more common in obese children, mandating close observation.

Associated comorbidities of OSAS include (Marcus et al. 2012; Koren et al. 2015):

- Cognitive deficits: learning, memory, language fluency, analytic thinking, school performance, math skills, executive function

- Behavioral abnormalities especially hyperactivity, depression, hypersomnolence, aggression
- Daytime sleepiness
- Hypertension
- Inflammation

Asthma

Respiratory symptoms including breathlessness and worsening of asthma in obese adolescents has been reported (Rastogi et al. 2015). Mechanisms include metabolic abnormalities and inflammation in addition to structural issues related to upper body adiposity (Rastogi et al. 2014; Strunk et al. 2015).

Renal Disease

Reduced estimated glomerular filtration rate has been documented in obese children as compared to children of normal weight in a study of 313 prepubertal children as young as 8 years old. Reduction in the estimated glomerular filtration rate correlated with increasing BMI (Correia-Costa et al. 2015).

ADHD

Unmedicated children with ADHD have been shown to have a 1.5 times increase in odds of being overweight as compared to children without ADHD (Waring and Lapane 2008; Davis 2010). A prospective study of 8106 children 7–8 years old showed that childhood ADHD symptoms significantly predicted adolescent obesity at age 16 years. Inattention was found to be a primary driver of interference with physical activity. Reduced physically active play in childhood in this study was also shown to be an early risk factor for symptoms of inattention in adolescence. Conclusions drawn by authors include the benefit of physically active play on children with ADHD and the need for monitoring of weight gain in children with ADHD as a preventive measure of overweight or obesity in adolescence (Khalife et al. 2014).

Vitamin D

It has been widely established that vitamin D deficiency is common in overweight and obese children, thought in part due to its lipophilic properties (Williams, Novick, and Lehman 2014). More recent studies show that although obese children have lower concentrations of total 25-hydroxy vitamin D, they have levels of bioavailable 25-hydroxy vitamin D that are comparable to normal weight children. This is due to decreased levels of vitamin D binding protein in obese children, which is thought to be associated with increased insulin resistance and upregulation of inflammatory cytokines. Vitamin D in childhood obesity remains an area of active study. Levels should be monitored regularly in overweight and obese children (Miraglia Del Giudice et al. 2015).

Skin Conditions

Acanthosis nigricans, associated with insulin resistance, is seen in approximately 1 in 10 obese Caucasian children and nearly one in two African American children (Williams, Novick, and Lehman 2014).

Peer Victimization (Bullying)

In addition to risk of serious physical comorbidities, obese children are common targets of criticism and peer victimization. This can come from parents, siblings, and other family members, as well as from peers. Teachers, physical education teachers, and coaches can also be sources of bullying towards overweight and obese children. Both direct and cyber bullying (Hamm et al. 2015) can shatter the self-esteem and self-confidence of the overweight or obese child. Multiple studies have shown that bullying is associated with serious detrimental mental and physical effects in children (Bogart et al. 2014) including suicidal ideation and completed suicide (Latzer and Stein 2013; Bell et al. 2011). Large prospective studies have shown high correlation between increased risk of age-related disease in adults who were bullied as children, including increased inflammatory markers such as C-reactive protein and obesity (Takizawa et al. 2015; Hawkes 2015).

A large multinational survey of adults identified weight-based bullying as the most prevalent reason for childhood bullying. Those surveyed identified parents and teachers as primary adults needed to intervene, and a majority also identified the child's healthcare provider, as important advocates who should take a role in intervention (Puhl et al. 2015).

Significant work is ongoing to develop anti-bullying laws and policy to establish consequences for those involved. Pediatricians and other clinicians who care for children should routinely and compassionately inquire about peer relationships, and add their efforts wherever possible to change this pervasive societal pattern.

Mental Health

Pediatric mental health issues, such as depression and low self-esteem, have been widely reported in overweight and obese preadolescents and adolescents. Major depression is estimated to occur in 20% of male and 30% of female adolescents in the highest obesity percentiles. In addition to bullying, triggers might include physical or sexual abuse, or harsh parenting styles. Signs of depression may be subtle and pass unnoticed if the child tries to cope alone. Food is an easy way of finding refuge as it can be both appealing and does not require deep explanation beyond the child's expression of hunger (Nemiary et al. 2012).

Treatment

There is no one treatment to completely "cure" obesity, although symptoms can be reduced to achieve a healthier lifestyle. Addressing mental health is a critical first step. Thorough psychological workup, including family and school factors, is often necessary to help understand the child's full situation. Physical rehabilitation is obviously crucial and should be accompanied with positive counseling and support of an experienced healthcare team. There are several modes of treatment to combat obesity; some of them are mentioned below. It is understood that early intervention is optimal, and that clinicians must be prepared to intervene at the earliest stages of overweight with an overarching goal of primary prevention.

Conventional Treatment

Once obesity is diagnosed, testing should be conducted to rule out the presence of serious comorbid diseases such as diabetes, hypertension, heart disease, joint, endocrine, or renal disease. Immediate medical issues should be addressed accordingly. Once the child has reached a level of stability, the actual obesity can be addressed. The main theme of the treatment is gradual sustained loss of the excess fat, which sounds simple, but in reality is a challenging undertaking for many patients and fraught with high likelihood of relapse. Bariatric surgery is not a standardized treatment in child and adolescent obesity unless the situation is life threatening. Although it has been shown in some studies to be effective in weight loss and correction of a range of metabolic abnormalities, it can be accompanied by a disproportionately high rate of complication. One of the problems with this surgery is its failure to address underlying causes of obesity. Full psychosocial evaluation and expert care is indicated if this treatment route is considered (Thakkar and Michalsky 2015; Ells et al. 2015).

LIFESTYLE MEASURES

Mainstream obesity treatment incudes a deceptively simple combination of reducing unhealthy habits and increasing healthy habits. For example, reducing non-nutritive food and beverages and introducing the intake of healthy food in age-appropriate portions, accompanied by reduction of sedentary activity and introduction of enjoyable physical activity.

Studies show that these simple measures are needed to lay a foundation for lasting change. A large population study of 8550 preschool-aged children showed that correlation with three basic household routines—regularly eating the evening meal as a family, adequate sleep (at least 10.5 hours per night), and limited screen time on weekdays (<2 hours)—was associated with an approximately 40% reduction in obesity prevalence compared to children exposed to none of these household routines regularly (Anderson and Whitaker 2010). A new concept in the literature is the "obesogenic home environment" consisting of limited fresh produce, higher intake of energy dense snacks, low rates of physical activity, and excessive screen time (Schrempft et al. 2015). Ongoing exposures to endocrine-disrupting chemicals, sleep fragmentation and deprivation (<9–11 hours per night), and high fructose foods and beverages have all been associated with treatment resistance in children (D'Aniello et al. 2015). Clinicians who are confident in several basic evidence-based recommendations can make an important initial impact, including counseling patients to:

- Eat breakfast
- Avoid fast food and frequent meals out of the home
- Avoid eating too quickly
- Watch portion size
- Eat only when actually hungry
- Reduce processed foods
- Add fresh vegetables and fruits, lean proteins, and sugar free beverages
- Avoid sugar sweetened beverages

SUGAR-SWEETENED BEVERAGES

In fact, sugar-sweetened beverages are the top source of energy intake in the United States and have been conclusively associated with obesity and increased incidence of type-2 diabetes in both adults and children. This category includes soft drinks, fruit drinks, energy drinks, and vitamin water drinks with sugar. The most common sweeteners include high fructose corn syrup, sucrose, or fruit juice concentrates. As an example, one typical can of soda contains about 150 calories and 40 grams of carbohydrate equivalent to approximately 10 teaspoons of sugar (Hu 2013). In one trial of 641 normal weight children reduction of only 104 kcal from sugar-sweetened beverages per day resulted in approximately 2.2 pounds less weight gain as opposed to controls over the 18-month study period (de Ruyter et al. 2012). The American Academy of Pediatrics has concluded that 100% fruit juice had no beneficial effect over whole fruit for infants < 6 months of age and children, and recommends limiting 100% fruit juice to 4–6 ounces daily for children 1–6 years of age and 8–12 ounces for older children (Committee on 2001). Sugar-sweetened beverage consumption has also been associated with earlier onset of menarche in a study of 5583 girls between the ages of 9 and 18.5 years independent of baseline BMI (Carwile et al. 2015). Consumption of artificially sweetened sodas, and caffeinated beverages, has also been associated with early menarche in a population sample of 2379 adolescent girls in the National Heart, Lung, and Blood Institute Growth and Health Study (Mueller et al. 2015). Multiple large studies in both children and adults show that decrease in sugar-sweetened beverage consumption alone is correlated in weight loss (Hu 2013).

Endorsement of reduction in consumption of sugar-sweetened beverages comes from the American Heart Association, the American Diabetes Association, American Academy of Pediatrics, World Health Organization, Institute of Medicine USDA, American Medical Association, and the Centers for Disease Control. Given the overwhelming body of evidence implicating sugar-sweetened beverages in pediatric obesity, it seems logical that one of the first treatment steps in pediatric obesity is to educate the child and family on the importance of reducing their intake and substituting with plain clean tap water. Use of diet soda has shown mixed results in obesity and is not recommended as a first-line approach in children. More studies are needed to examine the long-term metabolic and neurodevelopmental effects of its use in children and adolescents.

ACTIVITY AND SCREEN TIME

Basic recommendations in reduction of sedentary time and limiting screen time are also important. The American Academy of Pediatrics endorses no screen time for children under 2 years and no more than 2 hours of screen time for those over 2 years. This can be challenging depending on school and homework limitations. All televisions and monitors should be removed from sleeping areas and light at night should be eliminated.

Addition of regular enjoyable physical activity is important. A desired goal of 60 minutes of vigorous activity daily is the standard recommendation for children and adolescents. This may be challenging, and even predispose to injury in obese children initially. Supervision and guidance are needed to choose an appropriate activity, prevent injury, and to help ensure reasonable and successful goals are set and achieved. Team sports can be challenging depending on peer behavior, so options such as age-appropriate cross fit, personal training, martial arts, tai chi, and yoga may be good choices. Physical activity has also been shown to buffer the effect of chronic stress in overweight and obese adolescents (Yin et al. 2005). Small but encouraging studies have shown the benefit of resistance training on body composition and strength in obese children (Schranz, Tomkinson, and Olds 2013).

One study in 19 children, 8–12 years old, showed that twice weekly 75-minute exercise sessions that consisted of high repetition and moderate intensity resistance training resulted in significant increase in lean leg mass and leg strength compared to control group (Alberga et al. 2013).

Another study in 48 preadolescents used an 8-week training program consisting of closely supervised resistance training 3 days a week. Significant decrease in body fat, on average 2.6%, and increase in lean body mass of 5.3% were seen. No significant changes in weight, height, or body-mass-index were seen. Significant gains in strength were recorded with no adverse events. It is hypothesized that resistance training may be better tolerated than other types of exercise in certain obese children due to lack of aerobic capacity and fear of peer ridicule (McGuigan et al. 2009).

Another study of a 12-week resistance training program (3 days per week in 35 to 40-minute sessions in place of PE class) in 28 male and female Hispanic adolescents resulted in significant physical gains in strength and stamina and body composition, as well as significant gains in positive self-worth and body acceptance in both overweight and normal weight participants (Velez, Golem, and Arent 2010).

Yoga is another activity under active study in pediatric obesity. It can be considered both a mind and body therapy, and is comprised of a combination of poses or postures and controlled breathing exercises (McClafferty 2007). Yoga is used throughout the world to address stress, improve flexibility and fitness, and increase mindfulness and can be adapted in those with limited aerobic or physical ability to exercise. There are some small examples of yoga being successfully incorporated into pediatric obesity treatment programs. One example is a study in 20 obese adolescent boys who underwent yoga training three times per week (60 minutes) for 8 weeks. Treatment group showed significantly greater decrease in body fat, body weight, BMI, insulin resistance, and total cholesterol as compared to control group (Seo et al. 2012).

STRESS MANAGEMENT

Children can experience stress first hand, through their parents, or prenatally. Each pathway has been correlated with an increase in obesity, although it is still a relatively early area of study (Wilson and Sato 2014). Studies correlating paternal stress with childhood obesity have been shown to have a proportional element based on parental stress from more than one source. Examples of stressors include serious life events, parenting stress, perceived social support, and parental worries. Financial constraints, poor housing quality, violence in the neighborhood, racial or ethnic stress, and food insecurity are other familiar stressors associated with pediatric obesity.

Parental perceived stress was also positively correlated with fast-food consumption in this study of 2119 households with children aged 3–17 years (Parks et al. 2012). Chronic stress in caregivers of children with disabilities, such as autism, has also been associated with obesity in the children and deserves consideration from clinicians (Chen et al. 2015). Recognition and management of stressors are important for both normal weight and overweight or obese children. Stress-reduction techniques provide coping skills to help children manage situations both within and outside of their control and are highly adaptable. Clinicians treating children with obesity should ideally maximize support services and programs to reduce as many channels of family stress as possible during obesity treatment.

COORDINATION OF CARE, NATIONAL INITIATIVES

Consensus exists that integrated and coordinated care in multiple settings is needed to respond effectively to the pediatric obesity crisis. The AAP recommends an approach to preventing and treating obesity based on an incremental intervention of care outlined in four stages (Barlow and Expert Committee 2007). Stage 1 is Prevention Plus, which suggests delivery of basic counseling related to healthy nutrition and physical activity behaviors. Stage 2 is Structured Weight Management, requiring more frequent clinical visits and monitoring. Stage 3 is Comprehensive Multidisciplinary Intervention, involving a registered dietician and a behavioral medicine provider. Stage 4 is Tertiary Care Intervention, which may involve medication, very low calorie diet, and surgery depending on the individual. Multiple studies have identified clinicians' frustration and lack of comfort and sense of efficacy with obesity counseling. To this end, new techniques such as motivational interviewing are being tested (Barlow and Expert Committee 2007).

MOTIVATIONAL INTERVIEWING: A NEW TREATMENT APPROACH IN PEDIATRIC OBESITY

Motivational interviewing is a patient-centered counseling technique that helps the child and family identify and act on their own reasons for making behavior change. It takes into account readiness to change, uses non-judgmental questions and reflective listening to help child and family identify beliefs and values. The goals of this approach are to invoke motivation for change rather than use a directive approach. The basic technique includes (Resnicow, Davis, and Rollnick 2006; Schwartz 2010):

- Non-directive, open-ended questions.
- Reflective listening to build rapport and ideally help to resolve ambivalence.
- Comparison of stated values and current health practices; develop discrepancy.
- Assessment of importance of goals; for example, on a scale of 1–10.
- Assessment of confidence in achieving the goal: how confident are you that you can make this change?
- What would it take to get you to a higher number?
- Encourage goal setting.
- Focus on successes, expect challenges and setbacks.

A 2015 trial undertaken in 42 pediatric practices (645 children) through the AAP Pediatric Research in Office Settings Network over 2 years measured the impact of motivational interviewing on BMI in overweight children. Group 1 received usual care. Group 2 received four motivational interviewing sessions (by provider only) over 2 years. Group 3 patients received four motivational interviewing sessions from the provider, plus six sessions from a registered dietician. Motivational interviewing in Group 3 (provider plus registered dietician) resulted in a significant reduction in BMI percentile as compared to the other groups with a net difference between Group 1 usual care and Group 3 of 3.1 percentile units (Resnicow et al. 2015).

Questions remain as to how best to train practitioners and registered dieticians in motivational interviewing, how best to address overweight parents, and how to bring projects of this nature to scale. The AAP Change Talk website (http://www.kognito.com/changetalk/) offers training in motivational interviewing.

Another example in behavior change is seen in the Steps to Growing Up Healthy program, which is a prospective study designed to use a combination of brief motivational counseling "doses," brief motivational counseling plus monthly phone contact by community health workers, or brief motivational counseling plus monthly home visits. All groups are based on the use of specific and reachable goal setting and tracking based on primary recommendations of decreasing or eliminating sugar-sweetened beverages, decreasing screen time to less than 2 hours per day, and increasing physical activity to at least 60 minutes per day (Gorin et al. 2014; Ebbeling and Antonelli 2015).

POLICY CHANGES

Continued efforts on all levels are needed to make serious headway in pediatric obesity and to leverage the most effective preventive strategies given the complexity of the problem and the lack of progress on most fronts (Martin et al. 2014). The Affordable Care Act includes provisions for states that cover all U.S. Preventive Services Task Force grade A- and B-recommended preventive services. Some of the services included thereby are obesity screening and counseling for children, adolescents, and adults and breastfeeding counseling and gestational diabetes mellitus screening. Programs such as the Healthy Hunger-free Kids Act (2009–10), and continued improvements in the quality of programs such as the Women, Infants, and Children (WIC) program and the Supplemental Nutrition Assistance Program Education (SNAP-Ed) programs to include emphasis on energy balance and obesity prevention are urgently needed. Large coordinated studies such as the Childhood Obesity Research Demonstration (CORD) project which consists of three demonstration projects designed to approach the complex problem of childhood obesity across a spectrum of levels, settings, and public health interventions based on preventive approaches to the problem will help find solutions. Interventions in this program will target four key settings, based on accruing research about the strengths and weaknesses of earlier approaches. Current projects in planning include those to target (Joseph et al. 2015):

- Primary care clinics
- Early care and education centers
- Public schools
- Community institutions

Comprehensive approaches such as this will help catalyze solutions to complex problems such as: fair and appropriate insurance reimbursement for clinicians and inter-professional teams working with overweight and obese children; school based programs; increased research funding; and upgrading of government food programs.

Complementary and Integrative Therapies

The spirit of integrative care is inherent in the need for a full lifestyle approach to obesity prevention and treatment. Relatively few complementary approaches have been tried that are well supported by evidence in children. Mind–body approaches are some that show promise. For example, guided imagery was used successfully to reinforce a 12-week lifestyle behavior change program in a small randomized study of 35 obese Latino adolescents assigned to the treatment group. Participants received lifestyle education accompanied by a guided imagery program. Salivary cortisol was used to assess effect of guided imagery on stress reduction, which was significant in the treatment group. Significant reductions in leisure time and increase in physical activity in the treatment group were also observed. Guided imagery topics included: stress reduction, safe, relaxed place, conditioned relaxation, images and sensations related to hunger, visualization of participation in physical activity, and applying healthy eating habits, inner advisor offering guidance, inner warrior to recruit inner strength, discipline, courage, and self-confidence to meet inner and outer obstacles, visualizing future successes, and next healthy steps (Weigensberg et al. 2014).

MINDFULNESS

Small studies of mindfulness-based stress reduction in overweight adult women have shown promise using a combined mindfulness-based stress reduction and cognitive behavioral stress eating intervention (Corsica et al. 2014). Similar studies in children and families are needed to explore how best to leverage mind–body tools in this area (Dalen et al. 2015).

HYPNOSIS

The use of hypnosis is established for support of eating disorders and may prove to be effective in the treatment of pediatric obesity. Preliminary studies in adults show benefit, but studies are needed in children and adolescents (Entwistle et al. 2014).

OMEGA-3 FATTY ACIDS

Data from some animal studies shows benefit of omega-3 fatty acids on insulin resistance in metabolic syndrome and type-2 diabetes. Supplementation in humans has been conclusively shown to reduce serum triglycerides in the dose of 2–4 g per day in adults, and recent studies support the theory that marine origin omega-3 fatty acids have a positive effect on the dysregulation of inflammatory adipokines seen in obesity by modulating glucose intake and improving insulin response in adipose tissue (Siriwardhana, Kalupahana, and Moustaid-Moussa 2012).

The omega-3 fatty acids have also been shown to be upregulators of adiponectin, an anti-inflammatory insulin-sensitizing adipokine that regulates fat storage and utilization. This is one of the proposed mechanisms of the beneficial effect of the omega-3 fatty acids on insulin sensitivity and inflammation. They have also been shown to modulate adipocyte proliferation and differentiation. Research is very active in this area, with more human studies needed (Martinez-Fernandez et al. 2015).

Other complementary approaches, especially dietary supplements and acupuncture, although very popular in adults and in adolescents interested in weight loss, have a paucity of supporting evidence, especially in children (Esteghamati et al. 2015).

One exception showing promise is the dietary supplement curcumin, which is under active study for its anti-inflammatory and immunomodulatory effects. Animal trials and small human studies in adults show promise in reduction of inflammation and related insulin resistance in obesity and type-2 diabetes (Ganjali et al. 2014; Panzhinskiy et al. 2014).

PREVENTIVE MEASURES

Given the high rate of tracking of obesity from childhood to adolescence into adulthood, early preventive measures must be instituted. One of the first systematic reviews of preventive measures in early childhood obesity shows that multipronged approaches that address diet, activity, and behavior are most likely to be successful (Foster et al. 2015).

*Suggested Integrative Anticipatory Guidelines for Obesity Prevention by Age and Developmental Stage**

PRENATAL

- Optimize maternal weight as much as possible
- Addition of maternal DHA, minimum 200 mg/day (optimal dose unknown) (Haghiac et al. 2015)
- Avoid excessive maternal intake of sugar-sweetened beverages
- Normalize maternal vitamin D (Morales et al. 2015)
- Avoid preventable environmental exposures such as BPA and other known endocrine-disrupting chemicals (EDC)
- Address maternal stressors
- Encourage regular sleep cycle
- Avoid antibiotic use if possible

NEWBORN

Nutrition:

- Prioritize exclusive breastfeeding
- Allow child to set feeding pace and frequency; follow infant cues

Preventive measures:

- No television, no screen time
- Regular sleep schedule
- Minimize exposure to antibiotics if possible
- Minimize preventable environmental exposures to BPA and other endocrine-disrupting chemicals

Monitor and supplement as needed:

- Supplement maternal DHA, or provide infant DHA if not breastfeeding
- Vitamin D

* Adapted from: Brown et al. 2015; Daniels, Hassink, and Committee On Nutrition 2015; Martin-Biggers et al. 2015.

Clinician's initiatives:

- Regular monitoring of growth chart
- Preventive nutrition counseling and encouragement of family habit of physical activity
- Motivational interviewing techniques
- Monitor parental stress
- Introduce stress prevention measures, coping skills

6–12 MONTHS

Nutrition:

- Continue breastfeeding if possible
- Avoid early introduction of solids
- When ready for solids, introduce wide variety of fresh, organic (if possible) fruits and vegetables
- Vary tastes and textures, offer foods repeatedly in rotation if not liked on first several tries
- Establish routine meals and snack times

Prevention:

- No screen time
- Avoid antibiotic exposure (if possible)
- Minimize preventable environmental exposures to BPA and other EDC
- Address parental and caretaker stress
- Establish regular sleep patterns

Monitor and supplement as needed:

- DHA
- Vitamin D

Clinician's initiatives:

- Regular monitoring of growth chart, early intervention if concerned
- Preventive nutrition counseling and encouragement of physical activity
- Motivational interviewing techniques
- Monitor parental stress
- Introduce stress prevention measures and effective coping skills for caretakers

12–24 MONTHS

Nutrition:

- Avoid sugar-sweetened beverages and fast food
- Continue to offer variety of foods, tastes, textures

- Continue structured meal times, but avoid overly restrictive or harsh parenting around food
- Authoritative parenting preferred (respect's child's opinions, clear boundaries) (Rhee et al. 2006)
- Follow child's cues for hunger and satiety
- Parental modeling of healthy foods
- Avoid food as reward pattern

Prevention:

- Minimize preventable environmental exposures to BPA and other EDC
- Minimal to no screen time
- Avoid antibiotics (if possible)
- Address parental and caretaker stress
- Establish regular sleep patterns

Monitor and supplement as needed:

- DHA
- Vitamin D

Clinician's initiatives:

- Regular monitoring of growth chart, early intervention if concerned
- Preventive nutrition counseling and encouragement of physical activity
- Motivational interviewing techniques
- Monitor parental stress
- Introduce stress prevention measures, coping skills

24–48 MONTHS

Nutrition:

- Avoid sugar-sweetened beverages
- Expand food variety and textures
- Follow regular schedule for meals and snacks
- Continue parental modeling of healthy habits
- Avoid restrictive or harsh parenting style around meals and food
- Authoritative parenting preferred (respect's child's opinions, clear boundaries) (Rhee et al. 2006)
- Avoid food as reward

Prevention:

- Minimal screen time, less than 2 hours per day
- Active supervised play outdoors, daily minimum 60 minutes if possible
- Minimize preventable environmental exposures to BPA and other EDC

Monitor and supplement as needed:

- DHA
- Vitamin D

Clinician's initiatives:

- Regular monitoring of growth chart, early intervention if concerned
- Preventive nutrition counseling and encouragement of physical activity
- Motivational interviewing techniques
- Monitor parental stress
- Introduce stress-prevention measures, coping skills

4–12 YEARS

Nutrition:

- Maintain healthy food choices and regular meal times
- Introduce personal choice of healthy foods
- Maintain parental modeling of healthy habits
- Introduce meal and snack preparation skills
- Introduce gardening and farmer's markets if appropriate
- Preventive nutrition counseling
- Portion awareness

Prevention:

- Minimize screen time
- Physical activity 60 minutes per day, avoid sedentary summers
- Regular sleep schedule, minimize light at night
- Minimize preventable environmental exposures to BPA and other EDC
- Stress management, coping skills, awareness of peer victimization

Monitor and supplement as needed:

- DHA
- Vitamin D

Clinician's initiatives:

- Regular monitoring of growth chart, early intervention if concerned.
- Universal lipid screening between ages 9 to 11 years (Table 21.3).
- Total cholesterol and LDL cholesterol in childhood have been shown to be the best predictors of dyslipidemia and atherosclerosis in adulthood (Benuck 2015).
- Motivational interviewing techniques.
- Monitor for peer victimization.
- Monitor parental stress.
- Introduce stress prevention measures, coping skills.
- Family stress management.

Table 21.3 Cut Off Points in Children for Plasma Lipids, Lipoproteins, and Apolipoprotein (mg/dL)

Category	Acceptable	Borderline high	High
Total cholesterol	<170	170–199	≥200
LDL-C	<110	110–129	≥130
Non-HDL-C	<120	120–144	≥145
Apolipoprotein B	<90	90–109	≥110
Triglycerides			
0–9 years	<75	75–99	≥100
10–19 years	<90	90–129	≥130
	Acceptable	*Borderline low*	*Low*
HDL-C	>45	40–45	<40
Apolipoprotein A	>120	115–120	<115

Note: HDL-C, high-density lipoprotein cholesterol; LDL-C, low-density lipoprotein cholesterol.

Source: Adapted from Benuck, I. 2015. "Point: the rationale for universal lipid screening and treatment in children." *J Clin Lipidol* 9(5 Suppl): S93–100.

13–18 YEARS

Nutrition:

- Increasing autonomy around food choices
- Minimize fast food and meals eaten out
- Continue parental modeling of healthy nutrition behaviors
- Expand meal planning, preparation and grocery shopping participation
- Portion awareness

Prevention:

- Physical activity 60 minutes per day, avoid sedentary school breaks
- Manage screen time
- Regular protected sleep
- Minimize preventable environmental exposures to BPA and other EDC
- Stress management and cultivation of coping skills, awareness of peer victimization
- Family stress management

Clinician's initiatives:

- Regular monitoring of growth chart, early intervention if concerned.
- Preventive nutrition counseling and encouragement of physical activity.
- Universal lipid screening repeated between 17 and 19 years.
- Total cholesterol and LDL cholesterol in childhood have been shown to be the best predictors of dyslipidemia and atherosclerosis in adulthood (Benuck 2015).
- Motivational interviewing techniques.
- Monitor parental stress.
- Introduce stress-prevention measures, coping skills.

Emerging Interventions

One approach under study in obesity prevention and treatment includes a program to teach and encourage self-regulation in preschool students. A randomized controlled trial, the Growing Healthy study, will compare two obesity prevention programs in preschoolers in a Head Start preschool program versus controls. Both study arms will use a combined parent–child curriculum delivered over 8 weeks. Units include: Eating a Rainbow of Foods, Trying New Foods, Turning off the TV, Limiting Sugar Sweetened Beverages, Easy Healthy Meals at Home, Family Meals, and Meal Planning. Each teaching unit is followed up by telephone calls with master's level trained educators. One of these study arms will include the Incredible Years Series, which is a widely used program to teach and encourage self-regulation in preschool-aged children which will be directed toward stress management, impulse control, and learning delayed gratification. Parents learn to help children find ways to calm down without food, manage behavior without food rewards, and encourage healthy eating behaviors (Miller et al. 2012).

Smart phone apps are another type of intervention under study in childhood obesity to support behaviors to reduce overweight and obesity. Examples include personalized encouragement for self-determination skills, positive feedback, reminders about goal setting, and support in the event of a relapse in behavior. This is an area of developing technology and active research interest (Chaplais et al. 2015).

A third approach under study is web-based family education. For example, the Enabling Mothers to Prevent pediatric Obesity through Web-Based Education and Reciprocal Determinism (EMPOWER) study is a randomized, blinded, parallel-group study focused on four specific child behaviors (physical activity, fruit and vegetable consumption, sugar-free beverage intake, and screen time) and five maternal mediators of child behavior (environment, emotional coping, expectations, self-control, and self-efficacy) using a 2.5-hour web-based educational program. Results of this intervention in 44 participants (n = 22 in study group) showed improvement in fruit and vegetable intake even at 1-year follow-up (Knowlden and Sharma 2015).

A Healthy Teens program delivered through Facebook to Korean American adolescents offers a further example of social media in health education. Topics included discussion of goal setting, self-efficacy, vicarious experiences (observing success of others), motivation, positive feedback, healthy eating, and physical activity (Park, Nahm, and Rogers 2015).

Other randomized controlled trials using social media are underway (Jane et al. 2015). Exergames (combining web-based gaming with physical activity) is another emerging area in childhood obesity prevention that is garnering high research interest (Lamboglia et al. 2013), especially when used in a cooperative rather than a competitive model (Marker and Staiano 2015).

Metabolic Syndrome and Type-2 Diabetes

The metabolic syndrome is characterized by central obesity, dyslipidemia (particularly hypertriglyceridemia and low HDL cholesterol), hypertension, and impaired glucose tolerance. Criteria for the age-specific definition of metabolic syndrome in children by the International Diabetes Federation includes waist circumference and two or more other risk factor variables (Zimmet et al. 2007). Visceral abdominal fat, as opposed to subcutaneous abdominal fat, is significantly correlated with insulin resistance (Taksali et al. 2008). Prevalence of the metabolic syndrome is increasing globally, mirroring the upward trend of obesity in developed and developing countries (Gupta et al. 2013) and was found to be as high as 35.2% in obese Chinese adolescents in a cross-sectional study of 2761 students, with prevalence of 23.4% in the overweight category compared to 3.7% in normal weight students (Li et al. 2008). Similar prevalence was seen in Bolivian children, and a survey study of 793 Asian Indian adolescents reported metabolic syndrome prevalence of 29.0% in overweight students (Vikram et al. 2006).

A glucose challenge administered to 439 obese and overweight adolescents compared to controls showed that the prevalence of metabolic syndrome was one in two of severely obese study participants (Weiss et al. 2004).

In the study group, each half unit step up in BMI was associated with increased risk of metabolic syndrome and increasing insulin resistance. Pro-inflammatory markers such as C-reactive protein and interleukin-6 levels which were significantly elevated in the presence of insulin resistance and adiponectin levels (a positive biomarker for insulin sensitivity) decreased in this study population.

One of the most concerning elements of both obesity and the metabolic syndrome in children is the likelihood that they will persist into adulthood. The AAP guidelines recommend screening for diabetes using fasting blood glucose for all children 10 years and older who have BMI percentiles greater than 85%, weight for height, or weight greater than 120% of ideal height (Expert Panel on Integrated Guidelines for Cardiovascular Health et al. 2011; Benuck 2015).

Treatment Approaches to the Metabolic Syndrome

The mainstay of treatment of the metabolic syndrome is lifestyle modification including regular physical activity and maintaining optimal weight. This is reinforced by results from a unique and important randomized longitudinal atherosclerosis prevention trial in a large Finnish cohort of children. Participants were followed from 6 months through age 20 years, with treatment group who received repeated dietary interventions demonstrating a 41% reduction in metabolic syndrome between the ages of 15 and 20 years. The Special Turku Coronary Risk Factor Intervention Project for Children (STRIP) study involved dietary counseling in the treatment group at least biannually until the age of 20 years. Counseling centered on replacing saturated with unsaturated fats, salt reduction, and promotion of healthy whole foods, whole grains, fruits, and vegetables. The dietary intake and counseling were individualized and based on the Nordic nutrition recommendations (30% energy from fat, 10%–15% from protein, and 50%–60% from carbohydrates). Parents received the counseling until the child was aged 7 years, and going forward the child received direct counseling. In addition to the striking reduction in metabolic syndrome prevalence, earlier reports from the longitudinal study showed significant reduction in cardiovascular risk factors and blood pressure in the treatment group (Nupponen et al. 2015).

Mediterranean Diet

Although the benefits of the Mediterranean diet have been repeatedly shown to reduce cardiovascular risk factors in adults (Babio, Bullo, and Salas-Salvado 2009), few studies have examined its effect in children. One small study in 49 obese Mexican children and adolescents evaluated a 16-week Mediterranean diet. Patient caloric needs were individualized and followed a ratio of 55%–60% carbohydrates, no more than 10% refined and processed sugars, 25%–30% fats, and 15% protein. Treatment group was educated on the Mediterranean diet and received specific menus to guide them. All patients were seen every 3 weeks throughout the study to reinforce the assigned diet. Statistically significant improvements were seen in the treatment group in the following areas: BMI, fat mass, lean mass, fasting glucose, total cholesterol, triglycerides, and LDL-cholesterol levels. HDL-cholesterol levels rose significantly. As a group, the Mediterranean diet treatment arm showed a 45% decrease in metabolic syndrome measurements (p<0.05). Significant increase in the percentage of consumed fiber, protein, omega-9 fatty acids, zinc, selenium, vitamin E, and flavonoids were also noted. The authors also stressed the importance of healthy lifestyle habits, reduction of sedentary time, increase in physical activity as contributors to positive outcome (Velazquez-Lopez et al. 2014).

Cinnamon

Cinnamon is known to have potent anti-inflammatory properties and may improve fasting blood glucose levels by increasing insulin sensitivity. The mechanism at the molecular level is complex. In simplified terms, in vitro studies have shown that the action of cinnamon polyphenols increases the amount of insulin receptor and the amount of various substrates that enhance cellular uptake of glucose into the cell. Increased expression of anti-inflammatory cytokines has also been demonstrated, which act to prevent inflammation associated with adipose tissue (Rafehi, Ververis, and Karagiannis 2012). Cinnamon polyphenols also activate peroxisome proliferator-activated receptors (PPARs), which are intimately involved in the regulation of insulin sensitivity and adipogenesis (Rafehi, Ververis, and Karagiannis 2012). Cinnamon has been shown in animal studies to counteract gene expression of pro-inflammatory cytokines such as interleukin-6 and tumor necrosis factor-alpha, and to inhibit regulators of lipid metabolism and triglyceride transfer proteins (Rafehi, Ververis, and Karagiannis 2012). Although in vitro and animal studies are promising, clinical studies in humans have had mixed results and have shown high study design variability (Qin, Panickar, and Anderson 2010).

The risk of adverse effects from cinnamon used as a food or flavoring is low. More randomized controlled trials on its use are needed to determine its effect in metabolic syndrome and in type-2 diabetes, especially in the pediatric population (Rafehi, Ververis, and Karagiannis 2012). In addition to cinnamon, other widely used complementary botanicals that have been studied in the treatment of metabolic syndrome and type-2 diabetes include bitter gourd (*Momordica charantia*) (Habicht et al. 2014), and fenugreek. As with cinnamon, adult human studies show mixed results, and pediatric studies are lacking (Medagama and Bandara 2014).

Type-2 Diabetes

Pediatric risk factors for type-2 diabetes include central obesity (high waist-to-hip circumference ratio), hypertriglyceridemia, and family history of type-2 diabetes. The prevalence of type-2 diabetes is estimated to have increased threefold from 1999 to 2008 in U.S. children according to NHANES data, with prevalence estimated at approximately 12:100,000 (Arslanian 2000). Highest U.S. prevalence is found in African

American, Hispanic, Asian/Pacific Islanders, and American Indians, particularly Pima Indians in Arizona, where the prevalence is estimated at 22:1000 in adolescents (Fagot-Campagna et al. 2000). Globally, prevalence of type-2 diabetes in children is increasing in many developed and developing nations. The lowest incidence is in the Netherlands and Austria. The next highest after the U.S. and Canadian Indians was seen in Puerto Rico and the United Kingdom (Fazeli Farsani et al. 2013).

Risk factors for type-2 diabetes include obesity, family history of type-2 diabetes, hypertension, dyslipidemia, polycystic ovarian syndrome, and acanthosis nigricans (Reinehr 2013). Puberty is frequently a triggering factor of the disease. This has been shown in part to be a result of increased growth hormone secretion, which increases resistance to insulin. This corresponds with a peak in diagnosis of type-2 diabetes in mid-puberty (Pinhas-Hamiel et al. 2007). Younger obese children have also been shown to be hyperinsulinemic, and have been estimated to have a 40% lower insulin response in glucose metabolism than normal weight children (Weiss et al. 2004; May, Kuklina, and Yoon 2012).

Diagnosis of type-2 diabetes can be made in asymptomatic children by screening of blood or urine. Acanthosis nigricans is present in an estimated 50%–90% of children with the disease and should prompt screening if detected in an undiagnosed child or adolescent. Diagnosis of polycystic ovarian syndrome should also prompt diabetes screening.

A concerning issue in type-2 diabetes in children is the time dependent factor of complications such as cardiovascular and microvascular disease. Development of the disease at a younger age is predictive of significantly higher complications in those children with associated dyslipidemia and hypertension (Eppens et al. 2006).

Treatment

American Academy of Pediatric treatment guidelines are aimed at normalization of blood glucose levels and HBA1c, control of blood pressure and abnormal lipid levels. Lifestyle measures directed at weight loss are the mainstay of treatment approach. Often this requires an inter-professional team effort to progress in a safe manner that respects cultural and financial aspects and involves the whole family in sustainable change.

Pharmaceuticals are sometimes added as a bridging approach, although lifestyle measures should always be maximized. Mental health and socioeconomic constraints can compound the complexity of treatment necessitating extra support from the healthcare team. Primary prevention is critical to reduce the burden of this illness on children and adolescents (Reinehr 2013; Haemer et al. 2014).

As can be seen by review of the serious complication of overweight and obesity in children and adolescents, prevention is a priority. The majority of successful treatment programs emphasize a multifaceted approach addressing nutrition, lifestyle, physical activity, regular sleep, and family support. Some of the most successful programs include outreach counseling and the use of motivational interviewing to enhance self-efficacy and realistic goals setting.

It will take the coordinated efforts of an engaged society to reverse the obesity trend. Clinicians up to date on the research and able to counsel children and families effectively can have real impact on children's quality of life into adulthood (Juonala, Viikari, and Raitakari 2013).

References

111th Congress of the United States (2009–10). 2009–10. *Healthy, Hunger-Free Kids Act of 2010*.

Aggarwal, A., K. Puri, S. Thangada, N. Zein, and N. Alkhouri. 2014. "Nonalcoholic fatty liver disease in children: recent practice guidelines, where do they take us?" *Curr Pediatr Rev* 10(2): 151–61.

Agras, W. S., and A. J. Mascola. 2005. "Risk factors for childhood overweight." *Curr Opin Pediatr* 17(5): 648–52.

Alberga, A. S., B. C. Farnesi, A. Lafleche, L. Legault, and J. Komorowski. 2013. "The effects of resistance exercise training on body composition and strength in obese prepubertal children." *Phys Sportsmed* 41(3): 103–9. doi: 10.3810/psm.2013.09.2028.

Anderson, S. E., and R. C. Whitaker. 2009. "Prevalence of obesity among US preschool children in different racial and ethnic groups." *Arch Pediatr Adolesc Med* 163(4): 344–8. doi: 10.1001/archpediatrics.2009.18.

Anderson, S. E., and R. C. Whitaker. 2010. "Household routines and obesity in US preschool-aged children." *Pediatrics* 125(3): 420–8. doi: 10.1542/peds.2009-0417.

Arslanian, S. A. 2000. "Type 2 diabetes mellitus in children: pathophysiology and risk factors." *J Pediatr Endocrinol Metab* 13(Suppl 6): S1385–94.

Azad, M. B., S. L. Bridgman, A. B. Becker, and A. L. Kozyrskyj. 2014. "Infant antibiotic exposure and the development of childhood overweight and central adiposity." *Int J Obes (Lond)* 38(10): 1290–8. doi: 10.1038/ijo.2014.119.

Babio, N., M. Bullo, and J. Salas-Salvado. 2009. "Mediterranean diet and metabolic syndrome: the evidence." *Public Health Nutr* 12(9A): 1607–17. doi: 10.1017/S1368980009990449.

Barlow, S. E., and Expert Committee. 2007. "Expert committee recommendations regarding the prevention, assessment, and treatment of child and adolescent overweight and obesity: summary report." *Pediatrics* 120(Suppl 4): S164–92. doi: 10.1542/peds.2007-2329C.

Bass, R., and I. Eneli. 2015. "Severe childhood obesity: an under-recognised and growing health problem." *Postgrad Med J*. doi: 10.1136/postgradmedj-2014-133033.

Bell, L. M., J. A. Curran, S. Byrne, H. Roby, K. Suriano, T. W. Jones, and E. A. Davis. 2011. "High incidence of obesity co-morbidities in young children: a cross-sectional study." *J Paediatr Child Health* 47(12): 911–7. doi: 10.1111/j.1440-1754.2011.02102.x.

Benuck, I. 2015. "Point: the rationale for universal lipid screening and treatment in children." *J Clin Lipidol* 9(5 Suppl): S93–100. doi: 10.1016/j.jacl.2015.03.104.

Berardis, S., and E. Sokal. 2014. "Pediatric non-alcoholic fatty liver disease: an increasing public health issue." *Eur J Pediatr* 173(2): 131–9. doi: 10.1007/s00431-013-2157-6.

Berrington de Gonzalez, A., P. Hartge, J. R. Cerhan, A. J. Flint, L. Hannan, R. J. MacInnis, S. C. Moore, G. S. Tobias, H. Anton-Culver, L. B. Freeman, W. L. Beeson, S. L. Clipp, D. R. English, A. R. Folsom, D. M. Freedman, G. Giles, N. Hakansson, K. D. Henderson, J. Hoffman-Bolton, J. A. Hoppin, K. L. Koenig, I. M. Lee, M. S. Linet, Y. Park, G. Pocobelli, A. Schatzkin, H. D. Sesso, E. Weiderpass, B. J. Willcox, A. Wolk, A. Zeleniuch-Jacquotte, W. C. Willett, and M. J. Thun. 2010. "Body-mass index and mortality among 1.46 million white adults." *N Engl J Med* 363(23): 2211–9. doi: 10.1056/NEJMoa1000367.

Bogart, L. M., M. N. Elliott, D. J. Klein, S. R. Tortolero, S. Mrug, M. F. Peskin, S. L. Davies, E. T. Schink, and M. A. Schuster. 2014. "Peer victimization in fifth grade and health in tenth grade." *Pediatrics* 133(3): 440–7. doi: 10.1542/peds.2013-3510.

Brown, C. L., E. E. Halvorson, G. M. Cohen, S. Lazorick, and J. A. Skelton. 2015. "Addressing childhood obesity: opportunities for prevention." *Pediatr Clin North Am* 62(5): 1241–61. doi: 10.1016/j.pcl.2015.05.013.

Carwile, J. L., W. C. Willett, D. Spiegelman, E. Hertzmark, J. Rich-Edwards, A. L. Frazier, and K. B. Michels. 2015. "Sugar-sweetened beverage consumption and age at menarche in a prospective study of US girls." *Hum Reprod* 30(3): 675–83. doi: 10.1093/humrep/deu349.

Chaplais, E., G. Naughton, D. Thivel, D. Courteix, and D. Greene. 2015. "Smartphone interventions for weight treatment and behavioral change in pediatric obesity: a systematic review." *Telemed J E Health*. doi: 10.1089/tmj.2014.0197.

Chen, X., B. Gelaye, J. C. Velez, C. Barbosa, M. Pepper, A. Andrade, W. Gao, C. Kirschbaum, and M. A. Williams. 2015. "Caregivers' hair cortisol: a possible biomarker of chronic stress is associated with obesity measures among children with disabilities." *BMC Pediatr* 15: 9. doi: 10.1186/s12887-015-0322-y.

Cho, I., S. Yamanishi, L. Cox, B. A. Methe, J. Zavadil, K. Li, Z. Gao, D. Mahana, K. Raju, I. Teitler, H. Li, A. V. Alekseyenko, and M. J. Blaser. 2012. "Antibiotics in early life alter the murine colonic microbiome and adiposity." *Nature* 488(7413): 621–6. doi: 10.1038/nature11400.

Cibella, F., A. Bruno, G. Cuttitta, S. Bucchieri, M. R. Melis, S. De Cantis, S. La Grutta, and G. Viegi. 2015. "An elevated body mass index increases lung volume but reduces airflow in Italian schoolchildren." *PLoS One* 10(5): e0127154. doi: 10.1371/journal.pone.0127154.

Committee on Nutrition. 2001. "American Academy of Pediatrics: the use and misuse of fruit juice in pediatrics." *Pediatrics* 107(5): 1210–3.

Cornwell, T. B., A. R. McAlister, and N. Polmear-Swendris. 2014. "Children's knowledge of packaged and fast food brands and their BMI. Why the relationship matters for policy makers." *Appetite* 81: 277–83. doi: 10.1016/j.appet.2014.06.017.

Correia-Costa, L., A. C. Afonso, F. Schaefer, J. T. Guimaraes, M. Bustorff, A. Guerra, H. Barros, and A. Azevedo. 2015. "Decreased renal function in overweight and obese prepubertal children." *Pediatr Res*. doi: 10.1038/pr.2015.130.

Corsica, J., M. M. Hood, S. Katterman, B. Kleinman, and I. Ivan. 2014. "Development of a novel mindfulness and cognitive behavioral intervention for stress-eating: a comparative pilot study." *Eat Behav* 15(4): 694–9. doi: 10.1016/j.eatbeh.2014.08.002.

Council on School Health, and Committee on Nutrition. 2015. "Snacks, sweetened beverages, added sugars, and schools." *Pediatrics* 135(3): 575–83. doi: 10.1542/peds.2014-3902.

Cullen, K. W., T. A. Chen, J. M. Dave, and H. Jensen. 2015. "Differential improvements in student fruit and vegetable selection and consumption in response to the new national school lunch program regulations: a pilot study." *J Acad Nutr Diet* 115(5): 743–50. doi: 10.1016/j.jand.2014.10.021.

D'Aniello, R., J. Troisi, O. D'Amico, M. Sangermano, G. Massa, A. Moccaldo, L. Pierri, M. Poeta, and P. Vajro. 2015. "Emerging pathomechanisms involved in obesity." *J Pediatr Gastroenterol Nutr* 60(1): 113–9. doi: 10.1097/MPG.0000000000000559.

Dabelea, D., E. J. Mayer-Davis, S. Saydah, G. Imperatore, B. Linder, J. Divers, R. Bell, A. Badaru, J. W. Talton, T. Crume, A. D. Liese, A. T. Merchant, J. M. Lawrence, K. Reynolds, L. Dolan, L. L. Liu, R. F. Hamman, and Search for Diabetes in Youth Study. 2014. "Prevalence of type 1 and type 2 diabetes among children and adolescents from 2001 to 2009." *JAMA* 311(17): 1778–86. doi: 10.1001/jama.2014.3201.

Dalen, J., J. L. Brody, J. K. Staples, and D. Sedillo. 2015. "A conceptual framework for the expansion of behavioral interventions for youth obesity: a family-based mindful eating approach." *Child Obes*. doi: 10.1089/chi.2014.0150.

Daniels, S. R., S. G. Hassink, and Committee On Nutrition. 2015. "The role of the pediatrician in primary prevention of obesity." *Pediatrics* 136(1): e275–92. doi: 10.1542/peds.2015-1558.

Darmasseelane, K., M. J. Hyde, S. Santhakumaran, C. Gale, and N. Modi. 2014. "Mode of delivery and offspring body mass index, overweight and obesity in adult life: a systematic review and meta-analysis." *PLoS One* 9(2): e87896. doi: 10.1371/journal.pone.0087896.

Davis, C. 2010. "Attention-deficit/hyperactivity disorder: associations with overeating and obesity." *Curr Psychiatry Rep* 12(5): 389–95. doi: 10.1007/s11920-010-0133-7.

de Ruyter, J. C., M. R. Olthof, J. C. Seidell, and M. B. Katan. 2012. "A trial of sugar-free or sugar-sweetened beverages and body weight in children." *N Engl J Med* 367(15): 1397–406. doi: 10.1056/NEJMoa1203034.

Ebbeling, C. B., and R. C. Antonelli. 2015. "Primary care interventions for pediatric obesity: need for an integrated approach." *Pediatrics* 135(4): 757–8. doi: 10.1542/peds.2015-0495.

Ells, L. J., E. Mead, G. Atkinson, E. Corpeleijn, K. Roberts, R. Viner, L. Baur, M. I. Metzendorf, and B. Richter. 2015. "Surgery for the treatment of obesity in children and adolescents." *Cochrane Database Syst Rev* 6: CD011740. doi: 10.1002/14651858.CD011740.

Enax, L., B. Weber, M. Ahlers, U. Kaiser, K. Diethelm, D. Holtkamp, U. Faupel, H. H. Holzmuller, and M. Kersting. 2015. "Food packaging cues influence taste perception and increase effort provision for a recommended snack product in children." *Front Psychol* 6: 882. doi: 10.3389/fpsyg.2015.00882.

Entwistle, P. A., R. J. Webb, J. C. Abayomi, B. Johnson, A. C. Sparkes, and I. G. Davies. 2014. "Unconscious agendas in the etiology of refractory obesity and the role of hypnosis in their identification and resolution: a new paradigm for weight-management programs or a paradigm revisited?" *Int J Clin Exp Hypn* 62(3): 330–59. doi: 10.1080/00207144.2014.901085.

Eppens, M. C., M. E. Craig, J. Cusumano, S. Hing, A. K. Chan, N. J. Howard, M. Silink, and K. C. Donaghue. 2006. "Prevalence of diabetes complications in adolescents with type 2 compared with type 1 diabetes." *Diabetes Care* 29(6): 1300–6. doi: 10.2337/dc05-2470.

Esteghamati, A., T. Mazaheri, M. Vahidi Rad, and S. Noshad. 2015. "Complementary and alternative medicine for the treatment of obesity: a critical review." *Int J Endocrinol Metab* 13(2): e19678. doi: 10.5812/ijem.19678.

Expert Panel on Integrated Guidelines for Cardiovascular Health and Risk Reduction in Children and Adolescents, National Heart, Lung and Blood and Institute. 2011. "Expert panel on integrated guidelines for cardiovascular health and risk reduction in children and adolescents: summary report." *Pediatrics* 128(Suppl 5): S213–56. doi: 10.1542/peds.2009-2107C.

Fagot-Campagna, A., D. J. Pettitt, M. M. Engelgau, N. R. Burrows, L. S. Geiss, R. Valdez, G. L. Beckles, J. Saaddine, E. W. Gregg, D. F. Williamson, and K. M. Narayan. 2000. "Type 2 diabetes among North American children and adolescents: an epidemiologic review and a public health perspective." *J Pediatr* 136(5): 664–72.

Fazeli Farsani, S., M. P. van der Aa, M. M. van der Vorst, C. A. Knibbe, and A. de Boer. 2013. "Global trends in the incidence and prevalence of type 2 diabetes in children and adolescents: a systematic review and evaluation of methodological approaches." *Diabetologia* 56(7): 1471–88. doi: 10.1007/s00125-013-2915-z.

Ferolla, S. M., G. N. Armiliato, C. A. Couto, and T. C. Ferrari. 2015. "Probiotics as a complementary therapeutic approach in nonalcoholic fatty liver disease." *World J Hepatol* 7(3): 559–65. doi: 10.4254/wjh.v7.i3.559.

Foster, B. A., J. Farragher, P. Parker, and E. T. Sosa. 2015. "Treatment interventions for early childhood obesity: a systematic review." *Acad Pediatr* 15(4): 353–61. doi: 10.1016/j.acap.2015.04.037.

Francescatto, C., N. S. Santos, V. F. Coutinho, and R. F. Costa. 2014. "Mothers' perceptions about the nutritional status of their overweight children: a systematic review." *J Pediatr (Rio J)* 90(4): 332–43. doi: 10.1016/j.jped.2014.01.009.

Frasinariu, O. E., S. Ceccarelli, A. Alisi, E. Moraru, and V. Nobili. 2013. "Gut-liver axis and fibrosis in nonalcoholic fatty liver disease: an input for novel therapies." *Dig Liver Dis* 45(7): 543–51. doi: 10.1016/j.dld.2012.11.010.

Galley, J. D., M. Bailey, C. Kamp Dush, S. Schoppe-Sullivan, and L. M. Christian. 2014. "Maternal obesity is associated with alterations in the gut microbiome in toddlers." *PLoS One* 9(11): e113026. doi: 10.1371/journal.pone.0113026.

Ganjali, S., A. Sahebkar, E. Mahdipour, K. Jamialahmadi, S. Torabi, S. Akhlaghi, G. Ferns, S. M. Parizadeh, and M. Ghayour-Mobarhan. 2014. "Investigation of the effects of curcumin on serum cytokines in obese individuals: a randomized controlled trial." *ScientificWorld Journal* 2014: 898361. doi: 10.1155/2014/898361.

Gilmore, L. A., M. Klempel-Donchenko, and L. M. Redman. 2015. "Pregnancy as a window to future health: excessive gestational weight gain and obesity." *Semin Perinatol* 39(4): 296–303. doi: 10.1053/j.semperi.2015.05.009.

Goedert, J. J., X. Hua, G. Yu, and J. Shi. 2014. "Diversity and composition of the adult fecal microbiome associated with history of cesarean birth or appendectomy: analysis of the American Gut Project." *EBioMedicine* 1(2–3): 167–72. doi: 10.1016/j.ebiom.2014.11.004.

Gorin, A. A., J. Wiley, C. M. Ohannessian, D. Hernandez, A. Grant, and M. M. Cloutier. 2014. "Steps to Growing Up Healthy: a pediatric primary care based obesity prevention program for young children." *BMC Public Health* 14: 72. doi: 10.1186/1471-2458-14-72.

Grummer-Strawn, L. M., C. Reinold, N. F. Krebs, Centers for Disease Control and Prevention. 2010. "Use of World Health Organization and CDC growth charts for children aged 0–59 months in the United States." *MMWR Recomm Rep* 59(RR–9): 1–15.

Gupta, N., P. Shah, S. Nayyar, and A. Misra. 2013. "Childhood obesity and the metabolic syndrome in developing countries." *Indian J Pediatr* 80(Suppl 1): S28–37. doi: 10.1007/s12098-012-0923-5.

Gurnani, M., C. Birken, and J. Hamilton. 2015. "Childhood obesity: causes, consequences, and management." *Pediatr Clin North Am* 62(4): 821–40. doi: 10.1016/j.pcl.2015.04.001.

Habicht, S. D., C. Ludwig, R. Y. Yang, and M. B. Krawinkel. 2014. "Momordica charantia and type 2 diabetes: from in vitro to human studies." *Curr Diabetes Rev* 10(1): 48–60.

Haemer, M. A., H. M. Grow, C. Fernandez, G. J. Lukasiewicz, E. T. Rhodes, L. A. Shaffer, B. Sweeney, S. J. Woolford, and E. Estrada. 2014. "Addressing prediabetes in childhood obesity treatment programs: support from research and current practice." *Child Obes* 10(4): 292–303. doi: 10.1089/chi.2013.0158.

Haghiac, M., X. H. Yang, L. Presley, S. Smith, S. Dettelback, J. Minium, M. A. Belury, P. M. Catalano, and S. Hauguel-de Mouzon. 2015. "Dietary omega-3 fatty acid supplementation reduces inflammation in obese pregnant women: a randomized double-blind controlled clinical trial." *PLoS One* 10(9): e0137309. doi: 10.1371/journal.pone.0137309.

Hamm, M. P., A. S. Newton, A. Chisholm, J. Shulhan, A. Milne, P. Sundar, H. Ennis, S. D. Scott, and L. Hartling. 2015. "Prevalence and effect of cyberbullying on children and young people: a scoping review of social media studies." *JAMA Pediatr* 169(8): 770–7. doi: 10.1001/jamapediatrics.2015.0944.

Hawkes, N. 2015. "Bullying in childhood may be linked to heart disease risk, study says." *BMJ* 350: h2738. doi: 10.1136/bmj.h2738.

Holben, D. H., and C. A. Taylor. 2015. "Food insecurity and its association with central obesity and other markers of metabolic syndrome among persons aged 12 to 18 years in the United States." *J Am Osteopath Assoc* 115(9): 536–43. doi: 10.7556/jaoa.2015.111.

Hu, F. B. 2013. "Resolved: there is sufficient scientific evidence that decreasing sugar-sweetened beverage consumption will reduce the prevalence of obesity and obesity-related diseases." *Obes Rev* 14(8): 606–19. doi: 10.1111/obr.12040.

I'Allemand, D., S. Wiegand, T. Reinehr, J. Muller, M. Wabitsch, K. Widhalm, R. Holl, and A. PV-Study Group. 2008. "Cardiovascular risk in 26,008 European overweight children as established by a multicenter database." *Obesity (Silver Spring)* 16(7): 1672–9. doi: 10.1038/oby.2008.259.

Jane, M., J. Foster, M. Hagger, and S. Pal. 2015. "Using new technologies to promote weight management: a randomised controlled trial study protocol." *BMC Public Health* 15: 509. doi: 10.1186/s12889-015-1849-4.

Jenkin, G., N. Madhvani, L. Signal, and S. Bowers. 2014. "A systematic review of persuasive marketing techniques to promote food to children on television." *Obes Rev* 15(4): 281–93. doi: 10.1111/obr.12141.

Joseph, S., A. M. Stevens, T. Ledoux, T. M. O'Connor, D. P. O'Connor, and D. Thompson. 2015. "Rationale, design, and methods for process evaluation in the Childhood Obesity Research Demonstration Project." *J Nutr Educ Behav.* doi: 10.1016/j.jneb.2015.07.002.

Juonala, M., J. S. Viikari, and O. T. Raitakari. 2013. "Main findings from the prospective

Cardiovascular Risk in Young Finns Study." *Curr Opin Lipidol* 24(1): 57–64. doi: 10.1097/MOL.0b013e32835a7ed4.

Kelly, B., B. Freeman, L. King, K. Chapman, L. A. Baur, and T. Gill. 2015. "Television advertising, not viewing, is associated with negative dietary patterns in children." *Pediatr Obes*. doi: 10.1111/ijpo.12057.

Khalife, N., M. Kantomaa, V. Glover, T. Tammelin, J. Laitinen, H. Ebeling, T. Hurtig, M. R. Jarvelin, and A. Rodriguez. 2014. "Childhood attention-deficit/hyperactivity disorder symptoms are risk factors for obesity and physical inactivity in adolescence." *J Am Acad Child Adolesc Psychiatry* 53(4): 425–36. doi: 10.1016/j.jaac.2014.01.009.

Knowlden, A., and M. Sharma. 2015. "One-year efficacy testing of enabling mothers to prevent pediatric obesity through web-based education and reciprocal determinism (EMPOWER) randomized control trial." *Health Educ Behav*. doi: 10.1177/1090198115596737.

Koren, D., J. A. Chirinos, L. E. Katz, E. R. Mohler, P. R. Gallagher, G. F. Mitchell, and C. L. Marcus. 2015. "Interrelationships between obesity, obstructive sleep apnea syndrome and cardiovascular risk in obese adolescents." *Int J Obes (Lond)* 39(7): 1086–93. doi: 10.1038/ijo.2015.67.

Lamboglia, C. M., V. T. da Silva, J. E. de Vasconcelos Filho, M. H. Pinheiro, M. C. Munguba, F. V. Silva Junior, F. A. de Paula, and C. A. da Silva. 2013. "Exergaming as a strategic tool in the fight against childhood obesity: a systematic review." *J Obes* 2013: 438364. doi: 10.1155/2013/438364.

Latzer, Y., and D. Stein. 2013. "A review of the psychological and familial perspectives of childhood obesity." *J Eat Disord* 1: 7. doi: 10.1186/2050-2974-1-7.

Laurent, J. S., and J. Sibold. 2015. "Addictive-like eating, body mass index, and psychological correlates in a community sample of preadolescents." *J Pediatr Health Care*. doi: 10.1016/j.pedhc.2015.06.010.

Li, Y., X. Yang, F. Zhai, F. J. Kok, W. Zhao, J. Piao, J. Zhang, Z. Cui, and G. Ma. 2008. "Prevalence of the metabolic syndrome in Chinese adolescents." *Br J Nutr* 99(3): 565–70. doi: 10.1017/S0007114507797064.

Lupi, J. L., M. B. Haddad, J. A. Gazmararian, and K. J. Rask. 2014. "Parental perceptions of family and pediatrician roles in childhood weight management." *J Pediatr* 165(1): 99–103 e2. doi: 10.1016/j.jpeds.2014.02.064.

Marcus, C. L., L. J. Brooks, K. A. Draper, D. Gozal, A. C. Halbower, J. Jones, M. S. Schechter, S. D. Ward, S. H. Sheldon, R. N. Shiffman, C. Lehmann, K. Spruyt, and American Academy of Pediatrics. 2012. "Diagnosis and management of childhood obstructive sleep apnea syndrome." *Pediatrics* 130(3): e714–55. doi: 10.1542/peds.2012-1672.

Marker, A. M., and A. E. Staiano. 2015. "Better together: outcomes of cooperation versus competition in social exergaming." *Games Health J* 4(1): 25–30. doi: 10.1089/g4h.2014.0066.

Martin, A., D. H. Saunders, S. D. Shenkin, and J. Sproule. 2014. "Lifestyle intervention for improving school achievement in overweight or obese children and adolescents." *Cochrane Database Syst Rev* 3: CD009728. doi: 10.1002/14651858.CD009728.pub2.

Martin-Biggers, J., K. Spaccarotella, C. Delaney, M. Koenings, G. Alleman, N. Hongu, J. Worobey, and C. Byrd-Bredbenner. 2015. "Development of the Intervention Materials for the HomeStyles Obesity Prevention Program for Parents of Preschoolers." *Nutrients* 7(8): 6628–69. doi: 10.3390/nu7085301.

Martinez-Fernandez, L., L. M. Laiglesia, A. E. Huerta, J. A. Martinez, and M. J. Moreno-Aliaga. 2015. "Omega-3 fatty acids and adipose tissue function in obesity and metabolic syndrome." *Prostaglandins Other Lipid Mediat*. doi: 10.1016/j.prostaglandins.2015.07.003.

Marzouk, T. M., and W. A. Sayed Ahmed. 2015. "Effect of dietary weight loss on menstrual regularity in obese young adult women with polycystic ovary syndrome." *J Pediatr Adolesc Gynecol*. doi: 10.1016/j.jpag.2015.01.002.

Mason, S. M., R. F. MacLehose, S. L. Katz-Wise, S. B. Austin, D. Neumark-Sztainer, B. L. Harlow, and J. W. Rich-Edwards. 2015. "Childhood abuse victimization, stress-related eating, and weight status in young women." *Ann Epidemiol* 25(10): 760–766 e2. doi: 10.1016/j.annepidem.2015.06.081.

May, A. L., E. V. Kuklina, and P. W. Yoon. 2012. "Prevalence of cardiovascular disease risk factors among US adolescents, 1999–2008." *Pediatrics* 129(6): 1035–41. doi: 10.1542/peds.2011-1082.

McClafferty, H. H. 2007. "Integrative approach to obesity." *Pediatr Clin North Am* 54(6): 969–81; xi. doi: 10.1016/j.pcl.2007.10.006.

McGuigan, M. R., M. Tatasciore, R. U. Newton, and S. Pettigrew. 2009. "Eight weeks of resistance training can significantly alter body composition in children who are overweight or obese." *J Strength Cond Res* 23(1): 80–5.

McPherson, A. C., and S. Lindsay. 2012. "How do children with disabilities view 'healthy living'? A descriptive pilot study." *Disabil Health J* 5(3): 201–9. doi: 10.1016/j.dhjo.2012.04.004.

Medagama, A. B., and R. Bandara. 2014. "The use of complementary and alternative medicines (CAMs) in the treatment of diabetes mellitus: is continued use safe and effective?" *Nutr J* 13: 102. doi: 10.1186/1475-2891-13-102.

Menale, C., M. T. Piccolo, G. Cirillo, R. A. Calogero, A. Papparella, L. Mita, E. M. Del Giudice, N. Diano, S. Crispi, and D. G. Mita. 2015. "Bisphenol A effects on gene expression in adipocytes from children: association with metabolic disorders." *J Mol Endocrinol* 54(3): 289–303. doi: 10.1530/JME-14-0282.

Mencin, A. A., and J. E. Lavine. 2011. "Nonalcoholic fatty liver disease in children." *Curr Opin Clin Nutr Metab Care* 14(2): 151–7. doi: 10.1097/MCO.0b013e328342baec.

Metallinos-Katsaras, E., A. Must, and K. Gorman. 2012. "A longitudinal study of food insecurity on obesity in preschool children." *J Acad Nutr Diet* 112(12): 1949–58. doi: 10.1016/j.jand.2012.08.031.

Meule, A., T. Hermann, and A. Kubler. 2015. "Food addiction in overweight and obese adolescents seeking weight-loss treatment." *Eur Eat Disord Rev* 23(3): 193–8. doi: 10.1002/erv.2355.

Miller, A. L., M. A. Horodynski, H. E. Herb, K. E. Peterson, D. Contreras, N. Kaciroti, J. Staples-Watson, and J. C. Lumeng. 2012. "Enhancing self-regulation as a strategy for obesity prevention in Head Start preschoolers: the growing healthy study." *BMC Public Health* 12: 1040. doi: 10.1186/1471-2458-12-1040.

Miraglia Del Giudice, E., A. Grandone, G. Cirillo, C. Capristo, P. Marzuillo, A. Di Sessa, G. R. Umano, L. Ruggiero, and L. Perrone. 2015. "Bioavailable vitamin D in obese children: the role of insulin resistance." *J Clin Endocrinol Metab*: jc20152973. doi: 10.1210/jc.2015-2973.

Mor, A., S. Antonsen, J. Kahlert, V. Holsteen, S. Jorgensen, J. Holm-Pedersen, H. T. Sorensen, O. Pedersen, and V. Ehrenstein. 2015. "Prenatal exposure to systemic antibacterials and overweight and obesity in Danish schoolchildren: a prevalence study." *Int J Obes (Lond)*. doi: 10.1038/ijo.2015.129.

Morales, E., A. Rodriguez, D. Valvi, C. Iniguez, A. Esplugues, J. Vioque, L. S. Marina, A. Jimenez, M. Espada, C. R. Dehli, A. Fernandez-Somoano, M. Vrijheid, and J. Sunyer. 2015. "Deficit of vitamin D in pregnancy and growth and overweight in the offspring." *Int J Obes (Lond)* 39(1): 61–8. doi: 10.1038/ijo.2014.165.

Moran, L. J., S. K. Hutchison, R. J. Norman, and H. J. Teede. 2011. "Lifestyle changes in women with polycystic ovary syndrome." *Cochrane Database Syst Rev* (7): CD007506. doi: 10.1002/14651858.CD007506.pub3.

Mueller, N. T., D. R. Jacobs, Jr., R. F. MacLehose, E. W. Demerath, S. P. Kelly, J. G. Dreyfus, and M. A. Pereira. 2015. "Consumption of caffeinated and artificially sweetened soft drinks is associated with risk of early menarche." *Am J Clin Nutr* 102(3): 648–54. doi: 10.3945/ajcn.114.100958.

Nemiary, D., R. Shim, G. Mattox, and K. Holden. 2012. "The relationship between obesity and depression among adolescents." *Psychiatr Ann* 42(8): 305–308. doi: 10.3928/00485713-20120806-09.

Ng, M., T. Fleming, M. Robinson, B. Thomson, N. Graetz, C. Margono, E. C. Mullany, S.

Biryukov, C. Abbafati, S. F. Abera, J. P. Abraham, N. M. Abu-Rmeileh, T. Achoki, F. S. AlBuhairan, Z. A. Alemu, R. Alfonso, M. K. Ali, R. Ali, N. A. Guzman, W. Ammar, P. Anwari, A. Banerjee, S. Barquera, S. Basu, D. A. Bennett, Z. Bhutta, J. Blore, N. Cabral, I. C. Nonato, J. C. Chang, R. Chowdhury, K. J. Courville, M. H. Criqui, D. K. Cundiff, K. C. Dabhadkar, L. Dandona, A. Davis, A. Dayama, S. D. Dharmaratne, E. L. Ding, A. M. Durrani, A. Esteghamati, F. Farzadfar, D. F. Fay, V. L. Feigin, A. Flaxman, M. H. Forouzanfar, A. Goto, M. A. Green, R. Gupta, N. Hafezi-Nejad, G. J. Hankey, H. C. Harewood, R. Havmoeller, S. Hay, L. Hernandez, A. Husseini, B. T. Idrisov, N. Ikeda, F. Islami, E. Jahangir, S. K. Jassal, S. H. Jee, M. Jeffreys, J. B. Jonas, E. K. Kabagambe, S. E. Khalifa, A. P. Kengne, Y. S. Khader, Y. H. Khang, D. Kim, R. W. Kimokoti, J. M. Kinge, Y. Kokubo, S. Kosen, G. Kwan, T. Lai, M. Leinsalu, Y. Li, X. Liang, S. Liu, G. Logroscino, P. A. Lotufo, Y. Lu, J. Ma, N. K. Mainoo, G. A. Mensah, T. R. Merriman, A. H. Mokdad, J. Moschandreas, M. Naghavi, A. Naheed, D. Nand, K. M. Narayan, E. L. Nelson, M. L. Neuhouser, M. I. Nisar, T. Ohkubo, S. O. Oti, A. Pedroza, D. Prabhakaran, N. Roy, U. Sampson, H. Seo, S. G. Sepanlou, K. Shibuya, R. Shiri, I. Shiue, G. M. Singh, J. A. Singh, V. Skirbekk, N. J. Stapelberg, L. Sturua, B. L. Sykes, M. Tobias, B. X. Tran, L. Trasande, H. Toyoshima, S. van de Vijver, T. J. Vasankari, J. L. Veerman, G. Velasquez-Melendez, V. V. Vlassov, S. E. Vollset, T. Vos, C. Wang, X. Wang, E. Weiderpass, A. Werdecker, J. L. Wright, Y. C. Yang, H. Yatsuya, J. Yoon, S. J. Yoon, Y. Zhao, M. Zhou, S. Zhu, A. D. Lopez, C. J. Murray, and E. Gakidou. 2014. "Global, regional, and national prevalence of overweight and obesity in children and adults during 1980–2013: a systematic analysis for the Global Burden of Disease Study 2013." *Lancet* 384(9945): 766–81. doi: 10.1016/S0140-6736(14)60460-8.

Nobili, V., A. Alisi, C. Della Corte, P. Rise, C. Galli, C. Agostoni, and G. Bedogni. 2013. "Docosahexaenoic acid for the treatment of fatty liver: randomised controlled trial in children." *Nutr Metab Cardiovasc Dis* 23(11): 1066–70. doi: 10.1016/j.numecd.2012.10.010.

Nobili, V., A. Alisi, A. Vania, C. Tiribelli, A. Pietrobattista, and G. Bedogni. 2009. "The pediatric NAFLD fibrosis index: a predictor of liver fibrosis in children with non-alcoholic fatty liver disease." *BMC Med* 7: 21. doi: 10.1186/1741-7015-7-21.

Nobili, V., N. Alkhouri, A. Alisi, C. Della Corte, E. Fitzpatrick, M. Raponi, and A. Dhawan. 2015. "Nonalcoholic fatty liver disease: a challenge for pediatricians." *JAMA Pediatr* 169(2): 170–6. doi: 10.1001/jamapediatrics.2014.2702.

Nupponen, M., K. Pahkala, M. Juonala, C. G. Magnussen, H. Niinikoski, T. Ronnemaa, J. S. Viikari, M. Saarinen, H. Lagstrom, A. Jula, O. Simell, and O. T. Raitakari. 2015. "Metabolic syndrome from adolescence to early adulthood: effect of infancy-onset dietary counseling of low saturated fat: the Special Turku Coronary Risk Factor Intervention Project (STRIP)." *Circulation* 131(7): 605–13. doi: 10.1161/CIRCULATIONAHA.114.010532.

Ogden, C. L., M. D. Carroll, B. K. Kit, and K. M. Flegal. 2014. "Prevalence of childhood and adult obesity in the United States, 2011–2012." *JAMA* 311(8): 806–14. doi: 10.1001/jama.2014.732.

Panzhinskiy, E., Y. Hua, P. A. Lapchak, E. Topchiy, T. E. Lehmann, J. Ren, and S. Nair. 2014. "Novel curcumin derivative CNB-001 mitigates obesity-associated insulin resistance." *J Pharmacol Exp Ther* 349(2): 248–57. doi: 10.1124/jpet.113.208728.

Park, B. K., E. S. Nahm, and V. E. Rogers. 2015. "Development of a teen-friendly health education program on Facebook: lessons learned." *J Pediatr Health Care*. doi: 10.1016/j.pedhc.2015.06.011.

Parks, E. P., S. Kumanyika, R. H. Moore, N. Stettler, B. H. Wrotniak, and A. Kazak. 2012. "Influence of stress in parents on child obesity and related behaviors." *Pediatrics* 130(5): e1096–104. doi: 10.1542/peds.2012-0895.

Pearce, J., and S. C. Langley-Evans. 2013. "The types of food introduced during complementary feeding and risk of childhood obesity: a systematic review." *Int J Obes (Lond)* 37(4): 477–85. doi: 10.1038/ijo.2013.8.

Penfold, N. C., and S. E. Ozanne. 2015. "Developmental programming by maternal obesity in 2015: outcomes, mechanisms, and potential interventions." *Horm Behav.* doi: 10.1016/j. yhbeh.2015.06.015.

Pinhas-Hamiel, O., L. Lerner-Geva, N. M. Copperman, and M. S. Jacobson. 2007. "Lipid and insulin levels in obese children: changes with age and puberty." *Obesity (Silver Spring)* 15(11): 2825–31. doi: 10.1038/oby.2007.335.

Poti, J. M., K. J. Duffey, and B. M. Popkin. 2014. "The association of fast food consumption with poor dietary outcomes and obesity among children: is it the fast food or the remainder of the diet?" *Am J Clin Nutr* 99(1): 162–71. doi: 10.3945/ajcn.113.071928.

Powell, L. M., J. L. Harris, and T. Fox. 2013. "Food marketing expenditures aimed at youth: putting the numbers in context." *Am J Prev Med* 45(4): 453–61. doi: 10.1016/j. amepre.2013.06.003.

Puhl, R. M., J. D. Latner, K. O'Brien, J. Luedicke, M. Forhan, and S. Danielsdottir. 2015. "Cross-national perspectives about weight-based bullying in youth: nature, extent and remedies." *Pediatr Obes.* doi: 10.1111/ijpo.12051.

Qin, B., K. S. Panickar, and R. A. Anderson. 2010. "Cinnamon: potential role in the prevention of insulin resistance, metabolic syndrome, and type 2 diabetes." *J Diabetes Sci Technol* 4(3): 685–93.

Rafehi, H., K. Ververis, and T. C. Karagiannis. 2012. "Controversies surrounding the clinical potential of cinnamon for the management of diabetes." *Diabetes Obes Metab* 14(6): 493–9. doi: 10.1111/j.1463-1326.2011.01538.x.

Rastogi, D., K. Bhalani, C. B. Hall, and C. R. Isasi. 2014. "Association of pulmonary function with adiposity and metabolic abnormalities in urban minority adolescents." *Ann Am Thorac Soc* 11(5): 744–52. doi: 10.1513/AnnalsATS.201311-403OC.

Rastogi, D., S. Fraser, J. Oh, A. M. Huber, Y. Schulman, R. H. Bhagtani, Z. S. Khan, L. Tesfa, C. B. Hall, and F. Macian. 2015. "Inflammation, metabolic dysregulation, and pulmonary function among obese urban adolescents with asthma." *Am J Respir Crit Care Med* 191(2): 149–60. doi: 10.1164/rccm.201409-1587OC.

Reinehr, T. 2013. "Type 2 diabetes mellitus in children and adolescents." *World J Diabetes* 4(6): 270–81. doi: 10.4239/wjd.v4.i6.270.

Reinehr, T., C. Schmidt, A. M. Toschke, and W. Andler. 2009. "Lifestyle intervention in obese children with non-alcoholic fatty liver disease: 2-year follow-up study." *Arch Dis Child* 94(6): 437–42. doi: 10.1136/adc.2008.143594.

Resnicow, K., R. Davis, and S. Rollnick. 2006. "Motivational interviewing for pediatric obesity: conceptual issues and evidence review." *J Am Diet Assoc* 106(12): 2024–33. doi: 10.1016/j. jada.2006.09.015.

Resnicow, K., F. McMaster, A. Bocian, D. Harris, Y. Zhou, L. Snetselaar, R. Schwartz, E. Myers, J. Gotlieb, J. Foster, D. Hollinger, K. Smith, S. Woolford, D. Mueller, and R. C. Wasserman. 2015. "Motivational interviewing and dietary counseling for obesity in primary care: an RCT." *Pediatrics* 135(4): 649–57. doi: 10.1542/peds.2014-1880.

Rhee, K. E., J. C. Lumeng, D. P. Appugliese, N. Kaciroti, and R. H. Bradley. 2006. "Parenting styles and overweight status in first grade." *Pediatrics* 117(6): 2047–54. doi: 10.1542/peds.2005-2259.

Rietmeijer-Mentink, M., W. D. Paulis, M. van Middelkoop, P. J. Bindels, and J. C. van der Wouden. 2013. "Difference between parental perception and actual weight status of children: a systematic review." *Matern Child Nutr* 9(1): 3–22. doi: 10.1111/j.1740-8709.2012.00462.x.

Saari, A., L. J. Virta, U. Sankilampi, L. Dunkel, and H. Saxen. 2015. "Antibiotic exposure in infancy and risk of being overweight in the first 24 months of life." *Pediatrics* 135(4): 617–26. doi: 10.1542/peds.2014-3407.

Samuel, V. T., Z. X. Liu, X. Qu, B. D. Elder, S. Bilz, D. Befroy, A. J. Romanelli, and G. I. Shulman. 2004. "Mechanism of hepatic insulin resistance in non-alcoholic fatty liver disease." *J Biol Chem* 279(31): 32345–53. doi: 10.1074/jbc.M313478200.

Schranz, N., G. Tomkinson, and T. Olds. 2013. "What is the effect of resistance training on the strength, body composition and psychosocial status of overweight and obese children and adolescents? A systematic review and meta-analysis." *Sports Med* 43(9): 893–907. doi: 10.1007/s40279-013-0062-9.

Schrempft, S., C. H. van Jaarsveld, A. Fisher, and J. Wardle. 2015. "The obesogenic quality of the home environment: associations with diet, physical activity, TV viewing, and BMI in preschool children." *PLoS One* 10(8): e0134490. doi: 10.1371/journal.pone.0134490.

Schwartz, R. P. 2010. "Motivational interviewing (patient-centered counseling) to address childhood obesity." *Pediatr Ann* 39(3): 154–8. doi: 10.3928/00904481-20100223-06.

Seo, D. Y., S. Lee, A. Figueroa, H. K. Kim, Y. H. Baek, Y. S. Kwak, N. Kim, T. H. Choi, B. D. Rhee, K. S. Ko, B. J. Park, S. Y. Park, and J. Han. 2012. "Yoga training improves metabolic parameters in obese boys." *Korean J Physiol Pharmacol* 16(3): 175–80. doi: 10.4196/kjpp.2012.16.3.175.

Siriwardhana, N., N. S. Kalupahana, and N. Moustaid-Moussa. 2012. "Health benefits of n-3 polyunsaturated fatty acids: eicosapentaenoic acid and docosahexaenoic acid." *Adv Food Nutr Res* 65: 211–22. doi: 10.1016/B978-0-12-416003-3.00013-5.

Skinner, A. C., and J. A. Skelton. 2014. "Prevalence and trends in obesity and severe obesity among children in the United States, 1999–2012." *JAMA Pediatr* 168(6): 561–6. doi: 10.1001/jamapediatrics.2014.21.

Sorof, J., and S. Daniels. 2002. "Obesity hypertension in children: a problem of epidemic proportions." *Hypertension* 40(4): 441–7.

Spruyt, K., O. Sans Capdevila, L. D. Serpero, L. Kheirandish-Gozal, and D. Gozal. 2010. "Dietary and physical activity patterns in children with obstructive sleep apnea." *J Pediatr* 156(5): 724–30, 730 e1–730 e3. doi: 10.1016/j.jpeds.2009.11.010.

Strunk, R. C., R. Colvin, L. B. Bacharier, A. Fuhlbrigge, E. Forno, A. M. Arbelaez, K. G. Tantisira, and Childhood Asthma Management Program Research Group. 2015. "Airway obstruction worsens in young adults with asthma who become obese." *J Allergy Clin Immunol Pract* 3(5): 765–71 e2. doi: 10.1016/j.jaip.2015.05.009.

Takizawa, R., A. Danese, B. Maughan, and L. Arseneault. 2015. "Bullying victimization in childhood predicts inflammation and obesity at mid-life: a five-decade birth cohort study." *Psychol Med* 45(13): 2705–15. doi: 10.1017/S0033291715000653.

Taksali, S. E., S. Caprio, J. Dziura, S. Dufour, A. M. Cali, T. R. Goodman, X. Papademetris, T. S. Burgert, B. M. Pierpont, M. Savoye, M. Shaw, A. A. Seyal, and R. Weiss. 2008. "High visceral and low abdominal subcutaneous fat stores in the obese adolescent: a determinant of an adverse metabolic phenotype." *Diabetes* 57(2): 367–71. doi: 10.2337/db07-0932.

Taussig, M. D., K. P. Powell, H. A. Cole, S. K. Nwosu, T. Hunley, S. E. Romine, H. Iwinski, Jr., V. Talwalkar, T. Warhoover, S. A. Lovejoy, G. A. Mencio, J. E. Martus, J. Walker, T. Milbrandt, and J. G. Schoenecker. 2015. "Prevalence of hypertension in pediatric tibia vara and slipped capital femoral epiphysis." *J Pediatr Orthop*. doi: 10.1097/BPO.0000000000000569.

Thakkar, R. K., and M. P. Michalsky. 2015. "Update on bariatric surgery in adolescence." *Curr Opin Pediatr* 27(3): 370–6. doi: 10.1097/MOP.0000000000000223.

Turnbaugh, P. J., R. E. Ley, M. A. Mahowald, V. Magrini, E. R. Mardis, and J. I. Gordon. 2006. "An obesity-associated gut microbiome with increased capacity for energy harvest." *Nature* 444(7122): 1027–31. doi: 10.1038/nature05414.

Vehapoglu, A., M. Yazici, A. D. Demir, S. Turkmen, M. Nursoy, and E. Ozkaya. 2014. "Early infant feeding practice and childhood obesity: the relation of breast-feeding and timing of solid food introduction with childhood obesity." *J Pediatr Endocrinol Metab* 27(11–12): 1181–7. doi: 10.1515/jpem-2014-0138.

Velazquez-Lopez, L., G. Santiago-Diaz, J. Nava-Hernandez, A. V. Munoz-Torres, P. Medina-Bravo, and M. Torres-Tamayo. 2014. "Mediterranean-style diet reduces metabolic syndrome components in obese children and adolescents with obesity." *BMC Pediatr* 14: 175. doi: 10.1186/1471-2431-14-175.

Velez, A., D. L. Golem, and S. M. Arent. 2010. "The impact of a 12-week resistance training program on strength, body composition, and self-concept of Hispanic adolescents." *J Strength Cond Res* 24(4): 1065–73. doi: 10.1519/JSC.0b013e3181cc230a.

Vikram, N. K., A. Misra, R. M. Pandey, K. Luthra, J. S. Wasir, and V. Dhingra. 2006. "Heterogeneous phenotypes of insulin resistance and its implications for defining metabolic syndrome in Asian Indian adolescents." *Atherosclerosis* 186(1): 193–9. doi: 10.1016/j.atherosclerosis.2005.07.015.

Wang, J., B. Sun, M. Hou, X. Pan, and X. Li. 2013. "The environmental obesogen bisphenol A promotes adipogenesis by increasing the amount of 11beta-hydroxysteroid dehydrogenase type 1 in the adipose tissue of children." *Int J Obes (Lond)* 37(7): 999–1005. doi: 10.1038/ijo.2012.173.

Waring, M. E., and K. L. Lapane. 2008. "Overweight in children and adolescents in relation to attention-deficit/hyperactivity disorder: results from a national sample." *Pediatrics* 122(1): e1–6. doi: 10.1542/peds.2007-1955.

Weigensberg, M. J., C. J. Lane, Q. Avila, K. Konersman, E. Ventura, T. Adam, Z. Shoar, M. I. Goran, and D. Spruijt-Metz. 2014. "Imagine HEALTH: results from a randomized pilot lifestyle intervention for obese Latino adolescents using Interactive Guided ImagerySM." *BMC Complement Altern Med* 14: 28. doi: 10.1186/1472-6882-14-28.

Weiss, R., J. Dziura, T. S. Burgert, W. V. Tamborlane, S. E. Taksali, C. W. Yeckel, K. Allen, M. Lopes, M. Savoye, J. Morrison, R. S. Sherwin, and S. Caprio. 2004. "Obesity and the metabolic syndrome in children and adolescents." *N Engl J Med* 350(23): 2362–74. doi: 10.1056/NEJMoa031049.

Williams, R., M. Novick, and E. Lehman. 2014. "Prevalence of hypovitaminosis D and its association with comorbidities of childhood obesity." *Perm J* 18(4): 32–9. doi: 10.7812/TPP/14-016.

Wilson, S. M., and A. F. Sato. 2014. "Stress and paediatric obesity: what we know and where to go." *Stress Health* 30(2): 91–102. doi: 10.1002/smi.2501.

Witbreuk, M., F. J. van Kemenade, J. A. van der Sluijs, E. P. Jansma, J. Rotteveel, and B. J. van Royen. 2013. "Slipped capital femoral epiphysis and its association with endocrine, metabolic and chronic diseases: a systematic review of the literature." *J Child Orthop* 7(3): 213–23. doi: 10.1007/s11832-013-0493-8.

Yin, Z., C. L. Davis, J. B. Moore, and F. A. Treiber. 2005. "Physical activity buffers the effects of chronic stress on adiposity in youth." *Ann Behav Med* 29(1): 29–36. doi: 10.1207/s15324796abm2901_5.

Zimmet, P., K. G. Alberti, F. Kaufman, N. Tajima, M. Silink, S. Arslanian, G. Wong, P. Bennett, J. Shaw, S. Caprio, and I. D. F. Consensus Group. 2007. "The metabolic syndrome in children and adolescents—an IDF consensus report." *Pediatr Diabetes* 8(5): 299–306. doi: 10.1111/j.1399-5448.2007.00271.x.

22 Integrative Intake

The art of incorporating integrative medicine into the clinical visit requires a deliberate shift on the part of the practitioner. This entails broadening one's perspective, viewing the patient through a multifaceted lens, and recognizing the important connections between seemingly unrelated factors. Few conventional clinicians are trained to approach patients in this manner, which leverages both intuition and refined listening skills. Although initially the time investment needed for an expanded intake approach may seem daunting, when well practiced it can facilitate identification of hidden stressors, reveal unhealthy patterns, and may speed accurate diagnosis.

In the ideal world, an integrative intake interview might be allotted 90 minutes and cover every element of lifestyle. In reality, a fraction of that time may be available. In both situations the intake can be adapted to fit the needs of the patient and the constraints of the clinician. For example: a detailed intake form can be distributed to the patient ahead of the visit; new questions can be introduced into the conventional history designed to open the conversation to integrative topics; lifestyle and preventive health topics can be covered at sequential visits rather than bundled into one sitting; the practitioner may add an inter-professional team member whose role is focused on obtaining an in-depth lifestyle history and helping with behavioral change in a coaching role.

Goals

The main goals of an integrative medicine intake are to:

- Gather a sense of the whole person
- Identify habits, history, and lifestyle elements that may be influencing health
- Assess the individual's insight and understanding of their illness
- Acquire a sense of the patient's openness to new treatment options
- Determine readiness to change

Time spent in conversation allows the clinician to identify and appreciate the individual's strengths and motivation, and to understand past failures or obstacles that may impede desired behavior changes.

Setting the Tone

The tone of the visit is critical, as is allowing the patient to tell their story without repeated interruptions by the clinician.

Examples of setting the tone:

- Be mindfully present
- Greeting the patient by name
- Use eye contact, and a warm handshake or other appropriate greeting
- Identify and address any barriers in communication such as language or disability
- Comfortable seating and lighting
- A quiet, calm environment
- Clinician sitting and relaxed rather than standing as if poised to leave the room
- Non-obtrusive use of the computer

Active Listening

Active listening requires attention on several simultaneous levels to catch the underlying meanings and emotions behind the words. It is as important to note what is *not* being said as what is coming out in the conversation. Sometimes the most pressing concern of the patient is what they reveal last.

Mindful Presence

Maintaining mindful presence might entail expressing compassion and understanding, cultivating a feeling of being in tune with the patient, and projecting a positive and supportive feeling for the patient—even if they are struggling or have not followed the clinician's recommendations in the past. It can be very challenging to maintain a sense of mindful presence throughout a busy clinic day.

Some practitioners use a centering technique, breath work, mindful hand washing, or other deliberate pause between patients to help them stay present.

Typical Day

One approach is to have the patient or parent run through their "typical day" routine to provide a sense of background and lifestyle habits. This can help both patient and clinician quickly identify patterns such as: dietary preferences, recurring stressors, gaps in physical activity, sleep hygiene, and quantity and quality of daily media intake such as news, social media, or online gaming.

Comparison of a child's perception of their typical day with the parent's perception can lead to important new insights, especially if the child had not previously disclosed events such as domestic tension or recurring school or sibling bullying.

Detailed Intake Forms

A detailed intake form can allow the patient and family to systematically work through the topics of lifestyle: nutrition, dietary supplements, physical activity, stressors, sleep, environmental exposures, and prior integrative medicine use before the visit. When sent back by the patient ahead of time this has the benefit of allowing the clinician time for pre-review and to research any potential drug–supplement interactions. While some clinicians favor this approach, others prefer to gather the information face to face.

Adapted Standard History and Physical

A standard history and physical can also be used, with areas for added information such as stressors, dietary supplements, and other integrative elements.

Presenting Complaint

When establishing the presenting complaint, remember that the individual's main concern may not be the first thing they identify. Hesitation can occur for many reasons, including embarrassment, fear of being judged, and lack of trust. The clinician can help highlight the main concerns with open-ended questions and an engaged attitude. For example:

- What brings you in today?
- Is this your main concern?
- Is there anything else?
- Let me summarize your concerns ... am I understanding you correctly?

History of Present Illness

The history of the present illness gives a summary of the story leading up to the visit. Ideally the patient is doing the majority of the talking during the history taking.

Use of open-ended questions to gather more information is often more time efficient than directed questioning, for example:

- What else?
- Tell me more about that.
- What do you think the meaning of the illness or symptoms is?
- How did that make you feel?
- What's your biggest concern about what's going on right now?

Current Lifestyle Habits

Nutrition

- Review of typical breakfast, lunch, dinner, snacks, beverages.
- Meals regularly skipped?
- Recurring cravings?
- Who does the shopping, meal planning, cooking in the family?
- Family dynamic at meal time? Relaxed, stressed, high conflict?

Dietary Supplements, Including Botanicals

- Brand name?
- Why taking?
- Dose?
- Duration?
- Side effects experienced?

Physical Activity

- Types
- Frequency
- Duration
- Intensity
- Challenges
- Goals, short and long term

Mind–Body Skills

- Stressors—acute and chronic
- History of childhood adversity
- Stress management techniques
- Interest in learning new stress management skills
- Challenges in stress management
- Social support

Spirituality, Meaning and Purpose

- What is your biggest dream, goal?
- What is your biggest worry?
- What is most important to you in life?
- How do you cope when things get tough?

Sleep

- Quality
- Normal duration
- Regularity
- How often wake rested?
- Sleep aids used, prescriptions or supplements?
- Challenges and frustrations
- Goals

Environmental Health

- Awareness of potential exposures (air, land, water)
- Past history of known exposures
- Steps taken to reduce or eliminate exposures

Review of Current Symptoms

- General, including current stress level
- Head, ears, eyes, nose, throat (HEENT)
- Cardiovascular
- Pulmonary
- Gastrointestinal

- Genitourinary
- Musculoskeletal
- Neurologic
- Psychiatric
- Endocrine
- Hematologic
- Weight changes

Past Medical History

- Prenatal history, maternal stress, environmental exposures
- Birth history
- Illnesses
- Hospitalizations
- Surgeries
- Accidental injuries
- Chronic stressors
- Review of old records
- Review of existing laboratory values

Immunizations

- Up to date?
- Concerns?

Developmental History

- Developmental milestones on track?

Social History

- Support network
- Who lives at home?
- School friends?
- Extracurricular activities
- Relationship with teachers, coaches
- Who do you talk with about your problems?

Family History

- Allergies
- Arthritis
- Asthma, pneumonia
- Cancer
- Diabetes, Type 1, Type 2
- Gastrointestinal
- Kidney, urinary
- Liver

- Heart disease
- High blood pressure
- Headache, migraine
- Fibromyalgia
- Congenital or genetic illnesses
- Mental health, depression, anxiety, bipolar, suicide
- Substance abuse
- Other

Physical Exam

(Done with mindful intention)

- Vitals:
- Height (%)
- Weight (%)
- Head circumference (%)
- BMI-for-age
- Temperature
- Pulse
- Respiratory rate
- Blood pressure
- Eyes: conjunctiva, pupils, optic discs
- Ears, Nose, Throat: nasal mucosa, oral mucosa, teeth, oropharynx, tympanic membranes
- Neck: adenopathy, mobility, thyroid
- Chest: respirations, heart sounds, murmurs
- Cardiovascular: palpation of pulses, edema, perfusion
- Gastrointestinal: auscultation, masses, pain, hepato-splenomegaly, adenopathy
- Genitourinary: Tanner stage, adenopathy, hernia
- Musculoskeletal: gait, symmetry, range of motion, strength
- Back: symmetry, pain, range of motion
- Skin: rashes, dryness, masses, discoloration
- Neurologic: cranial nerves, reflexes, coordination, balance
- Psychologic: mood, interactivity, memory

Prioritization

Once the patient's concerns have been identified, it is necessary to prioritize their needs in terms of urgency, time, and desired outcome. This is often a negotiated discussion as priorities identified by clinician and patient may differ. This step can be simplified by understanding the patient's main goal in seeking care that day, and by fully understanding the desired outcome of the visit.

A collaborative approach to prioritizing next steps can help meet the patient's expectations, and can lighten the clinician's feeling of time pressure. For example, if the patient's primary need is to express worry, fear, or frustration, compassionate listening by the clinician may literally be the most important outcome of the visit rather than crafting a complex treatment plan.

If behavior change is a desired goal, it is also important to ask the patient where they feel most likely to succeed in changing, or which area of behavior change they would like to prioritize. It is not unusual for the patient's list of priorities to differ from the clinician's, another argument for a collaborative approach that respects the patient's readiness to change.

Closing the Interview

The ending of the interview is important and should reinforce the important information gathered, provide the patient with a feeling of personal connection, support, and a sense that their concerns were fully heard. It should provide a clear sense of next steps, and of setting an action plan in motion. Partnership, respect, hope and reassurance are critical components. Pediatrics is unique in that the clinician must connect with both the child and the parents in order to move forward successfully.

Creating an Integrative Treatment Plan

Once priorities have been identified, near and longer-term goals can be set.

In the near term, immediate steps are outlined, ideally paired with small, realistic goals to set the patient up for success. This typically includes direct suggestions by the clinician, and suggestions for steps the patient can take to begin to build a sense of self-efficacy. An example might be learning a mind–body skill such as breath work or progressive muscle relaxation to help address stress or sleep issues. Targeted areas would be those identified as high priority to the patient and could include any area covered in the intake, from diet to exercise to the addition of selected dietary supplements.

An expanded treatment plan is often prepared after the visit by the integrative clinician. This generally covers additional recommendations and resources. This plan may go into significant depth and can serve as a blueprint for the patient as they move towards optimum health. An expanded treatment plan typically covers both conventional and integrative suggestions, as follows.

Conventional Medicine

- Summaries and recommendations
- Suggested laboratory or imaging studies to clarify diagnosis
- Review of current medications, possible side effects and drug–supplement interactions

Integrative Medicine

Lifestyle Foundations

- Nutrition
- Dietary supplements
- Physical activity
- Mind–body medicine
- Sleep
- Environmental health

Complementary Approaches

- Botanicals
- Manual medicine (massage, osteopathy, craniosacral, chiropractic)
- Aromatherapy
- Whole medical systems (homeopathy, naturopathy, Ayurveda, traditional Chinese medicine)
- Bioenergetics

Motivational Interviewing Suggestions

What to work on first, why, and how the patient can position themselves for success.

Practice Models

Integrative clinicians use many practice models in both academic and community-based settings, therefore billing, coding, and malpractice models vary. One common approach is to use the Evaluation and Management (E&M) codes to accurately represent time use, paired with typical International Classification of Disease (ICD) codes. New codes are constantly evolving, for example the ICD 10 has a Z72 code labeled "Problems Related to Lifestyle" that includes lack of physical exercise, inappropriate diet and eating habits, sleep problems, and other similar categories.

A growing number of electronic medical records exist that can accommodate the integrative visit, yet modernization of insurance coding, billing, and reimbursement are still needed to prioritize fair reimbursement for time spent on preventive health and introduction of new skills. The value of an integrative approach in pediatrics is reinforced by the potential for early development of healthy habits, reduction in use of prescription medications, and cultivation of resiliency and self-efficacy.

When introducing the integrative approach, the clinician may want to focus on the one or two areas in which they feel best prepared to counsel a patient to avoid overwhelming the patient. Some clinicians may start with nutrition, or physical activity, and build on their strengths as they master other topics. Others may feel more confident introducing mind–body therapies. Momentum continues to build around the benefits of the inter-professional team approach that leverages the strengths of many disciplines and specialties, ideally in an integrative medical home where all services are available under one roof.

Clinician Self-Care

Given the depth of an integrative intake visit, a few moments of personal reflection and mindfulness after each visit, or at the end of the clinic day, can be extremely helpful to review the high points, savor the personal connection with patients, and to replenish one's well of energy.

23 Conclusion

The intent of the book has been to provide an overview of the emerging field of pediatric integrative medicine and to help the reader better understand which areas are supported by stronger research and where more data is needed. The field has significant potential to improve the quality of preventive health in children, an urgent priority given the serious diseases reaching down into ever-younger age groups with significant emotional and financial costs. Clinician self-care was added to reinforce emerging research that demonstrates how the health of the clinician impacts the health and wellbeing of their patient. Burnout has reached epidemic proportions in clinicians worldwide and must be addressed in a coordinated fashion that involves the individual, the organization, and the overarching culture of medicine. Integrative medicine provides a useful blueprint to craft a way forward, building on the unexpected blend of neuroscience and ancient meditation techniques that can help clinicians develop more skillful approaches to the daily stressors involved in authentic and caring patient interactions.

Foundations of health were covered with the goal of reviewing classic information and introducing emerging research in areas of nutrition science, selected dietary supplements, physical activity, mind–body therapies, sleep and environmental exposures, including how these foundational areas impact the prenatal environment and subsequently influence the child's lifelong health.

The complementary approaches were covered with an eye to expanding the clinician's worldview, if they were not already familiar with the fields, and to acknowledge the highly developed healing systems that exist throughout the world that can help enrich the practice of pediatrics in many ways. Learning to assess benefit and risk of complementary therapies, and to understand the background and incorporate the training of a range of inter-professional colleagues is the next frontier of medicine. The skillful clinician will appreciate this and move quickly to build strong collaborative inter-professional teams that will best serve the needs of the patient and their family.

Clinical applications were explored for a range of the most common pediatric conditions, yet still fall short on the distressing array of diseases faced by today's children, including chronic pain. The topics of allergy and asthma are among the most prevalent illnesses seen in children today; dermatologic conditions impact the child on levels that go far beyond the cosmetic; gut diseases similarly impact the child systemically, and emotionally, and require an approach that takes into account every element of a child's life and lifestyle. The upper respiratory illnesses are among the most common infectious diseases in the world, yet the conventional options to treat them in children can result in more harm than good. Review of expanded integrative treatment options for these common illnesses has the potential to keep a child out of danger's way while they maximize their full inherent healing potential.

A significant focus of the book was to highlight the rising prevalence of mental health conditions in children and adolescents, and to help equip clinicians to offer these children more than just another prescription. It is important for clinicians to be confident enough to move past the superficial in the mental health interview process so that they can fully understand the child's situation and stressors. Emerging research on the mental and physical implications of toxic stress means that clinicians must learn new approaches and be able to provide evidence-based counseling on stress reduction and self-regulation skills. Pediatric clinicians are a lynchpin of the child's care team, and as such must be ready to support the child's progress and rally the family and community to their cause.

Review of the increasingly common neurodevelopmental conditions, ADHD and autism, updates the reader on new research, and also on which treatments are without merit so they may knowledgeably advise families who may be willing to try anything to alleviate their child's suffering. The chapter on obesity and metabolic syndrome offers both an overview of the serious state of the worldwide obesity epidemic, and introduces an innovative approach to modern preventive care that incorporates emerging research with a whole child approach to anticipatory guidance. Finally, an example of an integrative intake is offered so that the clinician can begin to build new skills, or to deepen those already acquired, that will help them gain a multidimensional sense of the child and be ready to offer a full palate of evidence-based treatment options to help the child thrive.

Pediatric integrative medicine is a young field with incredible potential to help children and adolescents. It is being carried forward by some of the best and brightest colleagues I have ever had the privilege to work with and it is my hope that significant shifts will occur in healthcare policy and insurance reimbursement that will support ongoing successes in the field.

Hilary McClafferty, MD, FAAP

Index